BOC
Study Guide
5th edition

Clinical Laboratory
Certification Examinations

Oversight Editors

Patricia A. Tanabe, MPA, MLS(ASCP)^{CM}
Executive Director, ASCP Board of Certification

E. Blair Holladay, PhD, SCT(ASCP)^{CM}
Executive Vice President, ASCP

and the ASCP Board of Certification Staff

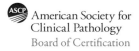 American Society for
Clinical Pathology
Board of Certification

Publishing Team
Erik N Tanck & Tae W Moon (design/production)
Joshua Weikersheimer (publishing direction)

Notice
Trade names for equipment and supplies described are included as suggestions only. In no way does their inclusion constitute an endorsement of preference by the Author or the ASCP. The Author and ASCP urge all readers to read and follow all manufacturers' instructions and package insert warnings concerning the proper and safe use of products. The American Society for Clinical Pathology, having exercised appropriate and reasonable effort to research material current as of publication date, does not assume any liability for any loss or damage caused by errors and omissions in this publication. Readers must assume responsibility for complete and thorough research of any hazardous conditions they encounter, as this publication is not intended to be all-inclusive, and recommendations and regulations change over time.

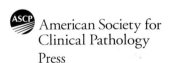 American Society for
Clinical Pathology
Press

Printed in Hong Kong

Reprinted 2010

14 13 12 11 10

Table of Contents

Table of Contents

Acknowledgments

The editors would like to thank *Melissa Meeks* and *Edith Miller* for their painstaking efforts in combining and reviewing this body of work in accordance with the ASCP Press and production staff. Special thanks are also extended to all our volunteers (former examination committee members and recently recruited volunteers) for their commitment in assisting us on this essential resource for laboratory science students and their professors.

Thank you to my family – *Adam*, *Peter* and *Joe*, for their support and understanding during this project.

– Patricia A. Tanabe, MPA, MLS(ASCP)^{CM}

Good luck with your board examination—my best to each of you as you embark on an exciting career in laboratory medicine.

– E. Blair Holladay, PhD, SCT(ASCP)^{CM}

Preface

The 5th edition of the *Board of Certification Study Guide for Clinical Laboratory Certification Examinations* contains over 2000 multiple choice questions. Unique to this study guide is the differentiation of questions appropriate for both the Medical Laboratory Technician and Medical Laboratory Scientist levels from questions that are appropriate for the Medical Laboratory Scientist level *only* (clearly marked MLS ONLY). The questions in this edition are arranged in chapters which correspond to the major content areas on the examination. Within each chapter, the questions are further grouped by topic. New to this edition are short answer explanations and references for each practice question. Questions with images will appear as they would on the certification examination. Laboratory results will be presented in both conventional and SI units.

The practice questions are presented in a format and style similar to the questions included on the Board of Certification certification examinations. **Please note: *None* of these questions will appear on any Board of Certification examination.**

These practice questions were compiled from previously published materials and submitted questions from recruited reviewers. (Note: These reviewers do not currently serve on any Examination Committee.)

This book is not a product of the Board of Certification, rather it is a product of the ASCP Press, the independent publishing arm of the American Society for Clinical Pathology. Use of this book does not ensure passing of an examination. The Board of Certification's evaluation and credentialing processes are entirely independent of this study guide; however, this book should significantly help you prepare for your BOC examination.

ur thanks to those who edited/ viewed questions for this book.

Blood Bank

Margaret G. Fritsma, MA, MT(ASCP) SBB, retired (co-Editor)
Formerly, Associate Professor
University of Alabama at Birmingham
Birmingham, AL

Joanne Kosanke, MT(ASCP)SBB^{CM} (co-Editor)
Manager, Immunohematology Reference Laboratory
American Red Cross Central Ohio Blood Services Region
Columbus, OH

Patricia J. Ellinger, MSEd, MASCP, MLS(ASCP)^{CM}SBB^{CM}
Laboratory Education and Training Consultant
Minneapolis, Minnesota

Deborah T. Firestone, EdD, MT(ASCP) SBB
Associate Dean
Stony Brook University
Stony Brook, NY

Carol McConnell, MS, MLS(ASCP)^{CM}
Laboratory Coordinator
St. Francis Memorial Hospital
San Francisco, CA

Chemistry

Polly Cathcart, MMSc, MT(ASCP)SC, retired
Formerly, Chemistry Supervisor
Piedmont Hospital
Atlanta, GA

Vicki S. Freeman, PhD, FACB, MLS(ASCP)^{CM}SC
Department Chair and
Distinguished Teaching Professor
University of Texas Medical Branch
Galveston, TX

Ross J. Molinaro, PhD, MT(ASCP), D(ABCC), FACB
Medical Director, Core Laboratory, Emory University Hospital Midtown & Assistant Professor, Pathology and Lab Medicine, Emory University School of Medicine
Emory University
Atlanta, GA

Christine Papadea, PhD, MT(ASCP)SC, retired
Formerly, Professor
Pathology and Laboratory Medicine, Medical University of South Carolina
Charleston, SC

Diane Wilson, PhD, MT(ASCP)
Program Director- Medical Technology
Morgan State University
Baltimore, MD

Hematology

Donna D. Castellone, MS, MT(ASCP)SH (Editor)
Clinical Project Manager/Hematology & Hemostasis
Siemens Healthcare Diagnostics
Tarrytown, NY

Sandra DiFalco, MS, MT(ASCP)
Education Coordinator

The Colorado Center for Medical Laboratory Science
Denver, CO

Kathy W. Jones, MS, MLS(ASCP)^{CM}
Faculty – Clinical Laboratory Science Program
Auburn University Montgomery
Montgomery, AL

Linda L. Myers, MEd, MT(ASCP)SH
Assistant Director Clinical Laboratory
St. Joseph Medical Center
Houston, TX

John K. Scariano, PhD, MT(ASCP)
Assistant Professor, Pathology & Internal Medicine
University of New Mexico School of Medicine
Albuquerque, NM

Ruth Scheib, MT(ASCP)SH
Medical Technologist
Cleveland Clinic
Cleveland, OH

Immunology

Barbara Anne Maier, MPA, MT(ASCP)SI, retired (Editor)
Formerly, Technical Specialist
Immunology, Serology & Flow Cytometry
Geisinger Medical Center
Danville, PA

Linda E. Miller, PhD, SI(ASCP)MB^{CM}
Professor of Clinical Laboratory Science
SUNY Upstate Medical University
Syracuse, NY

Kate Rittenhouse-Olson, PhD, SI(ASCP)
Professor, Director Biotechnology Program
University at Buffalo, The State University of New York
Buffalo, NY

Laboratory Operations

Ellen Boswell, MBA, MT(ASCP)SH
Director of Clinical Pathology Laboratory Operations
University of Virginia Medical Center
Charlottesville, VA

Cynthia S. Johns, MSA, MLS(ASCP)^{CM}SH^{CM}
Sr. IT Technical Specialist
Laboratory Corporation of America
Lakeland, FL

Ross J. Molinaro, PhD, MT(ASCP), D(ABCC), FACB
Medical Director, Core Laboratory, Emory University Hospital Midtown
Assistant Professor, Pathology and Lab Medicine, Emory University School of Medicine
Emory University
Atlanta, GA

Patricia A Myers, MT(ASCP)SM,SLS
Lead Technologist, Microbiology
Lancaster General Hospital
Lancaster, PA

Lynn Schwabe, MBA, CHE, MT(ASCP) (Editor-Safety)
Senior Director, Lab Services
NorthShore University HealthSystem, Evanston Hospital

Evanston, IL

Peggy Simpson, MS, MT(ASCP)
Administrative Director of Laboratories
Danville Regional Medical Center
Danville, VA

Microbiology

Yvette S. McCarter, PhD, D(ABMM) (Editor)
Director, Clinical Microbiology Laboratory
University of Florida Health Science Center - Jacksonville
Jacksonville, FL

JoAnn P. Fenn, MS, MT(ASCP)
Professor and Associate Division Head, Medical Laboratory Science, Department of Pathology
University of Utah School of Medicine
Salt Lake City, UT

Dawn S. Lumpkin, BA, MT(ASCP)SM,SV
Manager of Microbiology Services
HCA Midwest Division, Research Medical Center
Kansas City, MO

Karen Myers, MA, MT(ASCP)SC
The Colorado Center for Medical Laboratory Science
Denver, CO

Patty Newcomb-Gayman, MT(ASCP)SM
Point of Care Testing Coordinator
Swedish Medical Center
Seattle, WA

Molecular Pathology

Stephen T. Koury, PhD, MT(ASCP) (Editor)
Research Assistant Professor
Department of Biotechnical and Clinical Laboratory Sciences, University at Buffalo
Buffalo, NY

Urinalysis and Body Fluids

Kristina Jackson Behan, PhD, MT(ASCP)
Associate Professor and Program Director
University of West Florida Clinical Laboratory Sciences Program
Pensacola, FL

Susan Strasinger, DA, MT(ASCP), retired
Formerly, Visiting Assistant Professor
University of West Florida
Pensacola, FL

The Importance of Certification, CMP, Licensure and Qualification

The practice of modern medicine would be impossible without the tests performed in the laboratory. A highly skilled medical team of pathologists, specialists, laboratory scientists, technologists, and technicians works together to determine the presence or absence of disease and provides valuable data needed to determine the course of treatment.

Today's laboratory uses many complex, precision instruments and a variety of automated and electronic equipment. However, the success of the laboratory begins with the laboratorians' dedication to their profession and willingness to help others. Laboratorians must produce accurate and reliable test results, have an interest in science, and be able to recognize their responsibility for affecting human lives.

Role of the ASCP Board of Certification

Founded in 1928 by the American Society of Clinical Pathologists (ASCP—now, the American Society for Clinical Pathology), the Board of Certification is considered the preeminent certification agency in the US and abroad within the field of laboratory medicine. Composed of representatives of professional organizations and the public, the Board's mission is to: "*Provide excellence in certification of laboratory professionals on behalf of patients worldwide.*"

The Board of Certification consists of more than 100 volunteer technologists, technicians, laboratory scientists, physicians, and professional researchers. These volunteers contribute their time and expertise to the Board of Governors and the Examination Committees. They allow the BOC to achieve the goal of excellence in credentialing medical laboratory personnel in the US and abroad.

The Board of Governors is the policy-making governing body for the Board of Certification and is composed of 25 members. These 25 members include technologists, technicians, and pathologists nominated by the ASCP and representatives from the general public as well as from the following societies: the American Association for Clinical Chemistry, the AABB, American College of Microbiology, American Society for Clinical Laboratory Science, the American Society of Cytopathology, the American Society of Hematology, the American Association of Pathologists' Assistants, Association of Genetic Technology, the National Society for Histotechnology, and the Clinical Laboratory Management Association (CLMA).

The Examination Committees are responsible for the planning, development, and review of the examination databases; determining the accuracy and relevancy of the test items; confirming the standards for each examination and performing job or practice analyses.

Certification

http://www.ascp.org/certification

Certification is the process by which a nongovernmental agency or association grants recognition of competency to an individual who has met certain predetermined qualifications, as specified by that agency or association. Certification affirms that an individual has demonstrated that he or she possesses the knowledge and skills to perform essential tasks in the medical laboratory. The ASCP Board of Certification certifies those individuals who meet academic and clinical prerequisites and who achieve acceptable performance levels on examinations.

In 2004, the ASCP Board of Certification implemented the **Certification Maintenance Program** (CMP), which mandates participation every 3 years for newly certified individuals in the US. The goal of this program is to demonstrate to the public that laboratory professionals are performing the appropriate and relevant activities to keep current in their practice. Please follow the steps outlined on the website to apply for CMP and retain your certification. (http://www.ascp.org/CMP)

United States Certification

http://www.ascp.org/certification

To apply for a Certification Examination follow these step-by-step instructions:

1   Identify the examination you are applying for and determine your eligibility.

2   Gather your required education and experience documentation.

3   Apply for the examination. We offer 2 options:

   a.   Apply online and pay by credit card.

   b.   Or download an application, pay by credit card, check or money order and mail to:

        ASCP Board of Certification
        3335 Eagle Way
        Chicago, IL 60678-1033

4   Schedule your examination at a Pearson Professional Center. Visit the Pearson site (http://www.pearsonvue.com/ascp) to identify a location and time that is convenient for you to take your ASCP examination.

International Certification

http://www.ascp.org/certification/International

ASCP offers its gold standard credentials in the form of international certification (ASCP^i) to eligible individuals. The ASCP^i credential certifies professional competency among new and practicing laboratory personnel in an effort to contribute globally to the highest standards of patient safety. Graduates of medical laboratory science programs outside the United States are challenged with content that mirrors the standards of excellence established by the US ASCP exams. The ASCP^i credential carries the weight of 80 years of expertise in clinical laboratory professional certification. Please visit the website to view the following:

1   Website information translated into a specific language.

2   Current listing of international certifications.

3   Eligibility guidelines.

4   Step-by-step instructions to apply for international certification.

State Licensure

http://www.ascp.org/licensure

State Licensure is the process by which a state grants a license to an individual to practice their profession in the specified state. The individual must meet the state's licensing requirements, which may include examination and/or experience. It is important to identify the state and examination to determine your eligibility and view the steps for licensure and/or certification. For a list of states that require licensure, please go to the website. (http://www.ascp.org/statelicensureagencies)

The ASCP Board of Certification (BOC) examinations have been approved for licensure purposes by the states of California and New York. The BOC examinations also meet the requirements for all other states that require licensure.

Qualification

http://www.ascp.org/qualification

A qualification from the Board of Certification recognizes the competence of individuals in specific technical areas. Qualifications are available in laboratory informatics, immunohistochemistry and flow cytometry. To receive this credential, candidates must meet the eligibility requirements and successfully complete an examination (QCYM, QIHC) or a work sample project (QLI). Candidates who complete the Qualification process will receive a Certificate of Qualification, which is valid for 5 years. The Qualification may be revalidated every 5 years upon receipt of completed application and fee. (Documentation of acceptable continuing education may be requested.)

Preparing for and Taking the BOC Certification Examination

Begin early to prepare for the Certification Examination. Because of the broad range of knowledge and skills tested by the examination, even applicants with college education and those completing formal laboratory education training programs will find that review is necessary, although the exact amount will vary from applicant to applicant. Generally, last-minute cramming is the least effective method for preparing for the examination. The earlier you begin, the more time you will have to prepare; and the more you prepare, the better your chance of successfully passing the examination and scoring well.

Study for the Test

Plan a course of study that allows more time for your weaker areas. Although it is important to study your areas of weakness, be sure to allow enough time to review all areas. It is better to spend a short time studying every day than to spend several hours every week or 2. Setting aside a regular time and a special place to study will help ensure studying becomes a part of your daily routine.

Study Resources

http://www.ascp.org/studymaterials

Competency Statements and Content Guidelines

http://www.ascp.org/contentguidelines

The Board of Certification has developed competency statements and content guidelines to delineate the content and tasks included in its tests. Current Content Guidelines for the Medical Laboratory Scientist (MLS) and Medical Laboratory Technician (MLT) examinations as well as other certification examinations offered by the ASCP BOC are available.

Study Guide

The questions in this study guide are in a format and style similar to the questions on the Board of Certification examinations. The questions are in a multiple choice format with 1 best answer. Work through each chapter and answer all the questions as presented. Next, review your answers against the answer key. Review the answer explanation for those questions, that you answered incorrectly. Lastly, each question is referenced if you require further explanation.

Textbooks

The references cited in this study guide (see pp 481-484) identify many useful textbooks. The most current reading lists for most of the examinations are available on the ASCP's website (http://www.ascp.org/readinglists). Textbooks tend to cover a broad range of knowledge in a given field. An added benefit is that textbooks frequently have questions at the end of the chapters that you can use to test yourself should you need further clarification on specific subject matter.

Online practice tests

http://www.ascp-practice.com

The online practice test is a subscription product. It includes 90-day online access to the practice tests, comprehensive diagnostic scores, and discussion boards. If you are an institutional purchaser that would like to pay by check or purchase order (minimum of 20 tests to use a check or purchase order), please download the order form from the website. Content-specific online practice tests can be purchased online.

Taking the Certification Examination

The ASCP Board of Certification (BOC) uses computer adaptive testing (CAT), which is criterion referenced. With CAT, provided you answer the question correctly, the next examination question has a slightly higher level of difficulty. The difficulty level of the questions presented to the examinee continues to increase until a question is answered incorrectly. At this point, a slightly easier question is presented. The importance of testing in an adaptive format is that each test is individually tailored to your ability level.

Each question in the examination pool is calibrated for difficulty and categorized into a subtest area, which corresponds to the content guideline for a particular examination. The weight (value) given to each question is determined by the level of difficulty. All examinations (with the exception of phlebotomy (PBT) and donor phlebotomy (DPT)) are scheduled for 2 hours and 30 minutes and have 100 questions. The PBT and DPT examinations are scheduled for 2 hours and have 80 questions. Your preliminary test results (pass/fail) will appear on the computer screen immediately upon completion of your examination. Detailed examination scores will be mailed within 10 business days after your examination, provided that the BOC has received all required application documents. Examination results cannot be released by telephone under any circumstances.

Your official detailed examination score report will indicate a "pass" or "fail" status and the specific scaled score on the total examination. A scaled score is statistically derived (in part) from the raw score (number of correctly answered questions) and the difficulty level of the questions. Because each examinee has taken an individualized examination, scaled scores are used so that all examinations may be compared on the same scale. The minimum passing score is 400. The highest attainable score is 999.

If you were unsuccessful in passing the examination, your scaled scores on each of the subtests will be indicated on the report as well. These subtest scores cannot be calculated to obtain your total score. These scores are provided as a means of demonstrating your areas of strengths and weaknesses in comparison to the minimum pass score.

Blood Bank

*The following items have been identified generally as appropriate for both entry level medical laboratory scientists and medical laboratory technicians. Items that are appropriate for medical laboratory scientists **only** are marked with an "MLS ONLY."*

Blood Products

1   The minimum hemoglobin concentration in a fingerstick from a male blood donor is:

    a   12.0 g/dL (120 g/L)
    ⓑ   12.5 g/dL (125 g/L)
    c   13.5 g/dL (135 g/L)
    d   15.0 g/dL (150 g/L)

2   A cause for permanent deferral of blood donation is:
MLS ONLY

    a   diabetes
    b   residence in an endemic malaria region
    ⓒ   history of jaundice of uncertain cause
    d   history of therapeutic rabies vaccine

3   Which of the following prospective donors would be accepted for donation?
MLS ONLY

    a   32-year-old woman who received a transfusion in a complicated delivery 5 months previously *— 6 month referral*
    b   19-year-old sailor who has been stateside for 9 months and stopped taking his anti-malarial medication 9 months previously *– 12 month referral*
    ⓒ   22-year-old college student who has a temperature of 99.2°F (37.3°C) and states that he feels well, but is nervous about donating   *(not over 99.5°)*
    d   45-year-old woman who has just recovered from a bladder infection and is still taking <u>antibiotics</u>

4   Which one of the following constitutes <u>permanent</u> rejection status of a donor?

    a   a tattoo 5 months previously
    b   recent close contact with a patient with viral hepatitis
    c   2 units of blood transfused 4 months previously
    ⓓ   confirmed positive test for HBsAg 10 years previously

5   According to AABB standards, which of the following donors may be accepted as a blood donor?
MLS ONLY

    a   traveled to an area endemic for malaria 9 months previously *– 12 months*
    ⓑ   spontaneous abortion at 2 months of pregnancy, 3 months previously *– >6 weeks*
    c   resides with a known hepatitis patient
    d   received a blood transfusion 22 weeks previously *– 6 months*

6   Below are the results of the history obtained from a prospective female blood donor:

     age: 16 *ok*

     temperature: 99.0°F (37.2°C) *≯ 99.5*

     Hct: 36% *>38% ✱*

     history: tetanus <u>toxoid</u> immunization 1 week previously *– no problem with synthetic or killed vaccines*

How many of the above results excludes this donor from giving blood for a routine transfusion?

    a none
    (b) 1
    c 2
    d 3

7   For apheresis donors who donate platelets more frequently than every 4 weeks, a platelet count
MLS ONLY   must be performed prior to the procedure and be at least:

    (a) $150 \times 10^3/\mu L$ ($150 \times 10^9/L$)
    b $200 \times 10^3/\mu L$ ($200 \times 10^9/L$)
    c $250 \times 10^3/\mu L$ ($250 \times 10^9/L$)
    d $300 \times 10^3/\mu L$ ($300 \times 10^9/L$)

8   Prior to blood donation, the intended venipuncture site must be cleaned with a scrub
solution containing:

    a hypochlorite
    b isopropyl alcohol
    c 10% acetone
    (d) PVP <u>iodine</u> complex *if allergic, chlorhexadrine and 70% ETOH*

9   All donor blood testing must include:

    a complete Rh phenotyping
    b anti-CMV testing
    c direct antiglobulin test
    (d) serological test for syphilis

10   During the preparation of Platelet Concentrates from Whole Blood, the blood should be:

    a cooled towards 6°C
    (b) cooled towards 20°-24°C *– optimum function*
    c warmed to 37°C
    d heated to 57°C

11   The most common cause of posttransfusion hepatitis can be detected in donors by testing for:
MLS ONLY
    a anti-HCV
    (b) HBsAg
    c anti-HAV IgM
    d anti-HBe

12   The Western blot is a confirmatory test for the presence of:

    a CMV antibody
    (b) anti-HIV-1
    c HBsAg
    d serum protein abnormalities

13   The test that is currently used to detect donors who are infected with the AIDS virus is:

    a anti-HBc
    (b) anti-HIV 1,2
    c HBsAg
    d ALT

14 A commonly used screening method for anti-HIV-1 detection is:

    a latex agglutination
    b radioimmunoassay (RIA)
    c thin-layer-chromatography (TLC)
    d enzyme-labeled immunosorbent assay (ELISA)

15 Rejuvenation of a unit of Red Blood Cells is a method used to:
MLS ONLY

    a remove antibody attached to RBCs
    b inactivate viruses and bacteria
    c restore 2,3-DPG and ATP to normal levels
    d filter blood clots and other debris

16 A unit of packed cells is split into 2 aliquots under <u>closed sterile conditions</u> at 8 AM. The expiration time for each aliquot is now:

    a 4 PM on the same day
    b 8 PM on the same day
    c 8 AM the next morning
    d the original date of the unsplit unit

17 A unit of Red Blood Cells expiring in 35 days is split into 5 small aliquots using a sterile pediatric quad set and a <u>sterile connecting device.</u> Each aliquot must be labeled as expiring in:

    a 6 hours
    b 12 hours   *sterile docking device – same exp date*
    c 5 days
    d 35 days

18 When platelets are stored on a rotator set on an open bench top, the ambient air temperature must be recorded:

    a once a day
    b twice a day   *
    c every 4 hours
    d every hour

19 Which of the following is the correct storage temperature for the component listed?

    a Cryoprecipitated AHF, 4°C   *–18° or lower*
    b Fresh Frozen Plasma (FFP), –20°C *–18 or lower*
    c Red Blood Cells, Frozen, –40°C   *≤ –65*
    d Platelets, 37°C   *20-24° C*

20 A unit of Red Blood Cells is issued at 9:00 AM. At 9:10 AM the unit is returned to the Blood Bank. The container has **not** been entered, but the unit has **not** been refrigerated during this time span. The best course of action for the technologist is to:

    a culture the unit for bacterial contamination
    b discard the unit if not used within 24 hours
    c store the unit at room temperature
    d record the return and place the unit back into inventory – *can be out of refrig for 30 minutes*

21 The optimum storage temperature for Red Blood Cells, Frozen is:
MLS ONLY   *(with glycerol)*

    a –80°C   *< –65*
    b –20°C
    c –12°C
    d 4°C

22   The optimum storage temperature for Red Blood Cells is:

      not frozen

      a −80°C
      b −20°C
      c −12°C
      ⓓ   4°C (1−6°C)

23   If the seal is entered on a unit of Red Blood Cells stored at 1°C to 6°C, what is the maximum allowable storage period, in hours?

      a   6
      ⓑ 24
      c 48
      d 72

24   The optimum storage temperature for cryoprecipitated AHF is:

      ⓐ −20°C
      b −12°C
      c   4°C
      d   22°C

25   Cryoprecipitated AHF must be transfused within what period of time following thawing and pooling?

      ⓐ   4 hours
      b   8 hours
      c   12 hours
      d   24 hours

26   Platelets prepared in a polyolefin type container, stored at 22°-24°C in 50 mL of plasma, and gently agitated can be used for up to:

      a   24 hours
      b   48 hours
      c   3 days
      ⓓ   5 days

27   The optimum storage temperature for platelets is:

      a −20°C
      b −12°C
      c   4°C
      ⓓ 22°C

28   According to AABB standards, Fresh Frozen Plasma must be infused within what period of time following thawing?

      ⓐ 24 hours
      b 36 hours
      ~~c~~ 48 hours
      d 72 hours

29   Cryoprecipitated AHF, if maintained in the frozen state at −18°C or below, has a shelf life of:

      a   42 days
      b   6 months
      ⓒ 12 months
      d 36 months

30   Once thawed, Fresh Frozen Plasma must be transfused within:

     a   4 hours
     b   8 hours
     c   12 hours
     (d) 24 hours

31   *MLS ONLY*   An important determinant of platelet viability following storage is:

     a   plasma potassium concentration
     (b) plasma pH
     c   prothrombin time
     d   activated partial thromboplastin time

32   In the liquid state, plasma must be stored at: *(thawed)*

     (a)   1°- 6°C
     b   22°C
     c   37°C
     d   56°C

33   *MLS ONLY*   During storage, the concentration of 2,3-diphosphoglycerate (2,3-DPG) decreases in a unit of:

     a   Platelets
     b   Fresh Frozen Plasma
     (c) Red Blood Cells
     d   Cryoprecipitated AHF

34   *MLS ONLY*   Cryoprecipitated AHF: *— used primarily for fibrinogen replacement. stored at RT; after thawing → 6 hours. 4 hours if pooled*

     (a) is indicated for fibrinogen deficiencies
     b   should be stored at 4°C prior to administration
     c   will not transmit hepatitis B virus
     (d̶) is indicated for the treatment of hemophilia B

35   *MLS ONLY*   Which apheresis platelets product should be irradiated?

     a   autologous unit collected prior to surgery
     b   random stock unit going to a patient with DIC
     (c) a directed donation given by a mother for her son → *related; lymphocytes can cause graft vs. host disease*
     d   a directed donation given by an unrelated family friend

36   Irradiation of a unit of Red Blood Cells is done to prevent the replication of donor:

     a   granulocytes
     (b) lymphocytes
     c   red cells
     d   platelets

37   Plastic bag overwraps are recommended when thawing units of FFP in 37°C water baths because they prevent:

     (a̶) the FFP bag from cracking when it contacts the warm water
     b   water from slowly dialyzing across the bag membrane   ***
     (c) the entry ports from becoming contaminated with water
     d   the label from peeling off as the water circulates in the bath

38   Which of the following blood components must be prepared within 8 hours after phlebotomy?

     a   Red Blood Cells   ** **
     (b) Fresh Frozen Plasma
     c   Red Blood Cells, Frozen
     d   Cryoprecipitated AHF

39 Cryoprecipitated AHF contains how many units of Factor VIII?
MLS ONLY

    a   40
    b   80
    c   130
    d   250

40 Which of the following blood components contains the most Factor VIII concentration relative
MLS ONLY to volume?

    a   Single-Donor Plasma
    b   Cryoprecipitated AHF
    c   Fresh Frozen Plasma
    d   Platelets

41 The most effective component to treat a patient with fibrinogen deficiency is:
MLS ONLY

    a   Fresh Frozen Plasma
    b   Platelets
    c   Fresh Whole Blood
    d   Cryoprecipitated AHF

42 A blood component prepared by thawing Fresh Frozen Plasma at refrigerator temperature and
removing the fluid portion is:

    a   Plasma Protein Fraction
    b   Cryoprecipitated AHF *— precipitate upon thawing*
    c   Factor IX Complex
    d   FP24

43 Upon inspection, a unit of platelets is noted to have visible clots, but otherwise appears normal.
The technologist should:

    a   issue without concern
    b   filter to remove the clots
    c   centrifuge to express off the clots
    d   quarantine for Gram stain and culture

44 According to AABB Standards, at least 90% of all Apheresis Platelets units tested shall contain a
MLS ONLY minimum of how many platelets?

    a 5.5×10^{10}
    b 6.5×10^{10}
    c 3.0×10^{11}
    d 5.0×10^{11}

45 According to AABB Standards, Platelets prepared from Whole Blood shall have at least:
MLS ONLY

    a 5.5×10^{10} platelets per unit in at least 90% of the units tested
    b 6.5×11^{10} platelets per unit in 90% of the units tested
    c 7.5×10^{10} platelets per unit in 100% of the units tested
    d 8.5×10^{10} platelets per unit in 95% of the units tested

46 Which of the following is proper procedure for preparation of Platelets from Whole Blood?

    a   light spin followed by a hard spin
    b   light spin followed by 2 hard spins
    c   2 light spins
    d   hard spin followed by a light spin

47 According to AABB standards, what is the minimum pH required for Platelets at the end of the
MLS ONLY storage period?

    a 6.0
    b 6.2
    c 6.8
    d 7.0

48 According to AABB standards, Platelets must be:
MLS ONLY
    a gently agitated if stored at room temperature
    b separated within 12 hours of Whole Blood collection
    c suspended in sufficient plasma to maintain a pH of 5.0 or lower
    d prepared only from Whole Blood units that have been stored at 4°C for 6 hours

49 A unit of Whole Blood-derived (random donor) Platelets should contain at least:

    a 1.0×10^{10} platelets
    b 5.5×10^{10} platelets
    c 5.5×10^{11} platelets
    d 90% of the platelets from the original unit of Whole Blood

50 Platelets prepared by apheresis should contain at least:

    a 1×10^{10} platelets
    b 3×10^{10} platelets
    c 3×10^{11} platelets
    d 5×10^{11} platelets

51 Leukocyte-Reduced Red Blood Cells are ordered for a newly diagnosed bone marrow candidate.
MLS ONLY What is the best way to prepare this product?

    a crossmatch only CMV-seronegative units
    b irradiate the unit with 1,500 rads
    c wash the unit with saline prior to infusion
    d transfuse through a Log^3 leukocyte-removing filter

52 Of the following blood components, which one should be used to prevent HLA alloimmunization
MLS ONLY of the recipient?

    a Red Blood Cells
    b Granulocytes
    c Irradiated Red Blood Cells
    d Leukocyte-Reduced Red Blood Cells

53 A father donating Platelets for his son is connected to a continuous flow machine, which uses the
principle of centrifugation to separate Platelets from Whole Blood. As the Platelets are harvested,
all other remaining elements are returned to the donor. This method of Platelet collection is
known as:

    a apheresis
    b autologous
    c homologous
    d fractionation

54 To qualify as a donor for autologous transfusion a patient's hemoglobin should be at least:

    a 8 g/dL (80 g/L)
    b 11 g/dL (110 g/L) within 72 hours
    c 13 g/dL (130 g/L)
    d 15 g/dL (150 g/L)

55 What is/are the minimum pretransfusion testing requirement(s) for autologous donations collected and transfused by the same facility?

  (a) ABO and Rh typing only – *autologous*
  b ABO/Rh type, antibody screen
  c ABO/Rh type, antibody screen, crossmatch
  d no pretransfusion testing is required for autologous donations

56 In a quality assurance program, Cryoprecipitated AHF must contain a minimum of how many international units of Factor VIII?
MLS ONLY

  a 60
  b 70
  (c) 80
  d 90

57 An assay of plasma from a bag of Cryoprecipitated AHF yields a concentration of 9 international units (IU) of Factor VIII per mL of Cryoprecipitated AHF. If the volume is 9 mL, what is the Factor VIII content of the bag in IU?
MLS ONLY

  a 9
  b 18
  c 27
  (d) 81

Blood Group Systems

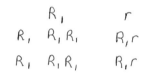

58 Refer to the following diagram:

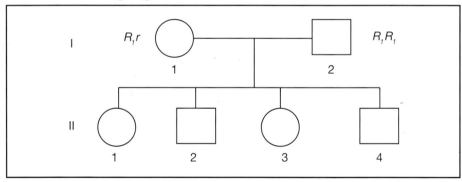

Given the most probable genotypes of the parents, which of the following statements best describes the most probable Rh genotypes of the 4 children?

  (a) 2 are R_1r, 2 are R_1R_1
  b 3 are R_1r, 1 is rr
  c 1 is R_0r, 1 is R_1r, 2 are R_1R_1
  d 1 is R_0r', 1 is R_1R_1, 2 are R_1r

59 The linked HLA genes on each chromosome constitute a(n):

  a allele – *gene mutation*
  b trait – *genetically determined characteristic; single or combined genes*
  c phenotype – *outward manifestation; physical*   *genotype – internal coding*
  (d) haplotype – *all located on one chromosome*

60   An individual's red blood cells give the following reactions with Rh antisera:

anti-D	anti-C	anti-E	anti-c	anti-e	Rh control
4+	3+	0	3+	3+	0

DCe/_ce

The individual's most probable genotype is:

a   DCe/DcE
b   DcE/dce   *DCe/dce ✳*
c   Dce/dce
d   DCe/dce   (circled)

61   A blood donor has the genotype: *hh*, AB. What is his red blood cell phenotype?

a   A
b   B
c   O – *will not produce A or B antigens without H*   (circled)
d   AB

62   An individual has been sensitized to the k antigen and has produced anti-k. What is her most probable Kell system genotype?

a   KK   (circled)
b   Kk
c   kk
d K_0K_0 = *K null*

63   Given the following typing results, what is this donor's racial ethnicity?

Le(a–b–); Fy(a–b–); Js(a+b+)

a   African American *Fy(a–b–)*   (circled)
b   Asian American
c   Native American
d   Caucasian

r' = dCe
r = dce

64   A mother has the red cell phenotype D+C+E–c–e+ with anti-c (titer of 32 at AHG) in her serum. The father has the phenotype D+C+E–c+e+. The baby is Rh-negative and not affected with hemolytic disease of the newborn. What is the baby's most probable Rh genotype?

a   r'r'   *dCe/dCe*   *dCe / dCe*   (circled)
b   r'r   *dCe/dce*
c R_1R_1 *DCe/DCe*
d R_1r *DCe/dce*
                 dce/dce

65   In an emergency situation, Rh-negative red cells are transfused into an Rh-positive person of the genotype CDe/CDe. The first antibody **most** likely to develop is:

a   anti-c   (circled)
b   anti-d
c   anti-e
d   anti-E

66   Most blood group systems are inherited as:

a   sex-linked dominant   *autosomal = not sex-linked*
b   sex-linked recessive
c   autosomal recessive
d   autosomal codominant   (circled)
                      XY   *XX*
67   The mating of an Xg(a+) man and an Xg(a–) woman will **only** produce:

a   Xg(a–) sons and Xg(a–) daughters
b   Xg(a+) sons and Xg(a+) daughters
c   Xg(a–) sons and Xg(a+) daughters   (circled)
d   Xg(a+) sons and Xg(a–) daughters

68   Refer to the following data:

anti-C	anti-D	anti-E	anti-c	anti-e
+	+	+	+	+

Given the reactions above, which is the most probable genotype?

a R_1R_1 DCe/DCe
b R_1r' DCe/dCe   DCE/Dce
c R_0r'' Dce/dcE
(d) R_1R_2 DCe/DcE

69   A patient's red cells type as follows:

anti-D	anti-C	anti-E
4+	0	0

Which of the following genotype would be consistent with these results?

(a) R_0R_0
b R_1r DCe/dce   Dce / Dce
c R_1R_2 DCe/DcE
d R_zr DCE/dce

70   The red cells of a nonsecretor (se/se) will most likely type as:

a   Le(a–b–) no lewis gene
b   Le(a+b+) lewis ~~non gene~~
(c)   Le(a+b–) ~~secre~~ non-secretor
d   Le(a–b+) lewis + secretor

71   Which of the following phenotypes will react with anti-f?   (ce) ✳

(a)   rr
b R_1R_1
c R_2R_2
d R_1R_2

72   A patient's red blood cells gave the following reactions:

anti-D	anti-C	anti-E	anti-c	anti-e	anti-f
+	+	+	+	+	0

The most probable genotype of this patient is:

(a) R_1R_2 DCE/Dce
b R_2r''
c R_zr
d R_zR_z

73   Anti-N is identified in a patient's serum. If random crossmatches are performed on 10 donor
MLS ONLY   units, how many would be expected to be compatible?

a   0
(b)   3
c   7
d   10

74   A woman types as Rh-positive. She has an anti-c titer of 32 at AHG. Her baby has a negative
DAT and is not affected by hemolytic disease of the newborn. What is the father's most likely
Rh phenotype?   c / c   DCe/DCE

~~a~~   rr
~~b~~   r''r
(c) R_1r
d R_2r

75   Which of the following red cell typings are most commonly found in the African American donor population?

    a Lu(a–b–)
    b Jk(a–b–)
    c Fy(a–b–)
    d K–k–

76   Four units of blood are needed for elective surgery. The patient's serum contains anti-C, anti-e, anti-Fy^a and anti-Jk^b. Which of the following would be the best source of donor blood?

    a test all units in current stock
    b test 100 group O, Rh-negative donors
    c test 100 group-compatible donors
    d rare donor file

77   A donor is tested with Rh antisera with the following results:

anti-D	anti-C	anti-E	anti-c	anti-e	Rh control
+	+	0	+	+	0

What is his most probable Rh genotype? DCe/Dce

    a R_1R_1
    b R_1r
    c R_0r
    d R_2r

78   A family has been typed for HLA because 1 of the children needs a stem cell donor. Typing results are listed below:

    father: A1,3;B8,35
    mother: A2,23;B12,18
    child #1:   A1,2;B8,12
    child #2:   A1,23;B8,18
    child #3:   A3,23;B18,?

What is the expected B antigen in child #3?

    a A1
    b A2
    c B12
    d B35

79   Which of the following is the best source of HLA-compatible platelets?
MLS ONLY
    a mother
    b father
    c siblings
    d cousins

80   A patient is group O, Rh-negative with anti-D and anti-K in her serum. What percentage of the
MLS ONLY   general Caucasian donor population would be compatible with this patient?

    a 0.5
    b 2.0
    c 3.0
    d 6.0

81 The observed phenotypes in a particular population are:

Phenotype	Number of persons
Jk(a+b–)	122
Jk(a+b+)	194
Jk(a–b+)	84

What is the gene frequency of Jk^a in this population?

a 0.31
b 0.45
c 0.55
d 0.60

82 In a random population, 16% of the people are Rh-negative (*rr*). What percentage of the Rh-positive population is heterozygous for *r*?

a 36%
b 48%
c 57%
d 66%

83 In relationship testing, a "direct exclusion" is established when a genetic marker is:

a absent in the child, but present in the mother and alleged father
b absent in the child, present in the mother and absent in the alleged father
c present in the child, absent in the mother and present in the alleged father
d present in the child, but absent in the mother and alleged father

84 Relationship testing produces the following red cell phenotyping results:

	ABO	**Rh**
alleged father:	B	D+C–c+E+e–
mother:	O	D+C+E–c–e+
child:	O	D+C+E–c+e+

What conclusions may be made?

a there is no exclusion of paternity
b paternity may be excluded on the basis of ABO typing
c paternity may be excluded on the basis of Rh typing
d paternity may be excluded on the basis of both ABO and Rh typing

85 In a relationship testing case, the child has a genetic marker that is absent in the mother and cannot be demonstrated in the alleged father. What type of paternity exclusion is this known as?

a indirect
b direct
c prior probability
d Hardy-Weinberg

86 A patient is typed with the following results:

Patient's cells with		Patient's serum with	
anti-A	0	A_1 red cells	2+
anti-B	0	B red cells	4+
anti-A,B	2+	Ab screen	0

The most probable reason for these findings is that the patient is group:

a O; confusion due to faulty group O antiserum
b O; with an anti-A_1
c A_x; with an anti-A_1
d A_1; with an anti-A

87   Human blood groups were discovered around 1900 by:

    a Jules Bordet
    b Louis Pasteur
    (c) Karl Landsteiner
    d PL Mollison

88   Cells of the A_3 subgroup will:

    a react with *Dolichos biflorus*
    b bE– with anti-A
    (c) give a mixed-field reaction with anti-A,B
    d bE– with anti-H

89   The enzyme responsible for conferring H activity on the red cell membrane is alpha-:

    a galactosyl transferase
    b N-acetylgalactosaminyl transferase
    (c) L-<u>fucos</u>yl transferase
    d N-acetylglucosaminyl transferase

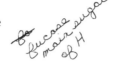 *fucose sugar main of H*

90   Even in the absence of prior transfusion or pregnancy, individuals with the Bombay phenotype (O_h) will always have naturally occurring:

    a anti-Rh   *no H on their cells (antigen), anti-H in their serum*
    b anti-K_o
    c anti-U
    (d) anti-H

91   The antibody in the Lutheran system that is best detected at lower temperatures is:

    (a) anti-Lu^a — *IgM*
    b anti-Lu^b
    c anti-Lu3   *IgG*
    d anti-Lu^{ab}

92   Which of the following antibodies is neutralizable by pooled human plasma?
MLS ØNLY

    a anti-Kn^a
    (b) anti-Ch
    c anti-Yk^a
    d anti-Cs^a

93   Anti-Sd^a is strongly suspected if: *Read up on anti-Sd^a HLA Antibodies*

    a the patient has been previously transfused
    (b) the agglutinates are mixed-field and refractile
    c the patient is group A or B
    d only a small number of panel cells are reactive

94   HLA antibodies are:

    a naturally occurring
    (b) induced by multiple transfusions
    c directed against granulocyte antigens only
    d frequently cause hemolytic transfusion reactions

95   Genes of the major histocompatibility complex (MHC):

    a code for HLA-A, HLA-B, and HLA-C antigens only
    b are linked to genes in the ABO system
    c are the primary genetic sex-determinants
    (d) contribute to the coordination of cellular and humoral immunity   *Self versus non-self*

96 Isoimmunization to platelet antigen HPA-1a and the placental transfer of maternal antibodies
MLS
ONLY would be expected to cause newborn:

    a erythroblastosis
    b leukocytosis
    c leukopenia
    d thrombocytopenia

97 Saliva from which of the following individuals would neutralize an auto anti-H in the serum of a
group A, Le(a–b+) patient?

    a group A, Le(a–b–)
    b group A, Le(a+b–)   *group O = most H*
    c group O, Le(a+b–)   *Le(a-b+) assures secretor*
    d group O, Le(a–b+)

98 Inhibition testing can be used to confirm antibody specificity for which of the
following antibodies?

    a anti-Lu^a ✳
    b anti-M
    c anti-Le^a *saliva soluble; anti-Le^a added = neutralization*
    d anti-Fy^a *Le^a+ cells = non-reactive*

99 Which of the following Rh antigens has the highest frequency in Caucasians?

    a D *85%*
    b E *30%*
    c c *80%*
    d e *98%* ✳

100 Anti-D and anti-C are identified in the serum of a transfused pregnant woman, gravida 2, para
MLS
ONLY 1. Nine months previously she received Rh immune globulin (RhIG) after delivery. Tests of the
patient, her husband, and the child revealed the following:

	anti-D	anti-C	anti-E	anti-c	anti-e
patient	0	0	0	+	+
father	+	0	0	+	+
child	+	0	0	+	+

The most likely explanation for the presence of anti-C is that this antibody is:

    a actually anti-C^w
    b from the RhIG dose
    c actually anti-G
    d naturally occurring

101 The phenomenon of an Rh-positive person whose serum contains anti-D is best explained by:
MLS
ONLY
    a gene deletion
    b missing antigen epitopes
    c trans position effect
    d gene inhibition

102 When the red cells of an individual fail to react with anti-U, they usually fail to react with:
MLS
ONLY
    a anti-M
    b anti-Le^b
    c anti-S
    d anti-P$_1$

103 Which of the following red cell antigens are found on glycophorin-A?

    a M, N = *glycophorin - A*
    b Le^a, Le^b
    c S, s
    d P, P_1, P^k

104 Paroxysmal cold hemoglobinuria (PCH) is associated with antibody specificity toward which of the following?

    a Kell system antigens
    b Duffy system antigens
    c P antigen = *PCH*
    d I antigen

105 Which of the following is a characteristic of anti-i? = *IM*

    a associated with warm autoimmune hemolytic anemia
    b found in the serum of patients with infectious mononucleosis
    c detected at lower temperatures in the serum of normal individuals
    d found only in the serum of group O individuals

106 In a case of cold autoimmune hemolytic anemia, the patient's serum would most likely react 4+ at immediate spin with:

    a group A cells, B cells and O cells, but not his own cells
    b cord cells but not his own or other adult cells
    c all cells of a group O cell panel and his own cells
    d only penicillin-treated panel cells, not his own cells

107 Cold agglutinin syndrome is associated with an antibody specificity toward which of the following?

    a Fy:3
    b P   *Anti - I = cold autoimmune hemolytic anemia*
    c I
    d Rh:1

108 Which of the following is a characteristic of anti-i?

    a often associated with hemolytic disease of the newborn
    b reacts best at room temperature or 4°C
    c reacts best at 37°C
    d is usually IgG

109 The Kell (K1) antigen is: *Kell: strongly immunogenic*

     9% of population
    a absent from the red cells of neonates   *on neonate RBC's*
    b strongly immunogenic   *NOT destroyed by enzymes*
    c destroyed by enzymes
    d has a frequency of 50% in the random population

110 In chronic granulomatous disease (CGD), granulocyte function is impaired. An association exists
MLS ONLY between this clinical condition and a depression of which of the following antigens?

    a Rh
    b P
    c Kell
    d Duffy

111 The antibodies of the Kidd blood group system:

   (a) react best by the indirect antiglobulin test
   b are predominantly IgM
   c often cause allergic transfusion reactions
   d do not generally react with antigen-positive, enzyme-treated RBCs

Kidd: delayed transfusion reactions
IgG → AHG
like enzymes

112 Proteolytic enzyme treatment of red cells usually destroys which antigen?

   a Jk^a
   b E
   (c) Fy^a
   d k

Duffy → destroyed by enzymes

113 Anti-Fy^a is:

   a usually a cold-reactive agglutinin
   b more reactive when tested with enzyme-treated red blood cells
   (c) capable of causing hemolytic transfusion reactions
   d often an autoagglutinin

114 Resistance to malaria is best associated with which of the following blood groups?

   a Rh
   b I/i
   c P
   (d) Duffy

115 What percent of group O donors would be compatible with a serum sample that contained anti-X
MLS
ONLY and anti-Y if X antigen is present on red cells of 5 of 20 donors, and Y antigen is present on
   red cells of 1 of 10 donors?

   a 2.5
   b 6.8
   c 25.0
   (d) 68.0

.25 × .10 = .75 × .90 = 67.5
×100

116 How many Caucasians in a population of 100,000 will have the following combination
MLS
ONLY of phenotypes?

System	Phenotype	Frequency (%)
ABO	O	45
Gm	Fb	48
PGM1	2-1	37
EsD	2-1	18

   a 1
   b 14
   c 144
   (d) 1,438

117 What is the approximate probability of finding compatible blood among random Rh-positive units
MLS
ONLY for a patient who has anti-c and anti-K? (Consider that 20% of Rh-positive donors lack c and 90%
   lack K)

   a 1%
   b 10%
   (c) 18%
   d 45%

118 A 25-year-old Caucasian woman, gravida 3, para 2, required 2 units of Red Blood Cells. The antibody screen was positive and the results of the antibody panel are shown below:

| | | | | | | | | | | | | | | EM | |
Cell	D	C	ⓒ	E	e	K	Jkᵃ	Jkᵇ	Leᵃ	Leᵇ	M	N	P₁	37°C	AHG
1	+	+	0	0	+	+	+	+	0	+	+	+	+	0	0
2	+	+	0	0	+	0	+	0	0	+	+	0	0	0	0
3	+	0	+	+	0	0	+	+	0	+	+	+	+	0	1+
4	+	+	+	0	+	0	0	+	0	+	+	0	+	0	1+
5	0	0	+	0	+	0	+	+	0	+	+	0	0	0	1+
6	0	0	+	+	+	0	+	0	+	0	+	+	0	0	1+
7	0	0	+	0	+	+	+	+	+	0	+	+	+	0	1+
8	0	0	+	0	+	0	0	+	0	+	0	+	+	0	1+
												auto		0	0

_____

EM = enhancement media

What is the most probable genotype of this patient?

- **a** rr   dce/dce
- **b** r′r′   dCe/dCe
- **c** R₀r   Dce/dce
- **d** R₁R₁   DCe/DCe ＊ *codes for little c*

(d) circled

$$r = dce \qquad R_0 = Dce$$
$$r' = dCe \qquad R_1 = DCe$$
$$r'' = dcE \qquad R_2 = DcE$$
$$r^Y = dCE \qquad R_z = DCE$$

Physiology and Pathophysiology

119 A man suffering from gastrointestinal bleeding has received 20 units of Red Blood Cells in the last 24 hours and is still oozing post-operatively. The following results were obtained:

PT:	20 seconds (control: 12 seconds)
APTT:	43 seconds (control: 31 seconds)
platelet count:	160 × 10³/µL (160 × 10⁹/L) *ok*
Hgb:	10 g/dL (100 g/L) *ok*
Factor VIII:	85% *ok*

massive transfusion = platelets + FFP

What blood product should be administered?

- (a) Fresh Frozen Plasma
- **b** Red Blood Cells
- **c** Factor VIII Concentrate
- **d** Platelets

120 Transfusion of which of the following is needed to help correct hypofibrinogenemia due to DIC?

- **a** Whole Blood
- **b** Fresh Frozen Plasma
- (c) Cryoprecipitated AHF
- **d** Platelets

Cryo = fibrinogen replacement

121 A blood component used in the treatment of hemophilia A is:

- (a) Factor VIII Concentrate
- **b** Fresh Frozen Plasma
- **c** Platelets
- **d** Whole Blood

122 Which of the following blood components is most appropriate to transfuse to an 8-year-old male
MLS ONLY   hemophiliac who is about to undergo minor surgery?

    a Cryoprecipitated AHF
    b Red Blood Cells
    c Platelets
    (d) Factor VIII Concentrate

123 A unit of Fresh Frozen Plasma was inadvertently thawed and then immediately refrigerated at 4°C
MLS ONLY   on Monday morning. On Tuesday evening this unit may still be transfused as a replacement for:

    a all coagulation factors
    b Factor V - ↓
    c Factor VIII - ↓
    (d) Factor IX - *no harm*

124 A newborn demonstrates petechiae, ecchymosis and mucosal bleeding. The preferred blood
MLS ONLY   component for this infant would be: *thrombocytopenia symptoms*

    a Red Blood Cells
    b Fresh Frozen Plasma
    (c) Platelets -
    d Cryoprecipitated AHF

125 Which of the following would be the best source of Platelets for transfusion in the case of
MLS ONLY   alloimmune neonatal thrombocytopenia?

    a father
    (b) mother
    c pooled platelet-rich plasma
    d polycythemic donor

126 An obstetrical patient has had 3 previous pregnancies. Her first baby was healthy, the second was
jaundiced at birth and required an exchange transfusion, while the third was stillborn. Which of
the following is the most likely cause?

    a ABO incompatibility
    b immune deficiency disease
    c congenital spherocytic anemia
    (d) Rh incompatibility

127 A specimen of cord blood is submitted to the transfusion service for routine testing. The following
MLS ONLY   results are obtained:

anti-A:	anti-B:	anti-D:	Rh-control:	direct antiglobulin test:
4+	negative	3+	negative	2+

It is known that the father is group B, with the genotype of *cde/cde*. Of the following 4 antibodies,
which 1 is the most likely cause of the positive direct antiglobulin test?

    a anti-A
    b anti-D
    (c) anti-c
    d anti-C

128 ABO-hemolytic disease of the newborn:

    a usually requires an exchange transfusion
    b most often occurs in first born children
    c frequently results in stillbirth
    (d) is usually seen only in the newborn of group O mothers

129 Which of the following antigens is **most** likely to be involved in hemolytic disease of the newborn?

    a Le^a
    b P₁ } *IgM*
    c M
    d Kell

130 ABO hemolytic disease of the fetus and newborn (HDFN) differs from Rh HDFN in that:

    a Rh HDFN is clinically more severe than ABO HDFN
    b the direct antiglobulin test is weaker in Rh HDFN than ABO
    c Rh HDFN occurs in the first pregnancy
    d the mother's antibody screen is positive in ABO HDN

131 The following results were obtained:
MLS ONLY

	anti-A	anti-B	anti-D	Weak D	DAT	Ab screen	
infant	0	0	0	NT	4+	NT	*O –*
mother	4+	0	0	0	NT	anti-D	*A –*

NT = not tested

Which of the following is the most probable explanation for these results?

    a ABO hemolytic disease of the fetus and newborn
    b Rh hemolytic disease of the fetus and newborn; infant has received intrauterine transfusions
    c Rh hemolytic disease of the fetus and newborn, infant has a false-negative Rh typing
    d large fetomaternal hemorrhage

132 A group A, Rh-positive infant of a group O, Rh-positive mother has a weakly positive direct antiglobulin test and a moderately elevated bilirubin 12 hours after birth. The most likely cause is:

    a ABO incompatibility
    b Rh incompatibility
    c blood group incompatibility due to an antibody to a low frequency antigen
    d neonatal jaundice **not** associated with blood group

133 In suspected cases of hemolytic disease of the newborn, what significant information can be
MLS ONLY obtained from the baby's blood smear?

    spherocytes = HDN

    a estimation of WBC, RBC, and platelet counts
    b marked increase in immature neutrophils (shift to the left)
    c a differential to estimate the absolute number of lymphocytes present
    d determination of the presence of spherocytes

134 The Liley method of predicting the severity of hemolytic disease of the newborn is based on the amniotic fluid:

    Liley graph = OD @ 450 nm

    a bilirubin concentration by standard methods
    b change in optical density measured at 450 nm
    c Rh determination
    d ratio of lecithin to sphingomyelin

    HDN = +DAT
    hgb ↓14 (14–20 normal)

135 These laboratory results were obtained on maternal and cord blood samples:

    mother: A–
    baby: AB+, DAT: 3+ cord hemoglobin: 10 g/dL (100 g/L)

Does the baby have HDN?

    a no, as indicated by the cord hemoglobin
    b yes, although the cord hemoglobin is normal, the DAT indicates HDN
    c yes, the DAT and cord hemoglobin level both support HDN
    d no, a diagnosis of HDN cannot be established without cord bilirubin levels

136 The main purpose of performing antibody titers on serum from prenatal immunized women is to:

  a determine the identity of the antibody
  (b) identify candidates for amniocentesis or percutaneous umbilical blood sampling
  c decide if the baby needs an intrauterine transfusion
  d determine if early induction of labor is indicated

137 Which unit should be selected for exchange transfusion if the newborn is group A, Rh-positive and the mother is group A, Rh-positive with anti-c?

  (a) A, CDe/CDe
  b A, cDE/cDE
  c O, cde/cde
  d A, cde/cde

138 A mother is group A, with anti-D in her serum. What would be the preferred blood product if an intrauterine transfusion is indicated?

  a O, Rh-negative Red Blood Cells
  (b) O, Rh-negative Red Blood Cells, Irradiated
  c A, Rh-negative Red Blood Cells
  d A, Rh-negative Red Blood Cells, Irradiated

139 Laboratory studies of maternal and cord blood yield the following results:

Maternal blood	**Cord blood**
O, Rh-negative	B, Rh-positive
anti-E in serum	DAT = 2+
	anti-E in eluate

If exchange transfusion is necessary, the best choice of blood is:

  a B, Rh-negative, E+
  b B, Rh-positive, E+
  c O, Rh-negative, E–
  (d) O, Rh-positive, E–

140 A blood specimen from a pregnant woman is found to be group B, Rh-negative and the serum contains anti-D with a titer of 512. What would be the most appropriate type of blood to have available for a possible exchange transfusion for her infant?

  (a) O, Rh-negative
  b O, Rh-positive
  c B, Rh-negative
  d B, Rh-positive

141 Blood selected for exchange transfusion must:

  (a) lack red blood cell antigens corresponding to maternal antibodies
  b be <3 days old
  c be the same Rh type as the baby
  d be ABO compatible with the father

142 When the main objective of an exchange transfusion is to remove the infant's antibody-sensitized red blood cells and to control hyperbilirubinemia, the blood product of choice is ABO compatible:

  a Fresh Whole Blood
  b Red Blood Cells (RBC) washed
  (c) RBC suspended in Fresh Frozen Plasma ✳
  d heparinized Red Blood Cells

143   To prevent graft-vs-host disease, Red Blood Cells prepared for infants who have received intrauterine transfusions should be:

    a   saline-washed
    b   irradiated
    c   frozen and deglycerolized
    d   group- and Rh-compatible with the mother

144   Which of the following is the preferred specimen for the initial compatibility testing in exchange transfusion therapy?

MLS ONLY

    a   maternal serum
    b   eluate prepared from infant's red blood cells
    c   paternal serum
    d   infant's postexchange serum

145   Rh-Immune Globulin is requested for an Rh-negative mother who has the following results:

	D	D control	Weak D	Weak D control
mother's postpartum sample:	0	0	$1+^{mf}$	0

mf = mixed field

What is the most likely explanation?

    a   mother is a genetic weak D
    b   mother had a fetomaternal hemorrhage of D+ cells
    c   mother's red cells are coated weakly with IgG
    d   anti-D reagent is contaminated with an atypical antibody

146   The following results are seen on a maternal postpartum sample:

	D	D control	Weak D	Weak D control
mother's postpartum sample:	0	0	$1+^{mf}$	0

mf = mixed field

The most appropriate course of action is to:

    a   report the mother as Rh-negative
    b   report the mother as Rh-positive
    c   perform an elution on mother's RBCs
    d   investigate for a fetomaternal hemorrhage

147   What is the most appropriate interpretation for the laboratory data given below when an Rh-negative woman has an Rh-positive child?

Rosette fetal screen using enzyme-treated D+ cells

mother's sample:	1 rosette/3 fields
positive control:	5 rosettes/3 fields
negative control:	no rosettes observed

quantitative: mild bleed = 1 rosette per 3 fields = 1 unit rhogam (normal bleed)

    a   mother is not a candidate for RhIg
    b   mother needs 1 vial of RhIg
    c   mother needs 2 vials of RhIg
    d   the fetal-maternal hemorrhage needs to be quantitated

148 Refer to the following information:

Postpartum	anti-D	Rh control	Weak D	Weak D control	Rosette fetal screen
mother	0	0	+ micro	0	20 rosettes/5 fields
newborn	4+	0	NT	NT	NT

NT = not tested

What is the best interpretation for the laboratory data given above?

  a mother is Rh-positive
  b mother is weak D+
  (c) mother has had a fetal-maternal hemorrhage
  d mother has a positive DAT

149 A weakly reactive anti-D is detected in a postpartum specimen from an Rh-negative woman.
MLS ONLY During her prenatal period, all antibody screening tests were negative. These findings indicate:

  a that she is a candidate for Rh immune globulin
  b that she is **not** a candidate for Rh immune globulin
  (c) a need for further investigation to determine candidacy for Rh immune globulin
  d the presence of Rh-positive cells in her circulation

150 The results of a Kleihauer-Betke stain indicate a fetomaternal hemorrhage of 35 mL of whole blood. How many vials of Rh immune globulin would be required?

  a 1 *vial = 30 mls whole blood protection / 15 mls RBC's*
  (b) 2
  c 3
  d 4

151 A fetomaternal hemorrhage of 35 mL of fetal Rh-positive packed RBCs has been detected in an Rh-negative woman. How many vials of Rh immune globulin should be given?

  a 0
  b 1
  c 2
  (d) 3 *– 15 mls RBC's*

152 Criteria determining Rh immune globulin eligibility include:

  a mother is Rh-positive
  b infant is Rh-negative
  (c) mother has not been previously immunized to the D antigen
  d infant has a positive direct antiglobulin test

153 While performing routine postpartum testing for an Rh immune globulin (RhIG) candidate, a
MLS ONLY weakly positive antibody screening test was found. Anti-D was identified. This antibody is most likely the result of:

  a massive fetomaternal hemorrhage occurring at the time of this delivery
  (b) antenatal administration of Rh immune globulin at 28 weeks gestation
  c contamination of the blood sample with Wharton jelly
  d mother having a positive direct antiglobulin test

154 Rh immune globulin administration would **not** be indicated in an Rh-negative woman who has a(n):

  a first trimester abortion
  b husband who is Rh-positive
  (c) anti-D titer of 1:4,096
  d positive direct antiglobulin test

155 A Kleihauer-Betke stain of a postpartum blood film revealed 0.3% fetal cells. What is the estimated volume (mL) of the fetomaternal hemorrhage expressed as whole blood?

a 5
(b) 15
c 25
d 35

% × 5,000 (*maternal blood volume*)
=

156 Based upon Kleihauer-Betke test results, which of the following formulas is used to determine the volume of fetomaternal hemorrhage expressed in mL of whole blood?

a % of fetal cells present × 30
(b) % of fetal cells present × 50
c % of maternal cells present × 30
d % of maternal cells present × 50

157 An acid elution stain was made using a 1-hour post-delivery maternal blood sample. Out of 2,000 cells that were counted, 30 of them appeared to contain fetal hemoglobin. It is the policy of the medical center to add 1 vial of Rh immune globulin to the calculated dose when the estimated volume of the hemorrhage exceeds 20 mL of whole blood. Calculate the number of vials of Rh immune globulin that would be indicated under these circumstances.

a 2
b 3
(c) 4
d 5

75 mls fetal blood = 75 ÷ 30 = 2.5 = ↑3 + 1 = (4)

158 The rosette test will detect a fetomaternal hemorrhage (FMH) as small as:

(a) 10 mL
b 15 mL
c 20 mL
d 30 mL

159 A 10 mL fetal maternal hemorrhage in an Rh-negative woman who delivered an Rh-positive baby
MLS ONLY means that the:

a mother's antibody screen will be positive for anti-D
(b) rosette test will be positive
c mother is not a candidate for Rh immune globulin
d mother should receive 2 doses of Rh immune globulin

160 Mixed leukocyte culture (MLC) is a biological assay for detecting which of the following?
MLS ONLY
a HLA-A antigens
b HLA-B antigens
(c) HLA-D antigens
d immunoglobulins

161 A 40-year-old man with autoimmune hemolytic anemia due to anti-E has a hemoglobin level of 10.8 g/dL (108 g/L). This patient will most likely be treated with:

a Whole Blood
b Red Blood Cells
c Fresh Frozen Plasma
(d) no transfusion

162 A patient in the immediate post bone marrow transplant period has a hematocrit of 21%. The red cell product of choice for this patient would be:

a packed
b saline washed
c microaggregate filtered
(d) irradiated

163   HLA antigen typing is important in screening for:

    a ABO incompatibility
    b a kidney donor
    c Rh incompatibility
    d a blood donor

164   DR antigens in the HLA system are:

MLS ONLY

    a significant in organ transplantation
    b not detectable in the lymphocytotoxicity test
    c expressed on platelets
    d expressed on granulocytes

165   Anti-E is identified in a panel at the antiglobulin phase. When check cells are added to the tubes, no agglutination is seen. The most appropriate course of action would be to:

    a quality control the AHG reagent and check cells and repeat the panel
    b open a new vial of check cells for subsequent testing that day
    c open a new vial of AHG for subsequent testing that day
    d record the check cell reactions and report the antibody panel result

Serology

166   A serological centrifuge is recalibrated for ABO testing after major repairs.

MLS ONLY

Time in seconds	15	20	25	30
is button delineated?	yes	yes	yes	yes
is supernatant clear?	no	yes	yes	yes
button easy to resuspend?	yes	yes	yes	no
strength of reaction?	+m	1+	1+	1+

Given the data above, the centrifuge time for this machine should be:

    a 15 seconds
    b 20 seconds
    c 25 seconds
    d 30 seconds

167   Which of the following represents an acceptably identified patient for sample collection and transfusion?

    a a handwritten band with patient's name and hospital identification number is affixed to the patient's leg
    b the addressographed hospital band is taped to the patient's bed
    c an unbanded patient responds positively when his name is called
    d the chart transported with the patient contains his armband not yet attached

168 Samples from the same patient were received on 2 consecutive days.
Test results are summarized below:

	Day #1	Day #2
anti-A	4+	0
anti-B	0	4+
anti-D	3+	3+
A₁ cells	0	4+
B cells	4+	0
Ab screen	0	0

How should the request for crossmatch be handled?

a crossmatch A, Rh-positive units with sample from day 1
b crossmatch B, Rh-positive units with sample from day 2
c crossmatch AB, Rh-positive units with both samples
d collect a new sample and repeat the tests

169 The following test results are noted for a unit of blood labeled group A, Rh-negative:

Cells tested with:

anti-A	anti-B	anti-D
4+	0	3+

What should be done next?

Test ABO and Rh reg units; notify blood bank if labeled wrong

a transfuse as a group A, Rh-negative
b transfuse as a group A, Rh-positive
c notify the collecting facility
d discard the unit

170 What information is essential on patient blood sample labels drawn for compatibility testing?

a biohazard sticker for AIDS patients
b patient's room number
c unique patient medical number
d phlebotomist initials

171 Granulocytes for transfusion should:

a be administered through a microaggregate filter
b be ABO compatible with the recipient's serum
c be infused within 72 hours of collection
d never be transfused to patients with a history of febrile transfusion reactions

172 A neonate will be transfused for the first time with group O Red Blood Cells. Which of the following is appropriate compatibility testing?

✳ no XM for babies if screen negative

a crossmatch with mother's serum
b crossmatch with baby's serum
c no crossmatch is necessary if initial plasma screening is negative
d no screening or crossmatching is necessary for neonates

173 A group B, Rh-negative patient has a positive DAT. Which of the following situations would occur?

✳ DAT positive pts

a all major crossmatches would be incompatible
b the weak D test and control would be positive
c the antibody screening test would be positive
d the forward and reverse ABO groupings would not agree

174 The following reactions were obtained:

Cells tested with:			Serum tested with:	
anti-A	anti-B	anti-A,B	A₁ cells	B cells
4+	3+	4+	2+	4+

The technologist washed the patient's cells with saline, and repeated the forward typing. A saline replacement technique was used with the reverse typing. The following results were obtained:

Cells tested with:			Serum tested with:	
anti-A	anti-B	anti-A,B	A₁ cells	B cells
4+	0	4+	0	4+

The results are consistent with:

handwritten: all positive → rouleaux (MM), washing cells → removes protein, saline replacement on serum

a acquired immunodeficiency disease
b Bruton agammaglobulinemia
c multiple myeloma
d acquired "B" antigen

175 What is the most likely cause of the following ABO discrepancy?

Patient's cells vs:		Patient's serum vs:	
anti-A	anti-B	A₁ cells	B cells
0	0	0	0

a recent transfusion with group O blood
b antigen depression due to leukemia
c false-negative cell typing due to rouleaux
d obtained from a heel stick of a 2-month old baby - *no antibodies until 3 months*

176 Which of the following patient data best reflects the discrepancy seen when a person's red cells demonstrate the acquired-B phenotype? - *no B in reverse grouping*

	Forward grouping	Reverse grouping
patient A	B	O
patient B	AB	A
patient C	O	B
patient D	B	AB

a A
b B
c C
d D

177 Which of the following is characteristic of Tn polyagglutinable red cells? *→ disease*

a if group O, they may appear to have acquired a group A antigen
b they show strong reactions when the cells are enzyme-treated
c they react with *Arachis hypogaea* lectin
d the polyagglutination is a transient condition

178 Mixed field agglutination encountered in ABO grouping with no history of transfusion would most likely be due to:

a Bombay phenotype (O_h)
b T activation
c A₃ red cells - *mixed field*
d positive indirect antiglobulin test

179 Which of the following is a characteristic of polyagglutinable red cells?

a can be classified by reactivity with *Ulex europaeus*
b are agglutinated by most adult sera
c are always an acquired condition
d autocontrol is always positive

180 Consider the following ABO typing results:

Patient's cells vs:		Patient's serum vs:	
anti-A	anti-B	A₁ cells	B cells
4+	0	1+	4+

Additional testing was performed using patient serum:

	IS	RT
screening cell I	1+	2+
screening cell II	1+	2+
autocontrol	1+	2+

What is the **most likely** cause of this discrepancy?

  a A₂ with anti-A₁
  b cold alloantibody
  ⓒ cold autoantibody   ✳
  d acquired-A phenomenon

181 Consider the following ABO typing results:
MLS ONLY

Patient's cells vs:		Patient's serum vs:	
anti-A	anti-B	A₁ cells	B cells
4+	0	1+	4+

Additional testing was performed using patient serum:

	IS	RT
screening cell I	1+	2+
screening cell II	1+	2+
autocontrol	1+	2+

What should be done next?

  a test serum against a panel of group O cells
  b neutralization
  ⓒ perform serum type at 37°C
  d elution

182 The following results were obtained on a patient's blood sample during routine ABO and Rh testing:

Cell testing:		Serum testing:	
anti-A:	0	A₁ cells:	4+
anti-B:	4+	B cells:	2+
anti-D:	0		
autocontrol:	0		

Select the course of action to resolve this problem:

  a draw a new blood sample from the patient and repeat all test procedures
  b test the patient's serum with A₂ cells and the patient's red cells with anti-A₁ lectin
  c repeat the ABO antigen grouping using 3× washed saline-suspended cells
  ⓓ perform antibody screening procedure at immediate spin using group O cells ✳

183 Which of the following explains an ABO discrepancy caused by problems with the patient's red blood cells?
MLS ONLY

  a an unexpected antibody
  b rouleaux
  c agammaglobulinemia
  ⓓ Tn activation

184 The test for weak D is performed by incubating patient's red cells with:

    a several different dilutions of anti-D serum
    b anti-D serum followed by washing and antiglobulin serum
    c anti-D^u serum
    d antiglobulin serum

185 Refer to the following data:
MLS
ONLY

Forward group:			Reverse group:		
anti-A	anti-B	anti-A$_1$ lectin	A$_1$ cells	A$_2$ cells	B cells
4+	0	4+	0	2+	4+

Which of the following antibody screen results would you expect with the ABO discrepancy seen above?

    a negative
    b positive with all screen cells at the 37°C phase
    c positive with all screen cells at the RT phase; autocontrol is negative
    d positive with all screen cells and the autocontrol cells at the RT phase

186 The following results were obtained when testing a sample from a 20-year-old, first-time blood donor:

Forward group:		Reverse group:	
anti-A	anti-B	A$_1$ cells	B cells
0	0	0	3+

What is the most likely cause of this ABO discrepancy?

    a loss of antigen due to disease
    b acquired B
    c phenotype O$_h$ "Bombay"
    d weak subgroup of A

187 A mother is Rh-negative and the father Rh-positive. Their baby is Rh-negative. It may be concluded that:

    a the father is homozygous for D
    b the mother is heterozygous for D
    c the father is heterozygous for D
    d at least 1 of the 3 Rh typings must be incorrect

188 Some blood group antibodies characteristically hemolyze appropriate red cells in the presence of:

    a complement
    b anticoagulants
    c preservatives
    d penicillin

189 Review the following schematic diagram:

    PATIENT SERUM + REAGENT GROUP "O" CELLS
    INCUBATE → READ FOR AGGLUTINATION
    WASH → ADD AHG →  AGGLUTINATION OBSERVED

The next step would be to:

    a add "check cells" as a confirmatory measure
    b identify the cause of the agglutination
    c perform an elution technique
    d perform a direct antiglobulin test

190 The following results were obtained in pretransfusion testing:

	37°C	IAT
screening cell I	0	3+
screening cell II	0	3+
autocontrol	0	3+

The most probable cause of these results is:

a rouleaux
(b) a warm autoantibody
c a cold autoantibody
d multiple alloantibodies

191 A patient is typed as group O, Rh-positive and crossmatched with 6 units of blood. At the indirect antiglobulin (IAT) phase of testing, both antibody screening cells and 2 crossmatched units are incompatible. What is the most likely cause of the incompatibility?

(a) recipient alloantibody
b recipient autoantibody
c donors have positive DATs
d rouleaux

192 Refer to the following data:

hemoglobin: 7.4 g/dL (74 g/L)
reticulocyte count: 22%

Direct Antiglobulin Test		**Ab Screen – IAT**	
polyspecific:	3+	SC I:	3+
IgG:	3+	SC II:	3+
C3:	0	auto:	3+

Which clinical condition is consistent with the lab results shown above?

a cold hemagglutinin disease
(b) warm autoimmune hemolytic anemia
c penicillin-induced hemolytic anemia
d delayed hemolytic transfusion reaction

193 A patient received 2 units of Red Blood Cells and had a delayed transfusion reaction. Pretransfusion antibody screening records indicate no agglutination except after the addition of IgG sensitized cells. Repeat testing of the pretransfusion specimen detected an antibody at the antiglobulin phase. What is the most likely explanation for the original results?

a red cells were overwashed
b centrifugation time was prolonged
(c) patient's serum was omitted from the original testing
d antiglobulin reagent was neutralized

194 At the indirect antiglobulin phase of testing, there is no agglutination between patient serum and screening cells. One of 3 donor units was incompatible.

The most probable explanation for these findings is that the:

a patient has an antibody directed against a high incidence antigen
(b) patient has an antibody directed against a low incidence antigen
c donor has an antibody directed against donor cells
d donor has a positive antibody screen

pt serum with donor's cells
group O cells used in this crossmatch

195 The major crossmatch will detect a(n):

a group A patient mistyped as group O
b unexpected red cell antibody in the donor unit
c Rh-negative donor unit mislabeled as Rh-positive
(d) recipient antibody directed against antigens on the donor red cells

196 A 42-year-old female is undergoing surgery tomorrow and her physician requests that 4 units of Red Blood Cells be crossmatched. The following results were obtained:

	IS	37°C	IAT
screening cell I	0	0	0
screening cell II	0	0	0
screening cell III	0	0	0

Crossmatch	IS	37°C	IAT
donor 1:	2+	1+	1+
donors 2,3,4:	0	0	0

What is the most likely cause of the incompatibility of donor 1?

   a single alloantibody *in pt serum; donor cells have low incidence antigen*
   b multiple alloantibodies
   c Rh incompatibilities
   d donor 1 has a positive DAT

197 Which of the following would most likely be responsible for an incompatible antiglobulin crossmatch?

   a recipient's red cells possess a low frequency antigen
   b anti-K antibody in donor serum
   c recipient's red cells are polyagglutinable
   d donor red cells have a positive direct antiglobulin test

✱ Crossmatch = pt serum w/ donor cells
incompatibility due to cells (DAT or low-incidence antigen)

198 A reason why a patient's crossmatch may be incompatible while the antibody screen is negative is:

   a the patient has an antibody against a high-incidence antigen
   b the incompatible donor unit has a positive direct antiglobulin test
   c cold agglutinins are interfering in the crossmatch
   d the patient's serum contains warm autoantibody

199 A blood specimen types as A, Rh-positive with a negative antibody screen. 6 units of group A, Rh-positive Red Blood Cells were crossmatched and 1 unit was incompatible in the antiglobulin phase. The same result was obtained when the test was repeated. Which should be done **first**?

   a repeat the ABO grouping on the incompatible unit using a more sensitive technique
   b test a panel of red cells that possesses low-incidence antigens
   c perform a direct antiglobulin test on the donor unit
   d obtain a new specimen and repeat the crossmatch

200 During emergency situations when there is no time to determine ABO group and Rh type on a current sample for transfusion, the patient is known to be A, Rh-negative. The technologist should:

   a refuse to release any blood until the patient's sample has been typed
   b release A Rh-negative Red Blood Cells
   c release O Rh-negative Red Blood Cells
   d release O Rh-positive Red Blood Cells

201 A 29-year-old male is hemorrhaging severely. He is AB, Rh-negative. 6 units of blood are required STAT. Of the following types available in the blood bank, which would be most preferable for crossmatch?

   a AB, Rh-positive
   b A, Rh-negative
   c A, Rh-positive
   d O, Rh-negative

202 A patient is group A$_2$B, Rh-positive and has an antiglobulin- reacting anti-A$_1$ in his serum. He is in the operating room bleeding profusely and group A$_2$B Red Blood Cells are **not** available. Which of the following blood types is first choice for crossmatching?

   (a) B, Rh-positive
   b B, Rh-negative
   c A$_1$B, Rh-positive
   d O, Rh-negative

203 A 10% red cell suspension in saline is used in a compatibility test. Which of the following would most likely occur?

   a a false-positive result due to antigen excess
   b a false-positive result due to the prozone phenomenon
   c a false-negative result due to the prozone phenomenon
   (d) a false-negative result due to antigen excess

204 A patient serum reacts with 2 of the 3 antibody screening cells at the AHG phase. 8 of the 10 units crossmatched were incompatible at the AHG phase. All reactions are markedly enhanced by enzymes. These results are most consistent with:

   a anti-M *destroyed by enzyme*
   b anti-E *rh enhanced by enzymes; anti-C 80%, anti-E 20%*
   (c) anti-c
   d anti-Fy^a *destroyed by enzymes*

205 A patient received 4 units of blood 2 years previously and now has multiple antibodies. He has not been transfused since that time. It would be most helpful to:

   (a) phenotype his cells to determine which additional alloantibodies may be produced
   b recommend the use of directed donors, which are more likely to be compatible
   c use proteolytic enzymes to destroy the "in vitro" activity of some of the antibodies
   d freeze the patient's serum to use for antigen typing of compatible units

206 Autoantibodies demonstrating blood group specificity in warm autoimmune hemolytic anemia are associated more often with which blood group system?

   (a) Rh !!!
   b I   *   *Warm autoimmune antibodies → rh*
   c P
   d Duffy

207 An antibody that causes in vitro hemolysis and reacts with the red cells of 3 out of ten crossmatched donor units is most likely:

   (a) anti-Le^a *→ binds complement; 22% incidence*
   b anti-s
   c anti-k
   d anti-E

208 A patient's serum reacted weakly positive (1+^{w}) with 16 of 16 group O panel cells at the AHG test phase. The autocontrol was negative. Tests with ficin-treated panel cells demonstrated no reactivity at the AHG phase. Which antibody is most likely responsible for these results?

   (a) anti-Ch
   b anti-k
   c anti-e *enhanced (rh) → enzyme*
   d anti-Js^b

209 An antibody identification study is performed with the 5-cell panel shown below:

		Antigens 1	2	3	4	5	Test results
Panel cells	I	+	0	0	+	+	+
	II	0	0	+	0	+	0
	III	0	+	+	+	0	0
	IV	0	+	+	0	+	+
	V	+	+	+	0	0	+
						auto	0

An antibody against which of the following antigens could **not** be excluded?

(a) 1
b 2
c 3
d 4

210 A 25-year-old Caucasian woman, gravida 3, para 2, required 2 units of Red Blood Cells.
The antibody screen was positive and the results of the antibody panel are shown below:

Cell	D	C	c	E	e	K	Jk^a	Jk^b	Le^a	Le^b	M	N	P$_1$	EM 37°C	AHG
1	+	+	0	0	+	+	+	+	0	+	+	+	+	0	0
2	+	+	0	0	+	0	+	0	0	+	+	0	0	0	0
3	+	0	+	+	0	0	+	+	0	+	+	+	+	0	1+
4	+	+	+	0	+	0	0	+	0	+	+	0	+	0	1+
5	0	0	+	0	+	0	+	+	0	+	+	0	0	0	1+
6	0	0	+	+	+	0	+	0	+	0	+	+	0	0	1+
7	0	0	+	0	+	+	+	+	+	0	+	+	+	0	1+
8	0	0	+	0	+	0	0	+	0	+	0	+	+	0	1+
													auto	0	0

EM = enhancement media

Which of the following antibodies may be the cause of the positive antibody screen?

a anti-M and anti-K
(b) anti-c and anti-E
c anti-Jk^a and anti-c
d anti-P$_1$ and anti-c

211
MLS ONLY
A 25-year-old Caucasian woman, gravida 3, para 2, required 2 units of Red Blood Cells. The antibody screen was positive and the results of the antibody panel are shown below:

Cell	D	C	c	E	e	K	Jka	Jkb	Lea	Leb	M	N	P1	EM 37°C	AHG
1	+	+	0	0	+	+	+	+	0	+	+	+	+	0	0
2	+	+	0	0	+	0	+	0	0	+	+	0	0	0	0
3	+	0	+	+	0	0	+	+	0	+	+	+	+	0	1+
4	+	+	+	0	+	0	0	+	0	+	+	0	+	0	1+
5	0	0	+	0	+	0	+	+	0	+	+	0	0	0	1+
6	0	0	+	+	+	0	+	0	+	0	+	+	0	0	1+
7	0	0	+	0	+	+	+	+	+	0	+	+	+	0	1+
8	0	0	+	0	+	0	0	+	0	+	0	+	+	0	1+
													auto	0	0

EM = enhancement media

Which common antibody has **not** been ruled out by the panel?

a anti-C
b anti-Leb
c anti-Jka
(d) anti-E

212 In the process of identifying an antibody, the technologist observed 2+ reactions with 3 of the 10 cells in a panel after the immediate spin phase. There was no reactivity after incubation at 37°C and after the anti-human globulin test phase. The antibody most likely is:

a anti-P1 } both IgM, but P1 80% and Lea 22%
(b) anti-Lea
c anti-C
d anti-Fya

213 Transfusion of Ch+ (Chido-positive) red cells to a patient with anti-Ch has been reported to cause:

(a) no clinically significant red cell destruction
b clinically significant immune red cell destruction
c decreased ^{51}Cr red cell survivals   Ch+ (Chido) → clinically insignificant
d febrile transfusion reactions

214
MLS ONLY
Results of a serum sample tested against a panel of reagent red cells gives presumptive evidence of an alloantibody directed against a high incidence antigen. Further investigation to confirm the specificity should include which of the following?

a serum testing against red cells from random donors
(b) serum testing against red cells known to lack high incidence antigens (inhibition)
c serum testing against enzyme-treated autologous red cells
d testing of an eluate prepared from the patient's red cells

215 Refer to the following data:

Forward group:			Reverse group:		
anti-A	anti-B	anti-A$_1$ lectin	A$_1$ cells	A$_2$ cells	B cells
4+	0	4+	0	2+	4+

The ABO discrepancy seen above is most likely due to:

a anti-A$_1$
b rouleaux
(c) anti-H → *greatest amount on O cells, then A$_2$ cells*
d unexpected IgG antibody present

216 Refer to the following panel:

														EM	
Cell	D̸	C̸	c̸	E	e̸	K	Jk^a	Jk^b	Le^a	Le^b	M̸	N̸	P̸$_1$	37°C	AHG
1	+	+	0	0	+	+	+	+	0	+	+	+	+	0	2+
2	+	+	0	0	+	0	+	0	0	+	+	0	0	0	3+
3	+	0	+	+	0	0	+	+	0	+	+	+	+	1+	3+
4	+	+	+	0	+	0	0	+	0	+	+	0	+	0	0
5	0	0	+	0	+	0	+	+	0	+	+	0	0	0	2+
6	0	0	+	+	+	0	+	0	+	0	+	+	0	1+	3+
7	0	0	+	0	+	+	+	+	+	0	+	+	+	0	2+
8	0	0	+	0	+	0	0	+	0	+	0	+	+	0	0
														auto 0	0

EM = enhancement media

Based on the results of the above panel, the most likely antibodies are:

a anti-M and anti-K
(b) anti-E, anti-Jk^a and anti-K
c anti-Jk^a and anti-M
d anti-E and anti-Le^b

✱ *dosage   -HDN*

217 Which characteristics are true of **all 3** of the following antibodies: anti-Fy^a, anti-Jk^a, and anti-K?

(a) detected at IAT phase and may cause hemolytic disease of the fetus and newborn (HDFN) and transfusion reactions
b not detected with enzyme treated cells; may cause delayed transfusion reactions
c requires the IAT technique for detection; usually not responsible for causing HDFN
d may show dosage effect; may cause severe hemolytic transfusion reactions

HDN: Anti-Fy^a
Anti-Jk^a
Anti-K

218 Refer to the following cell panel:

Cell	D	C	c	E	e	K	Jkᵃ	Jkᵇ	Leᵃ	Leᵇ	M	N	P₁	AHG	Enzymes AHG
1	+	+	0	0	+	+	+	+	0	+	+	+	+	3+	4+
2	+	+	0	0	+	0	+	0	0	+	+	0	0	3+	4+
3	+	0	+	+	0	0	+	+	0	+	+	+	+	0	0
4	+	+	+	0	+	0	0	+	0	+	+	0	+	2+	3+
5	0	0	+	0	+	0	+	+	0	+	+	0	0	0	0
6	0	0	+	+	+	0	+	0	+	0	+	+	0	0	0
7	0	0	+	0	+	+	+	+	+	0	+	+	+	0	0
8	0	0	+	0	+	0	0	+	0	+	0	+	+	0	0
													auto	0	0

Based on these results, which of the following antibodies is **most** likely present?

ⓐ anti-C
b anti-E
c anti-D
d anti-K

219 A pregnant woman has a positive antibody screen and the panel results are given below:

Cell	D	C	c	E	e	K	Jkᵃ	Jkᵇ	Fyᵃ	Fyᵇ	Leᵃ	Leᵇ	M	N	P₁	EM 37°C	AHG	Enzyme AHG
1	+	+	0	0	+	+	+	+	0	+	0	+	+	+	+	0	0	0
2	+	+	0	0	+	0	+	0	+	0	0	+	+	0	0	1+	2+	0
3	+	0	+	+	0	0	+	+	+	+	0	+	+	+	+	0	1+	0
4	+	+	+	0	+	0	0	+	0	+	0	+	+	0	+	0	0	0
5	0	0	+	0	+	0	+	+	+	+	0	+	+	0	0	0	1+	0
6	0	0	+	+	+	0	+	0	0	0	+	0	+	+	0	0	0	0
7	0	0	+	0	+	+	+	+	0	+	+	0	+	+	+	0	0	0
8	0	0	+	0	+	0	0	+	+	0	0	+	0	+	+	1+	2+	0
															auto	0	0	0

EM = enhancement media

What is the association of the antibody(ies) with hemolytic disease of the newborn (HDN)?

a usually fatal HDFN
ⓑ may cause HDFN
c is not associated with HDFN
d HDFN cannot be determined

220 Which of the following tests is most commonly used to detect antibodies attached to a patient's red blood cells in vivo?

ⓐ direct antiglobulin
b complement fixation
c indirect antiglobulin
d immunofluorescence

221 Anti-I may cause a positive direct antiglobulin test (DAT) because of:

    a anti-I agglutinating the cells
    b C3d bound to the red cells – *cold agglutinin* ✱
    c T-activation
    d C3c remaining on the red cells after cleavage of C3b

222 Which direct antiglobulin test results are associated with an anamnestic antibody response in a
MLS ONLY recently transfused patient?

Test result	Polyspecific	IgG	C3	Control
result A	$+^{mf}$	$+^{mf}$	0	0
result B	1+	0	1+	0
result C	2+	2+	0	0
result D	4+	4+	4+	0

mf=mixed field

    a result A
    b result B
    c result C
    d result D

223 In the direct (DAT) and indirect (IAT) antiglobulin tests, false-negative reactions may result if the:

    a patient's blood specimen was contaminated with bacteria
    b patient's blood specimen was collected into tubes containing silicon gel
    c saline used for washing the serum/cell mixture has been stored in glass or metal containers
    d addition of AHG is delayed for 40 minutes or more after washing the serum/cell mixture

224 Polyspecific reagents used in the direct antiglobulin test should have specificity for:

    a IgG and IgA
    b IgG and C3d
    c IgM and IgA
    d IgM and C3d

225 In the direct antiglobulin test, the antiglobulin reagent is used to:

    a mediate hemolysis of indicator red blood cells by providing complement
    b precipitate anti-erythrocyte antibodies
    c measure antibodies in a test serum by fixing complement
    d detect preexisting antibodies on erythrocytes

226 AHG (Coombs) control cells:

    a can be used as a positive control for anti-C3 reagents
    b can be used only for the indirect antiglobulin test
    c are coated only with IgG antibody
    d must be used to confirm all positive antiglobulin reactions

227 A 56-year-old female with cold agglutinin disease has a positive direct antiglobulin test (DAT). When the DAT is repeated using monospecific antiglobulin sera, which of the following is most likely to be detected?

    a IgM
    b IgG
    c C3d   ✱
    d C4a

228 The mechanism that best explains hemolytic anemia due to penicillin is:
MLS ONLY
    a drug-dependent antibodies reacting with drug-treated cells
    b drug-dependent antibodies reacting in the presence of drug
    c drug-independent with autoantibody production
    d nonimmunologic protein adsorption with positive DAT

229 Use of EDTA plasma prevents activation of the classical complement pathway by:

    a causing rapid decay of complement components
    b chelating Mg^{++} ions, which prevents the assembly of C6   ✳
    c chelating Ca^{++} ions, which prevents assembly of C1
    d preventing chemotaxis

230 Which of the following medications is most likely to cause production of autoantibodies?

    a penicillin
    b cephalothin
    c methyldopa – *drug that produces autoantibodies*
    d tetracycline

231 Serological results on an untransfused patient were:

MLS
ONLY

    antibody screen: negative at AHG
    direct antiglobulin test: 3+ with anti-C3d
    eluate: negative

These results are most likely due to:

    a warm autoimmune hemolytic anemia
    b cold agglutinin syndrome – *anti-I*
    c paroxysmal cold hemoglobinura
    d drug induced hemolytic anemia

232 The drug <u>cephalosporin</u> can cause a positive direct antiglobulin test with hemolysis by which of the following mechanisms?

    a drug-dependent antibodies reacting with drug-treated cells
    b drug-dependent antibodies reacting in the presence of a drug – *in vitro reaction*
    c drug-independent with autoantibody production
    d nonimmunologic protein adsorption with positive DAT

233 Crossmatch results at the antiglobulin phase were negative. When 1 drop of check cells was added, no agglutination was seen. The **most** likely explanation is that the:

    a red cells were overwashed
    b centrifuge speed was set too high
    c residual patient serum inactivated the AHG reagent   ✶
    d laboratorian did not add enough check cells

234 Which of the following might cause a false-negative indirect antiglobulin test (IAT)?

    a over-reading
    b IgG-coated screening cells
    c addition of an extra drop of serum
    d too heavy a cell suspension

235 The purpose of testing with anti-A,B is to detect:

    a anti-A_1
    b anti-A_2 *A_x react more strongly with anti-A,B*
    c subgroups of A
    d subgroups of B

236 What is the most appropriate diluent for preparing a solution of 8% bovine albumin for a red cell control reagent?

    a deionized water
    b distilled water
    c normal saline
    d Alsever solution

237 Which of the following antigens gives enhanced reactions with its corresponding antibody following treatment of the red cells with proteolytic enzymes?

    a Fy^a
    b E *enzymes weaken Fya and MNS system antigens*
    c S
    d M

238 In a prenatal workup, the following results were obtained:

Forward Group:				**Reverse Group:**	
anti-A	anti-B	anti-D	Rh control	A$_1$ cells	B cells
4+	2+	4+	0	0	3+

DAT: negative
antibody screen: negative

ABO discrepancy was thought to be due to an antibody directed against a component of the typing sera. Which test would resolve this discrepancy?

    a A$_1$ lectin
    b wash patient's RBCs and repeat testing
    c anti-A,B and extend incubation of the reverse group
    d repeat reverse group using A$_2$ cells

239 Refer to the following panel:

											EM	
Cell	D	C	c	E	e	K	Jk^a	Jk^b	Fy^a	Fy^b	37°C	AHG
1	+	+	0	0	+	+	+	+	+	+	0	2+
2	+	+	0	0	+	0	+	0	+	+	0	2+
3	+	0	+	+	0	0	0	+	+	+	1+	3+
4	+	+	0	0	+	0	0	+	0	+	0	0
5	0	0	+	0	+	0	+	+	+	+	0	2+
6	0	0	+	+	+	0	+	0	+	0	1+	3+
7	0	0	+	0	+	+	0	+	+	0	0	2+
8	0	0	+	0	+	0	0	+	0	+	0	0
										auto	0	0

EM = enhancement media

Based on the results of the above panel, which technique would be most helpful in determining antibody specificity?   *Duffy↓*   *E enhanced*

    a proteolytic enzyme treatment
    b urine neutralization
    c autoadsorption
    d saliva inhibition

240 Of the following, the most useful technique(s) in the identification and classification of high-titer, low-avidity (HTLA) antibodies is/are:

    a reagent red cell panels
    b adsorption and elution
    c titration and inhibition
    d cold autoadsorption

241 To confirm a serum antibody specificity identified as anti-P_1, a neutralization study was performed and the following results obtained:

	P_1+ RBCs
serum + P_1 substance:	negative
serum + saline:	negative

read about neutralization
positive saline control (agglutination)
neg = antibody present
antibody combines w/
substance, not with RBC's
no agglutination

What conclusion can be made from these results?

  a anti-P_1 is confirmed
  b anti-P_1 is ruled out
  c a second antibody is suspected due to the results of the negative control
  (d) anti-P_1 cannot be confirmed due to the results of the negative control

242 What happens to an antibody in neutralization study when a soluble antigen is added to the test?
MLS ONLY

  (a) inhibition
  b dilution
  c complement fixation
  d hemolysis

243 To confirm the specificity of anti-Le^b, an inhibition study using Lewis substance was performed with the following results:

	Le(b+) cells
tubes with patient serum + Lewis substance:	0
tubes with patient serum + saline control:	+

What conclusion can be made from these results?

  a a second antibody is suspected due to the positive control
  (b) anti-Le^b is confirmed because the tubes with Lewis substance are negative
  c anti-Le^b is not confirmed because the tubes with Lewis substance are negative
  d anti-Le^b cannot be confirmed because the saline positive is control

244 Which of the following is the correct interpretation of this saliva neutralization testing?
MLS ONLY

Sample	**Indicator cells**		
	A	**B**	**O**
saliva plus anti-A:	+	0	0
saliva plus anti-B:	0	+	0
saliva plus anti-H:	0	0	0

  a group A secretor
  b group B secretor
  c group AB secretor
  (d) group O secretor

245 A person's saliva incubated with the following antibodies and tested with the appropriate A_2, O, and B indicator cells, gives the following test results:
MLS ONLY

Antibody specificity	Test results
anti-A	reactive
anti-B	inhibited
anti-H	inhibited

The person's red cells ABO phenotype is:

  a A
  b AB
  (c) B
  d O

246 An antibody screen performed using solid phase technology revealed a diffuse layer of red blood cells on the bottom of the well. These results indicate:

   (a) a positive reaction (*bottom*)
   b a negative reaction (*top*)
   c serum was not added
   d red cells have a positive direct antiglobulin test

247 On Monday, a patient's K <u>antigen</u> typing result was positive. Two days later, the patient's K typing was negative. The patient was transfused with 2 units of Fresh Frozen Plasma. The tech might conclude that the:

   a transfusion of FFP affected the K typing
   (b) wrong patient was drawn   ✳
   c results are normal
   d anti-K reagent was omitted on Monday

248 Which one of the following is an indicator of <u>polyagglutination?</u> *caused by RBC antigens becoming more exposed*

   a RBCs typing as weak D+
   b presence of red cell autoantibody
   c decreased serum bilirubin
   (d) agglutination with normal adult ABO compatible sera

249 While performing an antibody screen, a test reaction is suspected to be rouleaux. A saline replacement test is performed and the reaction remains. What is the best interpretation?

   a original reaction of rouleaux is confirmed
   b replacement test is invalid and should be repeated
   (c) original reaction was due to true agglutination
   d antibody screen is negative

250
MLS
ONLY
A 10-year-old girl was hospitalized because her urine had a distinct red color. The patient had recently recovered from an upper respiratory infection and appeared very pale and lethargic. Tests were performed with the following results:

hemoglobin:	5 g/dL (50 g/L) ↓
reticulocyte count:	15% ↑
DAT:	weak reactivity with poly-specific and anti-C3d; anti-IgG was negative
antibody screen:	negative
Donath-Landsteiner test:	positive; P– cells showed no hemolysis

diagnostic for PCH

The patient probably has:

   (a) paroxysmal cold hemoglobinuria (PCH)
   b paroxysmal nocturnal hemoglobinuria (PNH)
   c warm autoimmune hemolytic anemia
   d hereditary erythroblastic multinuclearity with a positive acidified serum test (HEMPAS)

251 Which of the following is useful for removing IgG from red blood cells with a positive DAT to perform a phenotype?

   a bromelin
   (b) chloroquine *diphosphate* OR EDTA *glycine acid*
   c LISS
   d DTT

252 A patient's serum contains a mixture of antibodies. One of the antibodies is identified as anti-D. Anti-Jk^a, anti-Fy^a and possibly another antibody are present. What technique(s) may be helpful to identify the other antibody(ies)?

   (a) enzyme panel; select cell panel
   b thiol reagents – *for IgM displacement*
   c lowering the pH and increasing the incubation time
   d using albumin as an enhancement media in combination with selective adsorption

253 A sample gives the following results:

Cells with:		Serum with:	
anti-A	3+	A₁ cells	2+
anti-B	4+	B cells	0

Which lectin should be used first to resolve this discrepancy?

a *Ulex europaeus*
b *Arachis hypogaea*
c *Dolichos biflorus* (circled)
d *Vicia graminea*

254 The serum of a group O, Cde/Cde donor contains anti-D. In order to prepare a suitable anti-D reagent from this donor's serum, which of the following cells would be suitable for the adsorption?

a group O, cde/cde cells
b group O, Cde/cde cells
c group A₂B, CDe/cde cells
d group A₁B, cde/cde cells (circled)

[handwritten: Must remove (~~adsorp~~ adsorb) group O antibodies and leave Anti-D; needs cells with A, B on them to attract Anti-A and anti-B and neg for D (dd)]

255 A 26-year-old female is admitted with anemia of undetermined origin. Blood samples are received with a crossmatch request for 6 units of Red Blood Cells. The patient is group A, Rh-negative and has no history of transfusion or pregnancy. The following results were obtained in pretransfusion testing:

	IS	37°C	IAT
screening cell I	0	0	3+
screening cell II	0	0	3+
autocontrol	0	0	3+
all 6 donors	0	0	3+

[handwritten: positive autocontrol @ IAT]

The best way to find compatible blood is to:

a do an antibody identification panel
b use the saline replacement technique
c use the pre-warm technique
d perform a warm autoadsorption (circled)

256 A patient's serum was reactive 2+ in the antiglobulin phase of testing with all cells on a routine
MLS ONLY
panel including their own. Transfusion was performed 6 months previously. The optimal adsorption method to remove the autoantibody is:

a autoadsorption using the patient's ZZAP-treated red cells (circled)
b autoadsorption using the patient's LISS-treated red cells
c adsorption using enzyme-treated red cells from a normal donor
d adsorption using methyldopa-treated red cells

257 In a cold autoadsorption procedure, pretreatment of the patient's red cells with which of the
MLS ONLY
following reagents is helpful?

a ficin (circled)
b phosphate-buffered saline at pH 9.0
c low ionic strength saline (LISS)
d albumin

258 The process of separation of antibody from its antigen is known as:

a diffusion
b adsorption – *antibody attaches to antigen*
c neutralization – *inactivates antibody*
d elution – *antibody released from antigen* (circled)

259 Which of the following is most helpful to confirm a weak ABO subgroup?

MLS ONLY

   a adsorption-elution
   b neutralization
   c testing with A1 lectin
   d use of anti-A,B

260 One of the most effective methods for the elution of warm autoantibodies from RBCs utilizes:

   a 10% sucrose
   b LISS
   c change in pH   ✱
   d distilled water

Transfusion Practice

261 How would the hematocrit of a patient with chronic anemia be affected by the transfusion of a unit of Whole Blood containing 475 mL of blood, vs 2 units of Red Blood Cells each with a total volume of 250 mL?

   a patient's hematocrit would be equally affected by the Whole Blood or the Red Blood Cells
   b Red Blood Cells would provide twice the increment in hematocrit as the Whole Blood
   c Whole Blood would provide twice the increment in hematocrit as the Red Blood Cells
   d Whole Blood would provide a change in hematocrit slightly less than the Red Blood Cells

262 After checking the inventory, it was noted that there were no units on the shelf marked "May Issue as Uncrossmatched: For Emergency Only." Which of the following should be placed on this shelf?

   a 1 unit of each of the ABO blood groups
   b units of group O, Rh-positive Whole Blood
   c units of group O, Rh-negative Red Blood Cells
   d any units that are expiring at midnight

263 The primary indication for granulocyte transfusion is:

MLS ONLY

   a prophylactic treatment for infection
   b additional supportive therapy in those patients who are responsive to antibiotic therapy
   c clinical situations where bone marrow recovery is not anticipated
   d severe neutropenia with an infection that is nonresponsive to antibiotic therapy

264 A 42-year-old male of average body mass has a history of chronic anemia requiring transfusion support. Two units of Red Blood Cells are transfused. If the pretransfusion hemoglobin was 7.0 g/dL (70 g/L), the expected posttransfusion hemoglobin concentration should be:

   a 8.0 g/dL (80 g/L)   ↑ hemoglobin 1.0 g/dl
   b 9.0 g/dL (90 g/L)   ✱
   c 10.0 g/dL (100 g/L)
   d 11.0 g/dL (110 g/L)

265 How many units of Red Blood Cells are required to raise the hematocrit of a 70 kg nonbleeding man from 24% to 30%?

   a 1   ↑ hct by 3%   ✱
   b 2
   c 3
   d 4

266 For which of the following transfusion candidates would CMV-seronegative blood be **most**
likely indicated?

MLS
ONLY

   a renal dialysis patients
   b sickle cell patient
   c bone marrow and hematopoietic cell transplant recipients
   d CMV-seropositive patients

267 Although ABO compatibility is preferred, ABO incompatible product may be administered
when transfusing:

MLS
ONLY

   a Single-Donor Plasma
   b Cryoprecipitated AHF
   c Fresh Frozen Plasma
   d Granulocytes

268 Transfusion of plateletpheresis products from HLA-compatible donors is the preferred
treatment for:

   a recently diagnosed cases of TTP with severe thrombocytopenia
   b acute leukemia in relapse with neutropenia, thrombocytopenia and sepsis
   c immune thrombocytopenic purpura
   d severely thrombocytopenic patients, known to be refractory to random donor platelets → *HLA causes refractoriness*

269 Washed Red Blood Cells are indicated in which of the following situations?

MLS
ONLY

   a an IgA-deficient patient with a history of transfusion-associated anaphylaxis
   b a pregnant woman with a history of hemolytic disease of the newborn
   c a patient with a positive DAT and red cell autoantibody
   d a newborn with a hematocrit of <30%

270 Which of the following is consistent with standard blood bank procedure governing the infusion
of fresh frozen plasma?

   a only blood group-specific plasma may be administered
   b group O may be administered to recipients of all blood groups
   c group AB may be administered to AB recipients only
   d group A may be administered to both A and O recipients

271 A patient who is group AB, Rh-negative needs 2 units of Fresh Frozen Plasma. Which of the
following units of plasma would be **most** acceptable for transfusion?

   a group O, Rh-negative
   b group A, Rh-negative
   c group B, Rh-positive
   d group AB, Rh-positive

272 What increment of platelets/uL (platelets/L), in the typical 70-kg human, is expected to result
from each single unit of Platelets transfused to a non-HLA-sensitized recipient?

   a 3,000- 5,000
   b 5,000-10,000 = *each unit of platelets* ✳
   c 20,000-25,000
   d 25,000-30,000

273 Platelet transfusions are of most value in treating:

MLS
ONLY

   a hemolytic transfusion reaction
   b posttransfusion purpura
   c functional platelet abnormalities
   d immune thrombocytopenic purpura

274 Washed Red Blood Cells would be the product of choice for a patient with:

MLS
ONLY
   a multiple red cell alloantibodies
   b an increased risk of hepatitis infection
   c warm autoimmune hemolytic anemic
   (d) anti-IgA antibodies

275 A patient received about 15 mL of compatible blood and developed severe shock, but no fever. If the patient needs another transfusion, what kind of red blood cell component should be given?

   a Red Blood Cells
   (b) Red Blood Cells, Washed →*wash IgA proteins away*
   c Red Blood Cells, Irradiated
   d Red Blood Cells, Leukocyte-Reduced

anaphylactic = no fever.
few mls infused → reaction

276 Fresh Frozen Plasma from a group A, Rh-positive donor may be safely transfused to a patient who is group:

   (a) A, Rh-negative
   b B, Rh-negative
   c AB, Rh-positive
   d AB, Rh-negative

277 A patient admitted to the trauma unit requires emergency release of Fresh Frozen Plasma (FFP). His blood donor card states that he is group AB, Rh-positive. Which of the following blood groups of FFP should be issued?

   a A
   b B
   (c) AB
   d O

278 Fresh Frozen Plasma:

   a contains all labile coagulative factors ~~except~~ *including* cryoprecipitated AHF
   b has a higher risk of transmitting hepatitis than does Whole Blood
   (c) should be transfused within 24 hours of thawing
   d need ~~not~~ be ABO-compatible

279 Ten units of group A platelets were transfused to a group AB patient. The pretransfusion platelet count was $12 \times 10^3/\mu L$ ($12 \times 10^9/L$) and the posttransfusion count was $18 \times 10^3/\mu L$ ($18 \times 10^9/L$). From this information, the laboratorian would most likely conclude that the patient:

   a needs group AB platelets to be effective
   b clinical data does not suggest a need for platelets
   (c) has developed antibodies to the transfused platelets
   d should receive irradiated platelets

280 Hypotension, nausea, flushing, fever and chills are symptoms of which of the following transfusion reactions?

   a allergic ———→ *no fever*
   b circulatory overload
   (c) hemolytic - *FEVER*
   d anaphylactic - *no fever*

281 A patient has become refractory to platelet transfusion. Which of the following are

MLS
ONLY
probable causes?

   a transfusion of Rh-incompatible platelets
   b decreased pH of the platelets
   c development of an alloantibody with anti-D specificity
   (d) development of antibodies to HLA antigen

282 A poor increment in the platelet count 1 hour following platelet transfusion is most commonly caused by:

  a splenomegaly
  b alloimmunization to HLA antigens
  c disseminated intravascular coagulation
  d defective platelets

283 Posttransfusion purpura is usually caused by:

  a anti-A
  b white cell antibodies
  c anti-HPA-1a (Pl^{A1})
  d platelet wash-out

284 An unexplained fall in hemoglobin and mild jaundice in a patient transfused with Red Blood Cells 1 week previously would most likely indicate:

  a paroxysmal nocturnal hemoglobinuria
  b posttransfusion hepatitis infection
  c presence of HLA antibodies
  d delayed hemolytic transfusion reaction

285 In a delayed transfusion reaction, the causative antibody is generally too weak to be detected in routine compatibility testing and antibody screening tests, but is typically detectable at what point after transfusion?

  a 3-6 hours
  b 3-7 days   *✳ secondary response*
  c 60-90 days
  d after 120 days

286 The most serious hemolytic transfusion reactions are due to incompatibility in which of the following blood group systems?

  a ABO
  b Rh
  c MN
  d Duffy

287 Severe intravascular hemolysis is most likely caused by antibodies of which blood group system?

  a ABO
  b Rh
  c Kell
  d Duffy

288 Which of the following blood group systems is most commonly associated with <u>delayed hemolytic transfusion reactions</u>?

  a Lewis
  b Kidd *—show dosage, weak, difficult to detect*
  c MNS
  d I

289 After receiving a unit of Red Blood Cells, a patient immediately developed flushing, nervousness, fever spike of 102°F (38.9°C), shaking, chills and back pain. The plasma hemoglobin was elevated and there was hemoglobinuria. Laboratory investigation of this adverse reaction would most likely show:

  a an error in ABO grouping
  b an error in Rh typing
  c presence of anti-Fy^a antibody in patient's serum
  d presence of gram-negative bacteria in blood bag

290   A trauma patient who has just received ten units of blood may develop:

    a   anemia
    b   polycythemia   ✳
    c   leukocytosis
    d   thrombocytopenia

291   Five days after transfusion, a patient becomes mildly jaundiced and experiences a drop in
MLS
ONLY   hemoglobin and hematocrit with no apparent hemorrhage. Below are the results of the
    transfusion reaction workup:

	anti-A	anti-B	anti-D	A_1 cells	B cells	Ab screen	DAT
patient pretransfusion	neg	4+	3+	4+	neg	neg	neg
patient posttransfusion	neg	4+	3+	4+	neg	1+	1+
donor #1	neg	neg	3+	4+	4+	neg	
donor #2	neg	4+	3+	4+	neg	neg	

    In order to reach a conclusion, the technician should first:

    a   retype the pre- and posttransfusion patient samples and donor #1
    b   request an EDTA tube be drawn on the patient and repeat the DAT
    c   repeat the pretransfusion antibody screen on the patient's sample
    d   identify the antibody in the serum and eluate from the posttransfusion sample

292   The most appropriate laboratory test for early detection of acute posttransfusion hemolysis is:

    a   a visual inspection for free plasma hemoglobin
    b   plasma haptoglobin concentration
    c   examination for hematuria
    d   serum bilirubin concentration

293   During initial investigation of a suspected hemolytic transfusion reaction, it was observed that
    the posttransfusion serum was yellow in color and the direct antiglobulin test was negative.
    Repeat ABO typing on the posttransfusion sample confirmed the pretransfusion results. What is
    the next step in this investigation?

    clerical ✓
    look at plasma color
    a   repeat compatibility testing on suspected unit(s)   *DAT*
    b   perform plasma hemoglobin and haptoglobin determinations   *repeat ABO*
    c   use enhancement media to repeat the antibody screen
    d   no further serological testing is necessary

294   Which of the following transfusion reactions is characterized by high fever, shock,
    hemoglobinuria, DIC and renal failure?

    a   bacterial contamination
    b   circulatory overload
    c   febrile
    d   anaphylactic —

295   Hemoglobinuria, hypotension and generalized bleeding are symptoms of which of the following
    transfusion reactions?

    a   allergic
    b   circulatory overload
    c   hemolytic
    d   anaphylactic

296 When evaluating a suspected transfusion reaction, which of the following is the ideal sample collection time for a bilirubin determination?

    a 6 hours posttransfusion *- peaks in 5-7 hours*
    b 12 hours posttransfusion
    c 24 hours posttransfusion
    d 48 hours posttransfusion

297 A patient's record shows a previous anti-Jk^b, but the current antibody screen is negative. What further testing should be done before transfusion?

    a phenotype the patient's red cells for the Jk^b antigen
    b perform a cell panel on the patient's serum
    c crossmatch type specific units and release only compatible units for transfusion
    d give Jk^b negative crossmatch compatible blood *– AHG XM*

298 A posttransfusion blood sample from a patient experiencing chills and fever shows distinct hemolysis. The direct antiglobulin test is positive (mixed field). What would be most helpful to determine the cause of the reaction?

    a auto control
    b elution and antibody identification
    c repeat antibody screen on the donor unit
    d bacteriologic smear and culture

299 A patient is readmitted to the hospital with a hemoglobin level of 7 g/dL (70 g/L) 3 weeks after receiving 2 units of red cells. The initial serological tests are:

    ABO/Rh: A+
    antibody screen: negative
    DAT: 1+ mixed field

Which test should be performed next?

    a antibody identification panel on the patient's serum
    b repeat the ABO type on the donor units
    c perform an elution and identify the antibody in the eluate
    d crossmatch the post reaction serum with the 3 donor units

300 In a delayed hemolytic transfusion reaction, the direct antiglobulin test is typically:

    a negative
    b mixed-field positive
    c positive due to complement
    d negative when the antibody screen is negative

301 *MLS ONLY* A patient has had massive trauma involving replacement of 1 blood volume with Red Blood Cells and crystalloid. She is currently experiencing oozing from mucous membranes and surgical incisions. Laboratory values are as follows:

    PT: normal
    APTT: normal
    bleeding time: prolonged
    platelet count: $20 \times 10^3/\mu L$ ($20 \times 10^9/L$)
    hemoglobin: 11.4 g/dL (114 g/L)

What is the blood component of choice for this patient?

    a Platelets
    b Cryoprecipitated AHF
    c Fresh Frozen Plasma
    d Prothrombin Complex

302 For a patient who has suffered an acute hemolytic transfusion reaction, the primary treatment goal should be to:

  a prevent alloimmunization
  b diminish chills and fever
  c prevent hemoglobinemia
  (d) reverse hypotension and minimize renal damage

303 A patient multiply transfused with Red Blood Cells developed a headache, nausea, fever and chills during his last transfusion. What component is most appropriate to prevent this reaction in the future?

  a Red Blood Cells
  b Red Blood Cells, Irradiated
  (c) Red Blood Cells, Leukocyte-Reduced
  d Red Blood Cells selected as CMV-reduced-risk

304 The use of Leukocyte-Reduced Red Blood Cells and Platelets is indicated for which of the following patient groups?

  a CMV-seropositive postpartum mothers
  b victims of acute trauma with massive bleeding
  (c) patients with history of febrile transfusion reactions
  d burn victims with anemia and low serum protein

305 Leukocyte-Poor Red Blood Cells would most likely be indicated for patients with a history of:

  (a) febrile transfusion reaction
  b iron deficiency anemia
  c hemophilia A
  d von Willebrand disease

306 Posttransfusion anaphylactic reactions occur most often in patients with:

  a leukocyte antibodies
  b erythrocyte antibodies
  (c) IgA deficiency
  d Factor VIII deficiency

307 Which of the following transfusion reactions occurs after infusion of only a few milliliters of blood and gives no history of fever?

  a febrile
  b circulatory overload
  (c) anaphylactic →no fever; small amount of blood
  d hemolytic

308 Fever and chills are symptoms of which of the following transfusion reactions?

  a citrate toxicity
  b circulatory overload
  c allergic
  (d) febrile

309 Hives and itching are symptoms of which of the following transfusion reactions?

  a febrile
  (b) allergic
  c circulatory overload
  d bacterial

310 A temperature rise of 1°C or more occurring in association with a transfusion, with no abnormal results in the transfusion reaction investigation, usually indicates which of the following reactions?

   ⓐ febrile
   b circulatory overload
   c hemolytic
   d anaphylactic

311 A 65-year-old woman experienced shaking, chills, and a fever of 102°F (38.9°C) approximately 40 minutes following the transfusion of a second unit of Red Blood Cells. The most likely explanation for the patient's symptoms is:

   a transfusion of bacterially contaminated blood
   b congestive heart failure
   c anaphylactic transfusion reaction
   ⓓ febrile transfusion reaction

312 A sickle cell patient who has been multiply transfused experiences fever and chills after receiving a unit of Red Blood Cells. Transfusion investigation studies show:

   DAT: negative
   plasma hemolysis: no hemolysis observed

The patient is most likely reacting to: *Leukoreduced = febrile reactions*

   a IgA
   b plasma protein
   c red cells
   ⓓ white cells or cytokines

313 Use of only male donors as a source of plasma intended for transfusion is advocated to reduce which type of reaction?

MLS ONLY

   a allergic
   ⓑ TRALI *—lung damage due to donor HLA or granulocyte-specific antibodies*
   c hemolytic *most often found in women who have had*
   d TACO (circulatory overload) *multiple babies*

314 Platelets are ordered for a patient who has a history of febrile reactions following red cell transfusions. What should be done to reduce the risk of another febrile reaction?

MLS ONLY

   a pretransfusion administration of Benadryl®
   b transfuse Irradiated Platelets
   c give Platelets from IgA-deficient donors
   ⓓ give Leukocyte-Reduced Platelets

315 Symptoms of dyspnea, cough, hypoxemia, and pulmonary edema within 6 hours of transfusion is most likely which type of reaction?

   a anaphylactic
   b hemolytic
   c febrile
   ⓓ TRALI

316 A patient with a coagulopathy was transfused with FP24 (plasma frozen within 24 hours of collection). After infusion of 15 mL, the patient experienced hypotension, shock, chest pain and difficulty in breathing. The most likely cause of the reaction is:

   ⓐ anti-IgA
   b bacterial contamination
   c intravascular hemolysis
   d leukoagglutinins

317 To prevent febrile transfusion reactions, which Red Blood Cell product should be transfused?

   a Red Blood Cells, Irradiated
   b CMV-negative Red Blood Cells
   c Red Blood Cells, Leukocyte-Reduced
   d IgA-deficient donor blood

318 During the issue of an autologous unit of Whole Blood, the supernatant plasma is observed to be dark red in color. What would be the best course of action?

   a the unit may be issued only for autologous use
   b remove the plasma and issue the unit as Red Blood Cells
   c issue the unit only as washed Red Blood Cells
   d quarantine the unit for further testing

319 Coughing, cyanosis and difficult breathing are symptoms of which of the following transfusion reactions?

   a febrile
   b allergic
   c circulatory overload
   d hemolytic

320 Which of the following is a nonimmunologic adverse effect of a transfusion?

   a hemolytic reaction
   b febrile nonhemolytic reaction
   c congestive heart failure
   d urticaria

321 Congestive heart failure, severe headache and/or peripheral edema occurring soon after transfusion is indicative of which type of transfusion reaction?

   a hemolytic
   b febrile
   c anaphylactic
   d circulatory overload

322 A patient with severe anemia became cyanotic and developed tachycardia, hypertension, and difficulty breathing after receiving 3 units of blood. No fever or other symptoms were evident. This is most likely what type of reaction?

   a febrile reaction
   b transfusion-associated circulatory overload (TACO)
   c anaphylactic reaction
   d hemolytic reaction

323 A patient became hypotensive and went into shock after receiving 50 mL of a unit of Red Blood Cells. She had a shaking chill and her temperature rose to 104.8°F (40.4 °C). A transfusion reaction investigation was initiated but no abnormal results were seen. What additional testing should be performed?

   a Gram stain and culture of the donor unit
   b lymphocytotoxicity tests for leukoagglutinins
   c plasma IgA level
   d elution and antibody identification

324 The most frequent transfusion-associated disease complication of blood transfusions is:

   a cytomegalovirus (CMV)
   b syphilis
   c hepatitis
   d AIDS

325 The purpose of a low-dose irradiation of blood components is to:
reduces T cell proliferation
    a prevent posttransfusion purpura
    b prevent graft-vs-host (GVH) disease
    c sterilize components
    d prevent noncardiogenic pulmonary edema

326 Which of the following patient groups is at risk of developing graft-vs-host disease?
MLS ONLY
    a full term infants
    b patients with history of febrile transfusion reactions
    c patients with a positive direct antiglobulin test
    d recipients of blood donated by immediate family members

327 Irradiation of donor blood is done to prevent which of the following adverse effects of transfusion?
    a febrile transfusion reaction
    b cytomegalovirus infection
    c transfusion associated graft-vs-host disease
    d transfusion related acute lung injury (TRALI)

328 Therapeutic plasmapheresis is performed in order to:
MLS ONLY
    a harvest granulocytes
    b harvest platelets
    c treat patients with polycythemia
    d treat patients with plasma abnormalities

329 Plasma exchange is recommended in the treatment of patients with macroglobulinemia in order to remove:
MLS ONLY
    a antigen
    b excess IgM – *Waldenstron's*
    c excess IgG
    d abnormal platelets

330 The most important step in the safe administration of blood is to:
    a perform compatibility testing accurately
    b get an accurate patient history
    c exclude disqualified donors
    d accurately identify the donor unit and recipient

1 **b**	59 **d**	117 **c**	175 **d**	233 **c**	291 **d**
2 **c**	60 **d**	118 **d**	176 **b**	234 **d**	292 **a**
3 **c**	61 **c**	119 **a**	177 **a**	235 **c**	293 **d**
4 **d**	62 **a**	120 **c**	178 **c**	236 **c**	294 **a**
5 **b**	63 **a**	121 **a**	179 **b**	237 **b**	295 **c**
6 **b**	64 **a**	122 **d**	180 **c**	238 **b**	296 **a**
7 **a**	65 **a**	123 **d**	181 **c**	239 **a**	297 **d**
8 **d**	66 **d**	124 **c**	182 **d**	240 **c**	298 **b**
9 **d**	67 **c**	125 **b**	183 **d**	241 **d**	299 **c**
10 **b**	68 **d**	126 **d**	184 **b**	242 **a**	300 **b**
11 **b**	69 **a**	127 **c**	185 **c**	243 **b**	301 **a**
12 **b**	70 **c**	128 **d**	186 **d**	244 **d**	302 **d**
13 **b**	71 **a**	129 **d**	187 **c**	245 **c**	303 **c**
14 **d**	72 **a**	130 **a**	188 **a**	246 **a**	304 **c**
15 **c**	73 **b**	131 **c**	189 **b**	247 **b**	305 **a**
16 **d**	74 **c**	132 **a**	190 **b**	248 **d**	306 **c**
17 **d**	75 **c**	133 **d**	191 **a**	249 **c**	307 **c**
18 **c**	76 **d**	134 **b**	192 **b**	250 **a**	308 **d**
19 **b**	77 **b**	135 **c**	193 **c**	251 **b**	309 **b**
20 **d**	78 **d**	136 **b**	194 **b**	252 **a**	310 **a**
21 **a**	79 **c**	137 **a**	195 **d**	253 **c**	311 **d**
22 **d**	80 **d**	138 **b**	196 **a**	254 **d**	312 **d**
23 **b**	81 **c**	139 **d**	197 **d**	255 **d**	313 **b**
24 **a**	82 **b**	140 **a**	198 **b**	256 **a**	314 **d**
25 **a**	83 **d**	141 **a**	199 **c**	257 **a**	315 **d**
26 **d**	84 **c**	142 **c**	200 **c**	258 **d**	316 **a**
27 **d**	85 **b**	143 **b**	201 **b**	259 **a**	317 **c**
28 **a**	86 **c**	144 **a**	202 **a**	260 **c**	318 **d**
29 **c**	87 **c**	145 **b**	203 **d**	261 **b**	319 **c**
30 **d**	88 **c**	146 **d**	204 **c**	262 **c**	320 **c**
31 **b**	89 **c**	147 **b**	205 **a**	263 **d**	321 **d**
32 **a**	90 **d**	148 **c**	206 **a**	264 **b**	322 **b**
33 **c**	91 **a**	149 **c**	207 **a**	265 **b**	323 **a**
34 **a**	92 **b**	150 **b**	208 **a**	266 **c**	324 **c**
35 **c**	93 **b**	151 **d**	209 **a**	267 **b**	325 **b**
36 **b**	94 **b**	152 **c**	210 **b**	268 **d**	326 **d**
37 **c**	95 **d**	153 **b**	211 **d**	269 **a**	327 **c**
38 **b**	96 **d**	154 **c**	212 **b**	270 **d**	328 **d**
39 **b**	97 **d**	155 **b**	213 **a**	271 **d**	329 **b**
40 **b**	98 **c**	156 **b**	214 **b**	272 **b**	330 **d**
41 **d**	99 **d**	157 **c**	215 **c**	273 **c**	
42 **b**	100 **c**	158 **a**	216 **b**	274 **d**	
43 **d**	101 **b**	159 **b**	217 **a**	275 **b**	
44 **c**	102 **c**	160 **c**	218 **a**	276 **a**	
45 **a**	103 **a**	161 **d**	219 **b**	277 **c**	
46 **a**	104 **c**	162 **d**	220 **a**	278 **c**	
47 **b**	105 **b**	163 **b**	221 **b**	279 **c**	
48 **a**	106 **c**	164 **a**	222 **a**	280 **c**	
49 **b**	107 **c**	165 **a**	223 **d**	281 **d**	
50 **c**	108 **b**	166 **b**	224 **b**	282 **b**	
51 **d**	109 **b**	167 **a**	225 **d**	283 **c**	
52 **d**	110 **c**	168 **d**	226 **c**	284 **d**	
53 **a**	111 **a**	169 **c**	227 **c**	285 **b**	
54 **b**	112 **c**	170 **c**	228 **a**	286 **a**	
55 **a**	113 **c**	171 **b**	229 **c**	287 **a**	
56 **c**	114 **d**	172 **c**	230 **c**	288 **b**	
57 **d**	115 **d**	173 **b**	231 **b**	289 **a**	
58 **a**	116 **d**	174 **c**	232 **b**	290 **d**	

Blood Products

1 **b** All donors, regardless of sex, require a minimum hemoglobin of 12.5 g/dL (125 g/L). The value must not be performed on an earlobe stick.
[AABB Standards 2008a, p70]

2 **c** Jaundice is a sign of liver impairment, which might be due to HBV or HCV. Infection with HBV and HCV is a cause for indefinite deferral.
[AABB Standards 2008a, p73; Kaplan 2003, pp497-500]

3 **c** The receipt of blood products is a
MLS ONLY 6-month deferral, the deferral for travel to areas endemic for malaria is 12 months regardless of antimalarial prophylaxis, and a person taking antibiotics may have bacteremia. The requirement for temperature is not over 37.5°C or 99.5°F.
[AABB Standards 2008a, pp70-74]

4 **d** A positive test for HbsAg at any time is an indefinite deferral.
[AABB Standards 2008a, pp70-74]

5 **b** A woman who had a spontaneous
MLS ONLY abortion at 2 months of pregnancy, 3 months previously would be acceptable. A donor is acceptable if she has not been pregnant in the previous 6 weeks.
[AABB Standards 2008a, pp70-74]

6 **b** The Hct must be >38%. A donor may be 16 unless state law differs. Temperature must not exceed 99.5°F/37.5°C, blood pressure must be <180 mm Hg systolic and <100 mm Hg diastolic, pulse 50-100 unless an athlete (which can be lower). Toxoids and vaccines from synthetic or killed sources have no deferral.
[AABB Standards 2008a, pp70-71]

7 **a** The minimum platelet count required
MLS ONLY for frequent repeat donors is $150 \times 10^3/\mu L$ ($150 \times 10^9/L$). A platelet count is not required prior to the first donation or if the interval between donations is at least 4 weeks.
[AABB Standards 2008a, p25]

8 **d** The scrub must use iodine, eg, PVP iodine complex. Donors who are sensitive to iodine can have the area cleaned with a preparation of 2% chlorhexidine and 70% isopropyl alcohol.
[AABB Tech Manual 2008b, pp193, 942]

9 **d** Testing for syphilis was the first mandated donor screening test for infectious disease and is still part of donor screening.
[AABB Tech Manual 2008b, ch8]

10 **b** Platelets are prepared and stored at 20°-24°C for optimum function.
[AABB Tech Manual 2008b, p198]

11 **b** The most common posttransfusion
MLS ONLY hepatitis is hepatitis B. The estimated risk of transmission is 1:220,000 units transfused. The risk of hepatitis C transmission is 1:1,800,000 units. Hepatitis B surface antigen (HBsAg) is a required donor test for detection of acute or chronic HBV infection.
[AABB Tech Manual 2008b, pp242, 260-73]

12 **b** Western blot uses purified HIV proteins to confirm reactivity in samples whose screening test for anti-HIV is positive.
[AABB Tech Manual 2008b, ch10]

13 **b** The causative agent for AIDS is the human immunodeficiency virus types 1 and 2.
[AABB Tech Manual 2008b, ch8]

14 **d** The enzyme-labeled immunosorbent assay (ELISA) method is a very sensitive method employed to screen donors for markers of transfusion-transmitted viruses.
[AABB Tech Manual 2008b, ch8]

15 **c** Rejuvenation of RBCs uses additives to
MLS ONLY restore or enhance 2,3-DPG and ATP levels.
[Harmening 2005, p11]

16 **d** Sterile docking devices allow entry into donor units without affecting the expiration date of the product.
[Harmening 2005, p286]

17 **d** Sterile docking devices allow entry into donor units without affecting the expiration date of the product.
[Harmening 2005, p286]

18 **c** If storage devices do not have automated temperature recording, temperature must be manually monitored every 4 hours.
[AABB Tech Manual 2008b, p284]

19 **b** Fresh Frozen Plasma is stored at −18°C or below for 12 months.
[AABB Standards 2008a, Reference Standard 5.1]

Answers–Blood Bank

20 **d**   Blood may be returned to the blood bank after issue provided that 1) the container has not been entered, 2) at least 1 sealed segment is attached to the container, 3) visual inspection of the unit is satisfactory and documented, and 4) the unit has been maintained at the appropriate storage or transport temperature. Studies have shown that refrigerated components retain an acceptable temperature of <10°C for up to 30 minutes after removal from the refrigerator.
[AABB Tech Manual 2008b]

21 **a**   Red Blood Cells, Frozen with 40%
MLS ONLY glycerol are stored at –65°C or lower.
[AABB Standards 2008a, Reference Standard 5.1]

22 **d**   Red Blood Cells are stored at 1°-6°C.
[AABB Standards 2008a, Reference Standard 5.1]

23 **b**   If the seal is broken during processing, components are considered to be prepared in an open system, rather than a closed system. The expiration time for Red Blood Cells in an open system is 24 hours.
[AABB Standards 2008a, Reference Standard 5.1]

24 **a**   Cryoprecipitated AHF is stored at –18°C or lower.
[AABB Standards 2008a, Reference Standard 5.1]

25 **a**   Cryoprecipitate must be transfused within 4 hours of pooling.
[Harmening 2005, p232]

26 **d**   Whole Blood-derived platelets are stored at 20°-24°C with continuous gentle agitation. Platelets prepared by the PRP method may be stored for up to 5 days.
[AABB Standards 2008a, Reference Standard 5.1]

27 **d**   The required temperature for storage of platelets is 20°-24°C.
[AABB Standards 2008a, Reference Standard 5.1]

28 **a**   Per AABB standards, thawed FFP should be stored at 1°-6°C for no more than 24 hours.
[AABB Standards 2008a, p68]

29 **c**   Cryoprecipitate has a shelf life of 12 months in the frozen state.
[Harmening 2005, p232]

30 **d**   Once thawed, FFP is stored at 1°-6°C for up to 24 hours.
[Marques 2007, p25]

31 **b**   The pH of platelets should be
MLS ONLY maintained at 6.2 or above throughout the storage period.
[AABB Standards 2008a, §5·7·5]

32 **a**   The required temperature for storage of thawed plasma is 1°-6°C.
[AABB Standards 2008a, Reference Standard 5.1]

33 **c**   2,3-DPG declines during storage of
MLS ONLY Red Blood Cells, causing a "shift-to-the-left" in the oxygen dissociation curve and an impaired ability to deliver oxygen to the tissues.
[Harmening 2005, p308]

34 **a**   Cryoprecipitate is used primarily for
MLS ONLY fibrinogen replacement. It is stored at room temperature (20°-24°C) after thawing and must be infused within 6 hours. If pooled with other cryo units, it must be infused within 4 hours.
[Harmening 2005, p308]

35 **c**   Blood products from blood relatives
MLS ONLY containing viable lymphocytes must be irradiated to inhibit the proliferation of T cells and subsequent GVHD.
[Harmening 2005, p227]

36 **b**   Irradiation inhibits proliferation of T lymphocytes.
[Harmening 2005, p23]

37 **c**   FFP thawed in a water bath should be protected so that entry ports are not contaminated with water. One can may use a plastic overwrap or keep ports above the water level.
[AABB Tech Manual 2008b, p191]

38 **b**   Fresh Frozen Plasma (FFP) must be separated and frozen within 8 hours of Whole Blood collection.
[Harmening 2005, p231]

39 **b**   Cryoprecipitate contains at least
MLS ONLY 80 units of AHF.
[Harmening 2005, p232]

40 **b**   Cryoprecipitated AHF contains at least
MLS ONLY 80 IU of Factor VIII concentrated in about 10 mL of plasma.
[Harmening 2005, p237]

41 **d**   Cryoprecipitate is indicated as a source
MLS ONLY of fibrinogen for hypofibrinogenemia. It contains a minimum of 150 mg of fibrinogen concentrated in a small volume of plasma.
[Harmening 2005, p308]

42 **b**   Cryoprecipitate is the fraction of plasma proteins that precipitate when FFP is slowly thawed at 1°-6°C.
[Harmening 2005, p232]

43 **d**   Clots in the unit may indicate contamination.
[Harmening 2005, p372]

44 **c**   Per AABB standards, at least 90% of
MLS ONLY platelet pheresis units sampled must contain at least 3.0×10^{11} platelets.
[AABB Standards 2008a, p36]

45 **a**   Per AABB standards, at least 90% of the
MLS ONLY platelet units prepared from Whole Blood that are sampled must contain at least 5.5×10^{10} platelets.
[AABB Standards 2008a, pp35-36]

46 **a**   Whole blood-derived Platelets are prepared by a light spin to separate the Red Blood Cells from the platelet-rich plasma (PRP), followed by a heavy spin of the PRP to concentrate the platelets.
[Harmening 2005, p230]

47 **b**   Per AABB standards, at least 90% of
MLS ONLY platelet units sampled must have a pH of at least 6.2 at the end of the allowable storage.
[AABB Standards 2008a, pp35-36]

48 **a**   Per AABB standards, store Platelets
MLS ONLY at 20°-24°C with continuous agitation. Platelets must be separated from Whole Blood units and maintained at a temperature of at least 20°C. The pH must be at least 6.2 at the end of the storage time.
[AABB Standards 2008a, p65]

49 **b**   Whole blood-derived (random donor) Platelets should contain at least 5.5×10^{10} platelets, be stored with continuous agitation at 20°-24°C, and have a pH of 6.2 or higher when tested at the end of the storage period.
[Harmening 2005, p230]

50 **c**   Apheresis (single donor) Platelets should contain at least 3.0×10^{11} platelets, be stored with continuous agitation at 20°-24°C, and have a pH of 6.2 or higher when tested at the end of the storage period.
[Harmening 2005, p230]

51 **d**   Newly diagnosed bone marrow
MLS ONLY candidates are at great risk for severe sequelae of CMV infections. Infection can best be reduced by using leukocyte-reduction filters. CMV-seronegative units are rarely used since leukocyte reducing via filtration is so effective. Washing does not remove as many leukocytes as filtering.
[Harmening 2005, p310]

52 **d**   Leukoreduction of blood products
MLS ONLY reduces donor leukocytes to less than 5×10^6 and decreases the risk of HLA alloimmunization.
[Marques 2007, p20]

53 **a**   The apheresis process is to remove whole blood, the desired component removed, and the remaining portion of blood returned to the donor/patient.
[AABB Practical Guide 2007, ch14]

54 **b**   Autologous donors have less stringent criteria than allogeneic donors. Donations must be collected at least 72 hours prior to surgery.
[AABB Standards 2008a, p22]

55 **a**   Only ABO and Rh is required with the patient's sample. Each autologous unit must be confirmed for ABO and Rh from an integrally attached segment.
[AABB Standards 2008a, p44]

56 **c**   FDA requires that 4 representative units
MLS ONLY be tested each month for Factor VIII levels of 80 IU or higher. If the average value is less than 80 IU of Factor VIII, corrective action must be taken.
[AABB Tech Manual 2008b, p224]

57 **d**   To determine the total IU of Factor
MLS ONLY VIII per bag of cryoprecipitate, multiple the assayed value/mL by the number of mL in the container.
[Harmening 2005, p32]

Blood Group Systems

58 **a**   The mother has a 50% chance of passing on R_1 and 50% chance of passing on r. The father will always pass on R_1. Statistically, 50% of the children will be R_1r and 50% of the them will be R_1R_1.
[Harmening 2005, p139]

59 **d** The entire set of HLA antigens located on one chromosome is a haplotype.
[Harmening 2005, p485]

60 **d** The patient lacks *E*. Since *C* and *c* are alleles, *C* is inherited from one parent and *c* from the other. Since the person is homozygous for *e*, one of the genes needs to code for ce (RHce) and the other Ce (RHCe). The *RHD* gene is more likely inherited with *Ce* than *ce*, so the person's most probable genotype is *DCe/dce*. This genotype is found in 31% of the white and 15% of the black populations.
[AABB Tech Manual 2008b, pp387-392]

61 **c** The A and B structures can not be developed since there is no H precursor substance due to the lack of the *H* gene in the blood donor.
[AABB Tech Manual 2008b, p362]

62 **a** This individual cannot have the k antigen on their cells. K_0K_0 is rare and no Kell system antigens are detected on the red blood cells. Those individuals usually produce antibodies that are reactive with all normal cells. *KK* is the most probable genotype.
[Harmening 2005, p176]

63 **a** Fy(a–b–) individuals are very rare with all populations other than the individual of African descent. 68% of African Americans are Fy(a–b–).
[AABB Tech Manual 2008b, p422]

64 **a** The baby is Rh-negative and lacks c, since there is no evidence of HDFN. Inheritance of no D and no c is denoted as *r'*. The baby must have inherited this gene from both parents, and is homozygous *r'r'*.
[AABB Tech Manual 2008b, pp387-396]

65 **a** The most common genotype in Rh-negative individuals is *rr*. Anti-e would not be formed because the recipient's red cells contain the e antigen. The first antibody most likely to develop would be anti-c.
[Harmening 2005, p137]

66 **d** Blood group genes are autosomal; they are not carried on the sex gene. Whenever the gene is inherited, the antigen is expressed on the red blood cells, which is known as codominant.
[Harmening 2005, p110]

67 **c** The Xg blood group system is unique in that the gene encodes on the X chromosome. A negative mother would not have the Xg(a) to pass on. A positive father would, however, transmit the Xg(a) to all his daughters.
[Harmening 2005, p198]

68 **d** All common Rh antigens are present on the red blood cells. R_1 (*DCe*) and R_2 (*DcE*) are frequent genotypes.
[Harmening 2005, p139]

69 **a** R_0R_0 is the only correct choice here. R_0 = D+C–E–c+e+.
[AABB Tech Manual 2008b, pp387-396]

70 **c** The Lewis antigens are developed by gene interaction. Both the *Lewis* and *Secretor* gene are required for red cells to type as Le(a–b+). If a person has a *Lewis* gene, but not *Secretor* gene, then the cells type as Le(a+b–). The Le(a–b–) phenotype is derived when the *Lewis* gene is absent and the *Secretor* gene may or may not be present. The Le(a+b–) phenotype occurs in 22% of the population, and Le(a–b–) occurs in 6%, so the most likely phenotype of a nonsecretor (se/se) is Le(a+b–).
[AABB Tech Manual 2008b, p374]

71 **a** Anti-f will react with cells that carry c and e on the same Rh polypeptide. No other listed genotypes produce an Rh polypeptide that carries both c and e.
[AABB Tech Manual 2008b, pp387-396]

72 **a** Nonreactivity with anti-f indicates the cells do not have an Rh polypeptide that possesses both c and e, which is necessary to type as f+. R_1R_2 is the most likely genotype.
[AABB Tech Manual 2008b, pp387-396]

73 **b** The N antigen is lacking in 30% of the Caucasian population.
MLS ONLY
[AABB Tech Manual 2008b, p415]

74 **c** The baby appears to lack c since no HDFN was evident. The mom is most likely R_1R_1, so had to pass R_1 onto the baby. The father must have passed on an Rh gene that also did not produce c. Given the choices, the father has to be R_1r.
[AABB Tech Manual 2008b, pp387-396]

75 **c** The Fy(a–b–) phenotype occurs in 68% of the population of African descent, but is extremely rare in the other ethnic backgrounds. Lu(a–b–), Jk(a–b–) and K–k– are very rare in all ethnic backgrounds.
[AABB Tech Manual 2008b, ch14]

76 **d** The frequency of compatible donors for this patient can be calculated by multiplying the percentage of the population that is e–C– × Fy(a–) × Jk(b–). The blood supplier's immunohematology reference laboratory may have units in stock or can request blood from other IRLs through the American Rare Donor Program.
[Harmening 2005, p217, 257]

77 **b** The most likely haplotype is DCe/dce.
[AABB Tech Manual 2008b, p391]

78 **d** From the first 2 children it can be determined the mom has the haplotypes A2B12 and A23F18. The dad has the haplotypes A1B3 and A3B35. The expected B antigen in child #3 is B35.
[Harmening 2005, p435]

79 **c** If an exact match of HLA-A and HLA-B
MLS ONLY antigens is necessary, siblings would be the most likely match, since siblings may have received the same haplotypes from the parents.
[AABB Tech Manual 2008b, p550]

80 **d** Determination of compatibility can be
MLS ONLY determined by multiplying the percentage of compatibility of each antigen. 46% of the population is group O, 15% are D–, and 91% are K–. $0.46 \times 0.15 \times 0.91 = 0.06$, or 6%.
[AABB Tech Manual 2008b, p348]

81 **c** Use the Hardy-Weinberg equation:
MLS ONLY $p^2 + 2pq + q^2 = 1.0$. In this example, p^2 is the homozygous population, Jk(a+b–). The square root of p^2 = p, which is the gene frequency of Jk^a in this population. Out of 400 people, 122, or 30% are homozygous. The square root of 0.30 = is 0.55.
[AABB Tech Manual 2008b, pp349-351]

82 **b** The Hardy-Weinberg equation states
MLS ONLY $(p + q)^2 = 1.0$. When the equation is expanded, it is $p^2 + 2pq + q^2 = 1.0$.
[AABB Tech Manual 2008b, pp349-351]

83 **d** When a marker is in a child that the mother and alleged father do not have, the alleged father can not be the biological father of the child. This is a direct exclusion.
[AABB Tech Manual 2008b, p352]

84 **c** The child's genotype does not include E. The alleged father is homozygous for E. If he was the father the child would also have E. The father can be excluded from paternity.
[Harmening 2005, p139]

85 **b** Direct exclusion of paternity is established when a genetic marker is present in the child but is absent from the mother and the alleged father.
[AABB Tech Manual 2008b, p352]

86 **c** A_x cells are more strongly reactive with anti-A,B than with anti-A and the plasma frequently has anti-A_1 present.
[AABB Tech Manual 2008b, p366]

87 **c** The ABO blood group system was discovered by Karl Landsteiner.
[Harmening 2005, p109]

88 **c** Mixed-field reactivity with anti-A and anti-A,B is a typical finding for A_3 subgroups.
[AABB Tech Manual 2008b, p366]

89 **c** Fucose is the immunodominant sugar for H.
[AABB Tech Manual 2008b, p372]

90 **d** Bombay phenotypes (O_h) lack H antigen on their red cells, and produce naturally occurring anti-H in their serum.
[Harmening 2005, p121]

91 **a** Most examples of anti-Lu^a agglutinate saline suspended cells. Most examples of anti-Lu^b are IgG and reacts at 37°C. Anti-Lu3 usually reacts at the AHG phase as does anti-Lu^{ab}.
[Harmening 2005, p185]

92 **b** Anti-Ch and anti-Rg react at IAT with
MLS ONLY trace amounts of C4 (a component of complement) present on normal RBCs. The Ch and Rg substance is found soluble in plasma. Neutralization studies with pooled plasma can help confirm the antibody reactivity in a patient's sample. If test procedures are used to coat cells with C4, a patient with anti-Ch or anti-Rg may agglutinate the cells directly.
[AABB Tech Manual 2008b, p429]

93   **b**   Anti-Sd^a is an antibody to a high-prevalence antigen, which varies in strength from person to person. Most examples of anti-Sd^a characteristically present as small, mixed-field, refractile agglutinates that may have a shiny appearance when observed microscopically after the antiglobulin test.
[Harmening 2005, p197]

94   **b**   HLA antibodies are formed in response to pregnancy, transfusion or transplantation and are therefore not naturally occurring. They are associated with febrile nonhemolytic transfusion reactions and TRALI. They are directed against antigens found on granulocytes and other cells such as platelets.
[AABB Tech Manual 2008b, p397]

95   **d**   MHC consists of both class I and class II HLA antigens. Discrimination of self from nonself is the primary function of the HLA system and involves many immune responses.
[AABB Tech Manual 2008b, p555]

96   **d**   HPA-1a is a platelet specific antigen,
MLS
ONLY   which is the most common cause of neonatal alloimmune thrombocytopenia. Treatment consists of IVIG.
[AABB Tech Manual 2008b, p534]

97   **d**   Group O have the most H substance in their saliva. The person must also be a secretor of ABH substances. Due to gene interaction between the secretor gene and Lewis gene, people who are Le(a–b+) assures H in their saliva.
[Harmening 2005, p112]

98   **c**   Lewis antigens are found soluble in saliva. If saliva containing Lewis substance is added to a sample with anti-Le^a, then neutralization occurs. Le(a+) indicator cells added to the test system would be nonreactive. A proper control system is required whenever neutralization studies are performed.
[Harmening 2005, p155]

99   **d**   The overall incidence of the e antigen is 98%. The overall incidence of c is 80%, D is 85% and E is 30%.
[Harmening 2005, p136]

100   **c**   The G antigen is normally present on
MLS
ONLY   red cells possessing either C or D. Anti-G reacts with panel cells that are D+ or C+ and the antibodies appear to be anti-C and anti-D. The G antigen is expressed on the child's D+ red blood cells.
[Harmening 2005, p144]

101   **b**   Individuals who are partial D are
MLS
ONLY   missing epitopes of the D antigen and can develop antibodies toward the epitopes they lack. Since all normal D antigens have all epitopes, the specificity of the person's antibody is anti-D.
[AABB Tech Manual 2008b, p395]

102   **c**   The U antigen is a high incidence
MLS
ONLY   antigen found on the RBCs of all individuals except 1% of African-Americans, who lack glycoprotein B and usually type S–s–U–.
[Harmening 2005, p168]

103   **a**   The M and N antigens are found on glycophorin A.
[Harmening 2005, p167]

104   **c**   Autoanti-P, a cold-reactive IgG autoantibody described as a biphasic hemolysin, is associated with paroxysmal cold hemoglobinuria.
[Harmening 2005, p172]

105   **b**   Patients with infectious monucleosis often demonstrate potent examples of anti-i that are transient in nature.
[Harmening 2005, p174]

106   **c**   Anti-I is commonly found in all individuals, but when it causes hemolysis, the titer may be high and react at all temperatures. Cold agglutinin syndrome is mainly found in lymphoproliferative diseases.
[Harmening 2005, p173]

107   **c**   Anti-I is associated with cold agglutinin syndrome.
[Harmening 2005, p174]

108   **b**   Anti-i is an IgM antibody that reacts with cord cells and i adult cells. It is not associated with hemolytic disease of the newborn since IgM antibodies do not cross the placenta.
[Harmening 2005, p174]

109   **b**   The Kell antigen is highly immunogenic. It is present on the red cells of up to 9% of adults and neonates, and is not affected by enzymes.
[Harmening 2005, p176]

110 **c** Red blood cells of individuals with the
MLS
ONLY McLeod phenotype lack Kx and Km and have
significant depression of other Kell antigens.
The McLeod phenotype has been found
in patients with chronic granulomatous
disease (CGD).
[Harmening 2005, p179]

111 **a** Antibodies in the Kidd blood group
system are IgG and react best at the
antiglobulin phase. These antibodies
are associated with delayed hemolytic
transfusion reactions and reactivity can
be enhanced by testing with enzyme
pretreated cells.
[Harmening 2005, p183]

112 **c** The Fy^a and Fy^b antigens are sensitive to
denaturation by proteolytic enzymes. Serum
containing anti-Fy^a reacts with untreated
Fy(a+) cells, but not with enzyme treated
Fy(a+) cells.
[Harmening 2005, p180]

113 **c** Anti-Fy^a is an IgG antibody that reacts
best at the AHG phase, does not react with
enzyme-treated red cells, is capable of
causing hemolytic disease of the newborn,
and is not known to be an autoagglutinin.
[Harmening 2005, pp180-181]

114 **d** The Duffy glycoprotein on red cells
is a receptor for the malarial parasite
Plasmodium vivax. Red cells with the
phenotype Fy(a–b–) are resistant to invasion
by *P vivax*.
[Harmening 2005, p182]

115 **d** 75% of donors would be compatible
MLS
ONLY with anti-X and 90% with anti-Y.
The frequency of compatibility for both
antigens is determined by multiplying
the 2 compatibility percentages:
0.75 × 0.90 = 0.675.
[AABB Tech Manual 2008b, p348]

116 **d** When the percentages of each
MLS
ONLY phenotype are multiplied together, the
incidence of the phenotype occurs in
1.438% of the population, so in a population
of 100,000, there would be 1,438 with
the phenotype.
[AABB Tech Manual 2008b, p348]

117 **c** Multiplication of the individual
MLS
ONLY compatibility frequencies results in the
percentage of compatible donors that would
lack both antigens. 0.20 × 0.90 = 0.18,
or 18%.
[AABB Tech Manual 2008b, p348]

118 **d** After performing rule outs, the most
likely antibody is anti-c. To form anti-c, the
patient would need to inherit a gene from
both parents that does not produce the c
antigen. The most common gene that codes
for no c antigen is denoted as R_1.
[Harmening 2005, p136]

Physiology and Pathophysiology

119 **a** Massive transfusion patients (2 or more
MLS
ONLY blood volumes) usually require platelets and
FFP but since his platelet count is adequate,
only FFP should be given at this time.
[Harmening 2005, p314]

120 **c** Cryoprecipitate is used primarily for
MLS
ONLY fibrinogen replacement. Fibrinogen level
is decreased in patients with DIC, due to
uncontrolled thrombin generation.
[Harmening 2005, pp232, 237, 308]

121 **a** Patients with severe hemophilia A may
have spontaneous hemorrhages that are
treated with Factor VIII concentrate.
[Harmening 2005, p308]

122 **d** Factor VIII concentrate is the
MLS
ONLY product of choice in the treatment of
classic hemophilia.
[Harmening 2005, p223]

123 **d** Factors V and VIII would be decreased
MLS
ONLY but IX would not be decreased.
[Harmening 2005, p307]

124 **c** These are symptoms of a low platelet
MLS
ONLY count. If the mother's platelet count is
normal, the newborn likely has neonatal
alloimmune thrombocytopenia (NAIT),
caused by maternal antibody to the infant's
platelet antigens.
[Harmening 2005, p306]

125 **b** When platelets are needed, maternal
MLS
ONLY platelets are often prepared for use at
cordocentesis or delivery. Platelets should be
washed to remove maternal antibody.
[AABB Tech Manual 2008b, p534]

126 d HDFN is caused by maternal antibody crossing the placenta and destroying fetal antigen-positive red cells. Unlike ABO antibodies, which are naturally-occurring and can affect the first pregnancy, Rh antibodies are not produced until the mother has been exposed to Rh-positive red cells, usually during delivery of the first Rh-positive child. Once immunized, subsequent pregnancies with Rh-positive infants are affected, usually with increasing severity.
[Harmening 2005, pp384, 392]

127 c HDFN is caused by maternal antibodies against antigens on fetal red cells inherited from the father. Since the father is homozygous for c, the baby's red cells have to be c+, and could react with maternal anti-c if present. The father is A–, D–, and C–, and cannot pass these antigens to the child.
[Harmening 2005, p384]

128 d ABO HDFN is a mild disease, not usually requiring transfusion. It may occur in any pregnancy in which there is ABO incompatibility. High-titered IgG antibodies are more frequently seen in group O mothers than in A or B mothers.
[Harmening 2005, pp391-392]

129 d HDFN is caused by maternal IgG antibodies. Outside the Rh system, the most clinically significant antibody for HDFN is anti-K. IgM antibodies do not cross the placenta.
[Harmening 2005, p385]

130 a ABO HDFN is a mild disease that may occur in any ABO-incompatible pregnancy, including the first, since the antibodies are naturally occurring. Rh HDFN does not occur until the mother has become immunized. Once this happens, subsequent pregnancies may be quite severely affected. The DAT is typically weak or even negative in ABO HDFN, and strongly positive in Rh HDFN.
[Harmening 2005, pp384, 391-392]

131 c The mother has anti-D; the baby has a positive DAT; yet the baby appears to be Rh-negative. Textbooks state that, if a baby has a strongly positive DAT, the baby's red cells may be so heavily coated with maternal antibody that the D antigen sites are blocked and cannot react with anti-D reagent, causing a false-negative Rh type. Since the infant is type O, ABO hemolytic disease of the fetus and newborn (HDFN) does not fit this example. If the fetus had received enough D– intrauterine transfusions to cause the red cells to type as D–, they would not demonstrate a 4+ positive DAT, as shown in this example. There is no indication of a fetomaternal hemorrhage.
[Harmening 2005, p289]

132 a ABO HDFN occurs most commonly in group A babies born to group O mothers and usually has a mild course. The DAT is typically weak or negative and jaundice develops 12-48 hours after birth. The mother and baby are both Rh-positive.
[Harmening 2005, pp391-392]

133 d Spherocytosis is characteristic of ABO HDFN but not Rh HDFN.
[Harmening 2005, p392]

134 b The change in optical density (absorbance) of amniotic fluid measured spectrophotometrically at 450 nm is calculated and plotted on the Liley graph according to the weeks gestation. The graph is divided into 3 zones, which predict the severity of HDFN and the need for intervention and treatment.
[Harmening 2005, p388]

135 c A positive DAT on cord blood demonstrates the presence of maternal antibody coating the baby's red cells and indicates hemolytic disease of the newborn. Normal cord hemoglobin in newborns ranges from 14-20 g/L. A cord hemoglobin value of 10 g/L indicates anemia and supports the diagnosis of HDFN.
[Harmening 2005, pp389-390]

136 b Antibody titers do not themselves predict the severity of HDFN or the treatment needed. Instead, titers above a critical level, usually 16-32, identify candidates for amniocentesis or PUBS to monitor the fetus and determine the course of treatment.
[Harmening 2005, pp387-388]

137 **a** Blood for an exchange transfusion should lack the antigen to any maternal antibodies that have entered the infant's circulation and are reactive at 37°C or AHG.
[Harmening 2005, p274]

138 **b** Fetuses undergoing intrauterine
MLS ONLY transfusion must receive irradiated blood products. The unit must lack the antigen that the mother has produced antibody against. Most centers treating HDN use group O Rh-negative RBCs for intrauterine transfusions.
[Harmening 2005, pp227, 390]

139 **d** Blood selected for exchange transfusion
MLS ONLY is usually crossmatched with the mother's blood, and should be ABO-compatible. It should be negative for the antigen that she has produced antibody against. Unless the HDFN is caused by anti-D, the baby's Rh type is selected. In this case, group O, baby's Rh type, E–, is the best choice for the exchange transfusion.
[Harmening 2005, p390]

140 **a** Blood selected for exchange transfusion should be ABO-compatible with the mother and baby, and antigen-negative. Prenatal antibody titers above 16 or 32 are considered significant, and the condition of the fetus should be monitored.
[Harmening 2005, pp387-390]

141 **a** Blood selected for exchange transfusion should be antigen-negative and ABO-compatible with the mother and baby. Red Blood Cells are usually less than 7 days old, CMV–, hemoglobin S–, and irradiated.
[AABB Tech Manual 2008b, pp647-648]

142 **c** For exchange transfusion, antigen-negative Red Blood Cells are typically resuspended in ABO-compatible thawed Fresh Frozen Plasma.
[AABB Tech Manual 2008b, p647]

143 **b** Blood selected for intrauterine transfusion and transfusion to premature infants should be irradiated to prevent graft-vs-host disease.
[Harmening 2005, p390]

144 **a** If the initial antibody screen, using
MLS ONLY either the mother's or baby's serum is positive, either antigen-negative or AHG-crossmatch-compatible units are selected until the antibody is no longer demonstrable in the baby's serum.
[AABB Standards 2008, §5·16·1]

145 **b** Care must be taken so that fetal Rh-positive RBCs in the maternal circulation are not interpreted as maternal, because the mother would be assumed erroneously to be weak D+.
[Harmening 2005, p391]

146 **d** The presence of D+ infant's red cells in the mother's circulation can cause the weak D test to show mixed-field agglutination. Care must be taken so that fetal Rh-positive RBCs in the maternal circulation are not interpreted as maternal, because the mother would be assumed erroneously to be weak D+.
[Harmening 2005, p391]

147 **b** The rosette test is a qualitative test. When enzyme-treated cells are used as indicator cells, a negative test (indicating there was not an excessive bleed) can have up to 1 rosette per 3 fields. The mother needs to receive 1 vial of RhIg for a normal bleed.
[AABB Tech Manual 2008b, pp935-936]

148 **c** The weak D result is most likely due to excessive bleed of fetal cells. Rosette results indicate a quantitative test for approximate volume of fetal-maternal bleed should be performed.
[AABB Tech Manual 2008b, pp631-632]

149 **c** About half of the antenatal dose of
MLS ONLY RhIG may still be present at delivery so the antibody screen may detect weak anti-D, which should not be interpreted erroneously as active rather than passive immunization.
[Harmening 2005, p390]

150 **b** One dose of RhIg will protect the mother from a bleed of 30 mL. The bleed was 35 mL, 2 vials of RhIg will be needed.
[AABB Tech Manual 2008b, pp631-632]

151 **d** One vial of Rh immune globulin protects against a fetomaternal hemorrhage of 15 mL of red cells, or 30 mL of Whole Blood. Divide the volume of fetomaternal hemorrhage (35 mL) by 15; round down to 2, then add 1 extra vial = 3 vials total.
[AABB Tech Manual 2008b, p632]

152 **c** RhIG should be given to nonimmunized D– females who are pregnant or have delivered a D+ infant.
[Harmening 2005, p234]

153   **b**   About half of the antenatal dose of
_{MLS ONLY} RhIG may still be present at delivery so the antibody screen may detect weak anti-D, which should not be interpreted erroneously as active rather than passive immunization.
[Harmening 2005, p390]

154   **c**   RhIG is of no benefit once a person has been actively immunized and has formed anti-D.
[Harmening 2005, p391]

155   **b**   The formula to calculate the percentage assumes the mother's blood volume as 5,000 mL. $0.003 \times 5,000$ mL=15mL.
[AABB Tech Manual 2008b, p632]

156   **b**   The percentage is cells/100, the mother's volume is assumed to be 5,000 mL. The percentage must be multiplied by 50 to determine total volume.
[AABB Tech Manual 2008b, p632]

157   **c**   Use the formula: (fetal cells counted/cells counted) × (maternal blood volume). Assume the mother's blood volume is 5,000 mL. In this example, 30 fetal cells/2,000 cells counted × 5,000 mL = 75 mL. RhIg protects against 30 mL. So 2.5 vials are needed, rounded up to 3 full vials. Add 1 vial for hospital policy and 4 vials are needed.
[AABB Tech Manual 2008b, p632]

158   **a**   The rosette test is a sensitive method to detect FMH of 10 mL or more.
[AABB Tech Manual 2008b, pp387-388]

159   **b**   The rosette screen will be positive
_{MLS ONLY} if there is a FMH of 10 mL or more. A Kleihauer-Betke or flow cytometry should be performed to quantitate the FMH and determine if additional doses of Rh immune globulin are needed to prevent immunization from occurring.
[AABB Tech Manual 2008b, pp631-632]

160   **c**   The mixed lymphocyte culture (MLC) is
_{MLS ONLY} used to detect genetic differences in the HLA D region antigens.
[AABB Tech Manual 2008b, p559]

161   **d**   Transfusion should generally be avoided except in cases of life-threatening anemia. A hemoglobin of 10.8 g/dL (108 g/L) is not life-threatening, especially if the patient is not actively bleeding.
[Harmening 2005, p411]

162   **d**   Bone marrow transplant patients are at risk for transfusion-associated graft-vs-host disease (TA-GVHD) and therefore should receive irradiated blood products.
[Harmening 2005, p227]

163   **b**   HLA antigen typing is important to consider before organ transplantation.
[Harmening 2005, p435]

164   **a**   DR antigens, also known as Class
_{MLS ONLY} II antigens, are significant in organ transplantation. These antigens are expressed on B lymphocytes, macrophages, monocytes and endothelial cells and are detected in the lymphocytotoxicity test.
[Harmening 2005, pp436, 444]

165   **a**   Negative check cells means the results of tubes with the negative reactions are invalid. The reactivity of the check cells should be verified with anti-IgG since anti-E was detected, indicating the anti-IgG was reactive. All tests that were nonreactive with the check cells requires repeat test performance.
[Harmening 2005, p102]

Serology

166   **b**   The listed criteria are typical for
_{MLS ONLY} serological calibration of a centrifuge. Optimum spin time is the least amount of time when all criteria are satisfied.
[AABB Tech Manual 2008b, pp980-981]

167   **a**   Samples must be labeled with 2 independent patient identifiers and the date of collection. This information should be identical to that on the patient's identification band and request.
[AABB Tech Manual 2008b, p439]

168   **d**   Results of ABO and Rh testing on a current specimen must always be compared to that of a previous transfusion record. Errors in typing or patient identification may be detected when discrepancies are found. Collection of a new sample allows determination of which sample was incorrectly collected.
[AABB Tech Manual 2008b, p451]

169 **c**   A serological test to confirm the ABO on all RBC units and Rh on units labeled as Rh-negative must be performed prior to transfusion. Any errors in labeling must be reported to the collection facility.
[AABB Tech Manual 2008b, p451]

170 **c**   Samples must be labeled with 2 independent patient identifiers and the date of collection. This information should be identical to that on the patients identification band and request. There must be a mechanism to identify the phlebotomist, but initialing the sample tubes is not required.
[AABB Standards 2008a, §5·11; [AABB Tech Manual 2008b, p441]

171 **b**   Granulocytes must be compatible with recipient's plasma. Granulocyte products have an expiration of 24 hours.
[AABB Standards 2008a, pp45-46, 55]

172 **c**   Because neonates are immunologically immature, alloimmunization to red cell antigens is very rare during the neonatal period. No crossmatching is required if the initial antibody screen performed with either the baby's or mother's plasma is negative.
[AABB Standards 2008a, §5·16; [AABB Tech Manual 2008b, pp459-460]

173 **b**   A positive DAT will interfere with weak D testing causing both the patient and control to demonstrate positive results. Any positive result in the control tube invalidates any results.
[AABB Tech Manual 2008b, p404]

174 **c**   Patients with multiple myeloma demonstrate rouleaux formation, which can cause the appearance of agglutination. If the cells are washed to remove residual plasma, and tests repeated, an accurate red cell typing is obtained. By performing a saline replacement with the reverse typing, true agglutination will remain when the cell buttons of the reverse cells are resuspended in saline.
[AABB Tech Manual 2008b, pp370-371]

175 **d**   ABO immunoglobulins develop at approximately 3 months of age, attain adult levels by age 10, and may, but not always, decline in titer in the elderly.
[AABB Tech Manual 2008b, p363]

176 **b**   Acquired B occurs in group A individuals and is due to deacetylation of the A antigen by bacterial enzymes. Detection of acquired B is dependent upon the source of anti-B used.
[AABB Tech Manual 2008b, p367]

177 **a**   Tn is caused from a somatic mutation and the phenomenon is persistent. Resolution of the red cell typing can be performed with enzyme-treated patient cells, since Tn is denatured by enzymes. Although the reactivity with anti-A may be weak, testing with anti-A_1 lectin gives strong reactivity, unlike subgroups of A, which are weakly reacting with anti-A and nonreactive with A_1 lectin.
[Harmening 2005, pp508-515]

178 **c**   Mixed-field reactivity is a characteristic of the A_3 subgroup. Transfusion history would be important to be sure it is not 2 cell populations.
[AABB Tech Manual 2008b, p366]

179 **b**   Polyagglutination is a property of the cells. Most adult plasma agglutinate the cells due to naturally occurring antibodies directed towards the crypt antigens.
[AABB Tech Manual 2008b, p370]

180 **c**   Presence of agglutination with A_1 cells, screening cells and autocontrol at IS and RT is indicative of a cold autoantibody.
[Harmening 2005, 128]

181 **c**   Warming serum and reagent red cells to 37°C before repeating ABO typing will decrease/eliminate reactivity of cold autoantibody.
MLS ONLY
[Harmening 2005, p128]

182 **d**   Unexpected reactivity with reverse cells should include a test with screen cells at immediate spin to determine if alloantibodies are present. Resolution of the ABO discrepancy can be performed with group B cells that lack the corresponding antigen for the identified alloantibody.
[AABB Tech Manual 2008b, pp371-372]

183 **d**   Most ABO discrepancies are due to problems in the reverse typing. Discrepancies stemming from the forward type or the patient's cells are usually due to Tn activation from a somatic mutation.
MLS ONLY
[Harmening 2005, p510]

184 **b** Although monoclonal anti-D react with most D+ red blood cells, cells with fewer antigen sites requires testing after the antiglobulin test. The test is referred to as a test for weak D.
[AABB Tech Manual 2008b, p394]

185 **c** The ABO discrepancy is most likely
MLS
ONLY due to anti-H in an A_1 individual. Anti-H reacts most strongly at room temperature with group O screening cells and weaker or negative at room temperature with autologous or donor group A_1 cells. As the branched H structures are converted to A, some group A_1 individuals may develop a clinically-insignificant anti-H recognizing H structures on group O and A_2 blood groups.
[Harmening 2005, pp116, 126]

186 **d** Some subgroups of A are only recognized because of their lack of anti-A in the reverse typing. Often, the donors are confirmed as subgroups of A by an adsorption-elution technique.
[AABB Tech Manual 2008b, p366]

187 **c** The mom does not have the *D* gene. The father would have to have inherited one gene that produces D and another gene that does not produce D. The mom and dad both passed on genes that do not produce D.
[AABB Tech Manual 2008b, pp387-936]

188 **a** Some blood group antibodies, in the presence of their corresponding antigen and complement, activate the complement cascade and demonstrate in-vitro hemolysis.
[Harmening 2005, p58]

189 **b** Agglutination at AHG phase indicates the presence of clinically significant antibody, indicating the need for antibody identification.
[Harmening 2005, p246]

190 **b** Presence of agglutination at AHG phase with both screening cells and autocontrol is indicative of warm autoantibody.
[Harmening 2005, p407]

191 **a** Presence of agglutination at AHG phase with screening cells and 2 out of 6 donor units indicates antibody in patient serum to antigen(s) on screening cells and donor cells. The presence of an autoantibody would most likely react with all cells, including the autologous control or DAT.
[Harmening 2005, p60..

192 **b** Reaction with anti-IgG in the DAT and with both screening cells and autocontrol at the AHG phase is indicative of a warm autoantibody.
[Harmening 2005, p407]

193 **c** Initial result was most likely a false-negative result due to the omission of patient serum. This would explain the initial negative result followed by the subsequent positive result.
[Harmening 2005, p102]

194 **b** The absence of agglutination at the AHG phase with screening cells and agglutination with one of 3 donor units is most likely due to an antibody to a low-incidence antigen.
[Harmening 2005, p271]

195 **d** The major crossmatch tests the recipient's plasma with donor's cells. This would detect any antibody in the recipient that would react with antigens on the donor's RBCs. If a patient were mistyped as a group O rather than group A, then group O cells would be selected for crossmatch and no incompatibility would be found.
[AABB Tech Manual 2008b, pp452-456]

196 **a** The patient has a negative antibody screen, but one unit is found to be incompatible. The antibody is most likely directed towards a low-incidence antigen.
[AABB Tech Manual 2008b, p455]

197 **d** Since crossmatching is a test between the patient's plasma and donor's cells, any incompatibility is due to the donor's red cells. If a patient is negative for clinically significant antibodies to common antigens, an incompatible unit by the antiglobulin test is due to either a positive DAT on the donors red cells or the patient has an antibody to a low-incidence antigen that the donor's cells possess.
[AABB Tech Manual 2008b, p455]

198 **b** If a patient is negative for clinically significant antibodies, and a single crossmatch is incompatible, the incompatibility is either due to donor cells with a positive DAT or the patient has an antibody to a low-incidence antigen that the donor's cells possess.
[AABB Tech Manual 2008b, p455]

199 **c** If a patient is negative for clinically significant antibodies, and a single crossmatch is incompatible, the incompatibility is either due to donor cells with a positive DAT or the patient has an antibody to a low-incidence antigen that the donor's cells possess.
[AABB Tech Manual 2008b, p455]

200 **c** Emergent release of blood can not use previous records. Blood typing must be performed on the current sample. In this case, group O Rh-negative is the best choice since there is evidence the patient is Rh-negative.
[AABB Tech Manual 2008b, p455]

201 **b** When group specific units of Red Blood Cells are not available, group compatible units are selected. Since the patient is AB, group A would be selected to conserve group O units for group O patients. Rh-negative patients should receive Rh-negative units of red blood cells.
[Harmening 2005, p269]

202 **a** This patient has an anti-A_1, which eliminates A_1B cells immediately. Rh-negative units should be conserved for Rh-negative patients when Rh-positive units are available. Selection of group B units provides compatible units quickly.
[AABB Tech Manual 2008b, p368]

203 **d** The strength of agglutination is dependent upon optimal antigen to antibody ratio. Excessive amount of antigen does not allow maximal uptake of antibody per red cell and therefore agglutination is negatively affected leading to weaker or negative results.
[Harmening 2005, p63]

204 **c** Rh antibodies show enhanced reactivity
MLS ONLY with enzyme pretreated cells. The M and Fy^a antigens are cleaved from enzyme pretreated cells and therefore there would be no reaction between enzyme pretreated cells and serum containing anti-M or anti-Fy^a. The incidence of the c antigen is 80% in whites and 96% of blacks. The incidence of the E antigen is 29% in whites and 22% in blacks. Increased reactivity with enzyme pretreated cells and incompatible results with 8 of 10 donor units is most likely due to anti-c.
[Harmening 2005, pp166-167, 180-181]

205 **a** Determining the patient's phenotype allows focusing identification procedures toward antibodies the patient can develop.
[AABB Tech Manual 2008b, p441]

206 **a** Warm autoantibodies often exhibit Rh specificity.
[Harmening 2005, p406]

207 **a** Lewis antibodies may bind complement and fresh serum that contains anti-Le^a may hemolyze Le(a+) red cells in vitro. Approximately 22% of the population is Le(a+).
[Harmening 2005, p153]

208 **a** The reactivity of anti-k and anti-Js^b with
MLS ONLY enzyme pretreated cells is unchanged and anti-e would show enhanced reactivity with enzyme treated cells. Chido antigens are sensitive to treatment with most enzymes and anti-Ch would therefore not react with enzyme pretreated cells. The Chido antigen is a high incidence antigen.
[Harmening 2005, pp142, 177, 200]

209 **a** Antibodies to antigens on cells 2, 3, 4, and 5 can be ruled out in tubes II and III, in which there was no reaction between patient serum and cells.
[Harmening 2005, pp250-252]

210 **b** Anti-K and anti-P_1 can be ruled out on
MLS ONLY cell 1 since there is no agglutination of cell 1 with the patient's sample. Anti-M and anti-Jk^a can be eliminated on cell 2, which has a double-dose antigen expression of both M and Jk^a.
[Harmening 2005, pp250-252]

211 **d** Antibodies to C, Le^b and Jk^a can be
MLS ONLY eliminated due to the lack of agglutination with panel cells 1 and 2. Panel cells 1 and 2 possessed the C, Le^b and Jk^a antigens. Only anti-E remains.
[Harmening 2005, pp250-252]

212 **b** Lewis antibodies are usually IgM and agglutinate saline suspended cells. Approximately 22% of the population is Le(a+), which would account for 3 out of 10 donor units being incompatible. Anti-P_1 is also an antibody that may react at immediate spin, but 79% of the white population and 94% of the black population are P_1+. Anti-C and anti-Fy^a are IgG antibodies that react at the antiglobulin phase.
[Harmening 2005, pp153, 171, 180-181]

213 a Chido antibodies are considered clinically insignificant.
[Harmening 2005, p200]

214 b Lack of agglutination between patient serum and with cells that lack one of the high incidence antigens would confirm the specificity of the antibody.
[Harmening 2005, p258]
MLS ONLY

215 c An ABO discrepancy in an A_1 individual, manifested by agglutination in the serum grouping with A_2 cells, is most likely due to anti-H. The greatest concentration of H substance is found on O cells, followed by A_2 cells. The least amount of H substance is found on A_1 and A_1B cells.
[Harmening 2005, p116]

216 b Reactivity at 37°C and AHG indicate the presence of an IgG antibody. Anti-M, although usually IgM, may be partly or wholly IgG. Anti-M is ruled out on cell 4. Anti-Le^b is usually IgM and can be ruled out on cells 4 and 8. This leaves anti-E, anti-Fy^a and anti-K.
[Harmening 2005, pp250-252]

217 a All 3 antibodies can cause HDFN and delayed transfusion reactions. Anti-Jk^a is associated with showing dosage.
[Harmening 2005, p177, 180-181, 183]

218 a Rh antibodies demonstrate enhanced reactivity with enzyme-pretreated cells. Antibodies in the Kell system do not have enhanced reactivity with enzyme-pretreated cells. Anti-E and -D are ruled out on cell 3, and anti-K is ruled out on cell 7.
[Harmening 2005, pp250-252]
MLS ONLY

219 b Anti-Fy^a may cause mild to rarely severe hemolytic disease of the fetus and newborn.
[Harmening 2005, pp250-252]
MLS ONLY

220 a The direct antiglobulin test (DAT) is used to identify red blood cells that have been coated with antibody in vivo.
[AABB Tech Manual 2008b, p278]

221 b In cold agglutinin syndrome, anti-I acts as a complement binding antibody with a high titer and high thermal amplitude. The complement cascade is activated and C3d remains on the red cell membrane of circulating cells.
[Harmening 2005, p172]

222 a An anamnestic response is a secondary response from memory cells. There will be an increase in antibody titer upon exposure; the antibody sensitizes incompatible cells circulating in the patient. The DAT appears mixed-field since the patient's own cells are not sensitized.
[AABB Tech Manual 2008b, p446]
MLS ONLY

223 d After washing cells for the DAT or IAT procedure, the AHG should be added immediately and read. Delay can cause a weakened or negative result due to dissociation of the bound IgG in the prolonged time before reagent is added.
[AABB Tech Manual 2008b, p446]

224 b Polyspecific AHG contains anti-IgG and anti-C3d.
[AABB Tech Manual 2008b, p471]

225 d Antiglobulin reagent is used to detect the presence of red cells, coated in vivo with IgG and/or C3d. Antiglobulin reagent may be polyspecific (contains an anti-IgG and anti-C3d) or monospecific (anti-IgG or anti-C3d).
[Harmening 2005, p98]

226 c AHG control cells are IgG-sensitized cells that react with the anti-IgG in the AHG reagent to demonstrate AHG was added and not neutralized by insufficient washing of the tests prior to its addition.
[AABB Tech Manual 2008b, p449]

227 c Cold agglutinin disease is associated with cold reactive antibodies that typically activate complement. Cells that do not undergo lysis due to complement activation have C3d attached to the red blood cells.
[AABB Tech Manual 2008b, p511]

228 a Detection of antibodies to penicillin requires treatment of test cells with penicillin and the subsequent testing of the patient's plasma and eluate. Test cells that have not been treated with penicillin do not react.
[AABB Tech Manual 2008b, pp515-518]
MLS ONLY

229 c EDTA chelates calcium preventing blood to clot. This chelation of calcium also will stop the complement cascade. Calcium ions are necessary for C1 to attach to IgG on the red blood cells.
[AABB Tech Manual 2008b, p500]

230 **c**   Methyldopa is frequently listed as the prototype for drug-independent antibody mechanism where autoantibody is present on the red cells and may also be present in the plasma.
[AABB Tech Manual 2008b, pp515-518]

231 **b**   Auto-antibody specificity in cold
<small>MLS ONLY</small> agglutinin syndrome is most often anti-I. This auto-antibody reacts optimally at 4°C, but also reacts between 25°C and 31°C. Auto anti-I can activate complement so C3d can be attached to patient cells. The eluate will be negative as C3d cannot be eluted from cells.
[Harmening 2005, pp398-400]

232 **b**   Second and third generation cephalosporins react when the drug is present in vitro. When serum, drug, and red cells are present, direct or indirect agglutination or lysis may be observed.
[AABB Tech Manual 2008b, pp515-518]

233 **c**   A negative reaction after the addition of check cells indicates AHG serum was not present. Inadequate washing of red cells may leave residual patient serum behind, which can neutralize AHG serum.
[Harmening 2005, p101]

234 **d**   Weak antibodies may be missed if there are excess RBC antigens as there may be too few antibodies to bind to red cell antigens.
[Harmening 2005, p102]

235 **c** A_x cells react more strongly with anti-A,B than with anti-A. If anti-A is nonreactive, A_x cells may be detected with anti-A,B.
[AABB Tech Manual 2008b, p366]

236 **c**   A solution of 8% bovine albumin can be prepared by diluting the more concentrated solution with normal saline. The formula to be used is: (volume1 × concentration1) = (volume2 × concentration2). A solution of 6%-8% albumin is used with some anti-D reagents as a control for spontaneous agglutination.
[AABB Tech Manual 2008b, pp726-727]

237 **b**   Rh antibodies show enhanced reactivity with enzyme pretreated cells. Treatment of red cells with enzymes weakens reactivity with antibodies in the MNS and Duffy systems.
[Harmening 2005, pp166-167, 180-181]

238 **b**   Patients may have antibodies to components of reagents. Washing the patient's cells prior to testing to remove their plasma from the cell suspension will resolve the reactivity with anti-B.
[AABB Tech Manual 2008b, p370]

239 **a**   Enzyme treatment would allow for differentiation of the remaining antibodies after rule outs. The Fy^a antigen would be denatured, allowing determination of whether anti-Jk^a and -K are present, and to confirm anti-E.
[Harmening 2005, p252]

240 **c**   Soluble forms of some blood group antigens can be prepared from other sources and used to inhibit reactivity of the corresponding antibody, such as the HTLA antibodies anti-Ch and anti-Rg. Most HTLA antibodies, although weakly reactive in undiluted serum, will continue to react weakly at higher dilutions.
[AABB Tech Manual 2008b, pp444-445]

241 **d**   For neutralization studies to be valid, the saline dilutional control must be reactive. Since neutralization studies involve adding a substance to the patient's plasma, nonreactivity in test tubes may be due to simple dilution. The saline control acts as the dilutional control and must be reactive. When the saline control is reactive, then if the tube with the substance is nonreactive, the interpretation that neutralization has occurred is made. If it is reactive, neutralization did not occur.
[AABB Tech Manual 2008b, p480]

242 **a**   In neutralization, a known source of a
<small>MLS ONLY</small> blood group soluble substance (for example, saliva, urine, or plasma) is incubated with a plasma antibody. During the incubation, the antibody combines with the soluble substance. The antibody is neutralized and inhibited from combining with the same blood group substance found on red blood cells when the blood cells are added to the system.
[Harmening 2005, p252]

Answers–Blood Bank

243 b Anti-Le^b is confirmed because the tubes with Lewis substance are negative. Nonreactivity of the serum with Le(b+) cells indicates the anti-Le^b in the serum was neutralized by the Lewis substance. The test is valid since the patient's serum with saline rather than substance added is still able to react with the Le(b+) cells.
[Harmening 2005, p155]

244 d
MLS
ONLY
Reactivity with anti-H is no longer demonstrable, which indicates H substance is present. There is no A or B substance in the saliva as evidenced by the ability of anti-A and anti-B reacting with respective cells. People with H substance and no A or B substance are group O secretors.
[AABB Tech Manual 2008b, p883]

245 c
MLS
ONLY
Secretor studies demonstrates the presence of a substance by the observation of neutralization of the corresponding antibody. Nonreactivity with B and O cells indicates B and H substances are present in the saliva so the red cells from this person are group B.
[AABB Tech Manual 2008b, p883]

246 a In the solid phase technology, the antibody screening cells are bound to the surface of the well. Antibody specific for antigen on the red blood cells attaches, resulting in a diffuse pattern of red blood cells in the well. A negative reaction would have manifested as a pellet of red blood cells in the bottom of the well.
[Harmening 2005, pp246-247]

247 b The K antigen is integral to the red cell membrane and would not change in a patient. Errors in typing or patient identification may be detected when discrepancies are found when comparing historical records.
[AABB Tech Manual 2008b, pp418-419]

248 d Polyagglutination is a property of the red blood cells. Structures on the red cells are altered due to bacterial enzymes or a somatic mutation, so crypt antigens not normally exposed on cells are now present. Antibodies to the exposed structures are naturally occurring in adult plasma.
[Harmening 2005, p528]

249 c Rouleaux will readily disperse in saline whereas true agglutination will remain after saline replacement.
[AABB Tech Manual 2008b, pp903-904]

250 a
MLS
ONLY
The Donath-Landsteiner test is diagnostic for PCH. The antibody is IgG and is biphasic: hemolysis occurs when the antibody is incubated with cells and cold temperatures and then incubated at 37°C. Often the antibody demonstrates specificity towards the high-incidence antigen P (not to be confused with P$_1$). The antibody screen is usually negative and the patient's red cells are coated with complement.
[AABB Tech Manual 2008b, pp383, 514]

251 b Two reagents used for removing IgG from red blood cells are chloroquine diphosphate (CDP) and EDTA glycine acid (EGA). Using either of these procedures is useful to reduce a patient's DAT and allow phenotyping with IAT reactive antisera.
[AABB Tech Manual 2008b, p894]

252 a Anti-Fy^a would not react with enzyme pretreated cells; a select cell panel would allow for individual reactivity of the remaining 2 antibodies. Thiol reagents would be used to disperse agglutination of IgM antibodies; the antibodies in question are IgG.
[Harmening 2005, p252]

253 c *Dolichos biflorus* plant seed extract forms complexes with N-acetylgalactosamine. When properly diluted, it can distinguish between A$_1$ donor cells and all other subgroups of A.
[AABB Tech Manual 2008b, p365]

254 d The serum of a group O individual contains anti-A, anti-B and anti-A,B. To prepare a suitable reagent, the ABO antibodies must be removed and anti-D left in the serum. The serum would need to be adsorbed with cells of the A$_1$B, cde/cde phenotype.
[Harmening 2005, p110]

255 d Since the auto control is positive after the AHG phase and no reactivity was detected at immediate spin, the serology is most consistent with a warm autoantibody. An adsorption with autologous cells to remove the antibody to used the adsorbed plasma for alloantibody detection is the next step.
[AABB Tech Manual 2008b, pp506-507]

256 a ZZAP is a reagent to remove IgG from the patient's own cells to allow better adsorption of IgG autoantibody from the patient's plasma onto the cells. The intent of the autoadsorption is to remove autoantibody to look for alloantibodies prior to transfusion.
[AABB Tech Manual 2008b, pp507-508]
MLS ONLY

257 a Treating autologous cells with a proteolytic enzyme such as ficin enhances the adsorption of the cold reactive antibody.
[AABB Tech Manual 2008b, pp512-513]
MLS ONLY

258 d An elution is the process of removal of antibody from red blood cells. The product of the elution method is an eluate. The eluate contains the antibody and can be used in antibody identification methods.
[Harmening 2005, p523]

259 a Adsorption and elution techniques are used to detect ABO antigens that are not detectable by direct agglutination. The cells are incubated with the antibody (anti-A or anti-B) to the antigen expected on the red blood cells. An elution method is performed and the antibody in the eluate is tested for recovering anti-A (or anti-B depending on the specificity that was used in the adsorption).
[AABB Tech Manual 2008b, p366]
MLS ONLY

260 c Antibody-antigen complexes are dependent upon a neutral pH. Extremes in pH causes dissociation. Both auto and alloantibodies are recovered in elutes prepared by reagent kits that alter the pH.
[AABB Tech Manual 2008b, pp919-922]

Transfusion Practice

261 b Each unit of Whole Blood or RBCs will increase the hematocrit by 3%-5%, so 2 units of RBCs will increase the hematocrit by twice as much as 1 unit of Whole Blood.
[Harmening 2005, p305]

262 c For emergency transfusions, group O– RBC units should be used.
[Harmening 2005, p314]

263 d Granulocyte transfusions may be indicated for severely neutropenic patients with infections not controlled by antibiotic therapy, who are expected to recover bone marrow production of white cells.
[AABB Tech Manual 2008b, pp596-597]
MLS ONLY

264 b Each unit of RBCs is expected to increase the hemoglobin level by 1-1.5 g/dL (10-15 g/L).
[Harmening 2005, p305]

265 b Each unit of RBCs is expected to increase the hematocrit level by 3%-5%, so it would take 2 units to raise the level 6%.
[Harmening 2005, p305]

266 c CMV-seronegative or leukoreduced blood products should be administered to immunocompromised patients, including bone marrow and hematopoietic cell transplant recipients.
[Harmening 2005, p310]
MLS ONLY

267 b Cryoprecipitate contains ABO antibodies so one should consider giving ABO compatible, especially when infusing large volumes.
[AABB Tech Manual 2008b, p467]
MLS ONLY

268 d Class I HLA antigens on platelets are a known cause for platelet refractoriness. Leukoreduction of blood products is used as a mechanism to reduce or prevent patients from developing antibodies.
[AABB Practical Guide 2007, ch11]

269 a Patients with IgA deficiency who have had anaphylactic transfusion reactions should receive washed RBCs. Anaphylactic reactions are typically caused by anti-IgA in the recipient. Washing removes plasma IgA from the donor unit. cells.
[Harmening 2005, p305]
MLS ONLY

270 d FFP should be ABO compatible with the recipient's RBCs. Avoid FFP with antibodies to A or B antigens the patient may have. Group A plasma has anti-B, and should only be transfused to A or O recipients.
[Harmening 2005, p307]

271 d FFP should be ABO compatible with the recipient's RBCs. Avoid FFP with ABO antibodies to A or B antigens the patient may have.
[Harmening 2005, p307]

272 b Each unit of platelets should increase the count 5,000-10,000/µL (5,000-10,000/L).
[Harmening 2005, p306]

Answers–Blood Bank

273 **c**   Functional abnormalities are frequent
MLS   in hypoproliferative thrombocytopenia.
ONLY   Decreased platelets is not an outcome
of a hemolytic transfusion reaction,
posttransfusion purpura is usually
self-limiting and is due to an antibody
to a specific platelet antigen, immune
thrombocytopenia purpura patients
have low platelet counts but rarely
have hemorrhage.
[AABB Tech Manual 2008b, p579]

274 **d**   Washing red blood cells with saline
MLS   removes donor plasma and IgA, and
ONLY   prevents anaphylactic reactions due to
anti-IgA in the recipient.
[Harmening 2005, p305]

275 **b**   Anaphylactic transfusion reactions are
distinguished from other types of reactions
by 1) the absence of fever, and 2) the
reactions are sudden in onset after infusion
of only a few mL of blood. Since the reaction
is due to anti-IgA, washing the donor red
blood cells to remove all plasma protein
is indicated. Alternatively, blood products
from IgA-deficient donors may be used.
[Harmening 2005, p342]

276 **a**   FFP should be ABO compatible with
the recipient's RBCs. Avoid FFP with ABO
antibodies to A or B antigens the patient
may have. Rh type is not significant.
[Harmening 2005, p307]

277 **c**   FFP should be ABO compatible with the
recipient's RBCs. If patient's type has not
been determined (currently), plasma lacking
anti-A and anti-B should be given.
[Harmening 2005, p307]

278 **c**   FFP contains all factors, including
cryoprecipitate. It does not have a
higher risk of transmitting hepatitis
than Whole Blood. It must be transfused
within 24 hours of thawing and must be
ABO compatible.
[Harmening 2005, p307]

279 **c**   Each unit of platelets should increase
the count 5,000-10,000 platelets/μL (5,000-
10,000/L). Platelet antibodies can diminish
this expected increment.
[Harmening 2005, p306]

280 **c**   Symptoms of hemolytic transfusion
reactions are fever, chills, flushing, chest and
back pain, hypotension, nausea, dyspnea,
shock, renal failure, and DIC. Circulatory
overload, allergic, and anaphylactic reactions
are not characterized by fever.
[Harmening 2005, p339]

281 **d**   Alloimmunization to the HLA results
MLS   in refractoriness to random donor platelet
ONLY   transfusions.
[Harmening 2005, p339]

282 **b**   Alloimmunization to the HLA results
MLS   in refractoriness to random donor platelet
ONLY   transfusions.
[Harmening 2005, p443]

283 **c**   Posttransfusion purpura (PTP) is
MLS   caused by platelet-specific alloantibody in a
ONLY   previously immunized recipient. Transfused
donor platelets in blood products are
destroyed, with concomitant destruction
of the recipient's own platelets, through
unknown mechanisms. The usual antibody
specificity is HPA-1a.
[Harmening 2005, pp345-346]

284 **d**   Previously immunized patients may
have an undetectable level of antibody.
Transfusion of antigen-positive donor
red cells may cause an anamnestic
response and result in a delayed hemolytic
transfusion reaction. Symptoms may be
mild, and present only as jaundice and
unexplained anemia.
[Harmening 2005, pp345-346]

285 **b**   Delayed hemolytic transfusion reactions
are caused by a secondary anamnestic
response in a previously alloimmunized
recipient. Unlike a primary response, a
secondary response is rapid. Antibody
may be detectable 3-7 days from the time
of transfusion.
[Harmening 2005, p340]

286 **a**   Antibodies in the ABO system may
activate complement and cause immediate
intravascular hemolysis if incompatible
blood is transfused. Antibodies in the Rh,
Duffy, and MN systems typically cause
extravascular hemolysis, which is usually
less severe.
[Harmening 2005, p338]

287   **a**   ABO antibodies activate complement and may cause intravascular hemolysis. Rh, Kell, and Duffy antibodies are primarily associated with extravascular hemolysis.
[Harmening 2005, pp109-110, 143, 177]

288   **b**   Antibodies in the Kidd system activate complement and may cause intravascular hemolysis. The antibodies often decline in vivo, are weak, show dosage, and are difficult to detect in vitro, making them prime candidates for causing anamnestic delayed hemolytic transfusion reactions.
[Harmening 2005, p183]

289   **a**   ABO antibodies activate complement and may cause intravascular hemolysis. The antibodies are naturally occurring against A and B antigens that the recipient lacks. Rh and Duffy antibodies may also cause hemolytic transfusion reactions, but the antibodies are the results of alloimmunization and not naturally present in recipients who lack the antigen. The incidence of septic transfusion reactions from bacterial contamination of Red Blood Cells is rare, about 1:500,000.
[Harmening 2005, pp109, 339, 344]

290   **d**   Patients receiving >1 blood volume replacement often develop thrombo-cytopenia and require platelet transfusion.
[Harmening 2005, p314]

291   **d**   A positive DAT in a posttransfusion
MLS
ONLY   blood sample usually indicates that the patient is producing alloantibody against an antigen present on the transfused donor red cells. An elution should be performed to remove the antibody from the red cells and identify it. Free antibody may also be present in the serum. If the antibody screen is positive, the antibody should be identified.
[Harmening 2005, p350]

292   **a**   Free hemoglobin released from destruction of transfused donor red cells will impart a distinct pink or red color in the posttransfusion sample plasma.
[Harmening 2005, p349]

293   **d**   The immediate steps required to investigate a transfusion reaction include a clerical check of records and labels, visual inspection of postreaction plasma for hemolysis, and direct antiglobulin test and repeat ABO typing on the postreaction sample. Additional investigation is performed when there is evidence of hemolysis, bacterial contamination, TRALI, or other serious adverse event.
[AABB Standards 2008a, §7.4.2]

294   **a**   In septic transfusion reactions, patients experience fever >101°F (38.3° C), shaking chills, and hypotension. In severe reactions, patients develop shock, renal failure, hemoglobinuria, and DIC.
[AABB Tech Manual 2008b, p729]

295   **c**   Clinical signs of a hemolytic transfusion reaction include fever and chills, and, in severe cases, DIC. Circulatory overload, allergic and anaphylactic reactions are not characterized by fever and DIC.
[Harmening 2005, pp338-343]

296   **a**   Bilirubin is a marker for red cell hemolysis. Bilirubin peaks at 5-7 hours after transfusion and is back to pretransfusion levels at 24 hours if liver function is normal.
[AABB Tech Manual 2008b, p723]

297   **d**   Delayed hemolytic transfusion reactions may occur in recipients who are previously immunized but who do not have detectable antibody, if they receive blood with the corresponding antigen. When there is a history of clinically significant antibodies, donor red cells should be phenotyped and antigen-negative blood selected. A complete antiglobulin crossmatch must be performed.
[Marques 2007, pp51-52, 77]

298   **b**   If the direct antiglobulin test is positive in a transfusion reaction investigation, the antibody should be eluted from the red cells and identified.
[Marques 2007, pp72-74]

299 **c** Lack of expected rise in hemoglobin after transfusion may be a sign of a delayed hemolytic transfusion reaction. If the DAT is positive, an elution should be performed to remove and identify the antibody coating the transfused donor red cells. In this case, the antibody is not detectable in the antibody screen, so a routine cell panel on the serum would not be helpful. Since the transfusion occurred 3 weeks previously, donor samples are not available for testing.
[Harmening 2005, pp340, 349-350]

300 **b** Delayed hemolytic transfusion reactions are associated with extravascular hemolysis, rather than intravascular. Alloantibody coats the transfused antigen-positive donor cells in the recipient's circulation, producing a mixed-field positive reaction in the DAT.
[Harmening 2005, pp340, 349-350]

301 **a** In massive transfusions, Platelets are
MLS
ONLY indicated if the platelet count is less than 50,000/µL (50,000/L).
[Harmening 2005, p314]

302 **d** Treatment of acute hemolytic transfusion reactions focuses on supportive measures and control of DIC, hypotension, and acute renal failure.
[Harmening 2005, p339]

303 **c** Red Blood Cells, Leukocyte-Reduced should be chosen, because febrile nonhemolytic transfusion reactions are either due to chemokines released from leukocytes in nonleukoreduced blood components or to patient antibodies directed towards donor HLA antigens on the leukocytes.
[Harmening 2005, p341]

304 **c** Leukocyte-Reduced RBCs and Platelets can be used to prevent further nonhemolytic transfusion reactions.
[Harmening 2005, p310]

305 **a** Leukocyte antibodies are a primary cause of febrile transfusion reactions. Leukocyte-reduced blood components reduce the risk of febrile nonhemolytic reactions.
[Harmening 2005, p341]

306 **c** Anaphylactic transfusion reactions are attributed to anti-IgA in IgA-deficient recipients.
[Harmening 2005, p342]

307 **c** Two distinguishing features of anaphylactic transfusion reactions are that symptoms occur with transfusion of only small amounts of blood, and the patient has no fever.
[Harmening 2005, p342]

308 **d** Febrile nonhemolytic transfusion reactions are defined as fever of 1°C or greater (over baseline temperature) during or after transfusion, with no other reason for the elevation than transfusion, and no evidence of hemolysis in the transfusion reaction investigation. Allergic reactions, citrate toxicity, and circulatory overload are not characterized by fever.
[Harmening 2005, p341]

309 **b** Allergic reactions are a type 1 immediate hypersensitivity reaction to an allergen in plasma. Most are mild reactions shown by urticaria (hives, swollen red wheals) which may cause itching.
[Harmening 2005, pp341-342]

310 **a** Febrile nonhemolytic transfusion reactions are defined as fever of 1°C or greater (over baseline temperature) during or after transfusion, with no other reason for the elevation than transfusion, and no evidence of hemolysis in the transfusion reaction investigation.
[Harmening 2005, p341]

311 **d** Febrile nonhemolytic transfusion reactions occur in about 1% of transfusions, making it one of the most common types of reaction. Neither transfusion-associated circulatory overload (TACO) or anaphylactic transfusion reactions are characterized by fever. Bacterially contaminated Red Blood Cells are rare, and rapidly produce severe symptoms upon transfusion.
[Harmening 2005, pp341-344]

312 **d** Febrile nonhemolytic transfusion reactions are caused by leukoagglutinins in the patient or cytokines released from donor leukocytes during storage. Since these reactions are not caused by red cell antibodies, transfusion investigation studies show no hemolysis or abnormal test results.
[Marques 2007, pp72-74]

313 **b**   TRALI is most commonly caused
_{MLS ONLY} by donor HLA or granulocyte-specific
antibodies that react with recipient antigens,
causing damage to the lung basement
membrane and bilateral pulmonary edema
within 6 hours of transfusion. Multiparous
females are more likely to have antibodies
than males. Using male donors as the sole
source of plasma products is a strategy for
reducing the risk of TRALI.
[AABB Tech Manual 2008b, pp733-735]

314 **d**   Prestorage leukoreduction reduces the
_{MLS ONLY} number of white cells in Apheresis Platelets
and RBCs, and significantly decreases the
risk of febrile reactions.
[AABB Tech Manual 2008b, p730]

315 **d**   Noncardiogenic pulmonary edema,
dyspnea, hypotension, and hypoxemia
occurring within 6 hours of transfusion are
clinical symptoms of TRALI.
[Marques 2007, p76]

316 **a**   Anaphylactic transfusion reactions are
severe reactions that occur after infusion of
a small amount of donor blood. Symptoms
are hypotension, shock, respiratory distress,
dyspnea, and substernal pain. Anaphylactic
reactions are usually caused by anti-IgA.
[Marques 2007, p75]

317 **c**   Leukoreduction of blood products
reduces the risk of febrile nonhemolytic
transfusion reactions, which are caused
by leukoagglutinins or cytokines from
white cells.
[Marques 2007, p20]

318 **d**   One reason to quarantine blood
components before transfusion is hemolysis
of the red cells. Hemolysis of red cells
is an indication of contamination or
improper storage.
[Harmening 2005, p289]

319 **c**   Transfusion-associated circulatory
overload (TACO) is hypervolemia
manifested by coughing, cyanosis, and
pulmonary edema.
[Harmening 2005, p343]

320 **c**   Transfusion-associated circulatory
overload (TACO) is hypervolemia caused
by blood transfusion in susceptible
patients. Hemolytic (antibody to red cell
antigen), febrile NHTR (leukoagglutinins or
cytokines), and allergic (reaction to allergens
in plasma) are immunologic reactions.
[AABB Tech Manual 2008b, pp725-731]

321 **d**   Transfusion-induced hypervolemia
causing edema and congestive heart failure
is a feature of transfusion-associated
circulatory overload (TACO). Hypervolemia
is not a complication of a hemolytic, febrile,
or anaphylactic transfusion reaction.
[Harmening 2005, pp338-343]

322 **b**   Hypervolemia due to transfusion
in susceptible patients, such as cardiac,
elderly, infants, or severely anemic, causes
circulatory overload (TACO) and associated
respiratory and cardiac problems.
[Harmening 2005, p343]

323 **a**   Septic transfusion reactions due to
contaminated blood products are manifested
by high fever, chills, hypotension, shock,
nausea, diarrhea, renal failure, and
DIC. Symptoms usually appear rapidly.
Transfusion reaction investigation shows
no evidence of unexpected blood group
antibodies. A Gram stain and blood culture
of the donor unit may detect the presence of
aerobic or anaerobic organisms.
[Harmening 2005, p344]

324 **c**   Hepatitis transmission is unlikely, but
has a higher risk of transmission through
blood transfusion than CMV (rare), syphilis
(no transfusion-transmitted cases reported
in >30 years), or HIV (1:2,300,000 units).
[AABB Tech Manual 2008b, pp242-251]

325 **b**   Irradiation inhibits proliferation of
T cells and subsequent GVHD.
[Harmening 2005, p227]

326 **d**   Blood from a family member may be
_{MLS ONLY} homozygous for a shared HLA haplotype,
allowing donor lymphocytes to engraft
in the recipient and cause transfusion-
associated GVHD.
[Harmening 2005, p347]

327 **c**   Gamma irradiation of blood products
prevents donor lymphocytes from
replicating after transfusion and causing
transfusion associated graft-vs-host disease
in susceptible patients.
[Harmening 2005, p347]

328 **d**   The most common use of therapeutic
_{MLS ONLY} plasmapheresis is to remove plasma
abnormalities, such as pathological
antibodies, immune complexes,
or cryoglobulins.
[AABB Practical Guide 2007, ch14]

Answers–Blood Bank

329 **b**   Macroglobulinemia, also known as

MLS ONLY Waldenström, is a syndrome with IgM
monoclonal paraprotein. Since IgM protein
is intravascular, plasma exchange provides
symptomatic relief.
[AABB Practical Guide 2007, ch14]

330 **d**   The major cause of transfusion-
associated fatalities is transfusion of blood
to the wrong patient.
[Harmening 2005, p264]

Chemistry

*The following items have been identified generally as appropriate for both entry level medical laboratory scientists and medical laboratory technicians. Items that are appropriate for medical laboratory scientists **only** are marked with an "MLS ONLY."*

Carbohydrates

1 Following overnight fasting, <u>hypoglycemia</u> in adults is defined as a glucose of:

   a ≤70 mg/dL (≤3.9 mmol/L)
   b ≤60 mg/dL (≤3.3 mmol/L)
   c ≤55 mg/dL (≤3.0 mmol/L)
   d ≤45 mg/dL (≤2.5 mmol/L)

   hypoglycemia = ≤ 45 mg/dL

2 The following results are from a 21-year-old patient with a back injury who appears otherwise healthy:

   whole blood glucose: 77 mg/dL (4.2 mmol/L)
   serum glucose: 88 mg/dL (4.8 mmol/L)
   CSF glucose: 56 mg/dL (3.1 mmol/L)

   The best interpretation of these results is that:

   a the whole blood and serum values are expected but the CSF value is elevated
   b the whole blood glucose value should be higher than the serum value
   c all values are consistent with a normal healthy individual
   d the serum and whole blood values should be identical

3 The preparation of a patient for standard glucose tolerance testing should include:

   a a high carbohydrate diet for 3 days
   b a low carbohydrate diet for 3 days
   c fasting for 48 hours prior to testing
   d bed rest for 3 days

4   If a fasting glucose was 90 mg/dL, which of the following 2-hour postprandial glucose results would most closely represent normal glucose metabolism?

  a   55 mg/dL (3.0 mmol/L)
  b   100 mg/dL (5.5 mmol/L)
  c   180 mg/dL (9.9 mmol/L)
  d   260 mg/dL (14.3 mmol/L)

  normal fasting: 70-110
  normal PPG: ≤ 140
  diabetes ≤ 200

5   A healthy person with a blood glucose of 80 mg/dL (4.4 mmol/L) would have a simultaneously determined cerebrospinal fluid glucose value of:

  a   25 mg/dL (1.4 mmol/L)
  b   50 mg/dL (2.3 mmol/L)
  c   100 mg/dL (5.5 mmol/L)
  d   150 mg/dL (8.3 mmol/L)

6   A 25-year-old man became nauseated and vomited 90 minutes after receiving a standard 75 g carbohydrate dose for an oral glucose tolerance test. The best course of action is to:

  a   give the patient a glass of orange juice and continue the test
  b   start the test over immediately with a 50 g carbohydrate dose
  c   draw blood for glucose and discontinue test
  d   place the patient in a recumbent position, reassure him and continue the test

7   Cerebrospinal fluid for glucose assay should be:

  a   refrigerated
  b   analyzed immediately
  c   heated to 56°C
  d   stored at room temperature after centrifugation

8   Which of the following 2 hour postprandial glucose values demonstrates unequivocal hyperglycemia diagnostic for diabetes mellitus?

  a   160 mg/dL (8.8 mmol/L)
  b   170 mg/dL (9.4 mmol/L)
  c   180 mg/dL (9.9 mmol/L)
  d   200 mg/dL (11.0 mmol/L)

9   Serum levels that define hypoglycemia in pre-term or low birth weight infants are:

  a   the same as adults
  b   lower than adults
  c   the same as a normal full-term infant
  d   higher than a normal full-term infant

10   A 45-year-old woman has a fasting serum glucose concentration of 95 mg/dL (5.2 mmol/L) and a 2-hour postprandial glucose concentration of 105 mg/dL (5.8 mmol/L). The statement which best describes this patient's fasting serum glucose concentration is:

  a   normal; reflecting glycogen breakdown by the liver
  b   normal; reflecting glycogen breakdown by skeletal muscle
  c   abnormal; indicating diabetes mellitus
  d   abnormal; indicating hypoglycemia

11   Pregnant women with symptoms of thirst, frequent urination or unexplained weight loss should have which of the following tests performed?

  a   tolbutamide test
  b   lactose tolerance test
  c   epinephrine tolerance test
  d   glucose tolerance test

12 In the fasting state, the arterial and capillary blood glucose concentration varies from the venous glucose concentration by approximately how many mg/dL (mmol/L)?

    a 1 mg/dL (0.05 mmol/L) higher
    b 5 mg/dL (0.27 mmol/L) higher
    c 10 mg/dL (0.55 mmol/L) lower
    d 15 mg/dL (0.82 mmol/L) lower

13 The conversion of glucose or other hexoses into lactate or pyruvate is called:

    a glycogenesis → *glucose conversion to glycogen for storage*
    b glycogenolysis → *glycogen conversion to glucose*
    c gluconeogenesis → *amino acid conversion to glucose*
    d glycolysis → *hydrolysis by enzyme of glucose into lactate or pyruvate*

14 Which one of the following values obtained during a glucose tolerance test are diagnostic of diabetes mellitus?

    a 2-hour specimen   = 150 mg/dL (8.3 mmol/L)
    b fasting plasma glucose = 126 mg/dL (6.9 mmol/L)
    c fasting plasma glucose = 110 mg/dL (6.1 mmol/L)
    d 2-hour specimen   = 180 mg/dL (9.9 mmol/L)

15 The glycated hemoglobin value represents the integrated values of glucose concentration during the preceding:

    a 1-3 weeks
    b 4-5 weeks
    c 6-8 weeks
    d 16-20 weeks

16 Monitoring long-term glucose control in patients with adult onset diabetes mellitus can best be accomplished by measuring:

    a weekly fasting 7 AM serum glucose
    b glucose tolerance testing
    c 2-hour postprandial serum glucose
    d hemoglobin A_{1c}

17 A patient with Type I, insulin-dependent diabetes mellitus has the following results:

Test	Patient	Reference Range
fasting blood glucose:	150 mg/dL (8.3 mmol/L)	70-110 mg/dL (3.9-6.1 mmol/L)
hemoglobin A_{1c}:	8.5%	4.0%-6.0%
fructosamine:	2.5 mmol/L	2.0-2.9 mmol/L

After reviewing these test results, the technologist concluded that the patient is in a:

    a "steady state" of metabolic control
    b state of flux, progressively worsening metabolic control
    c improving state of metabolic control as indicated by fructosamine
    d state of flux as indicted by the fasting glucose level

18 Total glycosylated hemoglobin levels in a hemolysate reflect the:

    a average blood glucose levels of the past 2-3 months
    b average blood glucose levels for the past week
    c blood glucose level at the time the sample is drawn
    d hemoglobin A_{1c} level at the time the sample is drawn

19 Which of the following hemoglobins has glucose-6-phosphate on the amino-terminal valine of the beta chain?

    a S
    b C
    c A_2
    d A_{1c}

20   A patient with hemolytic anemia will:

    (a) show a decrease in glycated Hgb value → *shows life of RBC*
    b show an increase in glycated Hgb value
    c show little or no change in glycated Hgb value
    d demonstrate an elevated Hgb A_1

21   In using ion-exchange chromatographic methods, falsely increased levels of Hgb A_{1c} might be demonstrated in the presence of:

    a iron deficiency anemia
    b pernicious anemia   ✷
    c thalassemias
    (d) Hgb S = ↑ *Hgb A1C*

22   An increase in serum <u>acetone</u> is indicative of a defect in the metabolism of:
                                 (ketone)

    (a) carbohydrates
    b fat
    c urea nitrogen
    d uric acid

23   An infant with diarrhea is being evaluated for a carbohydrate intolerance. His stool yields a positive copper reduction test and a pH of 5.0. It should be concluded that:

    (a) further tests are indicated
    b results are inconsistent—repeat both tests
    c the diarrhea is not due to carbohydrate intolerance
    d the tests provided no useful information

24   Blood samples were collected at the beginning of an exercise class and after thirty minutes of aerobic activity. Which of the following would be most consistent with the post-exercise sample?

    a normal lactic acid, low pyruvate
    b low lactic acid, elevated pyruvate
    c elevated lactic acid, low pyruvate
    (d) elevated lactic acid, elevated pyruvate – *products of glycolysis* ✷

25   What is the best method to diagnose lactase deficiency?

    (a) H_2 breath test – *Lactase deficiency*
    b plasma aldolase level   *(Lactose intolerance)*
    c LDH level
    d D-xylose test

Acid-Base Balance

26   The expected blood gas results for a patient in chronic renal failure would match the pattern of:

    (a) metabolic acidosis
    b respiratory acidosis
    c metabolic alkalosis
    d respiratory alkalosis

27   Severe diarrhea causes:

    (a) metabolic acidosis – *severe bicarbonate depletion*
    b metabolic alkalosis
    c respiratory acidosis
    d respiratory alkalosis

28   The following blood gas results were obtained:

pH:	7.18 ↓↓	7.35 - 7.45
PO$_2$:	86 mm Hg	80 - 110
PCO$_2$:	60 mm Hg ⋔	35 - 45
O$_2$ saturation:	92%	
HCO$_3$:	7921 mEq/L (21 mmol/L)↓	22-26
TCO$_2$:	23 mEq/L (23 mmol/L)	22 - 29
base excess:	−8.0 mEq/L (−8.0 mmol/L)	

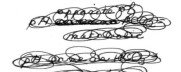

The patient's results are compatible with which of the following?

   a fever

   b uremia

   ⓒ emphysema

   d dehydration

pH opposite of PCO2 = respiratory
pH same as HCO3 = metabolic

29   Factors that contribute to a PCO$_2$ electrode requiring 60-120 seconds to reach equilibrium include the:

   ⓐ diffusion characteristics of the membrane   ✳

   b actual blood PO$_2$

   c type of calibrating standard (ie, liquid or humidified gas)

   d potential of the polarizing mercury cell

30   An emphysema patient suffering from fluid accumulation in the alveolar spaces is likely to be in what metabolic state?

   ⓐ respiratory acidosis

   b respiratory alkalosis

   c metabolic acidosis

   d metabolic alkalosis

31   At blood pH 7.40, what is the ratio of bicarbonate to carbonic acid?

   a 15:1

   ⓑ 20:1

   c 25:1

   d 30:1

20:1 ratio bicarb to carbonic acid

32   The reference range for the pH of arterial blood measured at 37°C is:

   a 7.28-7.34

   b 7.33-7.37

   ⓒ 7.35-7.45

   d 7.45-7.50

33   A 68-year-old man arrives in the emergency room with a glucose level of 722 mg/dL (39.7 mmol/L) and serum acetone of 4+ undiluted. An arterial blood gas from this patient is likely to be:

   ⓐ low pH

   b high pH

   c low PO$_2$

   d high PO$_2$

34   A patient is admitted to the emergency room in a state of metabolic <u>alkalosis.</u> Which of the following would be consistent with this diagnosis?

   ⓐ high TCO$_2$, increased HCO$_3$

   b low TCO$_2$, increased HCO$_3$ ✳

   c high TCO$_2$, decreased H$_2$CO$_3$

   d low TCO$_2$, decreased H$_2$CO$_3$

35   A person suspected of having metabolic alkalosis would have which of the following laboratory findings?

   a CO_2 content and PCO_2 elevated, pH decreased
   b CO_2 content decreased and pH elevated
   c CO_2 content, PCO_2 and pH decreased   ✳
   d CO_2 content and pH elevated

36   Metabolic acidosis is described as a(n):

   a   increase in CO_2 content and PCO_2 with a decreased pH
   b   decrease in CO_2 content with an increased pH   ✳
   c   increase in CO_2 with an increased pH
   d   decrease in CO_2 content and PCO_2 with a decreased pH

37   Respiratory acidosis is described as a(n):

   a   increase in CO_2 content and PCO_2 with a decreased pH
   b   decrease in CO_2 content with an increased pH
   c   increase in CO_2 content with an increased pH   ✳
   d   decrease in CO_2 content and PCO_2 with a decreased pH

38   A common cause of respiratory alkalosis is:

   a   vomiting
   b   starvation
   c   asthma   ✳
   d   hyperventilation

39   Acidosis and alkalosis are best defined as fluctuations in blood pH and CO_2 content due to changes in:

   a   Bohr effect
   b O_2 content
   c   bicarbonate buffer
   d   carbonic anhydrase

40   A blood gas sample was sent to the lab on ice, and a bubble was present in the syringe. The blood had been exposed to room air for at least 30 minutes. The following change in blood gases will occur:

   a CO_2 content increased/PCO_2 decreased
   b CO_2 content and PO_2 increased/pH increased
   c CO_2 content and PCO_2 decreased/pH decreased   ✳
   d PO_2 increased/HCO_3 decreased

41   The following laboratory results were obtained:

   Serum electrolytes
   sodium: 136 mEq/L (136 mmol/L)   135 -145
   potassium: 4.4 mEq/L (4.4 mmol/L)   3.4- 5.0
   chloride: 92 mEq/L (92 mmol/L)   98 -106
   bicarbonate: 40 mEq/L (40 mmol/L)   22-26
   Arterial blood
   pH: 7.32 ↓   7.35 - 7.45
   PCO_2:   79 mm Hg   35 - 45

   These results are most compatible with:

   a   respiratory alkalosis
   b   respiratory acidosis
   c   metabolic alkalosis
   d   metabolic acidosis

42   Select the test which evaluates renal tubular function.

 a IVP
 b creatinine clearance
 c osmolarity
 d microscopic urinalysis

43   A patient had the following serum results:

 Na⁺:   140 mEq/L (140 mmol/L)
 K⁺:   4.0 mEq/L (4.0 mmol/L)
 glucose: 95 mg/dL (5.2 mmol/L)
 BUN: 10 mg/dL (3.57 mmol/L)

 Which osmolality is consistent with these results?

 a 188
 b 204
 c 270
 d 390

osmolality calculation:

$$2.0\, Na + \frac{glucose}{20} + \frac{BUN}{3}$$

44   The degree to which the kidney concentrates the glomerular filtrate can be determined by:

 a urine creatine
 b serum creatinine
 c creatinine clearance
 d urine to serum osmolality ratio

45   Osmolal gap is the difference between:

 a the ideal and real osmolality values
 b calculated and measured osmolality values = *osmolal gap* ✱
 c plasma and water osmolality values
 d molality and molarity at 4°C

Electrolytes

46   The most important <u>buffer</u> pair in plasma is the:

 a phosphate/biphosphate pair
 b hemoglobin/imidazole pair
 c bicarbonate/carbonic acid pair
 d sulfate/bisulfate pair

47   Quantitation of Na⁺ and K⁺ by ion-selective electrode is the standard method because:

 a dilution is required for flame photometry
 b there is no lipoprotein interference
 c of advances in electrochemistry
 d of the absence of an internal standard

48   What battery of tests is most useful in evaluating an anion gap of 22 mEq/L (22 mmol/L)?

 a Ca^{++}, Mg^{++}, PO^{-4} and pH
 b BUN, creatinine, salicylate and methanol = *causes of ↑ anion gap* ✱
 c AST, ALT, LD and amylase
 d glucose, CK, myoglobin and cryoglobulin

49   A patient with myeloproliferative disorder has the following values:

Hgb: 13 g/dL (130 mmol/L) *(14-18)*
Hct: 38%   *(40-54)*
WBC: ↑↑ ↑   30 × 10³/µL (30 × 10⁹/L) *(4.5-11.5)*
platelets: ↑↑↑   1000 × 10³/µL (1000 × 10⁹/L)
serum Na⁺:   140 mEq/L (140 mmol/L) *135-145*
serum K⁺:   7 mEq/L (7 mmol/L) *3.5-5.0 (critical)*   ✳

The serum K⁺ should be confirmed by:

a   repeat testing of the original serum
b   testing freshly drawn serum
ⓒ   testing heparinized plasma   *✳ effect of plts on K⁺ in serum*
d   atomic absorption spectrometry

50   Most of the carbon dioxide present in blood is in the form of:

a   dissolved CO_2
b   carbonate
ⓒ   bicarbonate ion
d   carbonic acid

51   Serum "anion gap" is increased in patients with:

a   renal tubular acidosis
b   diabetic alkalosis
c   metabolic acidosis due to diarrhea   ✳
ⓓ   lactic acidosis

52   The anion gap is useful for quality control of laboratory results for:

a   amino acids and proteins
b   blood gas analyses
ⓒ   sodium, potassium, chloride, and total CO_2
d   calcium, phosphorus and magnesium

53   The buffering capacity of blood is maintained by a reversible exchange process between bicarbonate and:

a   sodium
b   potassium
c   calcium   ✳
ⓓ   chloride

54   In respiratory acidosis, a compensatory mechanism is the increase in:

a   respiration rate
b   ammonia formation
c   blood PCO_2
ⓓ   plasma bicarbonate concentration

55   Which of the following electrolytes is the chief plasma cation⁺ whose main function is maintaining osmotic pressure?

a   chloride
b   calcium
c   potassium
ⓓ   sodium

56   A potassium level of 6.8 mEq/L (6.8 mmol/L) is obtained. Before reporting the results, the first step the technologist should take is to:

ⓐ   check the serum for hemolysis
b   rerun the test
c   check the age of the patient
d   do nothing, simply report out the result

57 The solute that contributes the most to the total serum osmolality is:

    a glucose
    (b) sodium
    c chloride
    d urea

58 A sweat chloride result of 55 mEq/L (55 mmol/L) and a sweat sodium of 52 mEq/L (52 mmol/L) were obtained on a patient who has a history of respiratory problems. The best interpretation of these results is:

    a normal
    b normal sodium and an abnormal chloride test should be repeated
    c abnormal results
    (d) borderline results, the test should be repeated

< 60 mEq/L diagnostic
borderline range: 45-60 mEq/L
✱

59 Which of the following is true about direct ion selective electrodes for electrolytes?

    (a) whole blood specimens are acceptable
    b elevated lipids cause falsely decreased results
    c elevated proteins cause falsely decreased results
    d elevated platelets cause falsely increased results

✱

60 Sodium determination by indirect ion selective electrode is falsely decreased by:

    a elevated chloride levels
    (b) elevated lipid levels
    c decreased protein levels
    d decreased albumin levels

indirect interferences: ↑ lipid falsely ↓ Na with ↑ protein

61 A physician requested that electrolytes on a multiple myeloma patient specimen be run by direct ISE and not indirect ISE because:

    a excess protein binds Na in indirect ISE
    b Na is falsely increased by indirect ISE
    (c) Na is falsely decreased by indirect ISE
    d excess protein reacts with diluent in indirect ISE

✱

62 Which percentage of total serum calcium is nondiffusible protein bound?

    a 80%-90%
    b 51%-60%
    (c) 40%-50% *protein bound Calcium*
    d 10%-30%

63 Calcium concentration in the serum is regulated by:

    a insulin
    (b) parathyroid hormone
    c thyroxine
    d vitamin C

64 The regulation of calcium and phosphorous metabolism is accomplished by which of the following glands?

    a thyroid
    (b) parathyroid *– regulates Ca and phosphorous* *✱*
    c adrenal glands
    d pituitary

65 A patient has the following test results:

   increased serum calcium levels ↑
   decreased serum phosphate levels ↓
   increased levels of parathyroid hormone

   This patient most likely has:

   a hyperparathyroidism
   b hypoparathyroidism
   c nephrosis
   d steatorrhea

66 A hospitalized patient is experiencing increased neuromuscular irritability (tetany). Which of the following tests should be ordered immediately?

   a calcium = *tetany*
   b phosphate
   c BUN
   d glucose

67 Which of the following is most likely to be ordered in addition to serum calcium to determine the cause of tetany?

   a magnesium
   b phosphate
   c sodium
   d vitamin D

68 A reciprocal relationship exists between:

   a sodium and potassium   ↑ Na; ↓ Phosphate (PO_4)
   b calcium and phosphate
   c chloride and CO_2
   d calcium and magnesium

69 Fasting serum phosphate concentration is controlled primarily by the:

   a pancreas
   b skeleton
   c parathyroid glands
   d small intestine

70 A low concentration of serum phosphorus is commonly found in:

   a patients who are receiving carbohydrate hyperalimentation ✳
   b chronic renal disease
   c hypoparathyroidism
   d patients with pituitary tumors

71 The following laboratory results were obtained:

	Calcium	Alkaline Phosphate	Alkaline Phosphatase
serum:	increased	decreased	normal or increased
urine:	increased	increased	

   These results are most compatible with:

   a multiple myeloma
   b milk-alkali syndrome
   c sarcoidosis
   d primary hyperparathyroidism

Proteins and Other Nitrogen-Containing Compounds

72 The primary function of serum albumin in the peripheral blood is to:

a maintain colloidal osmotic pressure = *purpose of serum albumin*
b increase antibody production
c increase fibrinogen formation
d maintain blood viscosity

73 In a pleural effusion caused by *Streptococcus pneumoniae*, the protein value of the pleural fluid as
MLS ONLY compared to the serum value would probably be:

a decreased by 2
b decreased by ½
c increased by ½
d equal

74 The first step in analyzing a 24-hour urine specimen for quantitative urine protein is:

a subculture the urine for bacteria
b add the appropriate preservative
c screen for albumin using a dipstick
d measure the total volume

75 When performing a manual protein analysis on a xanthochromic spinal fluid, the
MLS ONLY technician should:

a perform the test as usual
b make a patient blank
c centrifuge the specimen
d dilute the specimen with deionized water

76 The direction in which albumin migrates (ie, toward anode or cathode) during electrophoretic
MLS ONLY separation of serum proteins, at pH 8.6, is determined by:

a the ionization of the amine groups, yielding a net positive charge
b the ionization of the carboxyl groups, yielding a net negative charge
c albumin acting as a zwitterion
d the density of the gel layer

77 The protein that has the highest dye-binding capacity is:
MLS ONLY
a albumin
b alpha globulin
c beta globulin
d gamma globulin

78 Refer to the following illustration:

The serum protein electrophoresis pattern shown below was obtained on cellulose acetate at pH 8.6.

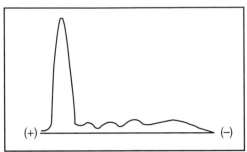

Identify the serum protein fraction on the left of the illustration.

  a gamma globulin
  b albumin
  c alpha-1 globulin
  d alpha-2 globulin

79 The biuret reaction for the analysis of serum protein depends on the number of:

  a free amino groups
  b free carboxyl groups
  c peptide bonds
  d tyrosine residues

80 In electrophoresis of proteins, when the sample is placed in an electric field connected to a buffer of pH 8.6, all of the proteins:

  a have a positive charge
  b have a negative charge
  c are electrically neutral
  d migrate toward the cathode

81 The relative migration rate of proteins on cellulose acetate is based on:

  a molecular weight
  b concentration
  c ionic charge
  d particle size

82 The cellulose acetate electrophoresis at pH 8.6 of serum proteins will show an order of migration beginning with the fastest migration as follows:

  a albumin, alpha-1 globulin, alpha-2 globulin, beta globulin, gamma globulin
  b alpha-1 globulin, alpha-2 globulin, beta globulin, gamma globulin, albumin
  c albumin, alpha-2 globulin, alpha-1 globulin, beta globulin, gamma globulin
  d gamma globulin, beta globulin, alpha-2 globulin, alpha-1 globulin, albumin

83 Which of the following amino acids is associated with sulfhydryl group?

  a cysteine
  b glycine
  c serine
  d tyrosine

84 Maple syrup urine disease is characterized by an increase in which of the following urinary
MLS
ONLY   amino acids?

    a phenylalanine
    b tyrosine
    c valine, leucine and isoleucine = *Maple Syrup disease*
    d cystine and cysteine

85 Increased serum albumin concentrations are seen in which of the following conditions?
MLS
ONLY
    a nephrotic syndrome
    b acute hepatitis
    c chronic inflammation
    d dehydration

86 The following data was obtained from a cellulose acetate protein electrophoresis scan:

    albumin area: 75 units
    gamma globulin area: 30 units
    total area: 180 units
    total protein: 6.5 g/dL (65 g/L)

$$\frac{180}{30} = \frac{6.5}{X}$$ ✳

The gamma globulin content in g/dL is:

    a 1.1 g/dL (11 g/L)
    b 2.7 g/dL (27 g/L)
    c 3.8 g/dL (38 g/L)
    d 4.9 g/dL (49 g/L)

87 A patient is admitted with biliary cirrhosis. If a serum protein electrophoresis is performed, which
MLS
ONLY   of the following globulin fractions will be most elevated?

    a alpha-1
    b alpha-2
    c beta
    d gamma

88 Which of the following serum protein fractions is most likely to be elevated in patients with
MLS
ONLY   nephrotic syndrome?

    a alpha-1 globulin
    b albumin
    c alpha-2 globulin
    d beta globulin and gamma globulin

89 Refer to the following illustration:

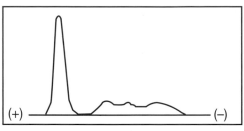

	Patient values	Reference values
total protein	7.3 g/dL (73 g/L)	6.0-8.0 g/dL (60-80 g/L)
albumin	4.2 g/dL (42 g/L)	3.6-5.2 g/dL (36-52 g/L)
alpha-1	0.0 g/dL (0 g/L	0.1-0.4 g/d (1-4 g/L)
alpha-2	0.9 g/dL (9 g/L)	0.4-1.0 g/dL (4-10 g/L)
beta	0.8 g/dL (8 g/L)	0.5-1.2 g/dL (5-12 g/L)
gamma	1.4 g/dL (14 g/L)	0.6-1.6 g/dL (6-16 g/L)

This electrophoresis pattern is consistent with:

a cirrhosis
b monoclonal gammopathy
c polyclonal gammopathy (eg, chronic inflammation)
d alpha-1 antitrypsin deficiency; severe emphysema

90 Refer to the following illustration:

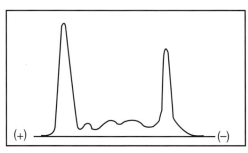

	Patient values	Reference values
total protein	8.9 g/dL (89 g/L)	6.0-8.0 g/dL (60-80 g/L)
albumin	4.8 g/dL (48 g/L)	3.6-5.2 g/dL (36-52 g/L)
alpha-1	0.3 g/dL (3 g/L)	0.1-0.4 g/d (1-4 g/L)
alpha-2	0.7 g/dL (7 g/L)	0.4-1.0 g/dL (4-10 g/L)
beta	0.8 g/dL (8 g/L)	0.5-1.2 g/dL (5-12 g/L)
gamma	2.3 g/dL (23 g/L)	0.6-1.6 g/dL (6-16 g/L)

The serum protein electrophoresis pattern is consistent with:

a cirrhosis
b acute inflammation
c monoclonal gammopathy
d polyclonal gammopathy (eg, chronic inflammation)

91 Refer to the following pattern:

MLS
ONLY

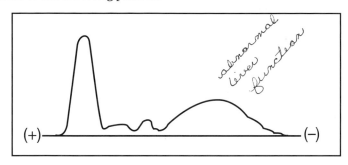

	Patient values	Reference values
total protein	6.1 g/dL (61 g/L)	6.0-8.0 g/dL (60-80 g/L)
albumin↓	2.3 g/dL (23 g/L)	3.6-5.2 g/dL (36-52 g/L)
alpha-1	0.2 g/dL (2 g/L)	0.1-0.4 g/d (1-4 g/L)
alpha-2	0.5 g/dL (5 g/L)	0.4-1.0 g/dL (4-10 g/L)
beta	1.2 g/dL (12 g/L)	0.5-1.2 g/dL (5-12 g/L)
gamma↑	1.9 g/dL (19 g/L)	0.6-1.6 g/dL (6-16 g/L)

This pattern is consistent with:

a cirrhosis
b acute inflammation
c polyclonal gammopathy (eg, chronic inflammation)
d alpha-1 antitrypsin deficiency; severe emphysema

92 A characteristic of the Bence Jones protein that is used to distinguish it from other urinary
MLS
ONLY
proteins is its solubility:

a in ammonium sulfate
b in sulfuric acid
c at 40°- 60°C
d at 100°C

93 The electrophoretic pattern of plasma sample as compared to a serum sample shows a:
MLS
ONLY
a broad prealbumin peak
b sharp fibrinogen peak
c diffuse pattern because of the presence of anticoagulants
d decreased globulin fraction

94 At a pH of 8.6 the gamma globulins move toward the cathode, despite the fact that they are
MLS
ONLY
negatively charged. What is this phenomenon called?

a reverse migration
b molecular sieve
c endosmosis
d migratory inhibition factor

95
Refer to the following illustration:

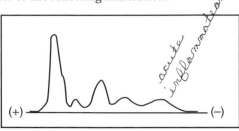

	Patient values	Reference values
total protein	7.8 g/dL (78 g/L)	6.0-8.0 g/dL (60-80 g/L)
albumin ↓	3.0 g/dL (30 g/L)	3.6-5.2 g/dL (36-52 g/L)
alpha-1	0.4 g/dL (4 g/L)	0.1-0.4 g/d (1-4 g/L)
alpha-2 ↑	1.8 g/dL (18 g/L)	0.4-1.0 g/dL (4-10 g/L)
beta	0.5 g/dL (5 g/L)	0.5-1.2 g/dL (5-12 g/L)
gamma	1.1 g/dL (11 g/L)	0.6-1.6 g/dL (6-16 g/L)

The serum protein electrophoresis pattern is consistent with:

a cirrhosis
b acute inflammation
c polyclonal gammopathy (eg, chronic inflammation)
d alpha-1-antitrypsin deficiency; severe emphysema

96
Refer to the following illustration:

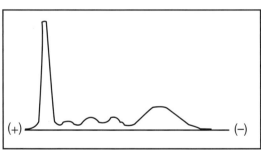

	Patient values	Reference values
total protein ↑	8.5 g/dL (85 g/L)	6.0-8.0 g/dL (60-80 g/L)
albumin	4.3 g/dL (43 g/L)	3.6-5.2 g/dL (36-52 g/L)
alpha-1	0.3 g/dL (3 g/L)	0.1-0.4 g/d (1-4 g/L)
alpha-2	0.7 g/dL (7 g/L)	0.4-1.0 g/dL (4-10 g/L)
beta	0.9 g/dL (9 g/L)	0.5-1.2 g/dL (5-12 g/L)
gamma ↑	2.3 g/dL (23 g/L)	0.6-1.6 g/dL (6-16 g/L)

The above serum protein electrophoresis pattern is consistent with:

a cirrhosis
b monoclonal gammopathy
c polyclonal gammopathy (eg, chronic inflammation)
d alpha-1-antitrypsin deficiency; severe emphysema

97
Analysis of CSF for oligoclonal bands is used to screen for which of the following disease states?

a multiple myeloma
b multiple sclerosis
c myasthenia gravis
d von Willebrand disease

98 The identification of Bence Jones protein is best accomplished by:

MLS
ONLY
  a a sulfosalicylic acid test
  b urine reagent strips
  (**c**) immunofixation
  d electrophoresis

99 Total iron-binding capacity measures the serum iron transporting capacity of:

  a hemoglobin
  b ceruloplasmin
  (**c**) transferrin
  d ferritin

100 The first step in the quantitation of serum iron is:

  a direct reaction with appropriate chromogen
  b iron saturation of transferrin
  c free iron precipitation
  (**d**) separation of iron from transferring

101 A patient's blood was drawn at 8 AM for a serum iron determination. The result was 85 µg/dL
MLS
ONLY
(15.2 µmol/L). A repeat specimen was drawn at 8 PM; the serum was stored at 4°C and run the next morning. The result was 40 µg/dL (7.2 µmol/L). These results are most likely due to:

  a iron deficiency anemia
  b improper storage of the specimen
  c possible liver damage
  (**d**) the time of day the second specimen was drawn

102 An elevated serum iron with normal iron binding capacity is most likely associated with:
MLS
ONLY
  a iron deficiency anemia
  b renal damage
  (**c**) pernicious anemia
  d septicemia

103 Decreased serum iron associated with increased TIBC is compatible with which of the following
MLS
ONLY
disease states?

  a anemia of chronic infection
  (**b**) iron deficiency anemia
  c chronic liver disease
  d nephrosis

104 A patient has the following results:
MLS
ONLY

	Patient values	Reference values
serum iron ↑	250 µg/dL (44.8 µmol/L)	60-150 µg/dL (10.7–26.9 µmol/L)
TIBC N	350 µg/dL (62.7 µmol/L)	300-350 µg/dL (53.7-62.7 µmol/L)

The best conclusion is that this patient has:

  a normal iron status
  b iron deficiency anemia
  c chronic disease
  (**d**) iron hemochromatosis

105 To assure an accurate ammonia level result, the specimen should be:

  a incubated at 37°C prior to testing
  b spun and separated immediately, tested as routine
  (**c**) spun, separated, iced, and tested immediately
  d stored at room temperature until tested

106 Erroneous ammonia levels can be eliminated by all of the following **except**:

    a assuring water and reagents are ammonia-free
    b separating plasma from cells and performing test analysis as soon as possible
    c drawing the specimen in a prechilled tube and immersing the tube in ice
    (d) storing the specimen protected from light until the analysis is done

107 A critically ill patient becomes comatose. The physician believes the coma is due to hepatic failure.
MLS
ONLY The assay most helpful in this diagnosis is:

    (a) ammonia
    b ALT
    c AST
    d GGT

108 A serum sample demonstrates an elevated result when tested with the Jaffe reaction.
This indicates:

    a prolonged hypothermia
    (b) renal functional impairment
    c pregnancy
    d arrhythmia

109 In order to prepare 100 mL of 15 mg/dL BUN (5.35 mmol/L) working standard from a stock
MLS
ONLY standard containing 500 mg/dL (178.5 mmol/L) of urea nitrogen, the number of mL of stock
solution that should be used is:

    (a) 3 mL
    b 5 mL
    c 33 mL
    d 75 mL

110 A patient with glomerulonephritis is most likely to present with the following serum results:
MLS
ONLY
    a creatinine decreased
    b calcium increased
    c phosphorous decreased
    (d) BUN increased

111 The principle excretory form of nitrogen is:
MLS
ONLY
    a amino acids
    b creatinine
    (c) urea
    d uric acid

112 In the Jaffe reaction, creatinine reacts with:
MLS
ONLY
    a alkaline sulfasalazine solution to produce an orange-yellow complex
    b potassium iodide to form a reddish-purple complex
    c sodium nitroferricyanide to yield a reddish-brown color
    (d) alkaline picrate solution to yield an orange-red complex

113 Creatinine clearance is used to estimate the:

    a tubular secretion of creatinine
    b glomerular secretion of creatinine
    c renal glomerular and tubular mass
    (d) glomerular filtration rate

114 A blood creatinine value of 5.0 mg/dL (442.0 µmol/L) is most likely to be found with which of the following blood values?

    a osmolality: 292 mOsm/kg
    b uric acid: 8 mg/dL (475.8 µmol/L)
    (c) urea nitrogen: 80 mg/dL (28.56 mmol/L)
    d ammonia: 80 µg/dL (44 µmol/L)

115 Technical problems encountered during the collection of an amniotic fluid specimen caused doubt as to whether the specimen was amniotic in origin. Which 1 of the following procedures would best establish that the fluid is amniotic in origin?

    a measurement of absorbance at 450 nm
    (b) creatinine measurement – *maternal urine versus amniotic fluid*
    c lecithin/sphingomyelin ratio
    d human amniotic placental lactogen (HPL)

116 Which of the following represents the end product of purine metabolism in humans?

    a AMP and GMP
    b DNA and RNA
    c allantoin
    (d) uric acid

117 Which of the following substances is the biologically active precursor of a fat soluble vitamin?

    a biotin
    (b) retinol – *Vitamin A*
    c folic acid
    d ascorbic acid

118 The troponin complex consists of:

    a troponin T, calcium and tropomyosin
    (b) troponin C, troponin I and troponin T
    c troponin I, actin, and tropomyosin
    d troponin C, myoglobin, and actin

119 The presence of C-reactive protein in the blood is an indication of:

    a a recent streptococcal infection
    b recovery from a pneumococcal infection
    (c) an inflammatory process
    d a state of hypersensitivity

120 Oligoclonal bands are present on electrophoresis of concentrated CSF and also on concurrently tested serum of the same patient. The proper interpretation is:

    a diagnostic for primary CNS tumor
    (b) diagnostic for multiple sclerosis
    c CNS involvement by acute leukemia
    d nondiagnostic for multiple sclerosis

121 Which of the following is an example of a peptide bond?

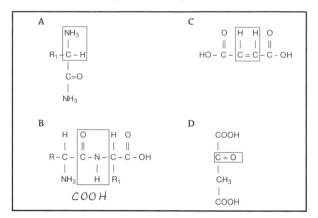

   a A
   b B
   c C
   d D

122 90% of the copper present in the blood is bound to:

   a transferrin
   b ceruloplasmin
   c albumin
   d cryoglobulin

123 Which of the following determinations is useful in prenatal diagnosis of open neural tube defects?

MLS ONLY

   a amniotic fluid alpha-fetoprotein
   b amniotic fluid estriol
   c maternal serum estradiol
   d maternal serum estrone

124 Below are the results of a protein electrophoresis:

MLS ONLY

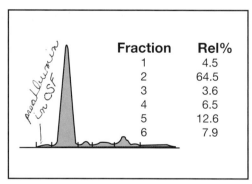

Fraction	Rel%
1	4.5
2	64.5
3	3.6
4	6.5
5	12.6
6	7.9

These results are consistent with a(n):

   a normal serum protein pattern
   b normal CSF protein pattern
   c abnormal serum protein pattern
   d abnormal CSF protein pattern

125 Serum concentrations of vitamin B_{12} are elevated in:

MLS ONLY

   a pernicious anemia in relapse
   b patients on chronic hemodialysis
   c chronic granulocytic leukemia
   d Hodgkin disease

126 Absorption of vitamin B_{12} requires the presence of:

MLS ONLY

  (**a**) intrinsic factor
  b gastrin
  c secretin
  d folic acid

127 The procedure used to determine the presence of neural tube defects is:

MLS ONLY

  a lecithin/sphingomyelin ratio
  b amniotic fluid creatinine
  c measurement of absorbance at 450 nm
  (**d**) alpha-fetoprotein

Heme Derivatives

128 The principle of the occult blood test depends upon the:

MLS ONLY

  a coagulase ability of blood
  b oxidative power of atmospheric oxygen
  c hydrogen peroxide in hemoglobin
  (**d**) peroxidase-like activity of hemoglobin

129 A breakdown product of hemoglobin is:

MLS ONLY

  a lipoprotein
  (**b**) bilirubin
  c hematoxylin
  d Bence Jones protein

130 Hemoglobin S can be separated from hemoglobin D by:

  (**a**) electrophoresis on a different medium and acidic pH   ✳
  b hemoglobin A_2 quantitation
  c electrophoresis at higher voltage
  d Kleihauer-Betke acid elution

131 On electrophoresis at alkaline pH, which of the following is the slowest migrating hemoglobin?

  a Hgb A
  b Hgb S
  (**c**) Hgb C – S – ⚡ F – A
  d Hgb F

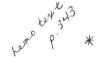 hemo text p. 343 ✳

132 The hemoglobin that is resistant to alkali (KOH) denaturation is:

MLS ONLY

  a A
  b A_2
  c C
  (**d**) F

133 The following bilirubin results are obtained on a patient:

> day 1: 4.3 mg/dL (73.5 μmol/L)
> day 2: 4.6 mg/dL (78.7 μmol/L)
> day 3: 4.5 mg/dL (77.0 μmol/L)
> day 4: 2.2 mg/dL (37.6 μmol/L)
> day 5: 4.4 mg/dL (75.2 μmol/L)
> day 6: 4.5 mg/dL (77.0 μmol/L)

Given that the controls were within range each day, what is a probable explanation for the result on day 4?

- **a** no explanation necessary
- **b** serum, not plasma, was used for testing
- **c** specimen had prolonged exposure to light
- **d** specimen was hemolyzed

134 Urobilinogen is formed in the:

- **a** kidney
- **b** spleen
- **c** liver
- **d** intestine

135 In bilirubin determinations, the purpose of adding a concentrated caffeine solution or methyl alcohol is to:
MLS ONLY

- **a** allow indirect bilirubin to react with color reagent
- **b** dissolve conjugated bilirubin
- **c** precipitate protein
- **d** prevent any change in pH

136 If the total bilirubin is 3.1 mg/dL (53.0 μmol/L) and the conjugated bilirubin is 2.0 mg/dL (34.2 μmol/L), the unconjugated bilirubin is:
MLS ONLY

- **a** 0.5 mg/dL (8.6 μmol/L)
- **b** 1.1 mg/dL (18.8 μmol/L)
- **c** 2.2 mg/dL (37.6 μmol/L)
- **d** 5.1 mg/dL (87.2 μmol/L)

137 The principle of the tablet test for bilirubin in urine or feces is:
MLS ONLY

- **a** the reaction between bile and 2,4-dichloronitrobenzene to a yellow color
- **b** the liberation of oxygen by bile to oxidize orthotolidine to a blue-purple color
- **c** chemical coupling of bile with a diazonium salt to form a brown color
- **d** chemical coupling of bilirubin with a diazonium salt to form a purple color

138 A serum sample was assayed for bilirubin at 10 AM, and the result was 12 mg/dL (205.6 μmol/L). The same sample was retested at 3 PM. The result now is 8 mg/dL (136.8 μmol/L). The most likely explanation for this discrepancy is:

- **a** the reagent has deteriorated
- **b** the sample was exposed to light
- **c** a calculation error in the first assay
- **d** the sample was not refrigerated

139 Serial bilirubin determinations are charted below.

Day	Collected	Assayed	Result
1	7 AM	8 AM	14.0 mg/dL (239.4 μmol/L)
2	7 AM	6 PM	9.0 mg/dL (153.9 μmol/L)
3	6 AM	8 AM	15.0 mg/dL (256.5 μmol/L)

The best explanation for the results is:

- **a** sample hemolysis and hemoglobin deterioration
- **b** sample exposure to light
- **c** sample left in warm location
- **d** reagent deterioration

140 In the liver, bilirubin is converted to:

MLS
ONLY

   a urobilinogen
   b urobilin
   c bilirubin-albumin complex
   d bilirubin diglucuronide

141 In which of the following disease states is conjugated bilirubin a major serum component?

MLS
ONLY

   a biliary obstruction
   b hemolysis
   c neonatal jaundice
   d erythroblastosis fetalis

142 Kernicterus is an abnormal accumulation of bilirubin in:

   a heart tissue
   b brain tissue
   c liver tissue
   d kidney tissue

143 In which of the following conditions does decreased activity of glucuronyl transferase result in increased unconjugated bilirubin and kernicterus in neonates?

MLS
ONLY

   a Gilbert disease
   b Rotor syndrome
   c Dubin-Johnson syndrome
   d Crigler-Najjar syndrome

144 A 21-year-old man with nausea, vomiting, and jaundice has the following laboratory findings:

MLS
ONLY

Test	Patient	Reference range
total serum bilirubin ↑↑	8.5 mg/dL (145.4 µmol/L)	0-1.0 mg/dL (0.0-17.1 µmol/L)
conjugated serum bilirubin ↑ ↑	6.1 mg/dL (104.3 µmol/L)	0-0.5 mg/dL (0.0-8.6 µmol/L)
urine urobilinogen	increased	
fecal urobilinogen	decreased	
urine bilirubin	positive	
AST ↑↑	300 U/L	0-50 U/L
alkaline phosphatase ↑	170 U/L	0-150 U/L

These can best be explained as representing:
   a unconjugated hyperbilirubinemia, probably due to hemolysis
   b unconjugated hyperbilirubinemia, probably due to toxic liver damage
   c conjugated hyperbilirubinemia, probably due to biliary tract disease
   d conjugated hyperbilirubinemia, probably due to hepatocellular obstruction

145 Biochemical profile:
MLS
ONLY

Test	Patient values	Reference range
total protein	7.3 g/dL (73 g/L)	6.0 - 8.0 g/dL (60-80 g/L)
albumin	4.1 g/dL (41 g/L)	3.5 - 5.0 g/dL (35-50 g/L)
calcium	9.6 mg/dL (2.4 mmol/L)	8.5 -10.5 mg/dL (2.1-2.6 mmol/L)
phosphorus	3.3 mg/dL (1.06 mmol/L)	2.5 - 4.5 mg/dL (0.80-1.45 mmol/L)
glucose	95 mg/dL (5.2 mmol/L)	65 - 110 mg/dL (3.6-6.1 mmol/L)
BUN	16 mg/dL (5.71 mmol/L)	10 - 20 mg/dL (3.57-7.14 mmol/L)
uric acid	6.0 mg/dL (356.9 µmol/L)	2.5 - 8.0 mg/dL (148.7-475.8 µmol/L)
creatinine	1.2 mg/dL (106.1 µmol/L)	0.7 - 1.4 mg/dL (61.9-123.8 µmol/L)
total bilirubin ↑↑	3.7 mg/dL (63.3 µmol/L)	0.2 - 0.9 mg/dL (3.4-15.4 µmol/L)
alkaline phosphatase ↑↑	275 U/L	30 - 80 U/L
lactate dehydrogenase	185 U/L	100- 225 U/L
AST ↑	75 U/L	10 - 40 U/L

The results the biochemical profile are most consistent with:

a viral hepatitis
b hemolytic anemia
c common bile duct stone
d chronic active hepatitis

146 A stool specimen that appears black and tarry should be tested for the presence of:

a occult blood
b fecal fat
c trypsin
d excess mucus

147 What substance gives feces its normal color?
MLS
ONLY
a uroerythrin
b urochrome
c urobilin
d urobilinogen

148 A condition in which erythrocyte protoporphyrin is increased is:
MLS
ONLY
a acute intermittent porphyria
b iron deficiency anemia
c porphyria cutanea tarda
d acute porphyric attack

149 Which of the following elevates carboxyhemoglobin?
MLS
ONLY
a nitrite poisoning
b exposure to carbon monoxide
c sulfa drug toxicity
d sickle cell anemia

150 The reason carbon monoxide is so toxic is because it:
MLS
ONLY
a is a protoplasmic poison
b combines with cytochrome oxidase
c has 200 times the affinity of oxygen for hemoglobin binding sites
d sensitizes the myocardium

151 Detection of carriers of hereditary coproporphyria should include analysis of:

MLS ONLY

   a 24-hour urine for porphobilinogen
   b fresh morning urine for delta-aminolevulinic acid
   c erythrocyte protoporphyrin
   d 24-hour urine for porphyrin

152 A fresh urine sample is received for analysis for "porphyrins" or "porphyria" without further information or specifications. Initial analysis should include:

MLS ONLY

   a porphyrin screen and quantitative total porphyrin
   b quantitative total porphyrin and porphobilinogen screen
   c porphyrin and porphobilinogen screen
   d porphobilinogen screen and ion-exchange analysis for porphobilinogen

153 Which of the following enzymes of heme biosynthesis is inhibited by lead?

MLS ONLY

   a aminolevulinate synthase
   b porphobilinogen synthase
   c uroporphyrinogen synthase
   d bilirubin synthetase

154 Serum haptoglobin:

MLS ONLY

   a is decreased in patients with tissue injury and neoplasia
   b is increased in patients with prosthetic heart valves
   c can be separated into distinct phenotypes by starch-gel electrophoresis
   d binds heme

haptoglobin → binds free hemoglobin in bloodstream

Enzymes

155 The most specific enzyme test for acute pancreatitis is:

   a acid phosphatase
   b trypsin
   c amylase
   d lipase – *longer ↑ than amylase*

156 Which of the following enzymes are used in the diagnosis of acute pancreatitis?

   a amylase (AMS) and lipase (LPS)
   b aspartate aminotransferase (AST) and alanine aminotransferase (ALT)
   c 5'-nucleotidase (5'N) and gamma-glutamyl transferase (GGT)
   d aspartate aminotransferase (AST) and lactate dehydrogenase (LD)

157 Which of the following enzymes catalyzes the conversion of starch to glucose and maltose?

   a malate dehydrogenase (MD)
   b amylase (AMS)
   c creatine kinase (CK)
   d isocitric dehydrogenase (ICD)

158 Which of the following sets of results would be consistent with macroamylasemia?

MLS ONLY

   a normal serum amylase and elevated urine amylase values
   b increased serum amylase and normal urine amylase values
   c increased serum and urine amylase values
   d normal serum and urine amylase values

159 A physician suspects his patient has pancreatitis. Which test(s) would be most indicative of this disease?

    a creatinine - *kidney*
    b LD isoenzymes - *muscle*
    c beta-hydroxybutyrate – *ketone/diabetis*
    (d) amylase

160 Aspartate amino transferase (AST) is characteristically elevated in diseases of the:

    (a) liver
    b kidney
    c intestine
    d pancreas

161 Amino transferase enzymes catalyze the:

    a exchange of amino groups and sulfhydryl groups between alpha-amino and sulfur-containing acids
    (b) exchange of amino and keto groups between alpha-amino and alpha-keto acids
    c hydrolysis of amino acids and keto acids
    d reversible transfer of hydrogen from amino acids to coenzyme

162 Aspartate aminotransferase (AST) and alanine aminotransferase (ALT) are both elevated in which of the following diseases?

    a muscular dystrophy
    (b) viral hepatitis
    c pulmonary emboli
    d infectious mononucleosis

163 The greatest activities of serum AST and ALT are seen in which of the following?

    (a) acute viral hepatitis
    b primary biliary cirrhosis
    c metastatic hepatic cirrhosis
    d alcoholic cirrhosis

164 Malic dehydrogenase is added to the aspartate aminotransaminase (AST) reaction to catalyze the
MLS ONLY conversion of:

    a alpha-ketoglutarate to aspartate
    b alpha-ketoglutarate to malate
    c aspartate to oxalacetate
    (d) oxalacetate to malate

165 Given the following results:
MLS ONLY

alkaline phosphatase:	slight increase ↑ (ALP)
aspartate amino transferase:	marked increase ↑↑↑ (AST)
alanine amino transferase:	marked increase ↑↑↑ (ALT)
gamma-glutamyl transferase:	slight increase ↑ (GGT)

This is most consistent with:

    (a) acute hepatitis
    b chronic hepatitis
    c obstructive jaundice
    d liver hemangioma

166 Which of the following clinical disorders is associated with the greatest elevation of lactate dehydrogenase isoenzyme 1?

    a pneumonia
    b glomerulonephritis
    c pancreatitis
    (d) pernicious anemia

167 The enzyme, which exists chiefly in skeletal muscle, heart, and brain, is grossly elevated in active muscular dystrophy, and rises early in myocardial infarction is:

    a lipase
    b transaminase
    c lactate dehydrogenase
    d creatine kinase

168 The enzyme present in almost all tissues that may be separated by electrophoresis into 5 components is:

    a lipase
    b transaminase
    c creatine kinase
    d lactate dehydrogenase

169 A common cause of a falsely increased LD_1 fraction of lactic dehydrogenase is:

    a specimen hemolysis
    b liver disease
    c congestive heart failure
    d drug toxicity

170 The presence of which of the following isoenzymes indicates acute myocardial damage?

    a CKMM
    b CKMB
    c CKBB
    d none

171 In which of the following conditions would a **normal** level of creatine kinase be found?

    a acute myocardial infarct
    b hepatitis
    c progressive muscular dystrophy
    d intramuscular injection

172 Of the following diseases, the one most often associated with elevations of lactate dehydrogenase isoenzymes 4 and 5 on electrophoresis is:

    a liver disease – LD 4+5
    b hemolytic anemia LD 1+2
    c myocardial infarction LD 1+2   ✳
    d pulmonary edema LD_3

173 When myocardial infarction occurs, the first enzyme to become elevated is:

    a CK
    b LD
    c AST
    d ALT

174 A scanning of a CK isoenzyme fractionation revealed 2 peaks: a slow cathodic peak (CKMM) and an intermediate peak (CKMB). A possible interpretation for this pattern is:

    a brain tumor – CKBB
    b muscular dystrophy – CKMM
    c myocardial infarction
    d viral hepatitis – none

175 An electrophoretic separation of lactate dehydrogenase isoenzymes that demonstrates an
MLS ONLY elevation in LD-1 and LD-2 in a "flipped" pattern is consistent with:

   (a) myocardial infarction
   b viral hepatitis
   c pancreatitis
   d renal failure

176 Increased total serum lactic dehydrogenase (LD) activity, confined to fractions 4 and 5 is most
MLS ONLY likely to be associated with:

   a pulmonary infarction
   b hemolytic anemia
   c myocardial infarction
   (d) acute viral hepatitis

177 A 10-year-old child was admitted to pediatrics with an initial diagnosis of skeletal muscle disease.
The best confirmatory tests would be:

   a creatine kinase and isocitrate dehydrogenase
   b gamma-glutamyl transferase and alkaline phosphatase
   (c) aldolase and creatine kinase
   d lactate dehydrogenase and malate dehydrogenase

178 In the immunoinhibition phase of the CKMB procedure:

   (a) M subunit is inactivated
   b B subunit is inactivated
   c MB is inactivated
   d BB is inactivated

179 The presence of increased CKMB activity on a CK electrophoresis pattern is most likely found in a
patient suffering from:

   a acute muscular stress following strenuous exercise
   b malignant liver disease
   (c) myocardial infarction
   d severe head injury

180 Refer to the following illustration:

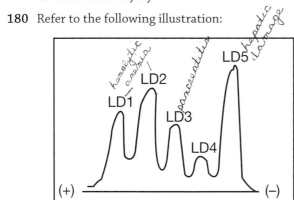

Which of the following is the most likely interpretation of the LD isoenzyme scan
illustrated above?

   a myocardial infarction
   b megaloblastic anemia
   c acute pancreatitis
   (d) viral hepatitis

181 Increased serum lactic dehydrogenase activity due to elevation of fast fraction (1 and 2) on electrophoretic separation is caused by:

  a nephrotic syndrome
  b hemolytic anemia
  c pancreatitis
  d hepatic damage

182 A serum sample drawn in the emergency room from a 42-year-old man yielded the following laboratory results:

	Patient	Reference range
CK:	185 U/L ↑	15-160 U/L
AST:	123 U/L ↑↑	0-48 U/L
CKMB:	6 U/L	2-12 U/L

Which of the following conditions might account for these values?

  a crush injury to the thigh — ↑ CK + AST
  b cerebrovascular accident — CKBB ↑
  c pulmonary infarction — CKBB↑
  d early acute hepatitis - AST ↑↑↑

183 Given the following results:

  alkaline phosphatase: ↑↑   marked increase   ALP
  aspartate amino transferase: ↑ slight increase A ST
  alanine amino transferase: ↑   slight increase ALT
  gamma-glutamyl transferase: marked increase GGT ↑↑↑

This is most consistent with:

  a acute hepatitis
  b osteitis fibrosa
  c chronic hepatitis
  d obstructive jaundice = ↑↑ ALP and GGT

184 Given the following results:

  alkaline phosphatase: ↑   slight increase
  aspartate aminotransferase: ↑ slight increase
  alanine aminotransferase: ↑   slight increase
  gamma-glutamyl transferase: slight increase ↑

This is most consistent with:

  a acute hepatitis
  b chronic hepatitis
  c obstructive jaundice
  d liver hemangioma

185 What specimen preparation is commonly used to perform the alkaline phosphatase isoenzyme determination? (ALP)

  a serum is divided into 2 aliquots, one is frozen and the other is refrigerated
  b serum is divided into 2 aliquots, one is heated at 56°C and the other is unheated
  c no preparation is necessary since the assay uses EDTA plasma
  d protein-free filtrate is prepared first

186 Regan isoenzyme has the same properties as alkaline phosphatase that originates in the:

  a skeleton
  b kidney
  c intestine
  d placenta

187 The **most** heat labile fraction of alkaline phosphatase is obtained from:

   a liver
   b bone
   c intestine
   d placenta

most heat stable = placenta → intestine → liver

PILB

188 The **most** sensitive enzymatic indicator for liver damage from ethanol intake is:

   a alanine aminotransferase (ALT)
   b aspartate aminotransferase (AST)
   c gamma-glutamyl transferase (GGT) = *liver damage from alcoholism* ✶
   d alkaline phosphatase

189 Isoenzyme assays are performed to improve:

   a precision
   b accuracy
   c sensitivity
   d specificity

190 The protein portion of an enzyme complex is called the:

   a apoenzyme – *protein enzyme*
   b coenzyme – *organic cofactor*
   c holoenzyme – *enzyme complex (apoenzyme + cofactor)* ✶
   d proenzyme – *component of an enzyme*

191 Which of the following chemical determinations may be of help in establishing the presence of seminal fluid?

   a lactic dehydrogenase (LD)
   b isocitrate dehydrogenase (ICD) ✶
   c acid phosphatase
   d alkaline phosphatase

192 Which of the following enzyme substrates is the most specific for prostatic acid phosphatase for
MLS ONLY quantitative endpoint reactions?

   a p-nitrophenylphosphate
   b thymolphthalein monophosphate
   c beta-naphthol-phosphate
   d beta-glycerophosphate

193 Lactate dehydrogenase, malate dehydrogenase, isocitrate dehydrogenase, and hydroxybutyrate
MLS ONLY dehydrogenase all:

   a are liver enzymes
   b are cardiac enzymes
   c catalyze oxidation-reduction reactions
   d are class III enzymes

Lipids and Lipoproteins

194 High levels of which lipoprotein class are associated with decreased risk of
MLS ONLY accelerated atherosclerosis?

   a chylomicrons
   b VLDL
   c LDL
   d HDL

195 The most consistent analytical error involved in the routine determination of HDL-cholesterol is caused by:

MLS ONLY

    a incomplete precipitation of LDL-cholesterol
    b coprecipitation of HDL- and LDL-cholesterol
    c inaccurate protein estimation of HDL-cholesterol
    d a small concentration of apoB-containing lipoproteins after precipitation

196 If the LDL-cholesterol is to be calculated by the Friedewald formula, what are the 2 measurements that need to be carried out by the same chemical procedure?

MLS ONLY

    a total cholesterol and HDL-cholesterol
    b total cholesterol and triglyceride
    c triglyceride and chylomicrons
    d apolipoprotein A and apolipoprotein B

197 The chemical composition of HDL-cholesterol corresponds to:

MLS ONLY

	Triglyceride	Cholesterol	Protein
a	60%	15%	10%
b	10%	45%	25%
c	5%	15%	50%
d	85%	5%	2%

198 In familial hypercholesterolemia, the hallmark finding is an elevation of:

MLS ONLY

    a low-density lipoproteins (LDL)
    b chylomicrons
    c high-density lipoproteins
    d apolipoprotein A_1

199 Premature atherosclerosis can occur when which of the following becomes elevated?

MLS ONLY

    a chylomicrons
    b prostaglandins
    c low-density lipoproteins – *transports cholesterol esters to cells for metabolism*
    d high-density lipoproteins

200 Transportation of 60%-75% of the plasma cholesterol is performed by:

MLS ONLY

    a chylomicrons — *transport triglycerides*
    b very low-density lipoproteins
    c low-density lipoproteins – *70%* > *of cholesterol*
    d high-density lipoproteins - *30%*

201 Which of the following diseases results from a familial absence of high density lipoprotein?

MLS ONLY

    a Krabbe disease
    b Gaucher disease
    c Tangier disease
    d Tay-Sachs disease

202 A 1-year-old girl with a hyperlipoproteinemia and lipase deficiency has the following lipid profile:

    cholesterol: 300 mg/dL (7.77 mmol/L)
    LDL: increased
    HDL: decreased
    triglycerides: 200 mg/dL (2.26 mmol/L)
    chylomicrons: present ✓

A serum specimen from this patient that was refrigerated overnight would most likely be:

    a clear
    b cloudy
    c creamy layer over cloudy serum
    d creamy layer over clear serum

203
MLS ONLY
Which of the following lipid results would be expected to be falsely elevated on a serum specimen from a nonfasting patient?

   a cholesterol
   b triglyceride
   c HDL
   d LDL

204
MLS ONLY
A 9-month-old boy from Israel has gradually lost the ability to sit up, and develops seizures. He has an increased amount of a phospholipid called GM_2-ganglioside in his neurons, and he lacks the enzyme hexosaminidase A in his leukocytes. These findings suggest:

   a Neimann-Pick disease
   b Tay-Sachs disease
   c phenylketonuria
   d Hurler syndrome

205
MLS ONLY
In amniotic fluid, the procedure used to determine fetal lung maturity is:

   a lecithin/sphingomyelin ratio
   b creatinine – *fetal age*
   c measurement of absorbance at 450 nm (*bilirubin*)
   d alpha-fetoprotein – *neural tube disorders*

206
MLS ONLY
Refer to the following illustration:

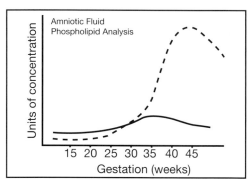

The class of phospholipid surfactants represented by the dotted line on the amniotic fluid analysis shown above is thought to originate in what fetal organ system?

   a cardiovascular
   b pulmonary
   c hepatic
   d placental

207
MLS ONLY
A fasting serum sample from an asymptomatic 43-year-old woman is examined visually and chemically with the following results:

initial appearance of serum:	milky – *↑ triglycerides + VLDL*
appearance of serum after overnight refrigeration:	cream layer over turbid serum – *chylomicrons*
triglyceride level:	2,000 mg/dL (22.6 mmol/L)
cholesterol level:	550 mg/dL (14.25 mmol/L)

This sample contains predominantly: ✳

   a chylomicrons, alone
   b chylomicrons and very low-density lipoproteins (VLDL)
   c very low-density lipoproteins (VLDL) and low-density lipoproteins (LDL)
   d high-density lipoproteins (HDL)

208 Chylomicrons are present in which of the following dyslipidemias?

    a familial hypercholesterolemia
    b hypertriglyceridemia
    c deficiency in <u>lipoprotein</u> <u>lipase</u> activity → *hydrolyzes chylomicrons + triglycerides*
    d familial hypoalphalipoproteinemia

209 The function of the major lipid components of the very low-density lipoproteins (VLDL) is
to transport:

    a cholesterol from peripheral cells to the liver *(HDL)*
    b cholesterol and phospholipids to peripheral cells *(LDL)*
    c exogenous triglycerides *(transported by chylomicrons)*
    d endogenous triglycerides *(transported by VLDL)*

210 Turbidity in serum suggests elevation of:

    a cholesterol
    b total protein
    c chylomicrons
    d albumin

Endocrinology and Tumor Markers

211 TSH is produced by the:

    a hypothalamus
    b pituitary gland   ✳
    c adrenal cortex
    d thyroid

212 A patient has the following thyroid profile:

total T_4: ↓	decreased
free T_4: ↓	decreased
thyroid peroxidase antibody:	positive
TSH: ✗ ↑	~~decreased~~ *increased*

This patient most probably has:

    a hyperthyroidism
    b hypothyroidism
    c a normal thyroid
    d Graves disease

213 A 45-year-old woman complains of fatigue, heat intolerance and hair loss. Total and free T_4 are abnormally low. If the TSH showed marked elevation, this would be consistent with:

    a Graves disease
    b an adenoma of the thyroid
    c thyrotoxicosis
    d primary hypothyroidism

214 The majority of thyroxine (T_4) is converted into the more biologically active hormone:

    a thyroglobulin
    b thyroid-stimulating hormone (TSH)
    c triiodothyronine (T_3)
    d thyrotropin-releasing hormone

215 A 2-year-old child with a decreased serum T_4 is described as being somewhat dwarfed, stocky, overweight, and having coarse features. Of the following, the most informative additional laboratory test would be the serum:

    a thyroxine binding globulin (TBG)
    b thyroid-stimulating hormone (TSH)
    c triiodothyronine (T_3)
    d cholesterol

216 Assays for free T_4 measure hormone not bound to thyroxine-binding prealbumin, thyroxine-
MLS
ONLY binding globulin and:

    a thyrotropin-releasing hormone
    b albumin
    c free T_3
    d thyroid-stimulating hormone

217 The recommended initial thyroid function test for either a healthy, asymptomatic patient or a patient with symptoms which may be related to a thyroid disorder is:

    a free thyroxine (free T_4)
    b thyroid-stimulating hormone (TSH)
    c total thyroxine (T_4)
    d triiodothyronine (T_3)

218 The screening test for congenital hypothyroidism is based upon:

    a TSH level in the newborn
    b thyroid-binding globulin level in the newborn
    c iodine level in the newborn   ✱
    d total thyroxine (T_4) level in the newborn

219 Which one of the following sets of results is consistent with primary hypothyroidism, (eg, Hashimoto thyroiditis):

Result	TSH ↑	T_4 (free thyroxine) ↓	Antimicrosomal antibody +
result A	decreased	decreased	positive
result B	increased	increased	positive
result C	normal	decreased	negative
result D	increased	decreased	positive

    a result A
    b result B
    c result C
    d result D

220 A 68-year-old female patient tells her physician of being "cold all the time" and recent weight gain, with no change in diet. The doctor orders a TSH level, and the laboratory reports a value of 8.7 μU/ mL (8.7 IU/L) (reference range = 0.5-5.0 μU/mL [0.5-5.0 IU/L]). This patient most likely has:

    a primary hypothyroidism
    b Graves disease
    c a TSH-secreting tumor
    d primary hyperthyroidism

221 Which of the following is secreted by the placenta and used for the early detection of pregnancy?

    a follicle-stimulating hormone (FSH)
    b human chorionic gonadotropin (HCG)
    c luteinizing hormone (LH)
    d progesterone

222 During pregnancy, the form of estrogen measured in urine is mostly:

MT
ONLY

   a estradiol
   b estriol - *urine*
   c estrone
   d pregnanediol

223 Refer to the following graph:

MLS
ONLY

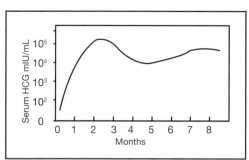

The HCG levels shown in the above graph most probably represent:

   a hydatidiform mole following miscarriage at 4 months
   b normal pregnancy - *HCG peaks at 8-10 weeks, then plateaus*
   c development of hydatidiform mole
   d miscarriage at 2 months with retained placenta

224 In amniotic fluid, the procedure used to detect hemolytic disease of the newborn is:

   a measurement of absorbance at 450 nm - *bilirubin*
   b creatinine
   c lecithin/sphingomyelin ratio
   d estriol

225 During a normal pregnancy, quantitative human chorionic gonadotropin (HCG) levels peak how many weeks after the last menstrual period?

   a 2-4
   b 8-10   ✱
   c 14-16
   d 18-20

226 "Laboratory A" measures maternal serum alpha-fetoprotein (MSAFP) at 16-18 weeks gestation as a screen for fetal disorders. The 16-week MSAFP median for Lab A is 32 µg/L. A 37-year-old woman has an MSAFP level of 34 µg/L at her 16th week. This result is consistent with:

MLS
ONLY

   a a normal MSAFP level for 16-week gestation
   b possible neural tube defect, including spina bifida
   c possible multiple birth (ie, twins)
   d possible trisomy disorder, including Down syndrome

227 Which of the following steroids is an adrenal cortical hormone?

   a angiotensinogen
   b aldosterone → *adrenal cortex*
   c epinephrine
   d growth hormone

228 What common substrate is used in the biosynthesis of adrenal steroids, including androgens and estrogens?

   a cortisol
   b catecholamines
   c progesterone
   d cholesterol

229 The biologically most active, naturally occurring <u>androgen</u> is:

    a androstenedione
    b cortisol
    c epiandrosterone
    d testosterone

230 Plasma for cortisol determinations were collected at 7 AM, after waking the patient, and at 10 PM that evening. The cortisol level of the morning sample was higher than the evening sample. This is consistent with:

    a a normal finding   ↑ in AM than PM   *
    b Cushing syndrome
    c Addison disease
    d hypopituitarism

231 <u>Night blindness</u> is associated with deficiency of which of the following vitamins?

    a A
    b C   *   A = night blindness
    c niacin B_1 = beriberi
    d thiamine   C = scurvy
                         D = rickets

232 Beriberi is associated with deficiency of vitamin: Niacin (B_3) = ~~pet~~ pellagra

    a A
    b C
    c niacin
    d thiamine (B_1) → alcoholism

233 Scurvy is associated with deficiency of which of the following vitamins?

    a A
    b C
    c niacin
    d thiamine

234 <u>Rickets</u> is associated with deficiency of which of the following vitamins?

    a B_1
    b C
    c niacin
    d D

235 Pellagra is associated with deficiency of which of the following vitamins?

    a A
    b B_1
    c thiamine
    d niacin

236 The major action of angiotensin II is:

    a increased pituitary secretion of vasopressin   *
    b increased vasoconstriction → stimulates adrenal cortex to make aldosterone
    c increased parathormone secretion by the parathyroid
    d decreased adrenal secretion of aldosterone

237 The urinary excretion product measured as an indicator of epinephrine production is:

    a dopamine
    b dihydroxyphenylalanine (DOPA)
    c homovanillic acid
    d vanillylmandelic acid (VMA) → epinephrine/norepinephrine

238 Which of the following hormones regulates normal blood calcium levels?

    a thyroxine
    b estriol
    c parathyroid hormone
    d growth hormone

PTH = calcium regulation of level

239 The most common form (95%) of congenital adrenal hyperplasia is 21-hydroxylase deficiency,
MLS ONLY which is detected by elevated plasma:

    a cortisol
    b aldosterone
    c 17-OH-progesterone
    d 11-deoxycortisol

240 A diagnosis of primary adrenal insufficiency requires demonstration of:

    a decreased urinary 17-keto- and 17-hydroxysteroids
    b decreased cortisol production
    c impaired response to ACTH stimulation
    d increased urinary cortisol excretion after metyrapone

ACTH stimulation = primary/ secondary adrenal insufficiency

241 The screen for adrenal cortical hyperfunction with the greatest sensitivity and specificity is:

    a 24-hour urine free cortisol
    b plasma cortisol
    c urinary 17-hydroxycorticosteroids
    d plasma corticosterone

242 A patient has signs and symptoms suggestive of acromegaly. The diagnosis would be confirmed if
MLS ONLY the patient had which of the following?

    a an elevated serum phosphate concentration
    b a decreased serum growth hormone releasing factor concentration
    c no decrease in serum growth hormone concentration 90 minutes after oral glucose administration
    d an increased serum somatostatin concentration

243 Estrogen and progesterone receptor assays are useful in identifying patients who are likely to
MLS ONLY benefit from endocrine therapy to treat which of the following?

    a ovarian cancer
    b breast cancer
    c endometriosis
    d amenorrhea

244 Which of the following sample collections would give an accurate assessment of potential excess cortisol production (hypercortisolism)?

    a collect a plasma sample as a baseline, and another one-hour after administration of metyrapone
    b collect a plasma sample at 8 AM only
    c collect a 24-hour urine free cortisol
    d collect a plasma sample at 8 AM and at 8 AM the next day

245 How is primary hypocortisolism (Addison disease) differentiated from secondary hypocortisolism
MLS ONLY (of pituitary origin)?

    a adrenal corticotropic hormone (ACTH) is decreased in primary and elevated in secondary
    b adrenal corticotropic hormone (ACTH) is elevated in primary and decreased in secondary
    c low aldosterone and hypoglycemia present with secondary hypocortisolism
    d normal cortisol levels and blood pressure with primary hypocortisolism

primary = ↓ACTH/↑ ↓ cortisol/↑ ACTH
secondary = ↓ cortisol/↓ ACTH

246 Aldosterone is released by the adrenal cortex upon stimulation by:

   a renin
   b angiotensinogen   LOOK UP FLOWCHART!!!
   c angiotensin I
   (d) angiotensin II

247 In developing the reference for a new EIA for CEA, the range for the normal population was
MLS ONLY broader than that published by the vendor. Controls are acceptable with a narrow coefficient of
   variation. This may be explained by:

   a positive interference by another tumor marker
   b population skewed to a younger age
   c improper temperature control during assay
   (d) inclusion of nonsmokers and smokers in the study population

248 Clinical assays for tumor markers are most important for:

   a screening for the presence of cancer
   (b) monitoring the course of a known cancer (*monitoring therapy, detecting*
   c confirming the absence of disease   *recurrence, prognosis;*
   (d) identifying patients at risk for cancer   *NOT for cancer screening*

249 Detection of which of the following substances is most useful to monitor the course of a patient
   with testicular cancer?

   (a) alpha-fetoprotein   *AFP = monitors testicular cancer*
   b carcinoembryonic antigen
   c prolactin
   d testosterone

250 Increased concentrations of alpha-fetoprotein (AFP) in adults are most characteristically
   associated with:

   (a) hepatocellular carcinoma   *AFP = liver cancer*
   b alcoholic cirrhosis
   c chronic active hepatitis
   d multiple myeloma

251 Carcinoembryonic antigen (CEA) is most likely to be produced in a malignancy involving the:

   a brain
   b testes   *CEA = colon*
   c bone
   (d) colon = CEA

252 Which of the following is useful in the detection and management of carcinoma of the prostate?

   (a) total prostate-specific antigen   *PSA = prostate*
   b prostatic acid phosphatase
   c human chorionic gonadotropin
   d alpha-fetoprotein

253 Which of the following statements most correctly describes the utility of clinical laboratory assays
   for tumor markers?

   a tumor markers are useful to screen asymptomatic patients for tumors
   b tumor markers are highly specific
   c tumor markers indicate the likelihood of an individual developing a tumor
   (d) tumor markers are useful in tracking the efficacy of treatment

254 Cancer antigen 125 (CA 125) is a tumor marker associated with:

   a breast carcinoma
   b colon cancer
   c lung cancer
   d ovarian and endometrial carcinoma

CA 125 = ovarian

255 In addition to carcinoma of the prostate, elevated prostate-specific antigen (PSA) can occur due to:

   a aspirin therapy
   b exogenous steroid use
   c benign prostatic hyperplasia
   d statin therapy (cholesterol lowering drug)

TDM and Toxicology

256 Blood specimens for digoxin assays should be obtained between 8 hours or more after drug administration because:

   a tissue and serum levels need to reach equilibrium
   b serum digoxin concentration will be falsely low prior to 6 hours
   c all of the digoxin is in the cellular fraction prior to 6 hours
   d digoxin protein-binding interactions are minimal prior to 6 hours

257 A drug has a half-life of 6 hours. If a dose is given every 6 hours, a steady-state drug level would usually be achieved in:

   a 3-5 hours
   b 10-12 hours
   c 24-42 hours
   d 48-50 hours

steady state → 4 to 7 doses

258 Free therapeutic drug levels are usually higher when serum protein concentrations are below normal. In which of the following conditions would this most likely occur?

   a acute inflammation
   b nephrotic syndrome
   c pregnancy
   d multiple myeloma

259 Which of the following factors is not relevant to therapeutic drug monitoring (TDM) of the aminoglycosides, antibiotics and vancomycin?

   a intestinal absorption
   b nephrotoxicity
   c ototoxicity
   d renal function

260 The drug procainamide is prescribed to treat cardiac arrhythmia. What biologically active liver metabolite of procainamide is often measured simultaneously?

   a phenobarbitol
   b quinidine
   c N-acetyl procainamide (NAPA) ✳
   d lidocaine

261 Cocaine is metabolized to:

   a carbamazepine
   b codeine ✳
   c hydrocodone
   d benzoylecgonine

262   The metabolite 11-nor-tetrahydrocannabinol-9-COOH can be detected by immunoassay 3-5 days after a single use of:

    a   methamphetamine
    b   cocaine
    c   benzodiazepine
    d   marijuana

263   A 3-year-old child was evaluated for abdominal pain and anorexia by a physician. A CBC revealed a hemoglobin of 9.8 g/dL (98 g/L) and basophilic stippling of the RBCs. The doctor should order further tests to check for poisoning from:

    a   arsenic
    b   iron
    c   mercury   ✳
    d   lead

264   Zinc protoporphyrin or free erythrocyte protoporphyrin measurements are useful to assess blood
MLS ONLY   concentrations of:

    a   lead
    b   mercury
    c   arsenic
    d   beryllium

265   A carbonate salt used to control manic-depressive disorders is:

    a   digoxin
    b   acetaminophen
    c   lithium
    d   phenytoin

266   An antiepileptic (or anticonvulsant) used to control seizure disorders is:

    a   digoxin
    b   acetaminophen
    c   lithium
    d   phenytoin

267   A drug that relaxes the smooth muscles of the bronchial passages is:

    a   acetaminophen
    b   lithium
    c   phenytoin
    d   theophylline

268   A cardiac glycoside that is used in the treatment of congenital heart failure and arrhythmias by increasing the force and velocity of myocardial contraction is:

    a   digoxin
    b   acetaminophen
    c   lithium
    d   phenytoin

269   A salicylate level is performed to detect toxicity caused by ingestion of excess:

    a   acetaminophen
    b   aspirin
    c   ibuprofen
    d   pseudoephedrine

270 Lithium therapy is widely used in the treatment of:

    a hypertension
    b hyperactivity
    c aggression
    d manic-depressive (bipolar) disorder

271 Serum and urine copper levels are assayed on a hospital patient with the following results:

	Patient values	**Reference values**
serum Cu: ↓	20 µg/dL (3.1 µmol/L)	70-140 µg/dL (11.0–22.0 µmol/L)
urine Cu: ↑	83 µg/dL (13.0 µmol/L)	<40 µg/dL (<63 µmol/L)

This is most consistent with:

    a normal copper levels
    b Wilms tumor
    c Wilson disease
    d Addison disease

272 An active metabolite of amitriptyline is:

    a nortriptyline
    b protriptyline
    c butriptyline
    d norbutriptyline

273 Phenobarbital is a metabolite of:

    a primidone
    b phenytoin
    c amobarbital
    d secobarbital

274 Testing for the diagnosis of lead poisoning should include:

    a erythrocyte protoporphyrin (EPP)
    b urine delta-aminolevulinic acid
    c whole blood lead
    d zinc protoporphyrin (ZPP)

Quality Assessment

275 Blood received in the laboratory for blood gas analysis must meet which of the following requirements?

    a on ice, thin fibrin strands only, no air bubbles
    b on ice, no clots, fewer than 4 air bubbles
    c on ice, no clots, no air bubbles
    d room temperature, no clots, no air bubbles

276 After a difficult venipuncture requiring prolonged application of the tourniquet, the serum K^+ was found to be 6.8 mEq/L (6.8 mmol/L). The best course of action is to:

    a repeat the test using the same specimen
    b adjust the value based on the current serum Na^+
    c repeat the test using freshly drawn serum
    d cancel the test

prolonged tourniquet:
↑ protein/albumin,
K+, Ca+, hemoglobin

277 Serum from a patient with metastatic carcinoma of the prostate was separated from the clot and
stored at room temperature. The following results were obtained:

MLS
ONLY

	Patient value	Reference range
Ca⁺⁺	10.8 mg/dL (2.7 mmol/L)	8.8-10.3 mg/dL (2.2-2.6 mmol/L)
LD	420 U/L	50-150 U/L
acid phosphatase	0.1 U/L	0-5.5 U/L

The technician should repeat the:

a LD using diluted serum
b acid phosphatase with freshly drawn serum
c LD with fresh serum
d tests using plasma

278 A lipemic serum is separated and frozen at −20°C for assay at a later date. One week later, prior to
performing an assay for triglycerides, the specimen should be:

MLS
ONLY

a warmed to 37°C and mixed thoroughly
b warmed to 15°C and centrifuged
c transferred to a glycerated test tube
d discarded and a new specimen obtained

279 The different water content of erythrocytes and plasma makes true glucose concentrations in
whole blood a function of the:

MLS
ONLY

a hematocrit
b leukocyte count
c erythrocyte count
d erythrocyte indices

280 In a specimen collected for plasma glucose analysis, sodium fluoride:

a serves as a coenzyme of hexokinase
b prevents reactivity of non-glucose reducing substances
c precipitates proteins
d inhibits glycolysis

281 As part of a hyperlipidemia screening program, the following results were obtained on a
25-year-old woman 6 hours after eating:

triglycerides: 260 mg/dL (2.86 mmol/L)
cholesterol: 120 mg/dL (3.12 mmol/L)

Which of the following is the **best** interpretation of these results?

a both results are normal, and not affected by the recent meal
b cholesterol is normal, but triglycerides are elevated, which may be attributed to the recent meal
c both results are elevated, indicating a metabolic problem in addition to the nonfasting state
d both results are below normal despite the recent meal, indicating a metabolic problem

282 Blood was collected in a serum separator tube on a patient who has been fasting since midnight.
The time of collection was 7 AM. The laboratory test which should be recollected is:

a triglycerides
b iron
c LD
d sodium

283 Arterial blood that is collected in a heparinized syringe but exposed to room air would be most consistent with the changes in which of the following specimens?

Specimen	PO$_2$	PCO$_2$	pH
A	elevated	decreased	elevated
B	decreased	elevated	decreased
C	unchanged	elevated	unchanged
D	decreased	decreased	decreased

   (a) specimen A
   b specimen B
   c specimen C
   d specimen D

284 Specimens for blood gas determination should be drawn into a syringe containing:
MLS
ONLY
   a no preservative
   (b) heparin
   c EDTA
   d oxalate

285 Unless blood gas measurements are made immediately after sampling, in vitro glycolysis of the blood causes a:

   a rise in pH and PCO$_2$
   b fall in pH and a rise in PO$_2$
   c rise in pH and a fall in PO$_2$
   (d) fall in pH and a rise in PCO$_2$

286 Which of the following serum constituents is unstable if a blood specimen is left standing at room temperature for 8 hours before processing?

   a cholesterol
   b triglyceride
   c creatinine
   (d) glucose

287 An arterial blood specimen submitted for blood gas analysis was obtained at 8:30 AM but was not received in the laboratory until 11AM. The technologist should:

   a perform the test immediately upon receipt
   b perform the test only if the specimen was submitted in ice water
   c request a venous blood specimen
   (d) request a new arterial specimen be obtained

288 In monitoring glomerular function, which of the following tests has the highest sensitivity?
MLS
ONLY
   a urine sodium
   b BUN/creatinine ratio
   (c) creatinine clearance
   d urea clearance

Laboratory Mathematics

289 If the pK$_a$ is 6.1, the CO$_2$ content is 25 mM/L, the salt equals the total CO$_2$ content minus
MLS
ONLY the carbonic acid; the carbonic acid equals 0.03 × PCO$_2$ and PCO$_2$ = 40 mm Hg, it may be concluded that:

   a pH = 6.1 + log [(40–0.03)/(0.03)]
   b pH = 6.1 + log [(25–0.03)/(0.03)]
   c pH = 6.1 + log [(25–1.2)/(1.2)]
   d pH = 6.1 + log [(1.2)/(1.2–25)]

290 A 24-hour urine specimen (total volume = 1,136 mL) is submitted to the laboratory for quantitative urine protein. Calculate the amount of protein excreted per day, if the total protein is 52 mg/dL. *52 mg/dl = .52 mg/ml • 1,136 ml = 590.72*

(a) 591 mg
b 487 mg
c 220 mg
d 282 mg

291 The following results were obtained:

urine creatinine:	90 mg/dL (7956 μmol/L)
serum creatinine:	0.90 mg/dL (79.6 μmol/L)
patient's total body surface:	1.73 m² (average = 1.73 m²)
total urine volume in 24 hours:	1500 mL

* Given the above data, the patient's creatinine clearance, in mL/min, is:

(a) 104
b 124
c 144   *C = UV/P*
d 150

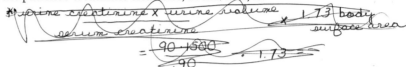

$$= \frac{90 \cdot 1500}{.90} \cdot 1.73$$

292 A 45-year-old male of average height and weight was admitted to the hospital for renal function studies. He had the following lab results:

urine creatinine:	120 mg/dL (10680 μmol/L)
serum creatinine:	1.5 mg/dL (132.6 μmol/L)
total urine volume in 24 hours:	1800/mL

Calculate the creatinine clearance for this patient in mL/min.

(a) 100
b 144
c 156
d 225

293 One international unit of enzyme activity is the amount of enzyme that will, under specified reaction conditions of substrate concentration, pH and temperature, cause utilization of substrate at the rate of:

a 1 mol/min
b 1 mmol/min
(c) 1 μmol/min
d 1 nmol/min

MLS ONLY

294 The bicarbonate and carbonic acid ratio is calculated from an equation by:

MLS ONLY

a Siggaard-Andersen
b Gibbs-Donnan
c Natelson
(d) Henderson-Hasselbalch

295 ^{125}I has a physical half-life of 60.0 days. A sample tested today had activity of 10,000 CPM/mL. How many days from today will the count be 1250 CPM/mL?

MLS ONLY

a 60
(b) 180
c 240
d 1250

296 In spectrophotometric determination, which of the following is the formula for calculating the absorbance of a solution?

MLS ONLY

   a (absorptivity × light path)/concentration
   b (absorptivity × concentration)/light path
   c absorptivity × light path × concentration   *or* $absorptivity = \dfrac{absorbance}{light\ path\ \times\ concentration}$
   d (light path × concentration)/absorptivity

297 Which of the following is the formula for calculating absorbance given the percent transmittance (%T) of a solution?

   a $1 - \log(\%T)$
   b $\log(\%T) \div 2$
   c $2 \times \log(\%T)$
   d $2 - \log(\%T)$

✳ ✳

298 Which of the following is the Henderson-Hasselbalch equation?

   a $pK_a = pH + \log([acid]/[salt])$
   b $pK_a = pH + \log([salt]/[acid])$
   c $pH = pK_a + \log([acid]/[salt])$
   d $pH = pK_a + \log([salt]/[acid])$

✳ ✳

299 The creatinine clearance (mL/min) is equal to:

   a urinary creatinine (mg/L)/[volume of urine (mL/min) × plasma creatinine (mg/L)]
   b [urinary creatinine (mg/L) × volume (mL/min)] ÷ plasma creatinine (mg/L)]
   c urinary creatinine (mg/L) ÷ [volume of urine (mL/hour) × plasma creatinine (mg/L)] ✳✳
   d [urinary creatinine (mg/L) × volume (mL/hour)] ÷ plasma creatinine (mg/L)

300 An adult diabetic with renal complications has the following results:

MLS ONLY

sodium:	133 mEq/L (133 mmol/L)
glucose:	487 mg/dL (26.8 mmol/L)
BUN:	84 mg/dL (30.0 mmol/L)
creatinine:	5 mg/dL (442.0 µmol/L)

On the basis of these results, the calculated serum osmolality is:

   a 266 mOsm/kg
   b 290 mOsm/kg
   c 323 mOsm/kg
   d 709 mOsm/kg

$V = \dfrac{\#}{1440}$

$C = \dfrac{UV}{P}$

$\dfrac{90 \cdot 1.04}{.90}$

$V = \dfrac{\#}{1440}$

(292) $\dfrac{1800}{1440} = 1.25$

$\dfrac{120 \cdot 1.25}{1.5} = 100$

301 Refer to the following illustration:

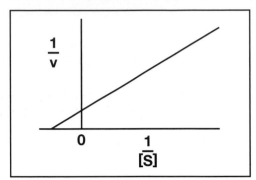

The above figure shows the reciprocal of the measured velocity of an enzyme reaction plotted against the reciprocal of the substrate concentration.

True statements about this figure include:

a   the intercept of the line on the abscissa (x-axis) can be used to calculate the V_{max}
b   the straight line indicates that the enzyme reaction proceeds according to zero order kinetics
c   the intercept on the abscissa (x-axis) can be used to calculate the Michaelis-Menten constant
d   the fact that the substrate concentration is plotted on both sides of the zero point indicates that the reaction is reversible

302 The following results were obtained in a creatinine clearance evaluation:

urine concentration:	84 mg/dL
urine volume:	1,440 mL/24 hr
serum concentration:	1.4 mg/dL
body surface area:	1.60 m² (average = 1.73 m²)

The creatinine clearance in mL/min is:

a   6
b   22
c   60
ⓓ   65

303 In the International System of Units, serum urea is expressed in millimoles per liter.

urea:	NH_2CONH_2
atomic weight:	N = 14, C = 12, O = 16, H = 1

A serum urea nitrogen concentration of 28 mg/dL would be equivalent to what concentration of urea?

a   4.7 mEq/L
b   5.0 mEq/L
c   10.0 mEq/L
d   20.0 mEq/L

304 The urea nitrogen concentration of a serum sample was measured to be 15 mg/dL.

urea:	NH_2CONH_2
atomic weight:	N = 14, C = 12, O = 16, H = 1

The urea concentration of the same sample, in mg/dL, is:

a   15
b   24
c   32
d   40

305 The osmol gap is defined as measured Osm/kg minus the calculated Osm/kg. Normally, the osmol gap is less than:

MLS
ONLY

  a   10
  b   20
  c   40
  d   60

306 Normally the bicarbonate concentration is about 24 mEq/L and the carbonic acid concentration is about 1.2; pK = 6.1, log 20 = 1.3. Using the equation pH = pK + log [salt]/[acid], calculate the pH.

  a   7.28
  b   7.38
  (c)   7.40   7.35 to 7.45
  d   7.42

$$6.1 + 1.3(24/1.2)$$

Instrumentation

307 Stray light can be detected in a spectrophotometer by utilizing a:

MLS
ONLY

  a   mercury vapor lamp
  b   holmium oxide glass
  c   potassium dichromate solution
  d   sharp cutoff filter

308 In the atomic absorption method for calcium, lanthanum is used:

MLS
ONLY

  a   as an internal standard
  b   to bind calcium
  c   to eliminate protein interference
  d   to prevent phosphate interference

309 Which of the following methods is susceptible to the solvent displacing effect that results in falsely decreased electrolyte values?

  (a)   indirect ion-selective electrodes
  b   direct ion-selective electrodes   *
  c   spectrophotometric
  d   fluorescence

310 Upon development of a thin-layer chromatogram for drug analysis all drug spots (including the standards) had migrated with the solvent front. The most probable cause for this would be:

MLS
ONLY

  a   environmental temperature too warm
  b   incorrect aqueous to nonaqueous solvent mixture
  c   too much sample applied
  d   chromatogram dried too quickly

311 To detect barbiturate abuse when analyzing urine specimens, immunoassay is the method of choice for screening. The method of choice for confirmation is:

  a   nephelometry
  b   thin-layer chromatography
  (c)   gas chromatography/mass spectrometry   * *
  d   ultraviolet absorption spectroscopy

312 Reverse phase high-performance liquid chromatography is being increasingly utilized in therapeutic drug monitoring. The term reverse phase implies that the column eluant is:

MLS
ONLY

  a   pumped up the column
  b   more polar than the stationary phase
  c   always nonpolar
  d   less polar than the stationary phase

313 When separating serum proteins by cellulose acetate electrophoresis, using Veronal ™ buffer at pH 8.6, beta globulin migrates:

   a faster than albumin
   b slower than gamma globulin
   c faster than gamma globulin
   d faster than alpha-2 globulin

*[handwritten: protein electrophoresis migration ** pH-8.6]*

314 Hemoglobin S can be separated from hemoglobin D by which of the following methods?

   a agar gel electrophoresis at pH 5.9
   b thin-layer chromatography
   c alkali denaturation
   d ammonium precipitation

315 What is the proper pH for the buffered solution used to perform serum protein electrophoresis?

   a 5.6
   b 7.6
   c 8.6   *
   d 9.6

316 The buffer pH most effective at allowing amphoteric proteins to migrate toward the cathode in an electrophoretic system would be:

   a 4.5
   b 7.5
   c 8.6
   d 9.5

317 On electrophoresis, transient bisalbuminemia or a grossly widened albumin zone is
MLS ONLY associated with:

   a dirty applicators
   b presence of therapeutic drugs in serum sample
   c endosmosis
   d prestaining with tracer dye

318 Which of the following serum proteins migrate with the beta-globulins on cellulose acetate at
MLS ONLY pH 8.6?

   a ceruloplasmin
   b hemoglobin
   c haptoglobin
   d C3 component of complement

319 An electrode has a silver/silver chloride anode and a platinum wire cathode. It is suspended in KCl solution and separated from the blood to be analyzed by a selectively permeable membrane. Such an electrode is used to measure which of the following?

   a pH
   b PCO_2
   c PO_2
   d HCO_3

*[handwritten: PO_2 = silver anode w/ KCl *]*

320 Hydrogen ion concentration (pH) in blood is usually determined by means of which of the following electrodes?

   a silver
   b glass= *pH* *
   c platinum
   d platinum-lactate

321 An automated method for measuring chloride which generates silver ions in the reaction is:

   a coulometry – *electrochemical; amount of electricity between two electrodes*
   b mass spectroscopy ⟩ *separation techniques*
   c chromatography
   d polarography – *electrochemical; measures current*

322 Coulometry is often used to measure:

   (a) chloride in sweat
   b the pH in saliva   ✳
   c bicarbonate in urine
   d ammonia in plasma | BLOOD GAS ANALYSIS |

323 In a pH meter reference electrodes may include:

   (a) silver-silver chloride
   b quinhydrone
   c hydroxide
   d hydrogen

324 Amperometry is the principle of the:
MLS ONLY
   a PCO_2 electrode
   (b) PO_2 electrode
   c pH electrode
   d Ionized calcium electrode

325 Most automated blood gas analyzers directly measure:

   a pH, HCO_3 and % O_2 saturation
   (b) pH, PCO_2 and PO_2 HCO_3 + TCO_2 *calculated*
   c HCO_3, PCO_2 and PO_2
   d pH, PO_2 and % O_2 saturation

326 Blood PCO_2 may be measured by:

   a direct colorimetric measurement of dissolved CO_2
   (b) a self-contained potentiometric electrode
   c measurement of CO_2-saturated hemoglobin   ✳
   d measurement of CO_2 consumed at the cathode

327 Valinomycin enhances the selectivity of the electrode used to quantitate:

   a sodium
   b chloride   *Valinomycin = potassium*
   (c) potassium
   d calcium

328 Which blood gas electrode is composed of silver/silver chloride reference electrode and glass?

   (a) PO_2
   b pH   ?
   (c) PCO_2 .
   d HCO_3

329 Most chemical methods for determining total protein utilize which of the following reactions?

   a molybdenum blue
   b ferri-ferrocyanide
   c resorcinol-HCl
   (d) biuret

330 Bromcresol purple at a pH of 5.2 is used in a colorimetric method to measure:

    ⓐ albumin
    b globulin
    c Bence Jones protein
    d immunoprotein

331 Magnesium carbonate is added in an iron binding capacity determination in order to:

    a allow color to develop
    b precipitate protein
    c bind with hemoglobin iron
    ⓓ remove excess unbound iron

332 The most specific method for the assay of glucose utilizes:

    ⓐ hexokinase
    b glucose oxidase
    c glucose-6-phosphatase
    d glucose dehydrogenase

333 Which of the following would be an example of a glucose-specific colorimetric method?
MLS
ONLY

    a alkaline ferricyanide
    b glucose oxidase
    c hexokinase
    d o-toluidine

334 Increased concentrations of ascorbic acid inhibit chromogen production in which of the following
MLS
ONLY glucose methods?

    a ferricyanide
    b ortho-toluidine
    c glucose oxidase (peroxidase)
    d hexokinase

335 In the hexokinase method for glucose determination, the actual end product measured is the:
MLS
ONLY

    a amount of hydrogen peroxide produced
    b NADH produced from the reduction of NAD
    c amount of glucose combined with bromcresol purple
    d condensation of glucose with an aromatic amine

336 Which of the following calcium procedures utilizes lanthanum chloride to eliminate interfering substances?

    a o-cresolphthalein complexone
    b precipitation with chloranilic acid
    c chelation with EDTA
    ⓓ atomic absorption spectrophotometry

337 Before unconjugated bilirubin can react with Ehrlich diazo reagent, which of the following must be added?

    a acetone
    b ether
    c distilled water
    ⓓ caffeine

338 The most widely used methods for bilirubin measurement are those based on the:

    a Jaffe reaction
    b Schales and Schales method
    c 8-hydroxyquinoline reaction
    ⓓ Jendrassik-Grof method

339 In the Malloy and Evelyn method for the determination of bilirubin, the reagent that is reacted with bilirubin to form a purple azobilirubin is:

  a dilute sulfuric acid
  b diazonium sulfate
  c sulfobromophthalein
  (d) diazotized sulfanilic acid

340 In the Jendrassik-Grof method for the determination of serum bilirubin concentration, quantitation is obtained by measuring the green color of:

  (a) azobilirubin
  b bilirubin glucuronide
  c urobilin
  d urobilinogen

341 In the Jendrassik-Grof reaction for total bilirubin, bilirubin reacts with diazotized sulfanilic acid to form:

  a diazo bilirubin
  b biliverdin
  (c) azobilirubin
  d bilirubin glucuronide

342 In the assay of lactate dehydrogenase, which of the following products is actually measured?

  (a) NADH
  b ATP
  c lactic acid
  d pyruvic acid

343 In the assay of lactate dehydrogenase (LD), the reaction is dependent upon which of the following coenzyme systems?

  (a) NAD/NADH
  b ATP/ADP
  c Fe^{++}/Fe^{+++}
  d Cu/Cu^{++}

344 Refer to the following illustration:

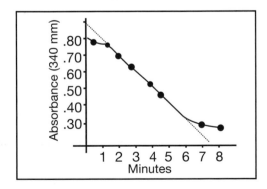

This illustration represents the change in absorbance at 340 nm over a period of 8 minutes in an assay for lactate dehydrogenase.

True statements about this figure include:

  a the reaction follows zero order kinetics between 5 and 8 minutes
  b the reaction is proceeding from lactate to pyruvate
  c nonlinearity after 6 minutes is due to substrate exhaustion
  d the change in absorbance is due to reduction of NAD to NADH

345 In competitive inhibition of an enzyme reaction, the:

MLS ONLY

   a inhibitor binds to the enzyme at the same site as does the substrate
   b inhibitor often has a chemical structure different to that of the substrate
   c activity of the reaction can be decreased by increasing the concentration of the substrate
   d activity of the reaction can be increased by decreasing the temperature

346 Refer to the following illustration:

MLS ONLY

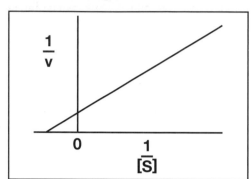

The figure above shows the reciprocal of the measured velocity of an enzyme reaction plotted against the reciprocal of the substrate concentration. True statements about this figure include:

   a the intercept of the line on the ordinate (y-axis) can be used to calculate the V_{max}
   b the straight line indicates that the enzyme reaction proceeds according to zero order kinetics
   c the intercept on the ordinate (y-axis) can be used to calculate the Michaelis-Menten constant
   d the fact the substrate concentration is plotted on both sides of the zero point indicates that the reaction is reversible

347 The International Federation for Clinical Chemistry (IFCC) recommends the use of methods such as the Bessey-Lowry-Brock method for determining alkaline phosphatase activity. The substrate used in this type of method is:

   a monophosphate
   b phenylphosphate
   c disodium phenylphosphate
   d para-nitrophenylphosphate

348 The illustration below represents a Lineweaver-Burk plot of 1/v vs 1/[S] in an enzyme reaction and the following assumptions should be made:

MLS ONLY

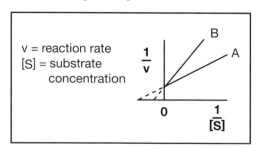

The enzyme concentration was the same for reactions A and B
The substrate concentration was in excess for reactions A and B
Reaction A occurred under ideal conditions

Which of the following statements about reaction B is true?

   a it illustrates noncompetitive inhibition
   b it illustrates competitive inhibition
   c it illustrates neither competitive nor noncompetitive inhibition
   d it could be the result of heavy metal contamination

349 Which of the following is a glycolytic enzyme that catalyzes the cleavage of fructose-1, 6-diphosphate to glyceraldehyde-3-phosphate and dihydroxyacetone phosphate?

   a aldolase
   b phosphofructokinase
   c pyruvate kinase
   d glucose-6-phosphate dehydrogenase

350 The substance that is measured to estimate the serum concentration of triglycerides by **most** methods is:

   a phospholipids
   (b) glycerol
   c fatty acids
   d pre-beta lipoprotein

351 Which of the following methods for quantitation of high-density lipoprotein is **most** suited for clinical laboratory use?

   a Gomori procedure
   (b) homogeneous
   c column chromatography
   d agarose gel electrophoresis

352 A chemiluminescent EIA:

   a measures absorption of light
   b is less sensitive than radioisotopic reactions
   c is monitored by the use of a gamma counter
   (d) is quantitated by the amount of light produced by the reaction

353 The osmolality of a urine or serum specimen is measured by a change in the:

   (a) freezing point
   b sedimentation point
   c midpoint
   d osmotic pressure

354 Which of the following applies to cryoscopic osmometry?

   (a) temperature at equilibrium is a function of the number of particles in solution
   b temperature plateau for a solution is horizontal
   c freezing point of a sample is absolute
   d initial freezing of a sample produces an immediate solid state

355 Assay of transketolase activity in blood is used to detect deficiency of:
MLS
ONLY
   a thiamine
   b folic acid
   c ascorbic acid
   d riboflavin

356 In amniotic fluid, the procedure used to detect Rh isosensitization is:
MLS
ONLY
   a human amniotic placental lactogen (HPL)
   b alpha-fetoprotein
   c measurement of absorbance at 450 nm
   d creatinine

Answer Key–Chemistry

1 d	59 a	117 b	175 a	233 b	291 a	349 a
2 c	60 b	118 b	176 d	234 d	292 a	350 b
3 a	61 c	119 c	177 c	235 d	293 c	351 b
4 b	62 c	120 d	178 a	236 b	294 d	352 d
5 b	63 b	121 b	179 c	237 d	295 b	353 a
6 c	64 b	122 b	180 d	238 c	296 c	354 a
7 b	65 a	123 a	181 b	239 c	297 d	355 a
8 d	66 a	124 b	182 a	240 c	298 d	356 c
9 b	67 a	125 c	183 d	241 a	299 b	
10 a	68 b	126 a	184 b	242 c	300 c	
11 d	69 c	127 d	185 b	243 b	301 c	
12 b	70 a	128 d	186 d	244 c	302 d	
13 d	71 d	129 b	187 b	245 b	303 c	
14 b	72 a	130 a	188 c	246 d	304 c	
15 c	73 b	131 c	189 d	247 d	305 a	
16 d	74 d	132 d	190 a	248 b	306 c	
17 c	75 b	133 c	191 c	249 a	307 d	
18 a	76 b	134 d	192 b	250 a	308 d	
19 d	77 a	135 a	193 c	251 d	309 a	
20 a	78 b	136 b	194 d	252 a	310 b	
21 d	79 c	137 d	195 d	253 d	311 c	
22 a	80 b	138 b	196 a	254 d	312 b	
23 a	81 c	139 b	197 c	255 c	313 c	
24 d	82 a	140 d	198 a	256 a	314 a	
25 a	83 a	141 a	199 c	257 c	315 c	
26 a	84 c	142 b	200 c	258 b	316 a	
27 a	85 d	143 d	201 c	259 a	317 b	
28 c	86 a	144 d	202 d	260 c	318 d	
29 a	87 d	145 c	203 b	261 d	319 c	
30 a	88 c	146 a	204 b	262 d	320 b	
31 b	89 d	147 c	205 a	263 d	321 a	
32 c	90 c	148 b	206 b	264 a	322 a	
33 a	91 a	149 b	207 b	265 c	323 a	
34 a	92 d	150 c	208 c	266 d	324 b	
35 d	93 b	151 b	209 d	267 d	325 b	
36 d	94 c	152 c	210 c	268 a	326 b	
37 a	95 b	153 b	211 b	269 b	327 c	
38 d	96 c	154 c	212 b	270 d	328 c	
39 c	97 b	155 d	213 d	271 c	329 d	
40 d	98 c	156 a	214 c	272 a	330 a	
41 b	99 c	157 b	215 b	273 a	331 d	
42 c	100 d	158 b	216 b	274 c	332 a	
43 c	101 d	159 d	217 b	275 c	333 b	
44 d	102 c	160 a	218 d	276 c	334 c	
45 b	103 b	161 b	219 d	277 b	335 b	
46 c	104 d	162 b	220 a	278 a	336 d	
47 c	105 c	163 a	221 b	279 a	337 d	
48 b	106 d	164 d	222 b	280 d	338 d	
49 c	107 a	165 a	223 b	281 b	339 d	
50 c	108 b	166 d	224 a	282 a	340 a	
51 d	109 a	167 d	225 b	283 a	341 c	
52 c	110 d	168 d	226 a	284 b	342 a	
53 d	111 c	169 a	227 b	285 d	343 a	
54 d	112 d	170 b	228 d	286 d	344 c	
55 d	113 d	171 b	229 d	287 d	345 a	
56 a	114 c	172 a	230 a	288 c	346 a	
57 b	115 b	173 a	231 a	289 c	347 d	
58 d	116 d	174 c	232 d	290 a	348 b	

Carbohydrates

1   **d**   Diagnosis of hypoglycemia in adults.
[Tietz 2006, p864]

2   **c**   Body fluid glucose reference ranges.
[Tietz 2006, pp871-872]

3   **a**   GTT diet preparation.
[Tietz 2006, p860]

4   **b**   Normal 2-hour postprandial value.
[Tietz 2006, p859]

5   **b**   Ratio of CSF glucose to blood glucose.
[Tietz 2006, pp871-872]

6   **c**   Use of partial GTT information.
[Tietz 2006, p859]

7   **b**   Effect of glycolysis on glucose.
[Tietz 2006, p869]

8   **d**   Unequivocal diagnosis of diabetes mellitus.
[Tietz 2006, p859]

9   **b**   Age effect on glucose.
[Tietz 2006, p460]

10   **a**   Factors contributing to FBS.
[Tietz 2006, p843]

11   **d**   Gestational diabetes.
[Tietz 2006, p843]

12   **b**   Arterial vs venous glucose values.
[Tietz 2006, p869]

13   **d**   Definition of glycolysis.
[Tietz 2006, p843]

14   **b**   Diagnosis of diabetes mellitus.
[Tietz 2006, p859]

15   **c**   Definition of glycated hemoglobin.
[Tietz 2006, p879]

16   **d**   Average glucose over time is best predictor.
[Tietz 2006, p879]

17   **c**   Role of fructosamine.
[Tietz 2006, p884]

18   **a**   Interpretation of glycated hemoglobin.
[Tietz 2006, p879]

19   **d**   Hgb A_{1C} structure.
[Tietz 2006, p879]

20   **a**   Glycated hemoglobin directly related to life of RBC.
[Tietz 2006, p880]

21   **d**   Interference Hgb A_{1C}.
[Tietz 2006, p882]

22   **a**   Acetone in carbohydrate metabolism.
[Tietz 2006, p876]

23   **a**   Copper reduction reaction detects many reducing substances.
[Bishop 2005, p275]

24   **d**   Products of glycolysis.
[Tietz 2006, p842]

25   **a**   Diagnosis of lactase deficiency.
[Tietz 2006, p1863]

Acid-Base Balance

26   **a**   Reduced excretion of acids.
[Tietz 2006, p1768]

27   **a**   Excessive loss of bicarbonate.
[Tietz 2006, p1768]

28   **c**   Diseases causing respiratory acidosis.
[Tietz 2006, p1774]

29   **a**   Blood gas instrumentation.
[Tietz 2006, p1009]

30   **a**   Diseases causing respiratory acidosis.
[Tietz 2006, p1774]

31   **b**   Normal ratio bicarbonate/carbonic acid.
[Tietz 2006, pp1759-1760]

32   **c**   Arterial pH reference range.
[Tietz 2006, p2289]

33   **a**   Interpretation of metabolic acidosis.
[Tietz 2006, p1772]

34   **a** HCO_3 and TCO_2 in metabolic alkalosis.
[Tietz 2006, p1774]

35   **d**   Levels of CO_2 and pH in metabolic alkalosis.
[Tietz 2006, p1774]

36   **d**   Component levels in metabolic acidosis.
[Tietz 2006, p1772]

37   **a**   Definition of respiratory acidosis.
[Tietz 2006, p1774]

38   **d**   Respiratory alkalosis caused by hyperventilation.
[Tietz 2006, p1775]

39   **c**   Chemical cause of alkalosis and acidosis.
[Tietz 2006, p1760]

40   **d**   Blood gas sample conditions.
[Tietz 2006, p1007]

41   **b**   Electrolyte/blood gas values in respiratory acidosis.
[Tietz 2006, p1775]

42   **c**   Best test for renal tubular function.
[Tietz 2006, pp821-822]

43   **c**   Osmolality empirical calculation.
[Tietz 2006, p992]

44   **d**   Kidney concentration determination.
[Tietz 2006, p992]

45   **b**   Definition of osmolal gap.
[Tietz 2006, p992]

Electrolytes

46   **c**   Most important buffer pair in plasma.
[Tietz 2006, p1759]

47   **c**   Ion selective electrode standard Na/K.
[Tietz 2006, p986]

48   **b**   Components of anion gap.
[Tietz 2006, pp1768-1771]

49   **c**   Effect of K^+ from platelets on serum K.
[Tietz 2006, p985]

50   **c**   Major component of CO_2 in blood.
[Tietz 2006, p1759]

51   **d**   Anion gap, lactic acidosis.
[Tietz 2006, pp1768-1771]

52   **c**   Calculation of anion gap.
[Tietz 2006, p1768]

53   **d**   Maintenance of buffering capacity of blood.
[Tietz 2006, p1761]

54   **d**   Compensatory mechanism in respiratory acidosis.
[Tietz 2006, p1774]

55   **d**   Cation in osmotic pressure.
[Tietz 2006, p992]

56   **a**   Effect of hemolysis on K.
[Tietz 2006, p985]

57   **b**   Largest solute in osmolality.
[Tietz 2006, p992]

58   **d**   Reference range sweat chloride.
[Tietz 2006, p2260]

59   **a**   Direct ISE method.
[Tietz 2006, pp987-988]

60   **b**   Interferences with indirect ISE methods.
[Tietz 2006, p987]

61   **c**   Interferences with indirect ISE methods.
[Tietz 2006, p987]

62   **c**   Protein-bound Ca^{++}.
[Tietz 2006, p1893]

63   **b**   Regulation of Ca^{++}.
[Tietz 2006, pp1891-1892]

64   **b**   Regulation of Ca^{++} and PO_{43}^- metabolism.
[Tietz 2006, pp1891-1892]

65   **a**   Hyperparathyroidism.
[Tietz 2006, pp1895-1896]

66   **a**   Tetany and calcium.
[Tietz 2006, p1893]

67   **a**   Tetany and magnesium.
[Tietz 2006, p1910]

68   **b**   Reciprocal relationship of Ca^{++} and phosphate.
[Tietz 2006, p1914]

69   **c**   Regulation of phosphate.
[Tietz 2006, p1914]

70   **a**   Most common cause of low phosphate.
[Tietz 2006, p1906]

71   **d**   Laboratory results in hyperthyroidism.
[Tietz 2006, pp1895, 1906]

Proteins and Other Nitrogen-Containing Compounds

72   **a**   Physiological feature of albumin.
[Tietz 2006, p546]

73 MLS ONLY   **b**   Abnormal accumulation of serous fluid due to an imbalance of fluid production and reabsorption. Fluid/serum protein ratio >0.5.
[Henry 2006, p441]

74   **d**   Basic principle of lab procedure timed urine.
[Kaplan 2003, p1098]

75 MLS ONLY   **b**   Spectral interference.
[Henry 2006, p428]

76 MLS ONLY   **b**   Principle of protein electrophoresis.
[Kaplan 2003, pp203-206]

77 MLS ONLY   **a**   Principle of protein electrophoresis.
[Tietz 2006, p548]

78 MLS ONLY   **b**   Concentration of albumin in serum.
[Kaplan 2003, p214]

79 MLS ONLY   **c**   Principle of biuret reaction.
[Tietz 2006, p586]

80 MLS ONLY   **b**   Principle of protein electrophoresis.
[Kaplan 2003, p214]

81 **c** Principle of electrophoresis on cellulose acetate.
MLS ONLY
[Kaplan 2003, p204]

82 **a** Separation based on charge.
MLS ONLY
[Kaplan 2003, p204]

83 **a** Biochemistry and structure of amino acids.
MLS ONLY
[Tietz 2006, p534]

84 **c** Abnormal metabolism of amino acids.
MLS ONLY
[Tietz 2006, p534]

85 **d** Loss of normal physiologic fluid balance.
MLS ONLY
[Henry 2006, p236]

86 **a** A ratio and proportion procedure is most useful for calculations in which concentrations are not changed, as in this case. Set up a ratio of total area (180) to gamma globulin area (30) in units, and total protein content (6.5) to gamma globulin content (x) in g/dL. Solve for x.
[Campbell 1997, p126]

87 **d** Elevated polyclonal gamma-globulins with beta-gamma bridging due to increased IgA.
MLS ONLY
[Henry 2006, p241]

88 **c** Due to loss of albumin in nephrotic syndrome, increased alpha-2 is a compensatory mechanism.
MLS ONLY
[Henry 2006, p237]

89 **d** Clinical correlation, deficiency of proteinase inhibitor.
MLS ONLY
[Henry 2006, p236]

90 **c** Abnormal protein of a malignant plasma cell.
MLS ONLY
[Henry 2006, p241]

91 **a** Abnormal liver function.
MLS ONLY
[Henry 2006, p241]

92 **d** Physical-chemical property.
MLS ONLY
[Henry 2006, p400]

93 **b** Anticoagulant prevents clotting.
MLS ONLY
[Henry 2006, p242]

94 **c** Effect of charge on cellulose acetate.
MLS ONLY
[Kaplan 2003, p206]

95 **b** Acute phase reactants.
MLS ONLY
[Henry 2006, p241]

96 **c** Immunoglobulin response in inflammation.
MLS ONLY
[Henry 2006, p241]

97 **b** Clinical correlation, autoimmune immunoglobulin G.
MLS ONLY
[Henry 2006, p242]

98 **c** Monoclonal free kappa or lambda light chains.
MLS ONLY
[Henry 2006, p400]

99 **c** Transport function of transferrin.
[Kaplan 2003,, p662]

100 **d** Principle of method of analysis.
[Tietz 2006, p1188]

101 **d** Diurnal variation of iron metabolism.
MLS ONLY
[Kaplan 2003, p662]

102 **c** Ineffective erythropoiesis, high iron turnover.
MLS ONLY
[Tietz 2006, p1190]

103 **b** Features of iron deficiency anemia.
MLS ONLY
[Tietz 2006, p1190]

104 **d** Features of iron overload hemochromatosis.
MLS ONLY
[Tietz 2006, p1190]

105 **c** Specimen requirements for analyte stability.
[Bishop 2005, p232]

106 **d** Specimen requirements for analyte stability.
[Bishop 2005, p232]

107 **a** Hyperammonemia to detect encephalopathy.
MLS ONLY
[Henry 2006, p266]

108 **b** Creatinine measurement. Kidney function test.
[Tietz 2006, p798]

109 **a** Dilutions. Laboratory calculation.
MLS ONLY
[Bishop 2005, p23]

110 **d** Correlation of disease and test result.
MLS ONLY
[Kaplan 2003, p448]

111 **c** Metabolic product of protein catabolism.
MLS ONLY
[Tietz 2006, p801]

112 **d** Description of the Jaffe reaction for creatinine.
MLS ONLY
[Tietz 2006, p798]

113 **d** Glomerular filtration rate is estimated by filtration markers such as creatinine clearance.
[Tietz 2006, p822]

114 **c** Abnormal results correlate with abnormal kidney function.
[Tietz 2006, pp801-803]

115 **b** Maternal urine instead of amniotic fluid.
MLS ONLY
[Bishop 2005, p556]

116 **d** Metabolism of purine bases.
MLS ONLY
[Bishop 2005, p484]

Answers–Chemistry

117 **b**   Retinol is one of the 3 biologically active
MLS   forms of fat-soluble vitamin A.
ONLY
[Kaplan 2003, p570]

118 **b**   Troponin complex (TIC triple complex)
MLS   consists of T, I and C.
ONLY
[Kaplan 2003, pp569-570]

119 **c**   Acute phase protein increased
MLS   in inflammation.
ONLY
[Bishop 2005, p198]

120 **d** β Oligoclonal proteins are produced
MLS   in multiple sclerosis and other
ONLY   demyelinating diseases.
[Bishop 2005, p562]

121 **b**   Structural definition of a peptide bond.
[Kaplan 2003, p1027]

122 **b**   Function of ceruloplasmin.
[Bishop 2005, p196]

123 **a**   Alpha-fetoprotein is the embryonic
MLS   form of albumin.
ONLY
[Kaplan 2003, p934]

124 **b**   Normal CSF includes prealbumin, the
MLS   fraction at 4.5%.
ONLY
[Henry 2006, p1415]

125 **c**   Other distractors are causes of B_{12}
MLS   deficiency.
ONLY
[Tietz 2006, p1105]

126 **a**   Biochemistry of absorption.
MLS   [Tietz 2006, p1101]
ONLY

127 **d**   Correlation of disease and prenatal
MLS   screening test.
ONLY
[Kaplan 2003, p934]

Heme Derivatives

128 **d**   Principle of the test reaction.
MLS   [Kaplan 2003, p536]
ONLY

129 **b**   Hemoglobin metabolism.
MLS   [Kaplan 2003, p497]
ONLY

130 **a**   Comparative mobilities due to
structures of Hgb variants.
[Henry 2006, p524]

131 **c**   Comparative mobilities due to
structures of Hgb variants.
[Henry 2006, p522]

132 **d**   Physical-chemical property of Hgb F.
MLS   [Henry 2006, p521]
ONLY

133 **c**   Light-exposed bilirubin is oxidized
(structurally altered).
[Bishop 2005, p483]

134 **d**   Biochemical pathway of bilirubin.
[Tietz 2006, p1195]

135 **a**   Principle of diazo reaction with
MLS   unconjugated bilirubin.
ONLY
[Tietz 2006, p1196]

136 **b**   Total bilirubin = (direct) conjugated
MLS   bilirubin + (indirect) unconjugated bilirubin
ONLY   3.1 – 2.0 = 1.1.
[Tietz 2006, p1196]

137 **d**   Principle of diazo reaction with
MLS   conjugated bilirubin.
ONLY
[Tietz 2006, p1197]

138 **b**   Light-exposed bilirubin is oxidized
(structurally altered).
[Bishop 2005, p483]

139 **b**   Light-exposed bilirubin is oxidized
(structurally altered).
[Bishop 2005, p483]

140 **d**   Metabolism of bilirubin in
MLS   the hepatocytes.
ONLY
[Tietz 2006, p1195]

141 **a**   Intrahepatic biliary atresia; conjugated
MLS   hyperbilirubinemia.
ONLY
[Tietz 2006, p1201]

142 **b**   Definition of kernicterus.
[Tietz 2006, p1201]

143 **d**   Correlation of disorder and abnormal
MLS   metabolism of bilirubin.
ONLY
[Tietz 2006, p1199]

144 **d**   Hepatocellular disorder and highly
MLS   elevated AST.
ONLY
[Henry 2006, pp273-275.

145 **c**   Post-hepatic biliary obstruction;
MLS   increased alkaline phosphatase.
ONLY
[Henry 2006, p275]

146 **a**   Bleeding from upper GI.
[Henry 2006, p272]

147 **c**   Bile pigments (uro-, meso-, stercobilin)
MLS   in feces.
ONLY
[Tietz 2006, p1195]

148 **b**   Correlation of disorder and high RBC
MLS   zinc protoporphyrin.
ONLY
[Kaplan 2003, p669]

149 **b**   Normal Hgb is changed to abnormal
MLS   derivative CO-Hgb.
ONLY
[Tietz 2006, p1296]

150 **c**   CO prevents heme iron from binding
MLS ONLY   with oxygen.
[Tietz 2006, p1296]

151 **b**   Deficiency of ALA synthase which
MLS ONLY   catalyzes the 1st step of porphyrin
synthesis.
[Tietz 2006, p1215]

152 **c**   Rapid initial screening should precede
MLS ONLY   complex testing.
[Tietz 2006, p1224]

153 **b**   Other distractors are not enzymes
MLS ONLY   affected by lead.
[Tietz 2006, p1211]

154 **c**   Haptoglobin phenotyping for rare
MLS ONLY   deficiency states.
[Tietz 2006, p561]

Enzymes

155 **d**   There is an increase in the serum levels
of amylase and lipase in acute pancreatitis.
However, the elevated level of lipase persists
longer than amylase. Elevated levels of
lipase and amylase are seen in other intra
abdominal conditions, but the frequency of
elevations is less with lipase than amylase.
[Bishop 2005, pp256-258]

156 **a**   Amylase and lipase are hydrolases
involved in the breakdown of starch and
glycogen, and lipid metabolism, respectively.
Both enzymes are primarily located in
the pancreas. Disorders of the pancreas
are characterized by elevated levels of the
enzymes. 5'-NT, GGT, AST and LD are
elevated in liver and hepatobiliary diseases.
[Bishop 2005, pp256-258]

157 **b**   In the amyloclastic, saccharogenic and
chromogenic methods for measurement of
amylase, the substrate, starch is converted
to glucose and maltose.
[Bishop 2005, p257]

158 **b**   Macroamylasemia is an asymptomatic
MLS ONLY   condition which results when the amylase
molecule and immunoglobulins combine to
form a complex. The complex is too large to
be filtered across the glomerulus. Lack of
renal clearance leads to an increased serum
amylase and a decreased urine amylase.
[Bishop 2005, p256]

159 **d**   Amylase is present primarily in the
pancreas. Pancreatitis results in the release
of the enzyme into the serum. Creatinine
is a nonprotein nitrogenous substance
and is measured for renal function. Beta-
hydroxybutyrate is measured for diabetic
acidosis and LD isoenzymes are evaluated
for disorders involving the heart and liver.
[Bishop 2005, p256]

160 **a**   Aspartate aminotransferase (AST) is
involved in the transfer of an amino group
between aspartate and alpha-keto acids. AST
is present in several tissues, with its highest
concentrations in cardiac tissue, liver and
skeletal muscle. Depending on the type of
liver disease, the levels may be 100× the
upper limits of normal (ULN).
[Bishop 2005, p250]

161 **b**   Aspartate aminotransferase (AST)
belongs to the class of transferase enzymes.
Specifically, AST catalyzes the transfer
of an amino group from aspartate to
alpha-ketoglutarate forming oxaloacetate
and glutamate.
[Bishop 2005, p250]

162 **b**   The transferases, alanine
aminotransferase (ALT) and AST are located
primarily in the liver. Elevated serum levels
of the enzymes are seen in hepatocellular
disorders. The levels may be 100 times
the upper limit of normal. The ALT level
is usually higher than AST. Increased
levels of AST are also seen in infectious
mononucleosis and muscular dystrophy, but
ALT is not elevated in the clinical disorders.
[Bishop 2005, pp250-251]

163 **a**   AST and ALT levels are the highest in
acute hepatocellular conditions, specifically
acute viral hepatitis. The levels may be 100
times the upper limit of normal. Slight
increases of the aminotranferases are seen in
cirrhosis and metastatic hepatic carcinoma.
[Bishop 2005, pp251, 485]

164 **d**   In the coupled reaction of AST
MLS ONLY   measurement, malate dehydrogenase
catalyzes the oxidation of oxaloacetate to
malate in the indicator reaction.
[Bishop 2005, p250]

165 **a**   In acute hepatocellular disorders, the
MLS ONLY   serum levels of AST and ALT can be 100
times the upper limit of normal. Slight
increases of the enzyme activities are seen
in chronic hepatitis, hemangioma, and
obstructive jaundice.
[Bishop 2005, p250, 485]

166 d Elevated serum levels of LD up to 50 times the upper limit of normal are seen with pernicious anemia. The ineffective erythropoiesis results in the release of large quantities of LD1 and LD2. Increased levels of LD1 and LD2 may be seen in renal disease, but the increase is not as great as for pernicious anemia. Slight increases of LD3 are seen in pulmonary conditions and pancreatitis.
[Bishop 2005, p249]

167 d Creatine kinase (CK) catalyzes the reversible phosphorylation of creatine. The highest levels of the enzyme are found in skeletal muscle, heart muscle and brain tissue. Increased serum enzyme activity is present in diseases involving the listed muscles and tissue. Lipase is measured for acute pancreatitis; the transaminase and lactate dehydrogenase (LD) are not markedly increased in muscular dystrophy.
[Bishop 2005, p244]

168 d Lactate dehydrogenase (LD) catalyzes the interconversion of lactic and pyruvic acids. Electrophoretically, using agarose or cellulose acetate medium, LD can be separated into 5 isoenzymes, LD1-LD5. CK and lipase have 3 isoenzymes; AST has 2.
[Bishop 2005, pp248-249]

169 a Erythrocytes contain 150 times more LD activity than serum, mostly LD1 and LD2. Rupture of the RBC membranes as in hemolysis will elevate the serum level of the enzyme. LD5 is increased in liver disorders and drug toxicity if the liver is involved.
[Bishop 2005, p250]

170 b The 3 CK isoenzymes are CK1 or CKBB, CK2 or CKMB, CK3 or CKMM. CKMB is primarily located in myocardial tissue. Damage to the myocardial will cause an elevation of the CKMB level.
[Burtis 2001, p357]

171 b Creatine kinase (CK) is located in brain tissue and heart and skeletal muscle. Diseases involving the tissue site will increase the level of the enzyme activity. CK activity is not increased in hepatitis.
[Burtis 2001, p357]

172 a Elevations of serum LD4 and LD5 fractions are seen in liver and skeletal muscle diseases because the isoenzymes are located in the tissues. LD1 and LD2 are elevated in hemolytic anemia and myocardial infarction. Increased levels of LD3 are observed in pulmonary edema.
[Burtis 2001, pp364-365]

173 a After an acute myocardial infarction (AMI), CK activity increases 4-6 hours after the symptoms, peaks at 12-24 hours and returns to normal within 48-72 hours. AST increases 6-8 hours after the infarction. Elevated levels of LD are noted 12-24 hours after the symptoms. ALT activity does not increase with a AMI.
[Bishop 2005, pp246, 248, 250]

174 c Although, CKMB activity is more specific for the myocardium, CKMM is present in both the skeletal and heart muscles. An increase of the isoenzyme activity may occur after a AMI. Only one peak would be present for a brain tumor and muscular dystrophy; no peaks would be present for hepatitis since the liver is not a tissue source of CK.
[Burtis 2001, p689]

175 a The major LDH isoenzymes in the
MLS ONLY serum of healthy persons are LD2, accounting for 29%-39% of the total activity and LD1=14%-26% of enzyme activity. In a myocardial infarction the pattern is changed. The activity of LD1 is greater than LD2. The ratio of LD1 to LD2 is >1. The normal ratio is 0.45-0.74.
[Burtis 2001, p365]

176 d LD4 and LD5 isoenzymes are located
MLS ONLY in the liver and skeletal muscle. LD5 is the predominate fraction in these tissues. Elevated levels of LD5 are seen with intrahepatic disorders. LD1 and LD2 are elevated in hemolytic anemia and myocardial infarction. LD3 fraction is increased with a pulmonary infarction.
[Bishop 2005, pp248-249]

177 c Increased levels of aldolase and CK are seen with skeletal muscle disease. The magnitude of the elevation is dependent on the type of skeletal muscle disease.
[Burtis 2001, pp357-359]

178 a In the immunoinhibition technique for CKMB determination, antibodies are directed against the M and B units of the enzymes. Anti-M inhibits all M activity but not B activity. CK activity is measured before and after inhibition. The activity remaining after inhibition is a result of the B subunit for BB and MB activity.
[Burtis 2001, p361]

179 c Of the 3 CK isoenzymes, CKMB is located in the myocardial. The fraction is elevated with an acute myocardial infarction (AMI). CKMM is elevated in acute muscular stress following strenuous exercise. CKBB is increased in brain injury.
[Burtis 2001, pp357-359]

180 d The LD isoenzymes as a percentage of total LD activity are LD1: 14%-26%, LD2: 29%-39%, LD3: 20%-26%, LD4: 8%-16% and LD5: 6%-16%. The scan indicates the fraction LD5 is increased. Elevated levels of LD5 are seen with viral hepatitis.
[Burtis 2001, pp362-365]

181 b The LD1 and LD2 fractions are increased in hemolytic anemia due to the intramedullary hemolysis. LD5 is increased with hepatic damage. LD3 may be increased with acute pancreatitis. The LD isoenzyme pattern in renal disease is very similar to a normal pattern except for the higher absolute values.
[Burtis 2001, pp362-363]

182 a Elevation of the levels of CK and AST is seen in muscle damage due to the crush injury to the thigh. AST levels can increase up to 4-8 times the upper limit of normal. Cerebrovascular accident and pulmonary infarction have increased CKBB levels. In acute hepatitis, the AST level may be 100 times the upper limit of normal.
[Bishop 2005, p244, 250]

183 d Obstructive jaundice is characterized by an increased ALP—3 times the upper limit of normal—and a marked increase in GGT. The aminotransferases are slightly elevated owing to the fact that they are sensitive for acute hepatocellular conditions.
[Bishop 2005, p252, 255]

184 b Chronic hepatitis is a chronic inflammation of the hepatocytes that persists for at least 6 months. The serum enzyme levels may be variable depending on the condition. ALT, AST and ALP may be increased by 2 times the upper limit of normal. GGT is slightly increased.
[Bishop 2005, pp490-491]

185 b The heat activation method of ALP isoenzyme separation involves heating an aliquot of the serum sample at 56°C for 10 minutes. An untreated aliquot of the sample along with the heated one are assayed for ALP activity.
[Burtis 2001, p368]

186 d The Regan isoenzyme is an abnormal ALP isoenzyme. The carcinoplacental ALP has properties similar to the placental enzyme, in that it is also heat stable (65°C, 30 min). It has been detected in lung, breast, ovarian and colon cancer.
[Burtis 2001, p368]

187 b The major serum ALP isoenzymes are located in the liver, bone, intestine and placenta. Placenta ALP is most heat stable followed by the intestinal, liver and bone fractions in decreasing order of stability.
[Bishop 2005, p252]

188 c GGT levels are elevated in alcoholism. The levels may range from 2-3 times the upper limit of normal. ALT, AST, and ALP may be increased depending on the alcohol damage to the liver.
[Bishop 2005, p255]

189 d Isoenzymes are multiple forms of an enzyme that possess the ability to catalyze a reaction, but differ in structure. For enzymes located in many tissue sites, an increased total enzyme activity cannot be associated with a specific clinical disorder. However, since the isoenzyme fractions are located in various tissue sources, measurement of the different fractions are considered a more specific indicator of various disorders than total levels.
[Burtis 2001, pp160-161]

190 a The holoenzyme is the active system formed by a protein portion called the apoenzyme and a cofactor which can be an activator if inorganic and a coenzyme if organic.
[Bishop 2005, p237]

191 c Approximately 20%-30% of the seminal fluid is prostatic fluid. The composition of the prostatic fluid is acid phosphatase, citric acid, and proteolytic enzymes. The activity of prostatic acid phosphatase may be measured in seminal fluid for medicolegal cases involving rape.
[Strasinger 2008, p200]

192 b
MLS ONLY Thymolphthalein monophosphate is the most specific substrate of choice for quantitative endpoint reactions; however, p-nitrophenylphosphate is the preferred substrate for continuous monitoring.
[Burtis 2001, p383]

193 c
MLS ONLY All of the enzymes are dehydrogenases which are oxidoreductases. The oxidoreductases catalyze oxidation reduction reaction between 2 substrates. The enzymes may be located in the liver and the heart; however, the enzymes are in class 1 and not class 3 according to the Enzyme Commission of the IUB system.
[Bishop 2005, p237]

Lipids and Lipoproteins

194 d
MLS ONLY High-density lipoprotein (HDL) is the smallest and most dense lipoprotein. Its role in lipid metabolism involves removing cholesterol from the peripheral cells and transporting it to the liver for further metabolism. Because of these actions, HDL is thought to be anti-atherogenic. Increased levels of LDL, VLDL and chylomicrons are associated with atherosclerosis.
[Bishop 2005, p287]

195 d
MLS ONLY Serum HDL has been routinely measured indirectly by a 2-step procedure. Precipitation of all of the non-HDL lipoproteins with a polyanion-divalent cation combination reagent and centrifugation to obtain the supernatant containing only HDL. The cholesterol bound to HDL is measured as HDL. One challenge regarding the method has been the selection of a precipitating reagent that would precipitate the apoB containing lipoproteins. Dextran sulfate with magnesium has proven to be very effective.
[Burtis 2001, p487]

196 a
MLS ONLY In the indirect measurement of LDL using the Friedewald equation, values are needed for the total cholesterol, HDL cholesterol and triglyceride. Because LDL and HDL are measured based on their cholesterol content, it is necessary to determine the total cholesterol and HDL cholesterol using the same cholesterol procedure.
[Burtis 2001, p488]

197 c
MLS ONLY High-density lipoprotein (HDL) is the smallest and most dense of the lipoproteins. This is evidenced by its lipid content of 20% and protein concentration of 50%.
[Bishop 2005, p286]

198 a
MLS ONLY Familial hypercholesterolemia is a genetic condition characterized by elevated serum cholesterol levels. In homozygotes and heterozygotes, the elevated cholesterol is associated with an increased LDL level. The lack or deficiency of the LDL receptors prevents the metabolism of LDL cholesterol, resulting in an increased LDL level.
[Bishop 2005, p295]

199 c
MLS ONLY Atherosclerosis is characterized by a thickening and hardening of the arterial walls by cholesterol plaques in the lining of the arteries. Elevated levels of cholesterol are associated with the development of the plaques. One of the roles of LDL is to transport cholesterol esters to the cells for metabolism. Elevated LDL levels are also associated with development of atherosclerosis.
[Bishop 2005, p502]

200 c
MLS ONLY Low-density lipoprotein (LDL) transports about 70% of the total plasma cholesterol. HDL transports only 30% of the cholesterol. Chylomicrons and VLDL transport triglycerides.
[Burtis 2001, p475]

201 c
MLS ONLY Tangier disease results from a defect in the catabolism of Apo A-I, an essential apoprotein for HDL. In homozygotes, the plasma level for HDL is practically zero. The reduced HDL levels result from increased HDL catabolism.
[Burtis 2001, p483]

202 d Lipid analysis using overnight refrigeration involves incubating the sample at 4°C overnight. The chylomicrons, present as a thick homogenous cream layer, may be observed floating at the plasma surface.
[Kaplan 2003, p625]

203 **b**   Food intake can cause a transient
MLS
ONLY increase in the triglyceride level by 50%.
The LDL and HDL levels may be decreased
by 10%-15 % depending on the fat content
of the meal.
[Burtis 2001, p489]

204 **b**   Tay-Sachs disease is a rare inherited
MLS
ONLY disorder characterized by the near-total
deficiency of the enzyme N-acetyl-
beta-hexosaminidase A. The enzyme
is responsible for the hydrolysis of the
beta (1,4)-glycosidic bond between
N-acetylgalactosamine and galactose in
GM2 ganglioside. Neimann-Pick disease and
Hurler's syndrome are lysosomal disorders
as is Tay-Sachs. Phenylketonuria results
from an absent enzyme, but is an inborn
error of metabolism.
[Burtis 2001, pp931-932]

205 **a**   The historical method to evaluate fetal
MLS
ONLY lung maturity is the lecithin/sphingomyelin
(L/S) ratio. Measurement of pulmonary
surfactant is done to evaluate fetal lung
maturity. Lecithin is the major component
of the lung surfactant. Sphingomyelin, a
non-lung phospholipid, has no role in the
surfactant system. It serves as a control
for the increase in lecithin that occurs
around the 34-36th week of gestation.
Other amniotic fluid evaluations include
measurement of creatinine for fetal age;
alpha-fetoprotein for neural tube disorder
and absorbance at 450nm-bilirubin for
fetal distress.
[Strasinger 2008, p240. [Burtis 2001, p919]

206 **b**   The scan shows an increase in the
MLS
ONLY phospholipids concentrations around
the 34-36th week of gestation. The
phospholipids are produced by the Type II
cells of the alveolar of the lungs.
[Bishop 2005, p557]

207 **b**   Mixed hyperlipoproteinemia or type
MLS
ONLY V hyperlipoproteinemia occurs primarily
in adulthood and is characterized by
markedly elevated triglycerides, elevated
very low-density lipoproteins (VLDL)
and chylomicrons. Because of the
markedly increased triglyceride level, the
specimen integrity is milky, and overnight
refrigeration shows a creamy layer over
turbid serum due to the chylomicrons
and triglycerides.
[Kaplan 2003, p623]

208 **c**   Lipoprotein lipase hydrolyzes
triglycerides and chylomicrons during
normal lipid metabolism. A deficiency
in lipoprotein lipase results in markedly
increased serum chylomicrons
and triglycerides.
[Burtis 2001, p481]

209 **d**   In the endogenous pathway for lipid
MLS
ONLY metabolism the hepatocytes can synthesize
triglycerides from carbohydrates and
fatty acids. The triglycerides are packaged
in VLDL, and ultimately delivered to
the circulation in that form. Exogenous
triglycerides are transported primarily by
chylomicrons. HDL transports cholesterol
from peripheral cells to the liver. LDL
transports cholesterol and phospholipids to
peripheral cells.
[Bishop 2005, pp288-289]

210 **c**   Elevated levels of chylomicrons in serum
or plasma will result in a turbid specimen.
The large size of the chylomicron will reflect
the light, causing a turbid appearance.
[Bishop 2005, p286]

Endocrinology and Tumor Markers

211 **b**   TSH produced by pituitary gland.
[Bishop 2005, p448]

212 **b**   Increased TSH, decreased free T_4 and
total T_4, positive microsomal Ab consistent
with primary hypothyroidism.
[Bishop 2005, pp449-451]

213 **d**   Increased TSH, decreased free
T_4 and total T_4, symptoms of cold
intolerance and hair loss are consistent
with hypothyroidism.
[Bishop 2005, pp449-451]

214 **c** T_3 is more biologically active, 80% of T_4
is converted into T_3.
[Bishop 2005, p446]

215 **b**   Congenital hypothyroidism presents
with very low thyroid hormones and is best
confirmed by serum TSH.
[Bishop 2005, pp664-665]

216 **b**   >99% of T_3 and T_4 are bound to
MLS
ONLY thyroxine-binding prealbumin, thyroxine-
binding globulin, and albumin.
[Bishop 2005, pp447-448]

217 **b**   TSH is the American Thyroid
Association's recommended screening test.
[Arneson 2007, p404]

218 d   Neonates are screened using total T_4.
[Arneson 2007, p402]

219 d   Hashimoto thyroiditis—the most common cause of hypothyroidism.
[Bishop 2005, pp450-451]

220 a   Age, sex, physical complaint, with elevated TSH point to primary hypothyroidism.
[Bishop 2005, pp450-451]

221 b   hCG is the primary marker for early pregnancy.
[Arneson 2007, pp429-431]

222 b
MLS
ONLY   During pregnancy, the largest fraction of estrogen in urine is estriol.
[Arneson 2007, p435]

223 b
MLS
ONLY   hCG levels peak at 8-10 weeks after the last menstrual period (LMP).
[Arneson 2007, p431.

224 a   The procedure "change in absorbance of amniotic fluid at 450 nm" used to detect hemolytic disease of newborn (HDN).
[Bishop 2005, pp555-557]

225 b   Serum hCG levels peak at 8-10 weeks.
[Arneson 2007, p431]

226 a   MoM calc = 34/32 = 1.06 (or <2).
MLS
ONLY   [Arneson 2007, p450]

227 b   Aldosterone is a hormone produced by the adrenal cortex.
[Bishop 2005, pp414-415]

228 d   All adrenal steroid hormones are enzymatically derived from cholesterol.
[Bishop 2005, p414]

229 d
MLS
ONLY   Testosterone is the most biologically active androgen in the embryonic stage and later effects sperm production and secondary sex characteristics.
[Bishop 2005, p436]

230 a   The normal variation of serum cortisol is higher at 8 AM than 4 PM.
[Arneson 2007, p383]

231 a   A deficiency of vitamin A leads to night blindness, and if prolonged total blindness.
[Bishop 2005, p620]

232 d   A deficiency of thiamine (vitamin B_1) known as beriberi, may be seen with chronic alcoholism in the U.S.
[Bishop 2005, p622]

233 b   A deficiency of ascorbic acid (vitamin C) is called scurvy.
[Bishop 2005, p626]

234 d   A deficiency of vitamin D in children leads to rickets.
[Bishop 2005, pp621-622]

235 d   A deficiency of niacin may be seen with chronic alcoholism, and is known as pellagra.
[Bishop 2005, p623]

236 b   Angiotensin II is a vasoconstrictor and stimulates the adrenal cortex to produce aldosterone.
[Arneson 2007, p388]

237 d   Vanillylmandelic acid (VMA) is the major metabolite of epinephrine and norepinephrine. VMA is measured in a 24-hour urine.
[Arneson 2007, p396.

238 c   Parathyroid hormone (PTH) and the hormone vitamin D play a dominant role in calcium regulation.
[Bishop 2005, pp458-461]

239 c
MLS
ONLY   95% of congenital adrenal hyperplasia is associated with a deficiency of 21-hydoxylase. Increased 17-OH progesterone is seen if measured by the laboratory.
[Bishop 2005, pp415-416]

240 c   ACTH stimulation tests, using synthetic ACTH, will differentiate primary from secondary adrenal insufficiency. Synthetic ACTH will not cause the adrenal gland to respond in primary insufficiency.
[Arneson 2007, pp384-385]

241 a   The 24-hour urine free coritsol is the most sensitive and specific screen for hypercortisolism.
[Bishop 2005, p420]

242 c
MLS
ONLY   Following an overnight fast, a 100 gram oral glucose load will cause a large drop in serum growth hormone in a normal individual, but will not suppress in patients with acromegaly.
[Bishop 2005, p404]

243 b
MLS
ONLY   About 55%-60% of patients whose breast tumors demonstrate estrogen receptors (ER) respond well to endocrine therapy.
[Bishop 2005, p613]

244 c   Due to circadian variation, the 24-hour UFC is an accurate measurement of active forms of cortisol.
[Bishop 2005, p420]

245 b Primary hypocortisolism = decreased
MLS ONLY cortisol/elevated ACTH; secondary
hypocortisolism = decreased cortisol/
decreased ACTH.
[Arneson 2007, p386]

246 d Angiotensin II directly stimulates the
adrenal cortex to release aldosterone.
[Bishop 2005, p415]

247 d Increased CEA levels are seen in
MLS ONLY patients with liver damage, heavy smokers
and following radiation and chemotherapy.
[Bishop 2005, p613]

248 b Tumor markers are useful for
monitoring therapy, detecting recurrence
and aiding in prognosis of tumors, but
are not useful for screening the general
population for cancer.
[Bishop 2005, pp608-609]

249 a Most testicular tumors are germ cell
tumors which are characterized by elevated
serum levels of alpha-fetoprotein (AFP).
Measurement of serum AFP is used in
the diagnosis, therapy and follow-up of
testicular cancer. The carcinoembryonic
antigen is a marker for colon cancer. The
serum levels of testosterone and prolactin
are not increased in testicular cancer.
[Kaplan 2003, p967]

250 a Alpha-fetoprotein (AFP) is an oncofetal
glycoprotein marker for hepatocellular
carcinoma. Elevated levels of AFP (<200 µg/L)
are seen in hepatitis and cirrhosis. However,
in hepatocellular carcinoma, the levels can
be greater than 1,000 µg/L.
[Burtis 2001, p403]

251 d The carcinoembryonic antigen (CEA) is
a marker for colon, gastrointestinal and lung
cancer. Elevated serum levels of CEA are
primarily seen with colon cancer. Although
the levels may be increased in individuals
with benign conditions, the level of CEA
elevation is greater for colon cancer.
[Burtis 2001, p403]

252 a tPSA along with DRE is the
recommended screen for prostate cancer in
males over 50 years of age.
[Bishop 2005, p608]

253 d Markers are good for monitoring
therapy and detecting recurrence of tumors.
[Arneson 2007, p469]

254 d CA 125 is elevated in 80% of epithelial
cell ovarian cancer.
[Bishop 2005, p612]

255 c PSA can be elevated due to BPH.
[Arneson 2007, p492]

TDM and Toxicology

256 a Intestinal absorption of digoxin
MLS ONLY is variable, and tissue uptake is slow;
therefore, serum levels are measured 8
hours after administration to permit tissue
and serum levels to equilibrate.
[Bishop 2005, pp577-578]

257 c A steady-state therapeutic drug
level is achieved between 4 and 7 doses.
Many variables affect when steady state
is achieved.
[Bishop 2005, p575; Arneson 2007, p506]

258 b Low serum protein means less of
MLS ONLY a drug is bound to protein. This may
occur due to nephrotic syndrome,
which causes significant protein loss
and hypoalbuminemia.
[Bishop 2005, p572]

259 a These drugs are not administered orally.
MLS ONLY [Bishop 2005, p579]

260 c NAPA is the active metabolite
of procainamide.
[Bishop 2005, pp578-579]

261 d The primary metabolite of cocaine
is benzoylecgonine, which is produced
by the liver and eliminated in the urine.
Benzoylecgonine is detected in drugs of
abuse screens for cocaine.
[Bishop 2005, pp600-601]

262 d 11-nor-THC-COOH is the urinary
metabolite of cannabinoids (marijuana
and hashish).
[Bishop 2005, p600]

263 d Lead interferes with heme synthesis,
which on a CBC may present as a decreased
hemoglobin, with basophilic stippling of
the red blood cells. These findings in a child
may indicate lead toxicity. Whole blood
lead is the recommended test; but urine
delta-aminolevulinic acid and RBC zinc
protoporphyrin are also useful assays.
[Bishop 2005, pp594-505; Arneson 2007, pp186-187.

264 a Erythrocyte zinc protoporphyrin is a
MLS ONLY useful screen for lead toxicity.
[Bishop 2005, p594]

265 c Lithium (carbonate) is used to treat
manic depression or bipolar disorder.
[Bishop 2005, p581; Arneson 2007, p515]

266 **d**   Phenytoin (trade name Dilantin™) is an anticonvulsant therapeutic drug used to treat seizure disorders.
[Bishop 2005, pp580-588; Arneson 2007, pp514-515]

267 **d**   The action of the drug theophylline is bronchodilation and smooth muscle relaxation.
[Arneson 2007, p515]

268 **a**   Digoxin at therapeutic serum levels (0.5-1.5 ng/mL) improves cardiac muscle contraction and rhythm.
[Arneson 2007, pp510-512]

269 **b**   Salicylate levels are used to determine if aspirin (acetylsalicylic acid) toxicity is present. Toxic serum or plasma levels are generally >300 μg/mL.
[Arneson 2007, pp517-518]

270 **d**   Lithium (carbonate) is used to treat manic depression or bipolar disorder.
[Bishop 2005, p581; Arneson 2007, p515]

271 **c**   Ceruloplasmin made by the liver, is the primary serum copper-bearing protein.
MLS ONLY
[Bishop 2005, p370]

272 **a**   Nortryptyline is an active metabolite of amitriptyline and must be included in analysis for tricyclic antidepressants (TCAs).
MLS ONLY
[Bishop 2005, p582]

273 **a**   Primidone is an inactive proform of phenobarbital.
MLS ONLY
[Bishop 2005, p580; Arneson 2007, p514]

274 **c**   Measurement of whole blood lead is the recommended test for children. In adults higher lead levels are significant; therefore other methods, such as erythrocyte protoporphyrin and delta-aminolevulinic acid, are acceptable for adults.
[Arneson 2007, pp188-189]

Quality Assessment

275 **c**   Preanalytical interferences with blood gases.
[Tietz 2006, pp1007-1008]

276 **c**   Use of tourniquet for over 1-3 minutes can cause elevation in protein and albumin, calcium, potassium, and hemoglobin.
MLS ONLY
[Clarke 2006, p5]

277 **b**   Serum for acid phosphatase measurement should not be stored at room temperature. This analyte requires special collection (citrate 10g/L) and storage (frozen) conditions to help stabilize the pH at about 6.2.
MLS ONLY
[Tietz 2006, p54]

278 **a**   Frozen samples should be allowed to thaw slowly at room temperature or in a 37°C water bath and should then be mixed thoroughly before analysis.
MLS ONLY
[Kaplan 2003, p78]

279 **a**   Water content is higher in plasma than in whole blood.
MLS ONLY
[Tietz 2006, p868]

280 **d**   Sodium fluoride exerts its preservative action by inhibiting the enzyme systems involved in glycolysis.
[Tietz 2006, p48]

281 **b**   A high-fat diet increases the serum concentrations of triglycerides. Fasting overnight for 10-14 hours is the optimal time for fasting around which to standardize blood collections, including lipids.
[Tietz 2006, p454]

282 **a**   A high-fat diet increases the serum concentrations of triglycerides. Fasting overnight for 10-14 hours is the optimal time for fasting around which to standardize blood collections, including lipids.
[Tietz 2006, p454]

283 **a**   The presence or exposure of excess gas (oxygen) in the syringe used to collect blood gas specimens will cause diffusion of carbon dioxide out of the specimen, oxygen into the specimen, and an increase in pH.
[Clarke 2006, p322]

284 **b**   Arterial specimens are best collected anaerobically with lyophilized heparin anticoagulant in sterile syringes.
MLS ONLY
[Tietz 2006, p1007]

285 **d**   Failure to adequately chill blood gas specimens if not immediately analyzed will allow glucose metabolism, which increases carbon dioxide and lowers pH.
[Clarke 2006, p322]

286 **d**   Glucose decreases at a rate of 5%-7% per hour in whole blood at room temperature. Glycolysis will continue until the specimen is processed by centrifugation, and serum and plasma is separated from the cellular components of blood.
[Clarke 2006, p6]

287   **d**   The use of an incorrect tube type or collection of a specimen at an inappropriate time may also require specimen recollection.
[Clarke 2006, p8]

288   **c**   Creatinine clearance offers the highest
MLS ONLY   sensitivity in monitoring glomerular function of the tests listed.
[Clarke 2006, p312]

Laboratory Mathematics

289   **c**   pH = 6.1 + log(salt/acid). Salt = total
MLS ONLY   carbon dioxide content – carbonic acid.
[Tietz 2006, p1002]

290   **a**   52 mg/dL = 0.52 mg/mL. Therefore 0.52 mg/mL × 1136 mL = 591 mg.
[Tietz 2006, p577]

291   **a**   Creatinine clearance = (urine creatinine × urine volume [mL/min]/serum creatinine) × 1.73 / total body surface.
[Clarke 2006, p43]

292   **a**   Creatinine clearance = (urine creatinine × urine volume [mL/min]/serum creatinine) × 1.73 / total body surface.
[Clarke 2006, p43]

293   **c**   In 1961, the enzyme commission
MLS ONLY   recommended the adoption of an international unit (IU) of enzyme activity. The IU was defined as the amount of enzyme that would convert 1 µmol of substrate per minute under standard conditions.
1 IU = µmol/min.
[Kaplan 2003, p1044]

294   **d**   pH = pK_a + log([salt]/[acid]); salt =
MLS ONLY   bicarbonate; acid = carbonic acid.
[Clarke 2006, p319]

295   **b**   t = 1.44 × t½ × ln(original activity /
MLS ONLY   remaining activity); t½ = half life.
[Clarke 2006, p42]

296   **c**   Absorbance = molar absorptivity
MLS ONLY   coefficient × light path × concentration. Therefore molar absorptivity = absorbance / light path × concentration.
[Kaplan 2003, p38]

297   **d**   Because the following relationship is true, A = light stopped and T = light passed through, A and T are inversely related. They are also logarithmically related, because the absorption of light is a logarithmic function.
[Campbell 1997, p212]

298   **d**   The Henderson-Hasselbalch equation describes the derivation of pH as a measure of acidity (using the acid dissociation constant, pK_a) in biological and chemical systems.
[Clarke 2006, p319]

299   **b**   Renal clearance tests are used to assess kidney function. Renal clearance of a substance is a rate measurement that expresses the volume of blood cleared of that substance (typically creatinine) per unit of time. The unit for the clearance is mL/ min. To calculate creatinine clearance, the following information is required: Serum concentration [S], urine concentration [U] (Note: the serum and urine concentration must be in the same units, for example, mg/L or mg/dL), and volume of urine excreted per minute (V) (volume of urine collected divided by the time period in minutes). The following formula can then be used: clearance (uncorrected for body mass) = [U] × V/[S].
[Kaplan 2003, p41]

300   **c**   Calculated osmolality (mOsm / kg) =
MLS ONLY   (2 × sodium [mEq/L]) + (glucose [mg/dL]/18) + (BUN [mg/dL]/ 2.8).
[Kaplan 2003, p267]

301   **c**   Reciprocal of substrate concentration
MLS ONLY   that produces 1/2 the maximal velocity (K_m) is displayed as the intercept of the x-axis on a Lineweaver-Burk transformation.
[Kaplan 2003, p1054]

302   **d**   Creatinine clearance = (urine
MLS ONLY   creatinine × urine volume [mL/min]/serum creatinine) × 1.73 / total body surface.
[Kaplan 2003, p41]

303   **c**
MLS ONLY   Urea/nitrogen factor =

$$\frac{\text{MW of urea (60)}}{2 \times \text{MW of nitrogen (28)}} = \frac{X \text{ g of urea}}{1 \text{ g of urea nitrogen}} = 2.14$$

The factor states that 2.14 g of urea is equivalent to 1 g of BUN. Convert BUN to urea, multiply by 2.14,

28 mg/dL BUN × 2.14 = 60 mg/dL urea

Convert to mEq/L by using the formula:

$$\frac{\text{mg/dL} \times}{\text{mg/mEq}} \quad \frac{10 \text{ dL}}{\text{L}} = \text{mEq/L}, \quad \frac{60 \text{ mg/dL x 10}}{60 \text{ mg/mEq}} = 10 \text{ mEq/L}$$

[Kaplan 2003, p36]

Answers–Chemistry

Answers–Chemistry

304 c
MLS
ONLY

Urea/nitrogen factor =

$$\frac{MW \text{ of urea (60)}}{2 \times MW \text{ of nitrogen}(28)} = \frac{x \text{ g of urea}}{1 \text{ g of urea nitrogen}} = 2.14$$

The factor states that 2.14 g of urea is equivalent to 1 g of BUN. Convert BUN to urea, multiply by 2.14,

15 mg/dL × 2.14 = 32 mg/dL

[Kaplan 2003, p36]

305 a   The difference between the actual
MLS
ONLY   osmolality commonly measured by freezing point depression and the calculated osmolality is referred to as the osmol gap. Normally, the osmol gap is <10 mOsm/kg.
[Tietz 2006, p1292]

306 c   Given the values of bicarbonate, carbonic acid, and the pK, the pH can be easily calculated using the Henderson-Hasselbalch equation. The Henderson-Hasselbalch equation describes the derivation of pH as a measure of acidity (using the acid dissociation constant, pK_a) in biological and chemical systems.
[Kaplan 2003, p39]

Instrumentation

307 d   Other distractors are methods to detect
MLS
ONLY   stray light.
[Kaplan 2003, p94]

308 d   In calcium analysis by AAS, lanthanum
MLS
ONLY   is added to bind with phosphate, thereby preventing interference by the formation of calcium phosphate.
[Bishop 2005, p98]

309 a   The electrolyte exclusion effect applies only to indirect methods and is caused by the solvent displacing effect of high concentrations of lipid and protein in the sample resulting in falsely decreased values.
[Tietz 2006, p987]

310 b   Principles of adsorption and selectivity
MLS
ONLY   in thin-layer chromatography.
[Kaplan 2003, p110]

311 c   In practice, a positive screening result for barbiturates obtained by immunoassay is confirmed by gas chromatography/mass spectrometry analysis of the urine specimen.
[Tietz 2006, p1327]

312 b   Retention of an analyte on a reversed-
MLS
ONLY   phase column depends on the relative amounts of polar and nonpolar character of the analyte. Retention on the reversed-phase packing material is favored by increased nonpolar content of the analyte, whereas residence in the mobile phase leading to early elution from the column is favored by an increased content of polar functionalities present on the analyte.
[Kaplan 2003, p137]

313 c   Protein electrophoresis migration.
[Tietz 2006, p128]

314 a   Separation of Hgb S from Hgb D.
[Tietz 2006, p1172]

315 c   Protein electrophoresis pH.
[Tietz 2006, p584]

316 a   Proteins are amphoteric substances; that is, they contain acidic and basic groups. Their overall (net) charge is highly positive at low pH values, 0 at a particular higher pH, and negative at still more alkaline pH values. At a pH of 4.5, the positively charged proteins will migrate toward the cathode in an electrophoretic system.
[Kaplan 2003, p204]

317 b   Occasionally, a split albumin zone is
MLS
ONLY   observed in the rare benign genetically relation condition of bisalbuminemia. However, transient bisalbuminemia or a grossly widened albumin zone could be due to albumin-bound medications.
[Tietz 2006, p127]

318 d   The C3 component of complement
MLS
ONLY   migrates with beta-globulins on electrophoresis.
[Tietz 2006, p567]

319 c PO_2 electrode.
[Tietz 2006, p104]

320 b   The pH electrode, a glass electrode, contains a specially designed thin piece of glass as a membrane. The glass membrane is made of silicon dioxide, added oxides and various metals. The membrane is selectively sensitive to hydrogen ions.
[Burtis 2001, p109]

321 a Coulometry is an electrochemical technique used to measure the amount of electricity passing between 2 electrodes in an electrochemical cell. An application of coulometry is the titration of chloride with silver ions generated by electrolysis from a silver wire at the anode. Polarography is also an electrochemical technique, but measures current. Mass spectroscopy and chromatography are separation techniques.
[Burtis 2001, p116]

322 a Coulometry is still used for chloride determinations in body fluids, such as sweat. However, chloride ion-selective electrodes (ISE) are commonly used today.
[Bishop 2005, p564; Arneson 2007, p118]

323 a The reference pH electrode is often constructed of Ag and AgCl.
[Bishop 2005, p102. [Arneson 2007, p304]

324 b The PO_2 electrode functions on
MLS ONLY the amperometric principle, which the measurement of electrical current at a constant voltage (or potential).
[Bishop 2005, p104. [Arneson 2007, p118]

325 b pH, PCO_2, and PO_2 are directly measured by modern blood gas analyzers; other parameters are calculated.
[Bishop 2005, p354. [Arneson 2007, p354]

326 b The PCO_2 electrode is a self-contained potentiometric cell. CO_2 gas from the sample or calibration matrix diffuses through the selective membrane and dissolves in the internal electrolyte layer. Carbonic acid is formed and dissociates, shifting the pH of the bicarbonate solution in the internal layer. This shift is related to the carbon dioxide in the sample.
[Tietz 2006, p99]

327 c Analyzers fitted with ion-selective electrodes usually contain potassium electrodes with liquid ion-exchange membranes that incorporate valinomycin. Valinomycin is a neutral carrier (ionophore) that binds potassium in the center of a ring of oxygen atoms.
[Clarke 2006, p100]

328 c PCO_2 electrode.
[Tietz 2006, p99]

329 d Total protein method.
[Tietz 2006, p587]

330 a Albumin method.
[Tietz 2006, p548]

331 d The total iron binding capacity (TIBC) is the amount of iron that transferrin and other minor iron binding proteins are capable of binding. In the measure of the TIBC, the molecules are saturated with iron (since they are only 30% saturated normally). Magnesium carbonate is used to remove the excess unbound by adsorption.
[Bishop 2005, p369]

332 a Most specific glucose method.
[Tietz 2006, p869]

333 b Other distractors are not glucose-
MLS ONLY specific methods.
[Tietz 2006, p870]

334 c Ascorbic acid interferes. This is
MLS ONLY a limitation of the glucose oxidase (peroxidase) reaction.
[Tietz 2006, p870]

335 b Principle of the hexokinase method.
MLS ONLY [Tietz 2006, p869]

336 d Atomic absorption spectrophotometry (AAS) measures calcium by detecting its atomic absorption by electromagnetic radiation. One limitation of this method is the nonspectral interference which occurs when phosphates are present and complex with calcium. The use of lanthanum chloride with the method has prevented the interference. Lanthanum chloride competes for the phosphate.
[Burtis 2001, p73]

337 d Unconjugated bilirubin solvent.
[Tietz 2006, p1196]

338 d Other distractors are not bilirubin methods.
[Bishop 2005, p482]

339 d The diazo method of Malloy and Evelyn involves bilirubin reacting with diazotized sulfanilic acid to form azobilirubin.
[Burtis 2001, p605]

340 a In the Jendrassik-Grof method for bilirubin measurement, the addition of caffeine plus diazotized sulfanilic acid and the serum produces azobilirubin. Ascorbic acid, alkaline tartrate and dilute HCl are added to the reaction mixture. The blue-green azobilirubin is measured. Bilirubin glucuronide, urobilin and urobilinogen are intermediaries in bilirubin metabolism. They are not measured by this method.
[Burtis 2001, p605]

Answers–Chemistry

341 c   Azobilirubin is the chromophore measured in the Jendrassik-Grof reaction. Azobilirubin is formed by bilirubin in the presence of diazotized-sulfanilic acid.
[Bishop 2005, p482. [Arneson 2007, p238]

342 a   LDH chemical reaction.
[Tietz 2006, p601]

343 a   Nicotinamide adenine dinucleotide is the coenzyme system for the LD assay. NADH is the reduced form and NAD is the oxidized form. The coenzymes serve as a substrate for dehydrogenases reactions. ATP/ADP and Cu/Cu^{++} are not coenzymes. Fe is an activator for enzymatic reactions.
[Burtis 2001, p364]

344 c   In the continuous monitoring method of the measurement of LD activity, the decrease in absorbance at each time interval indicates that the product formed (substrate converted) is constant up to 6 minutes. After 6 minutes, the substrate concentration is limited, and there is a decrease in the rate of product formation as indicated by the lack of linearity.
[Burtis 2001, p170]

345 a   Competitive inhibitors bind at the
MLS
ONLY   active site of enzymes and compete with the substrate for binding sites.
[Kaplan 2003, p1057]

346 a   Reciprocal of the maximal velocity
MLS
ONLY   (V_{max}) can be calculated and is displayed as the intercept of the y-axis on a Lineweaver-Burk transformation.
[Kaplan 2003, p1054]

347 d   Alkaline phosphatase catalyzes the hydrolysis of para-nitrophenyl phosphate, forming phosphate and free 4-nitrophenyl (4-npp) which, under alkaline conditions, has a very intense yellow color. IFCC recommended methods use 4-npp as the substrate.
[Tietz 2006, p609]

348 b   In competitive inhibition, the binding of
MLS
ONLY   the substrate is affected; thus, the apparent K_m will be higher while the V_{max} remains the same.
[Kaplan 2003, p1058]

349 a   Aldolase catalyzes the splitting of fructose-1,6-diphosphate to glyceraldehyde-3-phosphate and dihydroxyacetone phosphate, an important reaction in the glycolytic breakdown of glucose to lactate.
[Tietz 2006, p603]

350 b   There are several enzymatic methods for measuring serum triglyceride. The first step of the coupled reactions involves the hydrolysis of triglyceride by lipase to produce glycerol and fatty acids. Glycerol is a reactant in one of 2 enzymatic sequences for the final measurement of triglycerides.
[Burtis 2001, p487]

351 b   High-volume HDL method.
[Tietz 2006, p945]

352 d   Chemiluminescent labels are based on the emission of light produced during a chemical reaction. These labels are very useful because they provide very low levels of detection (2×10^{20} mol/L) with little or no background interference.
[Clarke 2006, p122]

353 a   Osmometry of serum and other body fluids is commonly measured by freezing-point depression, using a freezing point osmometer.
[Bishop 2005, pp118-119; Arneson 2007, p120]

354 a   The osmolality of a solution does not depend on the kind of particles but only on the number of particles, therefore it is called a colligative property.
[Kaplan 2003, p269]

355 a   Transketolase is decreased in thiamin
MLS
ONLY   deficiency. Low values of it have also been found in chronic alcoholism.
[Tietz 2006, p631]

356 c   The "optical density Delta 450"
MLS
ONLY   determination is a graphical calculation to estimate the amount of bilirubin in amniotic fluid. Bilirubin has a maximal absorbance at 450nm.
[Clarke 2006, p43]

Hematology

*The following items have been identified generally as appropriate for both entry level medical laboratory scientists and medical laboratory technicians. Items that are appropriate for medical laboratory scientists **only** are marked with an "MLS ONLY."*

[handwritten: Read up on: hexose monophosphate shunt, polypeptide chains of hemoglobin, iron forms, G-6-PD deficiency]

Erythrocytes: Physiology

1   The light-colored zone adjacent to the nucleus in a plasmacyte is the:

    a ribosome
    b chromatin
    c mitochondria
    d Golgi area

2   The following are compounds formed in the synthesis of heme:
MLS ONLY

      1 coproporphyrinogen ③
      2 porphobilinogen ①
      3 uroporphyrinogen ②
      4 protoporphyrinogen ④

[handwritten: por → uro → copro → proto]

    Which of the following responses lists these compounds in the order in which they are formed?

    a 4, 3, 1, 2
    b 2, 3, 1, 4
    c 4, 2, 3, 1
    d 2, 1, 3, 4

3   The majority of the iron in an adult is found as a constituent of:

    a hemoglobin *[handwritten: - 2/3 of iron stores]*
    b hemosiderin
    c myoglobin
    d transferrin

4   The main function of the hexose monophosphate shunt in the erythrocyte is to:

    a regulate the level of 2,3-DPG
    b provide reduced glutathione to prevent oxidation of hemoglobin ✳✳
    c prevent the reduction of heme iron
    d provide energy for membrane maintenance

5   Refer to the following illustration:

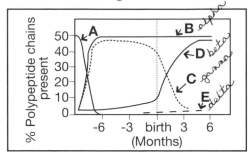

Which curve represents the production of alpha polypeptide chains of hemoglobin?

  a A
  b B
  c C
  d D

6   Refer to the following illustration:

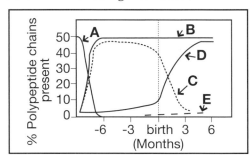

Which curve represents the production of beta polypeptide chains of hemoglobin?

  a B
  b C
  c E
  d D

7   Refer to the following illustration:

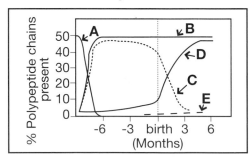

Which curve represents the production of gamma polypeptide chains of hemoglobin?

  a A
  b B
  c C
  d D

8   Refer to the following illustration:

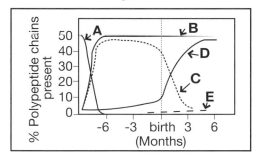

Which curve represents the production of delta polypeptide chains of hemoglobin?

  a   B
  b   C
  c   D
  (**d**)   E

conception: epsilon (drops)
early: alpha (continues)
*   gamma (drops off)*
late: beta (quick sustained)
just before birth: delta

9   Refer to the following illustration:

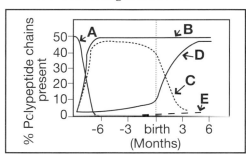

Which curve represents the production of epsilon polypeptide chains of hemoglobin?

  (**a**)   A
  b   B
  c   C
  d   D

10   In order for hemoglobin to combine reversibly with oxygen, the iron must be:

  a   complexed with haptoglobin
  b   freely circulating in the cytoplasm
  c   attached to transferrin
  (**d**)   in the ferrous state

11   In which of the following disease states are <u>teardrop cells</u> and <u>abnormal platelets</u> most characteristically seen?

  a   hemolytic anemia
  b   multiple myeloma
  c   G-6-PD deficiency
  (**d**)   myeloid metaplasia — *RBC morphology*

12   The characteristic erythrocyte found in <u>pernicious anemia</u> is:
_{MLS ONLY}   *impaired DNA synthesis*

  a   microcytic   **⁑**
  b   spherocytic
  c   hypochromic
  (**d**)   macrocytic

13   In the normal adult, the spleen acts as a site for:

    a storage of red blood cells
    b production of red blood cells
    c synthesis of erythropoietin
    ⓓ removal of imperfect and aging cells

14   After the removal of red blood cells from the circulation hemoglobin is broken down into:

    a iron, porphyrin, and amino acids
    ⓑ iron, protoporphyrin, and globin – *normal degradation products of hemoglobin*
    c heme, protoporphyrin, and amino acids
    d heme, hemosiderin, and globin

15   Heinz bodies are:

    a readily identified with polychrome stains
    b rarely found in glucose-6-phosphate dehydrogenase deficient erythrocytes
    c closely associated with spherocytes
    ⓓ denatured hemoglobin inclusions that are readily removed by the spleen
    formed with oxidation of Fe and formation of methemoglobin

16   Hemolysis in paroxysmal nocturnal hemoglobinuria (PNH) is:
_{MLS ONLY}

    a temperature-dependent
    b complement-independent
    c antibody-mediated
    ⓓ caused by a red cell membrane defect

17   Cells for the transport of O_2 and CO_2 are:

    ⓐ erythrocytes
    b granulocytes
    c lymphocytes
    d thrombocytes

18   Erythropoietin acts to:

    a shorten the replication time of the granulocytes
    ⓑ stimulate RNA synthesis of erythroid cells
    c increase colony-stimulating factors produced by the B-lymphocytes
    d decrease the release of marrow reticulocytes

19   What cell shape is **most** commonly associated with an increased MCHC?
    (hyperchromic)

    a teardrop cells
    b target cells
    ⓒ spherocytes
    d sickle cells

20   Which of the following is **most** closely associated with idiopathic hemochromatosis?
_{MLS ONLY}

    ⓐ iron overload in tissue
    b target cells
    c basophilic stippling
    d ringed sideroblasts

Erythrocytes: Disease States

21 A patient with <u>polycythemia vera</u> who is treated by phlebotomy is **most** likely to develop a
MLS
ONLY   deficiency of:

    a iron
    b vitamin B_{12}
    c folic acid
    d erythropoietin

22 The direct antiglobulin test is often positive in:
MLS
ONLY
    a congenital hemolytic spherocytosis
    b march hemoglobinuria
    c acquired hemolytic anemia – *positive DAT*
    d thalassemia major

23 The anemia of chronic infection is characterized by:
MLS
ONLY
    a decreased iron stores in the reticuloendothelial system
    b decreased serum iron levels
    c macrocytic erythrocytes
    d increased serum iron binding capacity

24 Factors commonly involved in producing anemia in patients with chronic renal disease include:
MLS
ONLY
    a marrow hypoplasia
    b inadequate erythropoiesis ← *uremia*
    c vitamin B_{12} deficiency
    d increased erythropoietin production

25 A 20-year-old woman with sickle cell anemia whose usual hemoglobin concentration is 8 g/dL
MLS
ONLY   (80 g/L) develops fever, increased weakness and malaise. The hemoglobin concentration is 4 g/dL
(40 g/L) and the reticulocyte count is 0.1%. The **most** likely explanation for her clinical picture is:

    a increased hemolysis due to hypersplenism
    b aplastic crisis
    c thrombotic crisis
    d occult blood loss

26 The hypoproliferative red cell population in the bone marrow of uremic patients is caused by:
MLS
ONLY
    a infiltration of bone marrow by toxic waste products
    b decreased levels of circulating erythropoietin
    c defective globin synthesis
    d overcrowding of bone marrow space by increased myeloid precursors

27 Which of the following characteristics are common to hereditary spherocytosis, hereditary
elliptocytosis, hereditary stomatocytosis, and paroxysmal nocturnal hemoglobinuria?

    a autosomal dominant inheritance
    b red cell membrane defects
    c positive direct antiglobulin test   ✳✳ *hereditary RBC membrane*
    d measured platelet count   *defects*

28 A 89-year-old Caucasian female was transferred to the hospital from a nursing facility for
treatment of chronic urinary tract infection with proteinuria. The patient presented with the
following laboratory data:

WBC:	$10.0 \times 10^3/\mu L$ ($10.0 \times 10^9/L$)
RBC:	$3.1 \times 10^6/\mu L$ ($3.1 \times 10^{12}/L$)
Hgb:	7.2 g/dL (72 g/L) ↓
Hct:	24%
MCV:	78 μm^3 (78 fL) ↓
MCH:	23 pg
MCHC:	31%
serum iron:	29 µg/dL (5.2 µmol/L)
TIBC:	160 µg/dL (28.6 µmol/L)
serum ferritin:	100 ng/mL (100 µg/L)

These data are most consistent with which of the following conditions?

a iron deficiency anemia
(b) anemia of chronic inflammation
c hemochromatosis
d acute blood loss

29 A patient is admitted with a history of chronic bleeding secondary to peptic ulcer. Hematology
workup reveals a severe microcytic, hypochromic anemia. Iron studies were requested. Which of
the following would be expected in this case?

	Serum iron	TIBC	Storage iron	
result A	decreased	increased	increased	
result B	increased	decreased	increased	
result C	decreased	increased	decreased	✳✳
result D	increased	normal	decreased	

a result A
b result B
(c) result C
d result D

Iron studies for microcytic hypochromic anemia
↓ serum and storage iron
↑ TIBC

30 Which of the following is **most** closely associated with iron deficiency anemia?

a iron overload in tissue
b target cells – *hemoglobinopathies (S+C)*
c basophilic stippling – *sideroblastic anemia*
(d) chronic blood loss

31 Which one of the following hypochromic anemias is usually associated with a normal free
erythrocyte protoporphyrin level?

a anemia of chronic disease
b iron deficiency
c lead poisoning
(d) thalassemia minor

32 Evidence indicates that the genetic defect in thalassemia usually results in:

✳

a the production of abnormal globin chains
(b) a quantitative deficiency in RNA resulting in decreased globin chain production
c a structural change in the heme portion of the hemoglobin
d an abnormality in the alpha- or beta-chain binding or affinity

33/ A 20-year-old African-American man has peripheral blood changes suggesting thalassemia minor.
MLS
ONLY The quantitative hemoglobin A_2 level is normal, but the hemoglobin F level is 5% (normal <2%).
This is most consistent with:

    a alpha thalassemia minor
    b beta thalassemia minor
    c delta-beta thalassemia minor
    d hereditary persistence of fetal hemoglobin

34/ Anemia secondary to uremia characteristically is:
MLS
ONLY

    a microcytic, hypochromic
    b hemolytic
    c normocytic, normochromic - *number of cells decreased*
    d macrocytic

35/ Which of the following sets of laboratory findings is consistent with hemolytic anemia?
MLS
ONLY

    a normal or slightly increased erythrocyte survival; normal osmotic fragility
    b decreased erythrocyte survival; increased catabolism of heme → *hemolytic anemia*
    c decreased serum lactate dehydrogenase activity; normal catabolism of heme
    d normal concentration of haptoglobin; marked hemoglobinuria

36 An enzyme deficiency associated with a moderate to severe hemolytic anemia after the patient
is exposed to certain drugs and characterized by red cell inclusions formed by denatured
hemoglobin is:

    a lactate dehydrogenase deficiency
    b G-6-PD deficiency   ✳ ✳
    c pyruvate kinase deficiency
    d hexokinase deficiency

37 Patients with A(-) type G-6-PD deficiency are **least** likely to have hemolytic episodes in which of
the following situations?

    a following the administration of oxidizing drugs
    b following the ingestion of fava beans
    c during infections   ?
    d spontaneously

38 A patient has a congenital nonspherocytic hemolytic anemia. After exposure to anti-malarial
drugs the patient experiences a severe hemolytic episode. This episode is characterized by red
cell inclusions caused by hemoglobin denaturation. Which of the following conditions is **most**
consistent with these findings?

    a G-6-PD deficiency
    b thalassemia major
    c pyruvate kinase deficiency
    d paroxysmal nocturnal hemoglobinuria

39/ All of the findings listed below may be seen in acquired hemolytic anemias of the autoimmune
MLS
ONLY variety. The one considered to be the **most** characteristic is:

    a increased osmotic fragility
    b leukopenia and thrombocytopenia
    c peripheral spherocytosis   ✳✳
    d positive direct antiglobulin test

40 Peripheral blood smears from patients with untreated pernicious anemia are characterized by:

    a pancytopenia and macrocytosis
    b leukocytosis and elliptocytosis
    c leukocytosis and ovalocytosis
    d pancytopenia and microcytosis

41   Laboratory tests performed on a patient indicate macrocytosis, anemia, leukopenia and thrombocytopenia. Which of the following disorders is the patient most likely to have?

     a   anemia of chronic disorder
     b   vitamin B_{12} deficiency – *pernicious anemia* *(pancytopenia + macrocytosis)*
     c   iron deficiency
     d   acute hemorrhage

42   A patient has the following laboratory data:
MLS ONLY

     RBC: $2.35 \times 10^6/\mu L$ (2.35×10^{12}/L)
     WBC: $3.0 \times 10^3/\mu L$ (3.0×10^9/L)
     Plt: $95.0 \times 10^3/\mu L$ (95.0×10^9/L)
     Hgb: 9.5 g/dL (95 g/L)
     Hct: 27%
     MCV: 115 μm^3 (115 fL)
     MCHC: 35%
     MCH: 40 pg

     Which of the following tests would contribute toward the diagnosis?

     a   reticulocyte count
     b   platelet factor 3
     c   serum B_{12} and folate
     d   leukocyte alkaline phosphatase

43   The characteristic morphologic feature in folic acid deficiency is:

     a   macrocytosis
     b   target cells
     c   basophilic stippling
     d   rouleaux formation

44   A 50-year-old patient was found to have the following lab results:
MLS ONLY

     Hgb: 7.0 g/dL (70 g/L)
     Hct: 20%
     RBC: $2.0 \times 10^6/\mu L$ (2.0×10^{12}/L)

     It was determined that the patient was suffering from <u>pernicious anemia</u>. Which of the following sets of results most likely was obtained from the same patient? *pancytopenia w/ low cell production*

	WBCs	Platelets	Reticulocytes
result A	17,500	350,000	5.2%
result B	7,500	80,000	4.1%
result C	5,000	425,000	2.9%
result D	3,500	80,000	0.8%

     a   result A
     b   result B
     c   result C
     d   result D

45   The most likely cause of the macrocytosis that often accompanies anemia of <u>myelofibrosis</u> is:

     a   folic acid deficiency – *accompanies myelofibrosis*
     b   increased reticulocyte count
     c   inadequate B_{12} absorption
     d   pyridoxine deficiency

46   Megaloblastic asynchronous development in the bone marrow indicates which one of
MLS ONLY the following?

     a   proliferation of erythrocyte precursors
     b   impaired synthesis of DNA – *Megaloblastic*
     c   inadequate production of erythropoietin
     d   deficiency of G-6-PD

47 Which of the following are found in association with megaloblastic anemia? *low platelet and WBC counts neutrophil*
    a neutropenia and thrombocytopenia
    b decreased LD activity
    c increased erythrocyte folate levels
    d decreased plasma bilirubin levels

48 Which of the following represents characteristic features of iron metabolism in patients with anemia of a chronic disorder?

	Serum iron	Transferrin saturation	TIBC
result A	normal	normal	normal
result B	increased	increased	normal or slightly increased
result C	normal	markedly increased	normal
result D	decreased	decreased	normal or decreased

    a result A
    b result B   ✳✳
    c result C
    d result D

49 A characteristic morphologic feature in hemoglobin C disease is:

    a macrocytosis
    b spherocytosis
    c rouleaux formation
    d target cells – *hemoglobin C*

50 Thalassemias are characterized by:

    a structural abnormalities in the hemoglobin molecule
    b absence of iron in hemoglobin
    c decreased rate of heme synthesis
    d decreased rate of globin synthesis

51 A patient has the following blood values:

    RBC: $6.5 \times 10^6/\mu L$ ($6.5 \times 10^{12}/L$)
    Hgb: 13.0 g/dL (130 g/L)
    Hct: 39.0%
    MCV: 65 μm^3 (65 fL)
    MCH: 21.5 pg
    MCHC: 33%

These results are compatible with:
    a iron deficiency
    b pregnancy
    c thalassemia minor
    d beta thalassemia major

52 Laboratory findings in hereditary spherocytosis do **not** include:

    a decreased osmotic fragility
    b increased autohemolysis corrected by glucose
    c reticulocytosis
    d shortened erythrocyte survival

53 Which of the following types of polycythemia is a severely burned patient **most** likely to have?

    a polycythemia vera
    b polycythemia, secondary to hypoxia
    c relative polycythemia associated with dehydration
    d polycythemia associated with renal disease

54   Which of the following is most likely to be seen in lead poisoning?

    a iron overload in tissue
    b codocytes
    ⓒ basophilic stippling
    d ringed sideroblasts

55   *MLS ONLY* Giant, vacuolated, multinucleated erythroid precursors are present in which of the following?

    a chronic myelocytic leukemia
    b myelofibrosis with myeloid metaplasia
    ⓒ erythroleukemia
    d acute myelocytic leukemia

56   *MLS ONLY* Which of the following is a significant feature of erythroleukemia/acute erythroid leukemia (DiGuglielmo syndrome)?

    a persistently increased M:E ratio
    ⓑ megaloblastoid erythropoiesis
    c marked thrombocytosis
    d decreased ferritin levels

57   *MLS ONLY* The M:E ratio in erythroleukemia is usually:

    a normal
    b high
    ⓒ low
    d variable

58   The characteristic morphologic feature in lead poisoning is:

    a macrocytosis
    b target cells (codocytes)
    ⓒ basophilic stippling
    d rouleaux formation

59   *MLS ONLY* Which of the following is increased in erythrocytosis secondary to a congenital heart defect?

    a arterial oxygen saturation
    b serum vitamin B_{12}
    c leukocyte alkaline phosphatase activity
    ⓓ erythropoietin

60   *MLS ONLY* A 40-year-old man had an erythrocyte count of $2.5 \times 10^6/\mu L$ ($2.5 \times 10^{12}/L$), hematocrit of 22% and a reticulocyte count of 2.0%. Which of the following statements best describes his condition?

    ⓐ the absolute reticulocyte count is $50 \times 10^3/\mu L$ ($50 \times 10^9/L$), indicating that the bone marrow is not adequately compensating for the anemia
    b the reticulocyte count is greatly increased, indicating an adequate bone marrow response for this anemia
    c the absolute reticulocyte count is $500 \times 10^3/\mu L$ ($500 \times 10^9/L$), indicating that the bone marrow is adequately compensating for the anemia
    d the reticulocyte count is slightly increased, indicating an adequate response to the slight anemia

61   *MLS ONLY* Which of the following is characteristic of polycythemia vera?

    a elevated urine erythropoietin levels
    b increased oxygen affinity of hemoglobin
    c "teardrop" poikilocytosis
    ⓓ decreased or absent bone marrow iron stores ✱✱

Erythrocytes: Laboratory Determinations

62   A 14-year-old boy is seen in the ER complaining of a sore throat, swollen glands and fatigue. The CBC results are:

WBC: $16.0 \times 10^3/\mu L$ ($16.0 \times 10^9/L$) ↑↑↑
RBC: $4.37 \times 10^6/\mu L$ ($4.37 \times 10^{12}/L$)
Hgb: 12.8 g/dL (128 g/L)
Hct: 38.4%
Plt: $180 \times 10^3/\mu L$ ($180 \times 10^9/L$)

Differential:

absolute neutrophils: $3.9 \times 10^9/L$
absolute lymphs: $6.0 \times 10^9/L$ ↑
absolute monos: $0.5 \times 10^9/L$
absolute atypical lymphs: $3.2 \times 10^9/L$ ↑

What is the most likely diagnosis?

a   acute lymphocytic leukemia
b   chronic lymphocytic leukemia
c   viral hepatitis
d   infectious mononucleosis

63   Which of the following technical factors will cause a decreased erythrocyte sedimentation rate?   *decreased ESR*

a   gross hemolysis
b   small fibrin clots in the sample   ✱✱
c   increased room temperature
d   tilting of the tube

64   Which of the RBC indices is a measure of the amount of hemoglobin in individual red blood cells?

a   MCHC
b   MCV
c   Hct   ✱✱
d   MCH

65   The RDW-CV and RDW-SD performed by automated cells counters are calculations that provide:

a   an index of the distribution of RBC volumes
b   a calculated mean RBC hemoglobin concentration
c   a calculated mean cell hemoglobin
d   the mean RBC volume

66   The erythrocyte sedimentation rate (ESR) can be falsely elevated by:

a   tilting the tube   *falsely elevated = acceleration of RBC fall*
b   refrigerated blood
c   air bubbles in the column   ✱ ✱
d   specimen being too old

67   A Wright-stained peripheral smear reveals the following:

_{MLS ONLY}

Erythrocytes enlarged 1½× to 2× normal size
Schüffner dots
Parasites with irregular "spread-out" trophozoites, golden-brown pigment
12 - 24 merozoites
Wide range of stages

This is consistent with *Plasmodium*:

a   *falciparum*
b   *malariae*
c   *ovale*
d   *vivax*

68   Which of the following is the formula for absolute cell count?

   a   number of cells counted/total count
   b   total count/number of cells counted
   c   10× total count
   d   % of cells counted × total count

69   Using a supra vital stain, the <u>polychromatic</u> red blood cells below would probably be:

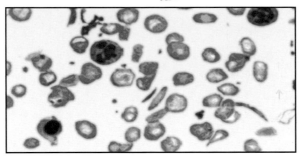

   a   rubricytes (polychromatophilic normoblast)
   b   reticulocytes
   c   sickle cells
   d   target cells

70   The laboratory tests performed on a patient indicate macrocytosis, anemia, leukopenia and thrombocytopenia. Which of the following disorders is the patient most likely to have?

   a   iron deficiency
   b   hereditary spherocytosis
   c   vitamin B_{12} deficiency
   d   acute hemorrhage

71   The mean value of a reticulocyte count on specimens of cord blood from healthy, full-term newborns is approximately:

   a   0.5%
   b   2.0%
   c   5.0%- *elevated in infants*
   d   8.0%

72   A red blood cell about 5 μm in diameter that stains bright red and shows no central pallor is a:

   a   spherocyte
   b   leptocyte
   c   microcyte
   d   macrocyte

73   The following results were obtained on a patient's blood:

Hgb:	11.5 g/dL (115 g/L)
Hct:	40%
MCV:	89 μm³ (89 fL)
MCH:	26 pg
MCHC:	29%

Examination of a Wright-stained smear of the same sample would most likely show:

   a   macrocytic, normochromic erythrocytes
   b   microcytic, hypochromic erythrocytes
   c   normocytic, hypochromic erythrocytes
   d   normocytic, normochromic erythrocytes

74 Evidence of active red cell regeneration may be indicated on a blood smear by:

    a basophilic stippling, nucleated red blood cells and polychromasia
    b hypochromia, macrocytes and nucleated red blood cells   ✶✶
    c hypochromia, basophilic stippling and nucleated red blood cells
    d Howell-Jolly bodies, Cabot rings and basophilic stippling

75 The smear represented below displays:

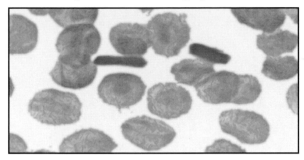

    a congenital ovalocytosis
    b hemoglobin C disease
    c poor RBC fixation
    d delay in smear preparation

76 The presence of excessive rouleaux formation on a blood smear is often accompanied by an increased:

    a reticulocyte count
    b sedimentation rate
    c hematocrit
    d erythrocyte count

77 The characteristic peripheral blood morphologic feature in multiple myeloma is:

    a cytotoxic T cells   ✶
    b rouleaux formation
    c spherocytosis
    d macrocytosis

78 In polycythemia vera, the hemoglobin, hematocrit, red blood cell count and red cell mass are:

    a elevated   ↑ RBC mass
    b normal   ↑ platelet count
    c decreased   ↑ LAP score

79 The M:E ratio in polycythemia vera is usually:

    a normal ↑ in both myeloid and erythrocyte precursors
    b high
  ~**c** low   ✶✶
    d variable

80 Many microspherocytes, schistocytes and budding off of spherocytes can be seen on peripheral blood smears of patients with:

    a hereditary spherocytosis
    b disseminated intravascular coagulation (DIC)
    c acquired autoimmune hemolytic anemia
    d extensive burns ✶✶

81   Which of the following is most closely associated with erythroleukemia?

     (a) ringed sideroblasts, nuclear budding and Howell-Jolly bodies
     b   disseminated intravascular coagulation
     c   micromegakaryocytes
     d   lysozymuria

82   The most characteristic peripheral blood smear finding in multiple myeloma is:

     a   plasmacytic satellitosis in the bone marrow
     b   many plasma cells in the peripheral blood
     c   many Mott cells in the peripheral blood
     (d) rouleaux formation of the red cells – *characteristic of MM*

83   The values below were obtained on an automated blood count system performed on a blood sample from a 25-year-old man:

	Patient	Normal
WBC	$5.1 \times 10^3/\mu L$ $(5.1 \times 10^9/L)$	$5.0\text{-}10.0 \times 10^3/\mu L$ $(5.0\text{-}10.0 \times 10^9/L)$
RBC	$2.94 \times 10^6/\mu L$ $(2.94 \times 10^{12}/L)$	$4.6\text{-}6.2 \times 10^6/\mu L$ $(4.6\text{-}6.2 \times 10^{12}/L)$
Hgb	13.8 g/dL (138 g/L)	14-18 g/dL (140-180 g/L)
Hct	35.4%	40%-54%
MCV	128 μm^3 (128 fL)	82-90 μm^3 (82-90 fL)
MCH	46.7 pg	27-31 pg
MCHC	40%	32%-36%

     These results are most consistent with which of the following?

     a   megaloblastic anemia
     b   hereditary spherocytosis
     (c) a high titer of cold agglutinins – *erroneous ↑ MCV and ↓ RBC due to clumping*
     d   an elevated reticulocyte count

84   A 56-year-old man was admitted to the hospital for treatment of a bleeding ulcer. The following
_{MLS ONLY} laboratory data were obtained:

     RBC: $4.2 \times 10^6/\mu L$ $(4.2 \times 10^{12}/L)$
     WBC: $5.0 \times 10^3/\mu L$ $(5.0 \times 10^6/L)$
     Hct: 30%
     Hgb: 8.5 g/dL (85 g/L)
     serum iron: 40 μg/dL (7.2 μmol/L) ↓   *↓ % transferrin saturation*
     TIBC: 460 μg/dL (82.3 μmol/L) ↑   *↑ FEP*
     serum ferritin: 12 ng/mL (12 μg/L) ↓   *↑ serum soluble transferrin receptor levels*

     Examination of the bone marrow revealed the absence of iron stores. This data is most consistent with which of the following conditions?

     (a) iron deficiency anemia
     b   anemia of chronic disease
     c   hemochromatosis
     d   acute blood loss

85 A 40-year-old Caucasian male was admitted to the hospital for treatment of anemia, lassitude,
MLS ONLY weight loss, and loss of libido. The patient presented with the following laboratory data:

WBC:	$5.8 \times 10^3/\mu L$ ($5.8 \times 10^9/L$)
RBC:	$3.7 \times 10^6/\mu L$ ($3.7 \times 10^{12}/L$)
Hgb:	10.0 g/dL (100 g/L)
Hct:	32%
MCV:	86 μm^3 (86 fL)
MCH:	26 pg
MCHC:	32%
serum iron:	220 µg/dL (39.4 µmol/L)
TIBC:	300 µg/dL (53.7 µmol/L)
serum ferritin:	2,800 ng/mL (2,800 µg/L)

Examination of the bone marrow revealed erythroid hyperplasia with a shift to the left of
erythroid precursors. Prussian blue staining revealed markedly elevated iron stores noted with
occasional sideroblasts seen. This data is most consistent with which of the following conditions?

a iron deficiency anemia
b anemia of chronic disease
c hemochromatosis
d acute blood loss

86 A common source of interference in the cyanmethemoglobin method is:

a hemolysis
b very high WBC count
c cold agglutinins
d clumped platelets

read up on!

87 A patient with beta-thalassemia characteristically has a(n):
MLS ONLY
a elevated A_2 hemoglobin ($\downarrow$ *in alpha-thalassemia*)
b low fetal hemoglobin
c high serum iron
d normal red cell fragility

88 With this blood picture, an additional test indicated is:

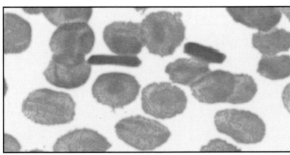

Hgb C crystals

a alkali denaturation
b alkaline phosphatase stain
c peroxidase stain
d hemoglobin electrophoresis

89 The most appropriate screening test for detecting hemoglobin F is:

a osmotic fragility
b dithionite solubility
c Kleihauer-Betke (*fetal hgb screen*)
d heat instability test

90   The most appropriate screening test for hemoglobin S is:

   a Kleihauer-Betke
   b dithionite solubility – *confirmed by electrophoresis*
   c osmotic fragility   *not to be used on newborns*
   d sucrose hemolysis   *needs correction for severe anemia*
      not specific for hemoglobin S
      (can cause other hgb variants to sickle)

91   Hematology standards include:

   a stabilized red blood cell suspension
   b latex particles
   c stabilized avian red blood cells
   d certified cyanmethemoglobin solution – *used for both hgb concentration calibration*

92   In an adult with rare homozygous delta-beta thalassemia, the hemoglobin produced is:
MLS ONLY

   a Hgb A
   b Hgb Bart
   c Hgb F – *100%*
   d Hgb H

93   Which of the following is **not** a characteristic of hemoglobin H?
MLS ONLY
                                                    oxygen affinity 10X higher than hgb A
   a it is a tetramer of beta chains
   b it is relatively unstable and thermolabile
   c electrophoretically, it represents a "fast" hemoglobin
   d its oxygen affinity is lower than that of hemoglobin A

94   In most cases of hereditary persistence of fetal hemoglobin (HPFH):
MLS ONLY

   a hemoglobin F is unevenly distributed throughout the erythrocytes
   b the black heterozygote has 75% hemoglobin F
   c beta and gamma chain synthesis is decreased
   d gamma chain production equals alpha chain production

95   Hemoglobin H disease results from:
MLS ONLY
   a absence of 3 of 4 alpha genes
   b absence of 2 of 4 alpha genes
   c absence of 1 of 1 alpha genes
   d absence of all 4 alpha genes

96   When using the turbidity (solubility) method for detecting the presence of hemoglobin S, an incorrect interpretation may be made when there is a(n):

   a concentration of less than 7 g/dL (70 g/L) hemoglobin
   b glucose concentration greater than 150 mg/dL (8.3 mmol/L)
   c blood specimen greater than 2 hours old
   d increased hemoglobin *?*

97   Refer to the following pattern:

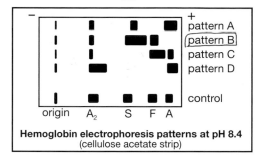

Hemoglobin electrophoresis patterns at pH 8.4
(cellulose acetate strip)

Which pattern is consistent with <u>beta-thalassemia major?</u>

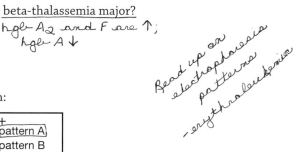

hgb A₂ and F are ↑;
hgb A ↓

Read up on electrophoresis patterns
– erythroleukemia

  a pattern A
  b pattern B
  c pattern C
  d pattern D

98   Refer to the following illustration:

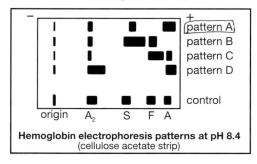

Hemoglobin electrophoresis patterns at pH 8.4
(cellulose acetate strip)

Which electrophoresis pattern is consistent with <u>sickle cell trait?</u>

  a pattern A
  b pattern B
  c pattern C
  d pattern D

99   A native of Thailand has a normal hemoglobin level. Hemoglobin electrophoresis on cellulose
MLS ONLY acetate shows 70% hemoglobin A and approximately 30% of a hemoglobin with the mobility of
hemoglobin A_2. This is most consistent with hemoglobin:

  a C trait
  b E trait
  c O trait
  d D trait

100 The laboratory findings on a patient are as follows:

    MCV: 55 μm³ (55 fL) ↓
    MCHC: 25% ↓
    MCH: 17 pg

A stained blood film of this patient would most likely reveal a red cell picture that is:

  a microcytic, hypochromic
  b macrocytic, hypochromic
  c normocytic, normochromic
  d microcytic, normochromic

101 A patient has the following laboratory results:

RBC:	$2.00 \times 10^6/\mu L$ ($2.00 \times 10^{12}/L$)
Hct:	24%
Hgb:	6.8 g/dL (68 g/L)
reticulocytes:	0.8%

$MCV = \dfrac{Hct \%}{RBC} \times 10$

$MCH = \dfrac{Hgb}{RBC} \times 10$

$MCHC = \dfrac{Hgb}{Hct \%} \times 100$

The mean corpuscular volume (MCV) of the patient is:

a 35 μm³ (35 fL)
b 83 μm³ (83 fL) $\dfrac{24}{2.0} \times 10$
c 120 μm³ (120 fL)
d 150 μm³ (150 fL)

102 The following results were obtained from a post-surgical patient receiving total parenteral nutrition:

Hospital day	17	18	19
Hgb	12.1 g/dL (121 g/L)	11.6 g/dL (116 g/L)	9.4 g/dL (94 g/L)
Hct	29.2%	29.4%	28.8%

The most consistent explanation for the above data is:

a acute surgical bleeder
b specimen on day 19 from wrong patient
c improperly mixed specimen on day 19
d lipid interference on days 17 and 18

103 A patient has a high cold agglutinin titer. Automated cell counter results reveal an elevated MCV, MCH and MCHC. Individual erythrocytes appear normal on a stained smear, but agglutinates are noted. The appropriate course of action would be to:

a perform the RBC, Hgb, and Hct determinations using manual methods
b perform the RBC determination by a manual method; use the automated results for the Hgb and Hct
c repeat the determinations using a microsample of diluted blood
d repeat the determinations using a prewarmed microsample of diluted blood

104 A blood sample from a patient with a high-titer cold agglutinin, analyzed at room temperature, with an electronic particle counter would cause an error in the:

a Hgb and MCV
b MCHC and WBC   ✳✳   ↑ MCHC
c WBC and RBC   falsely elevated ↑ MCV
-d MCV and MCHC   falsely ↓ decreased RBC

105 When using an electronic cell counter, which of the following results can occur in the presence of a cold agglutinin?

a increased MCV and decreased RBC
b increased MCV and normal RBC
- c decreased MCV and increased MCHC
d decreased MCV and RBC

106 In polycythemia vera, the leukocyte alkaline phosphatase activity is:

    a elevated
    b normal
    c decreased

107 Which of the following is the formula for mean corpuscular hemoglobin (MCH)?

    a Hct/(RBC × 1000)
    b Hgb/Hct
    c RBC/Hct
    d (Hgb × 10)/RBC

108 What is the MCH if the Hct is 20%, the RBC is $2.4 \times 10^6/\mu L$ ($2.4 \times 10^{12}/L$) and the Hgb is 5 g/ dL (50 g/L)?

    a 21 μm^3 (21 fL) $\dfrac{hgb}{RBC} \times 10 = \dfrac{5}{2.4} \times 10 =$
    b 23 μm^3 (23 fL)
    c 25 μm^3 (25 fL)
    d 84 μm^3 (84 fL)

109 What is the MCH if the Hct is 20%, the RBC is $1.5 \times 10^6/\mu L$ ($1.5 \times 10^{12}/L$) and the Hgb is 6 g/ dL (60 g/L)?

    a 28 μm^3 (28 fL) $\dfrac{6}{1.5} \times 10 =$
    b 30 μm^3 (30 fL)
    c 40 μm^3 (40 fL)
    d 75 μm^3 (75 fL)

110 Which of the following is the formula for MCHC?

    a (Hgb × 100)/Hct
    b Hgb/RBC
    c RBC/Hct
    d (Hct × 1000)/RBC

111 What is the MCHC if the Hct is 20%, the RBC is $2.4 \times 10^6/\mu L$ ($2.4 \times 10^{12}/L$) and the Hgb is 5 g/dL (50 g/L)?

    a 21%
    b 25% $\dfrac{hgb}{hct} \times 100 =$
    c 30%
    d 34%

112 What is the MCHC if the Hct is 20%, the RBC is $1.5 \times 10^6/\mu L$ ($1.5 \times 10^{12}/L$) and the Hgb is 6 g/dL (60 g/L)?

    a 28% $\dfrac{hgb}{hct\%} \times 100 = \dfrac{6}{20} \times 100 =$
    b 30%
    c 40%
    d 75%

113 Which of the following is the formula for mean corpuscular volume (MCV)?

    a (Hgb × 10)/RBC
    b Hgb/Hct
    c (Hct × 10)/RBC
    d RBC/Hct

114 Given the following data:

Hgb: 8 g/dL (80 g/L)
Hct: 28%
RBC: $3.6 \times 10^6/\mu L$ ($3.6 \times 10^{12}/L$)

The MCV is:

a $28\ \mu m^3$ (28 fL)
b $35\ \mu m^3$ (35 fL)
c $40\ \mu m^3$ (40 fL)
d $77\ \mu m^3$ (77 fL)

(hct) 28 / 3.6 (RBC) × 10 =

115 What is the MCV if the hematocrit is 20%, the RBC is $2.4 \times 10^6/\mu L$ ($2.4 \times 10^{12}/L$) and the hemoglobin is 5 g/dL (50 g/L)?

a   68 pg
b   83 pg
c 100 pg
d 120 pg

20 / 2.4 × 10 =

116 What is the MCV if the hematocrit is 20%, the RBC is $1.5 \times 10^6/\mu L$ ($1.5 \times 10^{12}/L$) and the hemoglobin is 6 g/dL (60 g/L)?

a   68 pg
b   75 pg
c 115 pg
d 133 pg

20 / 1.5 × 10 =

117 The principle confirmatory test for hereditary spherocytosis is:

a osmotic fragility *along with peripheral smear and RBC indices*
b sucrose hemolysis
c heat instability test
d Kleihauer-Betke

118 A screening test for paroxysmal nocturnal hemoglobinuria is:

a heat instability test
b sucrose hemolysis = *PNH; immunophenotyping best*
c osmotic fragility
d dithionite solubility

119 The Prussian blue staining of peripheral blood identifies:
(iron stain)

a Howell-Jolly bodies
b siderotic granules
c reticulocytes
d basophilic stippling

120 Supravital staining is important for reticulocytes since the cells must be living in order to stain the:

a remaining RNA in the cell ** *stain = new methylene blue*
b iron before it precipitates
c cell membrane before it dries out
d denatured hemoglobin in the cell

121 Which of the following is used for staining reticulocytes?

a Giemsa stain
b Wright stain
c new methylene blue
d Prussian blue

122 Which of the following stains is used to demonstrate iron, ferritin and hemosiderin?

    a peroxidase
    b Sudan black B
    c periodic acid-Schiff (PAS)
    d Prussian blue – *iron stores*

123 Which of the following stains can be used to differentiate siderotic granules (Pappenheimer bodies) from basophilic stippling?

    a Wright
    b Prussian blue
    c crystal violet
    d periodic acid-Schiff

124 A patient has pancytopenia, decreased total serum iron, decreased serum iron binding capacity, and shows a homogeneous fluorescence pattern with a high titer on a fluorescent anti-nuclear antibody test. This is suggestive of:

    a polycythemia vera
    b systemic lupus erythematosus – *homogenous fluorescent pattern (anti-DNA)*
    c iron deficiency anemia
    d hemoglobin SC disease

125 In an uncomplicated case of severe iron deficiency anemia, which of the following sets represents the typical pattern of results?

	Serum iron	Serum TIBC	% Saturation	Marrow % sideroblasts	Marrow iron stores	Serum ferritin	Hgb A$_2$
A	↓	↑	↓	↓	↑	↑	↑
B	↓	↓	↓	↓	↓	↓	↓
C	↓	↑	↓	↓	↓	↓	↓
D	↓	↓	↑	↑	↑	↑	↑

    increased = ↑ decreased = ↓

    a A
    b B
    c C
    d D

Iron deficiency anemia:
↓ RBC, hgb, MCV, MCH, MCHC, serum iron, serum ferritin % sat, bone marrow iron stores
↑ RDW, TIBC, FEP, serum transferrin

Leukocytes: Physiology

126 Inclusions in the cytoplasm of neutrophils as shown in the figure below are known as:

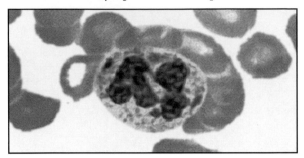

    a Auer bodies
    b Howell-Jolly bodies
    c Heinz bodies
    d Döhle bodies

127 An increased amount of cytoplasmic basophilia in a blood cell indicates:

    a increased cytoplasmic maturation
    b decreased cytoplasmic maturation
    c reduction in size of the cell
    d decreased nuclear maturation

128 The term "shift to the left" refers to:

    a a microscope adjustment
    b immature cell forms in the peripheral blood
    c a trend on a Levy-Jennings chart
    d a calibration adjustment on an instrument

129 A term that means varying degrees of leukocytosis with a shift to the left and occasional nucleated red cells in the peripheral blood is:

    a polycythemia vera
    b erythroleukemia
    c leukoerythroblastosis
    d megaloblastoid

130 Cells that produce antibodies and lymphokines are:

    a erythrocytes
    b granulocytes
    c lymphocytes
    d thrombocytes

131 The peripheral blood monocyte is an intermediate stage in the formation of the:

MLS
ONLY

    a plasmacyte
    b osteoclast
    c fibroblast
    d hairy cell

132 Specific (secondary) granules of the neutrophilic granulocyte:

    a appear first at the myelocyte stage
    b contain lysosomal enzymes
    c are formed on the mitochondria
    d are derived from azurophil (primary) granules

133 In normal adult bone marrow, the most common granulocyte is the:

   a basophil
   b myeloblast
   c eosinophil   ✸✶
   (d) metamyelocyte

134 Elevation of the total granulocyte count above $7.7 \times 10^3/\mu L$ ($7.7 \times 10^9/L$) is termed:

   a relative lymphocytosis
   b leukocytosis
   c relative neutrophilic leukocytosis
   (d) absolute neutrophilic leukocytosis

135 Elevation of the total white cell count above $12 \times 10^3/\mu L$ ($12 \times 10^9/L$) is termed:

   a relative lymphocytosis
   b absolute lymphocytosis
   (c) leukocytosis
   d relative neutrophilic leukocytosis

136 Elevation of the granulocyte percentage above 75% is termed:

   a absolute lymphocytosis
   b leukocytosis
   (c) relative neutrophilic leukocytosis
   d absolute neutrophilic leukocytosis

137 Elevation of the lymphocyte percentage above 47% is termed:

   (a) relative lymphocytosis
   b absolute lymphocytosis
   c leukocytosis
   d absolute neutrophilic leukocytosis

138 Terminal deoxynucleotidyl transferase (TdT) is a marker found on:

   a hairy cells
   b myeloblasts   *TdT staining = Lymphoblasts*
   c monoblasts
   (d) lymphoblasts

139 Multipotent stem cells are capable of producing:

   a daughter cells of only one cell line   *Multipotent stem cells =*
   b only T-lymphocytes and B-lymphocytes   *lymphoid and myeloid lines*
   c erythropoietin, thrombopoietin, and leukopoietin
   (d) lymphoid and myeloid stem cells

140 The Philadelphia chromosome is formed by a translocation between the:

   (a) long arm of chromosome 22 and long arm of chromosome 9 = *Philadelphia Chromosome*
   b long arm of chromosome 21 and long arm of chromosome 9   *22 + 9 Long arms*
   c long arm of chromosome 21 and short arm of chromosome 6
   d long arm of chromosome 22 and short arm of chromosome 6

141 Phagocytosis is a function of:

   a erythrocytes
   (b) granulocytes
   c lymphocytes
   d thrombocytes

142 Mechanism of cortisol-induced neutrophilia includes:

MLS
ONLY - (a) a shift in granulocytes from the marginating pool to the circulating pool
   b an increased exit of granulocytes from the circulation
   c a decrease exit of granulocytes from the bone marrow
   d granulocyte return from the tissues to the circulating pool

143 Which cells are involved in immediate hypersensitivity reactions?

MLS
ONLY - **a** eosinophils
   (b) basophils
   c plasma cells
   d reactive lymphocytes

144 The white cell feature most characteristic of pernicious anemia is:

   a eosinophilia
   b toxic granulation
   (c) hypersegmentation
   d atypical lymphocytes

Leukocytes: Disease States

145 Which of the following conditions is **not** associated with a high incidence of leukemia?

   a paroxysmal nocturnal hemoglobinuria
   b Fanconi anemia   *bone marrow disfunction*
   c aplastic anemia
   (d) megaloblastic anemia – *nutritional deficiency*

146 The M:E ratio in chronic myelocytic leukemia is usually:

   a normal
   (b) high
   c low
   d variable

147 In the French-American-British (FAB) classification, myelomonocytic leukemia would be:

MLS
ONLY **a** M1 and M2
   b M3
   c M4 – *mono*
   d M5

148 Abnormalities found in <u>erythroleukemia</u> include:

   a rapid DNA synthesis
   b marrow fibrosis
   (c) megaloblastoid development   ✳✳
   d increased erythrocyte survival

149 Neutropenia is **not** usually associated with:

   a viral infections
   (b) Hodgkin disease   ✳✳
   c select antibiotics
   d chemotherapy

150 <u>Auer rods</u> are **most** likely present in which of the following?

   a chronic myelocytic leukemia
   b myelofibrosis with myeloid metaplasia
   c erythroleukemia
   (d) acute myelocytic leukemia → *auer rods*

151 The following results were obtained on a 45-year-old man complaining of chills and fever:

WBC: $23.0 \times 10^3/\mu L$ ($23.0 \times 10^9/L$) ↑↑
LAP: 200↑
Philadelphia chromosome: negative
Differential

Segs: 60%
Bands: 21%
Lymphs: 11%
Monos: 3%
Metamyelos: 2%
Myelos: 3%
Toxic granulation, Döhle bodies and vacuoles

These results are consistent with:

a neutrophilic leukemoid reaction
b polycythemia vera
c chronic myelocytic leukemia
d leukoerythroblastosis in myelofibrosis

152 In an uncomplicated case of infectious mononucleosis, which of the following cells are affected?

a erythrocytes
b lymphocytes
c monocytes
d thrombocytes

153 The atypical lymphocyte seen in the peripheral smear of patients with infectious mono is probably derived from which of the following?

a T lymphocytes
b B lymphocytes
c monocytes
d mast cells

154 Which of the following cells is the atypical lymphocyte seen on the peripheral blood smear of patients with infectious mononucleosis?

a T lymphocytes
b B lymphocytes   ✳
c monocytes
d mast cells

155 The disease most frequently present in patients with atypical lymphocytosis and persistently negative tests is:

a toxoplasmosis
b cytomegalovirus (CMV) infection
c herpes virus infection
d viral hepatitis

156 Dwarf or micro megakaryocytes may be found in the peripheral blood of patients with:

a pernicious anemia
b DIC
c myelofibrosis with myeloid metaplasia
d chronic lymphocytic leukemia

157 Which of the following is associated with pseudo-Pelger-Huët anomaly?

a aplastic anemia
b iron deficiency anemia
c myelogenous leukemia
d Chédiak-Higashi syndrome

158 Auer bodies are:

   a a normal aggregation of lysosomes or primary (azurophilic) granules
   (b) predominately found in acute myelogenous leukemia
   c peroxidase negative
   d alkaline phosphatase positive

159 The absence of the Philadelphia chromosome in granulocytic leukemia suggests:

   (a) rapid progression of the disease
   b a polyclonal origin to the disease
   c excellent response to therapy
   d conversion from another myeloproliferative disorder

160 Increased numbers of basophils are often seen in:

   a acute infections
   (b) chronic myelocytic leukemia = ↑ basophils
   c chronic lymphocytic leukemia
   d erythroblastosis fetalis (hemolytic disease of the newborn)

161 A hypercellular marrow with an M:E ratio of 6:1 is most commonly due to:

   a lymphoid hyperplasia
   (b) granulocytic hyperplasia
   c normoblastic hyperplasia
   d myeloid hypoplasia

162 The following results were obtained:

   WBC: $5.0 \times 10^3/\mu L$ ($5.0 \times 10^9/L$)
   RBC: $1.7 \times 10^6/\mu L$ ($1.7 \times 10^{12}/L$) ↓
   MCV: 84 μm^3 (84 fL)
   Plt: $89 \times 10^3/\mu L$ ($89 \times 10^9/L$) ↓
   LAP: 142

Philadelphia chromosome: negative

Differential:

Segs:	16%
Bands:	22%
Lymphs:	28%
Monos:	16%
Eos:	1%
Basos:	1%
Metamyelos:	4%
Myelos:	3%
Promyelos:	4%
Blasts:	5%

1 megakaryoblast; 30 nucleated erythrocytes; teardrops; schistocytes; polychromasia; giant, bizarre platelets noted

This is consistent with:

   a idiopathic thrombocythemia
   b polycythemia vera
   c chronic myelocytic leukemia
   (d) leukoerythroblastosis in myelofibrosis

163 A 50-year-old man was admitted into the hospital with acute leukemia. Laboratory findings included the following:

Myeloperoxidase stain:	Blast cells negative
PAS stain:	Blast cells demonstrate a blocking pattern
Terminal deoxynucleotidyl transferase (TdT):	Blast cells positive
Surface immunoglobulin:	Blast cells negative
CD2:	Blast cells negative
Philadelphia chromosome:	Positive

These results are most consistent with:

a acute myelogenous leukemia
b chronic lymphocytic leukemia in lymphoblastic transformation
c T-cell acute lymphocytic leukemia
d chronic myelogenous leukemia in lymphoblastic transformation

164 A 30-year-old man who had been diagnosed as having leukemia 2 years previously was readmitted because of cervical lymphadenopathy. Laboratory findings included the following:

WBC:	$39.6 \times 10^3/\mu L$ ($39.6 \times 10^9/L$)
RBC:	$3.25 \times 10^6/\mu L$ ($3.25 \times 10^{12}/L$)
Hgb:	9.4 g/dL (94 g/L)
Hct:	28.2%
MCV:	$86.7 \ \mu m^3$ (86.7 fL)
MCH:	29.0 pg
MCHC:	33.4%
Plt:	$53 \times 10^3/\mu L$ ($53 \times 10^9/L$)
LAP:	11

Philadelphia chromosome: positive

Differential:

Polys:	7%
Lymphs:	4%
Monos :	2%
Eos:	3%
Basos:	48%
Myelos:	13%
Promyelos:	2%
Metamyelos:	8%
Blasts:	13%
NRBCs:	11

Bone marrow: 95% cellularity, 50% blast cells (some with peroxidase and SBB positivity)

These results are most consistent with:

a acute myeloid leukemia
b erythroleukemia
c chronic myelogenous leukemia (CML)
d CML in blast transformation

165　The following results were obtained on a 35-year-old woman complaining of fatigue and weight loss:

WBC:	$1.8 \times 10^3/\mu L$ ($1.8 \times 10^9/L$)
RBC:	$4.6 \times 10^6/\mu L$ ($4.6 \times 10^{12}/L$)
Plt:	$903 \times 10^3/\mu L$ ($903 \times 10^9/L$)
uric acid:	$6.4 \times mg/dL$ (380 µmol/L)
LAP:	0
Philadelphia chromosome:	positive

Differential:

Segs:	30%
Bands:	17%
Lymphs:	13%
Monos:	3%
Eos:	4%
Basos:	6%
Metamyelos:	3%
Myelos:	20%
Promyelos:	3%
Blasts:	1%

leukopenia
immature granulocytes at all stages with blasts
↓↓ LAP
(+) Philadelphia chromosome
long arms of Chromosomes 22 + 9

These results are consistent with:

a　neutrophilic leukemoid reaction
b　idiopathic thrombocythemia
c　chronic myelocytic leukemia
d　leukoerythroblastosis in myelofibrosis

166　Which is the most predominant form of secondary hematologic malignancy seen in patients with
　　multiple myeloma?

a　acute lymphoblastic leukemia
b　acute eosinophilic leukemia
c　acute myelomonocytic leukemia *→ possible progression of MM*
d　acute megakaryocytic leukemia

167　In chronic myelocytic leukemia, blood histamine concentrations tend to reflect the:

a　number of platelets present
b　serum uric acid concentrations
c　number of basophils present *– blood histamine*
d　the total number of granulocytes

168　Biochemical abnormalities characteristic of polycythemia vera include:

a　increased serum B_{12} binding capacity *erythroid versus myeloid*
b　hypouricemia
c　hypohistaminemia
d　decreased leukocyte alkaline phosphatase activity

169　Auer rods:

a　contain lactoferrin
b　are lysosome and acid phosphatase-positive
c　are found in the leukemic phase of lymphoma
d　are found in acute lymphocytic leukemia

170　50%-90% myeloblasts in a peripheral blood is typical of which of the following?

a　chronic myelocytic leukemia
b　myelofibrosis with myeloid metaplasia
c　erythroleukemia *50% RBC precursors*
d　acute myelocytic leukemia *> 20% myeloblasts*

171 The M:E ratio in acute myelocytic leukemia is usually:

    a normal
    (b) high
    c low
    d variable

172 Which of the following is most closely associated with <u>acute promyelocytic leukemia</u>?
MLS ONLY

    a ringed sideroblasts
    (b) disseminated intravascular coagulation (DIC)
    c micromegakaryocytes
    d Philadelphia chromosome

173 Which of the following is most closely associated with chronic myelomonocytic leukemia?

    a Philadelphia chromosome *CGL CML*
    b disseminated intravascular coagulation – *promyelocytic leukemia*
    c micromegakaryocytes – *myelofibrosis*   **✱✱**
    (d) lysozymuria – *CMML (chronic myelomonocytic leukemia)*

174 The absence of intermediate maturing cells between the blast and mature neutrophil commonly seen in acute myelocytic leukemia and myelodysplastic syndromes is called:

    a subleukemia
    b aleukemic leukemia
    (c) leukemic <u>hiatus</u> → *opening*   **✱✱**
    d leukemoid reaction

175 Which of the following is most closely associated with chronic myelogenous leukemia?

    a ringed sideroblasts
    b disseminated intravascular coagulation
    c micromegakaryocytes
    (d) Philadelphia chromosome

176 The bone marrow in the terminal stage of erythroleukemia is often indistinguishable from that seen in:
MLS ONLY

    a myeloid metaplasia
    b polycythemia vera
    (c) acute myelocytic leukemia
    d aplastic anemia

177 A block in the differentiation or maturation of, and an accretion of immature hematopoietic progenitors is a hallmark of: ?

    a chronic lymphocytic leukemia
    b myeloproliferative diseases
    c polycythemia vera
    (d) acute myelogenous leukemia

178 <u>All stages of neutrophils</u> are most likely to be seen in the peripheral blood of a patient with:

    (a) chronic myelocytic leukemia
    b myelofibrosis with myeloid metaplasia
    c erythroleukemia
    d acute myelocytic leukemia

179 All of the following conditions are myeloproliferative disorders **except**:

    a myelocytic leukemia
    (b) lymphocytic leukemia – NOT *a granulocytic precursor*
    c polycythemia vera   **✱**
    d idiopathic thrombocythemia

180 The following results were obtained on a 55-year-old man complaining of headaches and
     blurred vision:

     ↑ WBC: $19.0 \times 10^3/\mu L$ ($19.0 \times 10^9/L$)
     ↑ RBC: $7.2 \times 10^6/\mu L$ ($7.2 \times 10^{12}/L$)
     ↑↑ Plt: $1,056 \times 10^3/\mu L$ ($1056 \times 10^9/L$)
       uric acid: 13.0 mg/dL (0.76 mmol/L)
       O_2 saturation: 93%
       Rh[1]:   negative
       Red cell volume: 3,911 mL (normal = 1,600)
     Differential:
       Segs: 84%
       Bands: 10%
       Lymphs: 3%
       Monos: 2%
       Eos: 1%

     These results are consistent with:

     a neutrophilic leukemoid reaction
     (b) polycythemia vera – *proliferation of all cell lines*
     c chronic myelocytic leukemia
     d leukoerythroblastosis in myelofibrosis

181 A patient has a tumor that concentrates erythropoietin. He is most likely to have which of the
     following types of polycythemia?

     a polycythemia vera
     b polycythemia, secondary to hypoxia
     c benign familial polycythemia
     (d) polycythemia associated with renal disease

182 Which of the following types of polycythemia is most often associated with emphysema?

     a polycythemia vera
     (b) polycythemia, secondary to hypoxia
     c relative polycythemia associated with dehydration
     d polycythemia associated with renal disease

183 Hemorrhage in polycythemia vera is the result of:

     a increased plasma viscosity
     b persistent thrombocytosis
     c splenic sequestration of platelets
     (d) abnormal platelet function – *inhibits clotting*

184 A patient diagnosed with polycythemia vera 5 years ago now has a normal hematocrit, decreased
     hemoglobin and microcytic, hypochromic red cells. What is the most probable cause for the
     current blood situation?

     (a) phlebotomy
     b myelofibrosis
     c preleukemia
     d aplastic anemia

185   A patient has been treated for polycythemia vera for several years. His blood smear now shows:

   Oval macrocytes
   Howell-Jolly bodies
   Hypersegmented neutrophils
   Large, agranular platelets

   The most probable cause of this blood picture is:

   a iron deficiency
   b alcoholism
   c dietary B_{12} deficiency
   ⓓ chemotherapy – *toxic effects*

186   In infectious mononucleosis, lymphocytes tend to be:

   a small with little cytoplasm
   b normal
   c decreased in number
   ⓓ enlarged and indented by surrounding structures

187   In comparison to malignant lymphoma cells, reactive lymphocytes:

   a have a denser nuclear chromatin
   b are known to be T cells
   c have more cytoplasm and more mitochondria
   ⓓ are morphologically more variable throughout the smear

188   T-cell acute lymphocytic leukemia (ALL) is closely related to:

   a chronic lymphocytic leukemia (CLL)
   b autoimmune disease
   ⓒ lymphoblastic lymphoma *(B-cell)*
   d acute myelocytic leukemia (AGL)

189   In the French-American-British (FAB) classification, acute lymphocytic leukemia is divided into
groups according to:

   a prognosis
   b immunology
   c cytochemistry
   ⓓ morphology

190   Increased levels of TdT activity are indicative of:

   a Burkitt lymphoma
   b acute myelocytic leukemia
   ⓒ acute lymphocytic leukemia *(ALL → TdT activity)*
   d eosinophilia

191   Which of the following is true of acute lymphoblastic leukemia (ALL)?

   a occurs most commonly in children ~~1-2~~ *1-5* years of age   **✳✳**
   b patient is ~~a~~symptomatic *(lethargy, bone pain, fever)*
   ⓒ massive accumulation of primitive lymphoid-appearing cells in bone marrow occurs
   d children under 1 year of age have a ~~good~~ *poor* prognosis

192 A 50-year-old woman who has been receiving busulfan for three years for chronic myelogenous leukemia becomes anemic. Laboratory tests reveal:

Thrombocytopenia
Many peroxidase-negative blast cells in the peripheral blood
Bone marrow hypercellular in blast transformation
Markedly increased bone marrow TdT

Which of the following complications is this patient most likely to have?

a acute lymphocytic leukemia → *progresses in ⅓ of cases* **✳✳**
b acute myelocytic leukemia
c acute myelomonocytic leukemia
d busulfan toxicity

193 The most common form of childhood leukemia is:

a acute lymphocytic
b acute granulocytic   **✳✳**
c acute monocytic
d chronic granulocytic

194 Chronic lymphocytic leukemia is defined as a(n):

a malignancy of the thymus
b accumulation of prolymphocytes
c accumulation of hairy cells in the spleen
d accumulation of monoclonal B cells with a block in cell maturation

195 Hairy cell leukemia (leukemic reticuloendotheliosis) is:
MLS ONLY

a an acute myelocytic leukemia
b a chronic leukemia of myelocytic origin   **✳✳**
c a chronic leukemia of lymphocytic origin
d an acute myelocytic monocytic-type leukemia

196 Which of the following is **not** a characteristic usually associated with hairy cell leukemia?
decreased infection resistance
a pancytopenia
b mononuclear cells with ruffled edges
c splenomegaly
d increased resistance to infection

197 Morphologic variants of plasma cells do **not** include: ?

a flame cells
b morula cells
c grape cells
d Gaucher cells - *lipid storage disease*

198 Which of the following bone marrow findings favor the diagnosis of multiple myeloma?
MLS ONLY

a presence of Reed-Sternberg cells - *Hodgkin lymphoma*
b sheaths of immature plasma cells - *most common*
c presence of flame cells and Russell bodies
d presence of plasmacytic satellitosis

199 Which of the following have a B cell origin?
MLS ONLY

a Sézary syndrome
b malignant lymphoma, lymphoblastic type
c Sternberg sarcoma
d Waldenström macroglobulinemia - *lymphoplasmacytic lymphoma*

200 Which of the following cells is most likely identified in lesions of mycosis fungoides?

MLS ONLY

   ⓐ T lymphocytes
   b B lymphocytes
   c monocytes
   d mast cells

201 Of the following, the disease most closely associated with cytoplasmic granule fusion is:

   ⓐ Chédiak-Higashi syndrome – *giant fused lyso...* [LOOK-UP!]
   b Pelger-Huët anomaly
   c May-Hegglin anomaly
   d Alder-Reilly anomaly

202 Which of the following anomalies is an autosomal dominant disorder characterized by irregularly-sized inclusions in polymorphonuclear neutrophils, abnormal giant platelets and often thrombocytopenia?

   a Pelger-Huët
   b Chédiak-Higashi
   c Alder-Reilly
   ⓓ May-Hegglin – *giant platelets, ↓ PLT count, inclusions in PMNS*

203 Of the following, the disease most closely associated with granulocyte hyposegmentation is:

   a May-Hegglin anomaly
   ⓑ Pelger-Huët anomaly – *"aviator glasses"*
   c Chédiak-Higashi syndrome
   d Gaucher disease

204 Which of the following cell types is characteristic of Pelger-Huët anomaly is the:

   a band form
   ⓑ pince-nez form – *bilobed, dumbbell shaped, "aviator glasses*
   c normal neutrophil
   d myelocyte

205 Which of the following is associated with Chédiak-Higashi syndrome?

   ⓐ membrane defect of lysosomes
   b Döhle bodies and giant platelets
   c two-lobed neutrophils
   d mucopolysaccharidosis

206 Which of the following is associated with Alder-Reilly inclusions?

   a membrane defect of lysosomes
   b Döhle bodies and giant platelets
   c two-lobed neutrophils
   ⓓ mucopolysaccharidosis

207 Which of the following is associated with May-Hegglin anomaly?

   a membrane defect of lysosomes
   ⓑ Döhle bodies and giant platelets
   c chronic myelogenous leukemia
   d mucopolysaccharidosis

208 A differential was performed on an asymptomatic patient. The differential included 60% neutrophils: 55 of which had 2 lobes and 5 had 3 lobes. There were no other abnormalities. This is consistent with which of the following anomalies?

   ⓐ Pelger-Huët – *hyposegmentation*
   b May-Hegglin
   c Alder-Reilly
   d Chédiak-Higashi

209 The cytoplasmic abnormality of the white blood cell of Alder-Reilly anomaly is found in the:

   a endoplasmic reticulum
   (b) lysosomes ~~C·H~~
   c mitochondria
   d ribosomes

210 Of the following, the disease most closely associated with mucopolysaccharidosis is:

   a Pelger-Huët anomaly
   b Chédiak-Higashi syndrome
   c Gaucher disease
   (d) Alder-Reilly anomaly

211 Of the following, the disease most closely associated with <u>glucocerebrosidase deficiency</u> is:

   (a) Gaucher disease - *lipid storage*
   b Chédiak-Higashi syndrome
   c Pelger-Huët anomaly
   d May-Hegglin anomaly

212 Patients with chronic granulomatous disease suffer from frequent pyogenic infections due to
MLS
ONLY the inability of:

   a lymphocytes to produce bacterial antibodies
   b eosinophils to degranulate in the presence of bacteria
   (c) neutrophils to kill phagocytized bacteria
   d basophils to release histamine in the presence of bacteria

213 Of the following, the disease most closely associated with pale blue inclusions in granulocytes
   and giant platelets is:

   a Gaucher disease
   b Alder-Reilly anomaly
   (c) May-Hegglin anomaly
   d Pelger-Huët anomaly

Leukocytes: Laboratory Determinations

214 An oncology patient has the following results:

	Day 1	Day 3
WBC	$8.0 \times 10^3/\mu L$ $(8.0 \times 10^9/L)$	$2.0 \times 10^3/\mu L$ $(2.0 \times 10^9/L)$
RBC	$3.50 \times 10^6/\mu L$ $(3.50 \times 10^{12}/L)$	$3.45 \times 10^6/\mu L$ $(3.45 \times 10^{12}/L)$
Hgb	10.0 g/dL (100 g/L)	9.9 g/dL (99 g/L)
Hct	29.8%	29.5%
Plt	$180 \times 10^3/\mu L$ $(180 \times 10^9/L)$	$150 \times 10^3/\mu L$ $(150 \times 10^9/L)$

The most probable explanation is:
   (a) chemotherapy ↓ *WBC/RBC's same*
   b cold antibody
   c clotted specimen
   d inadequate mixing

215 A leukocyte count and differential on a 40-year-old Caucasian man revealed:

WBC: $5.4 \times 10^3/\mu L$ ($5.4 \times 10^9/L$)

Differential:

Segs:	20%
Lymphs:	58%
Monos:	20%
Eos:	2%

This data represents:

a absolute lymphocytosis
b relative neutrophilia
c absolute neutropenia
d leukopenia

216 A leukocyte count and differential on a 40-year-old Caucasian man revealed:

WBC: $5.4 \times 10^3/\mu L$ ($5.4 \times 10^9/L$)

Differential:

Segs:	20%
Lymphs:	58%
Monos:	20%
Eos:	2%

This represents:

a relative lymphocytosis
b absolute lymphocytosis
c relative neutrophilia
d leukopenia

217 In synovial fluid, the most characteristic microscopic finding in gout is:

a calcium pyrophosphate crystals
b cartilage debris
c monosodium urate crystals
d hemosiderin-laden macrophages

218 Given the following data:

WBC: $8.5 \times 10^3/\mu L$ ($8.5 \times 10^9/L$)

Differential:

Segs:	56%
Bands:	2%
Lymphs:	30%
Monos:	6%
Eos:	6%

Total count × % =
8.5 × .30 = 2.55 × 10³/µl

What is the absolute lymphocyte count?

a $170/\mu L$ ($0.17 \times 10^9/L$)
b $510/\mu L$ ($0.51 \times 10^9/L$)
c $2,550/\mu L$ ($2.55 \times 10^9/L$)
d $4,760/\mu L$ ($4.76 \times 10^9/L$)

219 Given the following data:

WBC: $8.5 \times 10^3/\mu L$ ($8.5 \times 10^9/L$)

Differential:

Segs:	56%
Bands:	2%
Lymphs:	30%
Monos:	6%
Eos:	6%

What is the absolute eosinophil count? $8.5 \times .06 = .51 \times 10^3/\mu l$

a $170/\mu L$ ($0.17 \times 10^9/L$)
b $510/\mu L$ ($0.51 \times 10^9/L$)
c $2,550/\mu L$ ($2.55 \times 10^9/L$)
d $4,760/\mu L$ ($4.76 \times 10^9/L$)

220 Which of the following is the formula for manual white cell count?

a   (number of cells counted × dilution × 10)/number of squares counted
b   (number of cells counted × dilution)/10 × number of squares counted
c   number of cells counted × dilution
d   number of cells counted × number of squares counted

221 If a WBC count is performed on a 1:10 dilution and the number of cells counted in 8 squares is 120, the total WBC count is:

a $1,200/\mu L$ ($1.2 \times 10^9/L$)
b $1,500/\mu L$ ($1.5 \times 10^9/L$)
c $12,000/\mu L$ ($12.0 \times 10^9/L$)
d $15,000/\mu L$ ($15.0 \times 10^9/L$)

$$\frac{\# \text{ of cells} \cdot \text{dilution} \cdot \text{depth factor}}{\# \text{ of squares}} =$$

$$\frac{120 \cdot 10 \cdot 10}{8} = 1500/\mu l$$

222 If a WBC count is performed on a 1:100 dilution and the number of cells counted in eight squares is 50, the total WBC count is:

a $5,000/\mu L$ ($5.0 \times 10^9/L$)
b $6,250/\mu L$ ($6.25 \times 10^9/L$)
c $50,000/\mu L$ ($50.0 \times 10^9/L$)
d $62,500/\mu L$ ($62.5 \times 10^9/L$)

$$\frac{50 \cdot 100 \cdot 10}{8} = 6,250/\mu l$$

X 223 An automated leukocyte count is $22.5 \times 10^9/\mu L$ ($22.5 \times 10^9/L$). The differential reveals 200 normoblasts/100 leukocytes. What is the actual leukocyte count per microliter?

a $7,500/\mu L$ ($7.5 \times 10^9/L$)
b $11,500/\mu L$ ($11.5 \times 10^9/L$)
c $14,400/\mu L$ ($14.4 \times 10^9/L$)
d $22,300/\mu L$ ($22.3 \times 10^9/L$)

$$\frac{22.5 \times 100}{200 + 100} = 7.5$$

X 224 A total leukocyte count is $10.0 \times 10^3/\mu L$ ($10.0 \times 10^9/L$) and 25 NRBCs are seen per 100 leukocytes on the differential. What is the corrected leukocyte count?

a $2,000/\mu L$ ($2.0 \times 10^9/L$)
b $8,000/\mu L$ ($8.0 \times 10^9/L$)
c $10,000/\mu L$ ($10.0 \times 10^9/L$)
d $12,000/\mu L$ ($12.0 \times 10^9/L$)

$$\frac{10 \times 100}{25 + 100} = 8$$

X 225 If the total leukocyte count is $20.0 \times 10^3/\mu L$ ($20.0 \times 10^9/L$) and 50 NRBCs are seen per 100 leukocytes on the differential, what is the corrected leukocyte count?

a $6,666/\mu L$ ($6.666 \times 10^9/L$)
b $10,000/\mu L$ ($10.0 \times 10^9/L$)
c $13,333/\mu L$ ($13.333 \times 10^9/L$)
d $26,666/\mu L$ ($26.666 \times 10^9/L$)

$$\frac{20 \times 100}{50 + 100} = 13.3$$

X **226** A blood smear shows 80 nucleated red cells per 100 leukocytes. The total leukocyte count is $18 \times 10^3/\mu L$ ($18 \times 10^9/L$). The true white cell count expressed in SI units is:

a $17.2 \times 10^3/\mu L$ ($17.2 \times 10^9/L$)
b $9.0 \times 10^3/\mu L$ ($9.0 \times 10^9/L$)
c $10.0 \times 10^3/\mu L$ ($10.0 \times 10^9/L$)
d $13.4 \times 10^3/\mu L$ ($13.4 \times 10^9/L$)

$$\frac{18 \times 100}{80 + 100} = 10.0$$

227 A mean cellular hemoglobin concentration (MCHC) over 36 g/dL (36 g/L) is frequently found in:

a hereditary spherocytosis
b lipemia (abnormally high plasma lipid)   ✳✳
c active cold agglutinin disease
d all of the above

228 An unexplained elevation of the prothrombin time (PT) in a 72-year-old smoker who has been diagnosed with chronic pulmonary obstructive disease is most likely due to:

a an elevated hematocrit
b a decreased hematocrit
c vitamin K deficiency   ✳
d decreased thrombin activity

abnormal hematocrit effects PT→
most adjust citrate

229 Which of the following statements about this field is **true**?

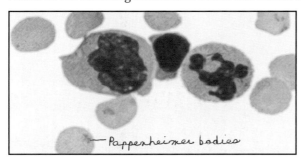

— *Pappenheimer bodies*

a reticulocytes are demonstrable
b toxic granulation is present
c the cell in the center is a basophilic normoblast
d the large cell on the left is a monocyte

230 The large nucleated cell in the lower right-hand side of the image below is a:

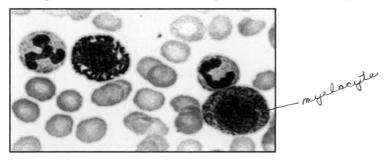

— *myelocyte*

a myelocyte
b metamyelocyte
c basophil
d plasma cell

231 In the image below, the small nucleated cell seen in the lower left corner is a:

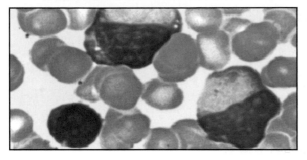

    a polychromatophilic normoblast (rubricyte)
    b mature lymphocyte
    c plasma cell
    d lymphoblast

232 The cells seen in the image below are most consistent with:
MLS
ONLY

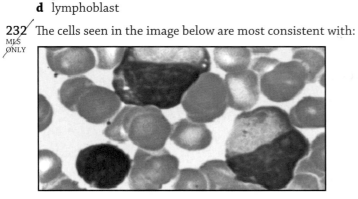

    a chronic myelogenous leukemia
    b infectious mononucleosis
    c acute lymphocytic leukemia
    d Sézary syndrome

233 Cell description:

    Size: 12 to 16 µm
    Nucleus: oval, notched, folded over to horseshoe shape
    Chromatin: fine lacy, stains light purple-pink
    Nucleoli: none present
    Cytoplasm: abundant, slate gray, with many fine lilac-colored granules

This cell is a:

    a promyelocyte
    b lymphocyte
    c neutrophil
    d monocyte

234 The large cell in the center of the image would be best described as a(n):

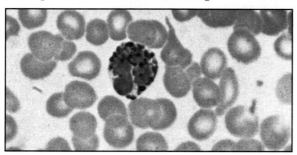

   a neutrophil
   b basophil
   c eosinophil
   d myelocyte

235 The large cell indicated by the arrow in image below is a:

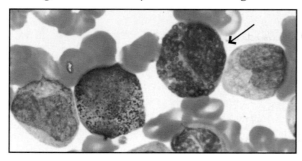

   a myeloblast
   b promyelocyte
   c myelocyte
   d metamyelocyte

236 A patient is diagnosed as having bacterial septicemia. Which of the following would best describe the expected change in his peripheral blood?

   a granulocytic leukemoid reaction
   b lymphocytic leukemoid reaction
   c neutropenia
   d eosinophilia

237 The most characteristic morphologic features of atypical lymphocytes include:

   a coarse nuclear chromatin and basophilic cytoplasm
   b blue-grey cytoplasm, fine nuclear chromatin   ✳
   c nucleoli and deep blue RNA-rich cytoplasm
   d a stretched nucleus and cytoplasmic indentations

238 A bone marrow shows <u>foam cells</u> ranging from 20-100 μm in size, vacuolated cytoplasm
MLS
ONLY containing sphingomyelin and is faintly PAS+. This cell type is most characteristic of:

   a Gaucher disease
   b myeloma with Russell bodies
   c DiGuglielmo disease
   d Niemann-Pick disease

239 Bone marrow examination reveals a hypercellular marrow consisting of probable lymphoblasts. The cells stain positively with anti-TdT and anti CD3 and CD7 antibodies; however, the lymphoblasts are negative for SIgs, CD19, CD10 (CALLA), Fc, and complement receptors. The most likely diagnosis is:

MLS ONLY

   a null-cell acute lymphocytic leukemia (non-B, non-T cell ALL)
   b chronic lymphocytic leukemia (CLL)
   ⓒ T-cell leukemia (T-ALL)
   d hairy-cell leukemia

240 In synovial fluid, the most characteristic finding in pseudogout is:

   ⓐ calcium pyrophosphate dihydrate crystals = *PSEUDOGOUT*
   b cartilage debris
   c monosodium urate crystals
   d hemosiderin-laden macrophages

241 In synovial fluid, the most characteristic finding in traumatic arthritis is:

   a monosodium urate crystals
   b cartilage debris
   c calcium pyrophosphate dihydrate crystals
   ⓓ hemosiderin-laden macrophages = *traumatic arthritis*

242 Which of the following stains is most frequently used to differentiate acute myelocytic from acute lymphocytic leukemia?

MLS ONLY

   a alkaline phosphatase
   b nonspecific esterase
   c acid phosphatase
   ⓓ peroxidase – *granulocyte line (myelocytic)*

243 The cell series most readily identified by a positive Sudan black B is:

MLS ONLY

   a erythrocytic
   ⓑ myelocytic = *Sudan black B*
   c plasmacytic
   d lymphocytic

244 Which cell type shows the most intense staining with peroxidase?

MLS ONLY

   ⓐ neutrophil = *most intense staining with peroxidase*
   b basophil
   c eosinophil (or lymphocyte)
   d monocyte

245 Which of the following may be used to stain neutral fats, phospholipids and sterols?

MLS ONLY

   a peroxidase
   ⓑ Sudan black B – *fats, phospholipids and sterols*
   c periodic acid-Schiff (PAS)
   d Prussian blue

246 The stain that selectively identifies phospholipid in the membranes of primary and secondary granules within myeloid cells is:

MLS ONLY

   ⓐ Sudan black B
   b leukocyte alkaline phosphatase (LAP)
   c periodic acid-Schiff (PAS)
   d peroxidase

247 Which substrate is used for the detection of specific esterase?

   a acetate
   (b) chloroacetate
   c pararosanilin acetate
   d phenylene diacetate

248 A useful chemical test for the diagnosis of hairy cell leukemia is the:

   a peroxidase test
   b Sudan black test
   c periodic acid-Schiff test
   (d) tartrate-resistant acid phosphatase test - TRAP *for hairy cell*

249 Cytochemical stains were performed on bone marrow smears from an acute leukemia patient.

All blasts were periodic acid-Schiff (PAS) negative. The majority of the blasts showed varying amounts of Sudan black B positivity. Some of the blasts stained positive for naphthol AS-D acetate esterase, some were positive for naphthol AS-D chloroacetate esterase, and some blasts stained positive for both esterases. What type of leukemia is indicated?

   a lymphocytic
   b myelogenous
   (c) myelomonocytic
   d erythroleukemia

250 Which of the following stains is closely associated with the lysosomal enzyme in primary (azurophilic) granules?

   (a) peroxidase
   b Sudan black B
   c periodic acid-Schiff (PAS)
   d Prussian blue

251 What feature would **not** be expected in pseudo-Pelger-Huët cells?

   a hyperclumped chromatin
   b decreased granulation
   (c) normal peroxidase activity (*hypergranular*)
   d abnormal neutrophils

252 A 30-year-old woman was admitted to the hospital for easy bruising and menorrhagia. Laboratory
MLS
ONLY findings included the following:

WBC:	$3.5 \times 10^3/\mu L$ ($3.5 \times 10^9/L$)
RBC:	$2.48 \times 10^6/\mu L$ ($2.48 \times 10^{12}/L$)
Plt:	$30 \times 10^3/\mu L$ ($30.0 \times 10^9/L$)
Hgb:	8.6 g/dL (86 g/L)
Hct:	25.0%
MCV:	100.7 μm^3 (100.7 fL)
MCH:	34.7 pg
MCHC:	34.3%
PT:	34.0 sec
APTT:	62.5 sec
TT:	15.0 sec
FSP:	>40 µg/mL (>40 mg/L)
fibrinogen:	315 mg/dL (3.15 g/L) (control 200–400 mg/dL [2.0–4.0 g/L])

Differential:

Polys:	3%
Lymphs:	%
Monos:	2%
Myelos:	4%
Abnormal immature:	58%
Blasts:	31%
nRBC:	1

Auer bodies, 1+ macrocytes, 1+ polychromasia

The cells identified as "abnormal immature" were described as having lobulated nuclei with
prominent nucleoli; the cytoplasm had intense azurophilic granulation over the nucleus, with
some cells containing 1-20 Auer bodies, frequently grouped in bundles. A 15-17 chromosomal
translocation was noted. Cells were SBB, peroxidase and NAS-D-chloroacetate positive, PAS
negative. Which of the following types of acute leukemia is most likely?

a myeloblastic
b promyelocytic
c myelomonocytic
d monocytic

253 Which of the following leukemias is characterized by immature cells that are Sudan black B
MLS
ONLY positive with discrete fine granules, peroxidase negative, PAS variable, strongly alpha naphthyl
acetate esterase positive, and muramidase positive?

a acute lymphocytic
b chronic lymphocytic
c acute myelocytic
d acute myelomonocytic

254 Chronic lymphocytic leukemia cells are most likely to express which of the following cell
MLS
ONLY surface markers?

a CD3, CD7, CD19 and CD20
b CD19, CD20, CD4 and CD5
c CD19, CD20, CD21, CD5
d CD13, CD33, CD107

255 Which of the following markers, typically detected in normal myeloid cells, are expressed on the
MLS
ONLY surface of hairy cell leukemia lymphocytes?

a CD3
b CD8
c CD11c
d CD103

256 In flow cytometric analysis, low angle or forward scatter of a laser light beam provides information that pertains to a cell's:

    a volume *(size)*
    b viability
    c granularity
    d lineage

257 In flow cytometric analysis, right angle (90 degrees) or side scatter of a laser light beam provides information that pertains to a cell's:

    a volume
    b viability
    c granularity *(complexity)*
    d lineage

258 A cell surface marker that is expressed on neoplastic plasma cells and is helpful in the diagnosis of
MLS ONLY myeloma is:

    a CD19
    b CD20
    c CD45
    d CD138

259 The (8;14) chromosomal translocation brings which of the following 2 genes in close proximity?
MLS ONLY

    a core binding factor alpha and the retinoic acid receptor
    b the Abelson tyrosine kinase and breakpoint cluster region
    c *c-myc* and the immunoglobulin heavy chain
    d core binding factor beta and the myosin heavy chain

260 Laboratory tests that are designed to aid in the diagnosis of chronic granulomatous disease rely
MLS ONLY upon the detection of the activity of:

    a MPO (myeloperoxidase)
    b PHOX (phagocyte oxidase proteins)
    c lysosomal proteinases
    d (G6PD) glucose-6-phosphate dehydrogenase

261 Which of the following laboratory results would be expected in a child with aryl sulfatase B
MLS ONLY deficiency (mucopolysaccharidosis type VI or Maroteaux-Lamy syndrome)?

    a giant platelets, thrombocytopenia and Döhle-body like inclusions in leukocytes
    b increased urinary excretion of glycosaminoglycans (chondroitin sulfate)
    c increased sensitivity of RBC and WBC to complement-mediated lysis
    d accumulation of glucocerebrosides and other lipids in splenic macrophages

Platelets: Physiology

262 vWF antigen can be found in which of the following?

    a myeloblast
    b monoblast
    c lymphoblast
    d megakaryoblast

263 Which of the following is characteristic of cellular changes as megakaryoblasts mature into megakaryocytes within the bone marrow?

    a progressive decrease in overall cell size
    b increasing basophilia of cytoplasm
    c nuclear division without cytoplasmic division
    d fusion of the nuclear lobes

264 Which of the following cells contain hemosiderin?

    a megakaryocyte
    b osteoclast
    c histiocyte (*macrophages*)
    d mast cell

265 Which of the following cells is the largest cell in the bone marrow:

    a megakaryocyte
    b histiocyte
    c osteoblast
    d mast cell

266 Normal platelets have a circulating life-span of approximately:

    a 5 days
    b 10 days (*9.5 days*)
    c 20 days
    d 30 days

267 Aspirin affects platelet function by interfering with platelets' metabolism of:
MLS ONLY
    a prostaglandins
    b lipids
    c carbohydrates
    d nucleic acids

268 The combination of increased <u>capillary fragility</u> and prolonged <u>bleeding time</u> suggests a
MLS ONLY deficiency in: *testing to evaluate vessel and platelet function*

    a thromboplastin
    b prothrombin
    c platelets
    d fibrinogen

269 Platelet activity is affected by:

    a calcium
    b aspirin - *affects platelet secretion*
    c hyperglycemia
    d hypoglycemia

270 Cells involved in hemostasis are:

    a erythrocytes
    b granulocytes
    c lymphocytes
    d thrombocytes

271 Alpha granules are found on the platelet in:
MLS ONLY
    a peripheral zone - *platelet adhesion and aggregation*
    b sol gel zone
    c organelle zone
    d membranes

Platelets: Disease States

272 Thrombocytopenia is a characteristic of:
MLS ONLY

    a classic von Willebrand disease

    b hemophilia A

    c Glanzmann thrombasthenia

    d May-Hegglin anomaly *= giant platelets* ✱

273 Which of the following is a true statement about acute idiopathic thrombocytopenic
MLS ONLY purpura (ITP)?

    a it is found primarily in adults

    b spontaneous remission usually occurs within several weeks; *children; not gender specific*

                                                                platelet destruction ↑

    c women are more commonly affected

    d peripheral destruction of platelets is decreased

274 Which of the following is the most common cause of an abnormality in hemostasis?
MLS ONLY

    a decreased plasma fibrinogen level

    b decreased Factor VIII level *- hemophilia*

    c decreased Factor IX level

    d quantitative abnormality of platelets

275 The following results were obtained:
MLS ONLY

WBC:	$1.8 \times 10^3/\mu L$ (1.8×10^9/L) ↓
Hgb:	8.9 g/dL (89 g/L) ↑
Hct:	27.4%
Plt:	$2,300 \times 10^3/\mu L$ (2.30×10^9/L) ↑
LAP:	90

Differential:

Segs:	70%
Bands:	10%
Lymphs:	18%
Monos:	2%

  Giant, bizarre platelets, rare megakaryocytes

  3+ Poikilocytosis, 2+ Anisocytosis

  1+ Schizocytosis

  This is consistent with:

    a neutrophilic leukemoid reaction *– ↑ WBC; leukemoid reaction left shift; ↑ LAP*

    b polycythemia vera *↑ WBC, ↑ LAP, ↑ plt* ✱

    c leukoerythroblastosis in myelofibrosis *– nRBC and immatures*

    d idiopathic thrombocythemia *- giant platelets*

276 A 53-year-old man was in recovery following a triple bypass operation. Oozing was noted from his
MLS ONLY surgical wound. The following laboratory data were obtained:

Hemoglobin:	12.5 g/dL (125 g/L)
Hematocrit:	37%
Prothrombin time:	12.3 seconds
APTT:	34 seconds
Platelet count:	$40.0 \times 10^3/\mu L$ (40.0×10^9/L)
Fibrinogen:	250 mg/dL (2.5 g/L)

  The most likely cause of bleeding would be:

    a dilution of coagulation factors due to massive transfusion

    b intravascular coagulation secondary to microaggregates

    c hypofibrinogenemia

    d dilutional thrombocytopenia

277 ADAMTS13 deficiency is responsible for thrombocytopenia found in:

   a TTP
   b DIC
   c HUS
   d ITP

278 Heparin induced thrombocytopenia (HIT) is an immune mediated complication associated with heparin therapy. Antibodies are produced against:

   a ACLA
   b PF4
   c AT
   d B2GP1

279 In polycythemia vera, the platelet count is:

   (a) elevated *WBC, plt and RBC's* ✳
   b normal
   c decreased
   d variable

280 Thrombocytosis would be indicated by a platelet count of:

   a $100 \times 10^3/\mu L$ (100×10^9/L)
   b $200 \times 10^3/\mu L$ (200×10^9/L)
   c $300 \times 10^3/\mu L$ (300×10^9/L)
   (d) $600 \times 10^3/\mu L$ (600×10^9/L)

281 A 60-year-old man has a painful right knee and a slightly enlarged spleen. Hematology results include:

hemoglobin:	15 g/dL (150 g/L)
absolute neutrophil count:	$10.0 \times 10^3/\mu L$ (10.0×10^9/L)
platelet count:	$900 \times 10^3/\mu L$ (900×10^9/L)
uncorrected retic count:	1%

normal red cell morphology and indices
a slight increase in bands
rare metamyelocyte and myelocyte
giant and bizarre-shaped platelets

This is most compatible with:

   a congenital spherocytosis
   b rheumatoid arthritis with reactive thrombocytosis
   c myelofibrosis
   (d) idiopathic thrombocythemia

282 Which of the following is characteristic of platelet disorders?

   a deep muscle hemorrhages

   b retroperitoneal hemorrhages *Factor disorders*

   (c) mucous membrane hemorrhages

   d severely prolonged clotting times

plt lack a substance to stick to vessel walls

283 Which of the following is characteristic of Bernard-Soulier syndrome?

   (a) giant platelets, *abnormal bleeding time, normal aggregation, ↓ plt count*

   b normal bleeding time   *✳*

   c abnormal aggregation with ADP

   d increased platelet count

284 Which of the following is associated with Glanzmann thrombasthenia? *lack a protein for plts to clump together*

MLS ONLY

   a normal bleeding time

   b normal EPI aggregation

   c abnormal initial wave ristocetin aggregation

   (d) abnormal ADP aggregation

285 The preferred blood product for a bleeding patient with Type I von Willebrand disease is:

MLS ONLY

   a Factor II, VII, IX, X concentrates

   b Platelet Concentrates

   c Fresh Frozen Plasma and Platelets

   (d) DDAVP

Platelets: Laboratory Determinations

286 A phase-platelet count is performed using a platelet Unopette™ (dilution = 1:100). 155 platelets are counted on one side of the hemacytometer in the center square millimeter, and 145 are counted on the other side in the same area. After making the appropriate calculations, the next step would be to:

   a repeat the procedure, using a 1:20 dilution with acetic acid

   (b) report the calculated value

   c collect a new specimen

   d repeat the procedure, using a 1:200 dilution with saline

287 The chamber counting method of platelet enumeration:

   (a) allows direct visualization of the particles being counted

   b has a high degree of precision

   c has a high degree of reproducibility

   d is the method of choice for the performance of 50-60 counts per day

288 Blood is diluted 1:200, and a platelet count is performed. 180 platelets were counted in the center square millimeter on one side of the hemacytometer and 186 on the other side. The total platelet count is:

   a $146 \times 10^3/\mu L$ ($146 \times 10^9/L$)

   b $183 \times 10^3/\mu L$ ($183 \times 10^9/L$)

   (c) $366 \times 10^3/\mu L$ ($366 \times 10^9/L$)

   d $732 \times 10^3/\mu L$ ($732 \times 10^9/L$)

289   A phase-platelet count was performed and the total platelet count was $356 \times 10^3/\mu L$ ($356 \times 10^9/L$). 10 fields on the stained blood smear were examined for platelets and the results per field were:

   16, 18, 15, 20, 19, 17, 19, 18, 20, 16   *blood smear platelet count =*
                                                average of 10 fields × 20,000

   The next step would be to:

   a report the phase-platelet count since it correlated well with the slide
   b repeat the phase-platelet count on a recollected specimen and check for clumping
   c check ten additional fields on the blood smear
   d repeat the platelet count using a different method

290   An automated platelet count indicates platelet clumping, which is confirmed by examining the smear. The technician should:

   a repeat the count on the same sample
   b report the automated count
   c perform a manual count
   d recollect in sodium citrate

291   The automated platelet count on an EDTA specimen is $58 \times 10^3/\mu L$ ($58 \times 10^9/L$). The platelet estimate on the blood smear appears normal, but it was noted that the platelets were surrounding the neutrophils. The next step should be to: *platelet ~~antibd~~ satellitosm →*
                                                                              recollect in sodium citrate

   a report the automated platelet count since it is more accurate than a platelet estimate
   b warm the EDTA tube and repeat the automated platelet count
   c rerun the original specimen since the platelet count and blood smear estimate do not match
   d recollect a specimen for a platelet count using a different anticoagulant

292   Which one of the following is a true statement about megakaryocytes in a bone marrow aspirate?
MLS
ONLY **a** an average of 5-10 should be found in each low power field (10×)
   b the majority of forms are the MK_1 stage
   c morphology must be determined from the biopsy section
   d quantitative estimation is done using the 100× oil immersion lens

293   Which of the following platelet responses is most likely associated with
MLS
ONLY Glanzmann thrombasthenia?

   a decreased platelet aggregation to ristocetin
   b defective ADP release; normal response to ADP
   c decreased amount of ADP in platelets
   d markedly decreased aggregation to epinephrine, ADP and collagen

294   A bleeding time is used to evaluate the activity of:

   a platelets
   b prothrombin
   c labile factor
   d Factor XIII

295   A patient has been taking aspirin regularly for arthritic pain. Which one of the following tests is most likely to be abnormal in this patient?

   a platelet count
   b template bleeding time – *aspirin effects plt function*
   c prothrombin time
   d activated partial thromboplastin time

296 A platelet count done by phase microscopy is $200 \times 10^3/\mu L$ ($200 \times 10^9/L$) (reference range 150-$450 \times 10^3/\mu L$ (150-$450 \times 10^9/L$). A standardized template bleeding time on the same person is 15 minutes (reference range 4.5 ± 1.5 minutes). This indicates that:

    a the Duke method should have been used for the bleeding time   *?*
    b the manual platelet count is in error
    ⓒ abnormal platelet function should be suspected – *accesses both function and number*
    d the results are as expected

297 Which of the following detects or measures platelet function?

    ⓐ bleeding time
    b prothrombin time
    c thrombin time
    d partial thromboplastin time

298 Platelet aggregation is dependent in vitro on the presence of:

    ⓐ calcium ions
    b sodium citrate
    c thrombin
    d potassium

Calcium - needed for platelet aggregation

299 Which of the following platelet responses is most likely associated with classic von
MLS ONLY Willebrand disease?

    ⓐ decreased platelet aggregation to ristocetin
    b normal platelet aggregation to ristocetin
    c absent aggregation to epinephrine, ADP and collagen
    d decreased amount of ADP in platelets

300 Which of the following platelet responses is most likely associated with hemophilia A (Factor VIII
MLS ONLY deficiency)?

    a defective ADP release; normal response to ADP
    b decreased amount of ADP in platelets
    c absent aggregation to epinephrine, ADP and collagen
    ⓓ normal platelet aggregation

301 Refer to the following diagram:
MLS ONLY

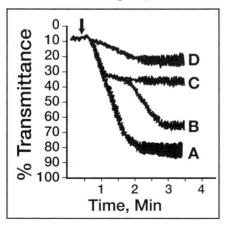

In the platelet aggregation curves shown above, the aggregating agent was added at the point indicated by the arrow. Select the appropriate aggregation curve for recent aspirin ingestion. (Aggregating agent is ADP or epinephrine.)

    a A
    b B
    c C
    d D

302 Platelet aggregation will occur with the end production of:

MLS
ONLY

   a cyclooxygenase

   b arachidonic acid

   c prostacyclin

   d thromboxane A_2

303 In von Willebrand disease, platelets give an abnormal aggregation result in the presence of:

MLS
ONLY

   a adenosine diphosphate

   b epinephrine

   c collagen

   d ristocetin

304 The following platelet aggregation tracing represents:

MLS
ONLY

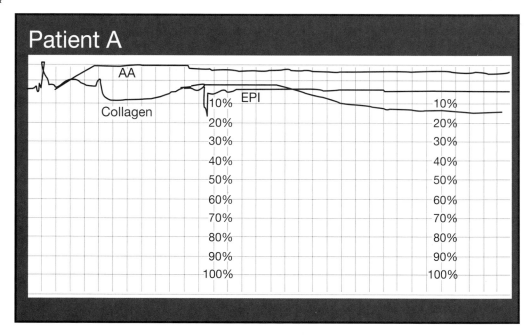

   a von Willebrand disease

   b storage pool disease

   c Glanzmann thrombasthenia

   d aspirin

Hemostasis

305 Coagulation factors affected by warfarin (Coumadin®) drugs are:

   a VIII, IX and X

   b I, II, V and VII

   c II, VII, IX and X *(Vitamin K dependent)*

   d II, V and VII

306　Which one of the following statements concerning Vitamin K is **not** true?

　　a　there are 2 sources of Vitamin K: vegetable and bacterial ✓
　　b　Vitamin K converts precursor molecules into functional coagulation factors ✓
　　c　heparin inhibits the action of Vitamin K – *coumadin*
　　d　Vitamin K is fat soluble ✓　　　　*Heparin inhibits X and thrombin*

307　Which of the following is Vitamin-K dependent?　*2, 7, 9, 10*

　　a　Factor XII
　　b　fibrinogen *I*
　　c　antithrombin III
　　d　Factor VII

308　Which of the following factors is used only in the extrinsic coagulation pathway?

　　a　II – *common*
　　b　V – *common*
　　c　VII
　　d　VIII – *intrinsic*

309　Hageman Factor (XII) is involved in each of the following reactions **except**:

　　a　activation of C1 to C1 esterase
　　b　activation of plasminogen
　　c　activation of Factor XI
　　d　transformation of fibrinogen to fibrin – *thrombin*

310　Prothrombin is:

　　a　a protein formed by the liver in the presence of Vitamin K
　　b　an enzyme that converts fibrinogen into fibrin threads
　　c　the end product of the reaction between fibrinogen and thrombin
　　d　a protein released by platelets during coagulation

311　Which of the following coagulation factors is considered to be labile?

　　a　II
　　b　V (*labile factor*)
　　c　VII
　　d　X

312　The most potent plasminogen activator in the contact phase of coagulation is:

　　a　kallikrein
　　b　streptokinase　　　　✳
　　c　HMWK
　　d　fibrinogen

313　Which of the following factor deficiencies is associated with either no bleeding or only a minor bleeding tendency, even after trauma or surgery?

　　a　Factor X
　　b　Factor XII　　　　✳
　　c　Factor XIII
　　d　Factor V

314　Which of the following is a characteristic of Factor XII deficiency?

　　a　negative bleeding history
　　b　normal clotting times
　　c　~~decreased~~ risk of thrombosis　✳
　　d　epistaxis

315 The 2 factors that differentiate liver disease from Vitamin K deficiency are:

    a II and VII
    b IX and VII   ✳
    c VIII and IX
    d V and VII– *Vit K*   *both ↓ in liver disease*
    not Vit K dependent

316 Which one of the following factors typically shows an increase in liver disease?
                                     affects all Vit K
                                     dependent factors

    a Factor VII
    b Factor VIII – *acute phase reactant ↑ in liver*
                           disease
    c Factor IX
    d Factor X

317 A patient has a normal prothrombin time and a prolonged activated partial thromboplastin time (APTT) using a kaolin activator. The APTT corrects to normal when the incubation time is increased. These results suggest that the patient has:

    a hemophilia A (Factor VIII deficiency)   *prolonged APTT with normal PT*
    b Hageman Factor (XII) deficiency   *= intrinsic factors 8, 9, 11, PK*
    c Fletcher Factor deficiency (prekallikrein)
    d Factor V deficiency

318 The results on a patient are:

Test	Patient results	Reference range
PT	18.5 sec	11.0-13.5 sec −
APTT	47.5 sec	24-35 sec −
thrombin time	14.0 sec	12-19 sec
ATIII	82%	70%-130%
protein C	54%	77%-167% −
protein S	48%	65%-140% −
activated protein C resistance	2.6	>2.1

                                                      ?

These results reflect:

    a thrombophilia
    b Factor IX deficiency
    c heparin
    d warfarin

319 A 4-year-old boy presents with chronic ear infections and is on prophylactic antibiotics. He presents with bleeding. Factor assays reveal: *interrupts normal flora*

Test	Patient results	Reference range
Factor VIII	100%	50%-150%
Factor V	75%	50%-150%
Factor IX	38%	50%-150%
Factor II	22%	50%-150%

Possible causes are:

    a Factor II deficiency
    b lupus anticoagulant
    c hemophilia
    d Vitamin K deficiency

320 A hemophiliac male and a normal female can produce a:

Factor VIII lies on the X chromosomes

    a female carrier
    b male carrier
    c male hemophiliac
    d normal female

321 The following laboratory data were obtained from a 27-year-old man with a long history of
MLS
ONLY abnormal bleeding:

prothrombin time:	normal
activated partial thromboplastin time:	markedly prolonged
Factor VIII coagulant activity:	markedly decreased
Factor VIII related antigen:	normal
platelet count:	normal
template bleeding time:	normal

Which of the following disorders does this man most likely have:

    a classic hemophilia
    b von Willebrand disease
    c Christmas disease
    d disseminated intravascular coagulation (DIC)

322 The following laboratory data were obtained from a 40-year-old woman with a long history of
MLS
ONLY abnormal bleeding:

prothrombin time:	normal
activated partial thromboplastin time:	prolonged
Factor VIII-coagulant activity:	decreased
Factor VIII-related antigen:	markedly decreased
platelet count:	normal
template bleeding time:	prolonged

Which of the following disorders does this woman most likely have:

    a classic hemophilia
    b von Willebrand disease
    c Christmas disease
    d disseminated intravascular coagulation (DIC)

323 Hemophilia B is a sex-linked recessive disorder that presents with a decrease in Factor:
MLS
ONLY
    a VIII
    b IX
    c X
    d XI

324 To distinguish between hemophilia and von Willebrand disease, a patient with von Willebrand will
MLS
ONLY present with which of the following test results?

Results	APTT	Platelet screen	Ristocetin cofactor
result A	abnormal	normal	normal
result B	normal	abnormal	normal
result C	abnormal	abnormal	abnormal
result D	normal	normal	abnormal

    a result A
    b result B
    c result C
    d result D

325 Patient presents with bleeding 48 hours post tooth extraction. Results are as follows:

Test	Patient results	Reference range
PT	11.5 sec	10-13 sec
APTT	32.5 sec	23-35 sec
fibrinogen	345 mg/dL (3.45 g/L)	200-400 mg/dL (2.0–4.0 g/L)
platelets	$324 \times 10^3/\mu L$ (324×10^9/L)	$150-450 \times 10^3/\mu L$ ($150–450 \times 10^9$/L)

all normal

Possible causes are a deficiency in:

a plasminogen
b Factor XIII
c alpha$_2$ anti-plasmin
d Factor XII

326 Plasma from a patient with lupus coagulation inhibitor can show:

a a prolonged APTT and normal PT
b a prolonged thrombin time
c no change with platelet neutralization
d complete correction when incubated with normal plasma — *mixing study doesn't correct*

327 The activation of plaminogen to plasmin resulting in the degradation of fibrin occurs by
MLS ONLY

a PAI-1
b alpha$_2$ antiplasmin
c tPA
d alpha$_2$ macroglobulin

328 A deficiency of protein C is associated with which of the following?
MLS ONLY

a prolonged activated partial thromboplastin time (APTT)
b decreased fibrinogen level (<100 mg/dL [<1.0 g/L])
c increased risk of thrombosis
d spontaneous hemorrhage

329 Biological assays for antithrombin III (AT III) are based on the inhibition of:
MLS ONLY

a Factor VIII
b heparin
c serine proteases
d anti-AT III globulin

330 A patient presents with a low Protein S activity, antigen and free antigen. The C4b binding protein
MLS ONLY is normal. This is classified as:

a no deficiency
b Type I
c Type II
d Type III

331 APC resistance is confirmed by the molecular test for
MLS ONLY

a PAI 1 4G/5G
b MTHFR
c FVL
d G20210A

332 Acute disseminated intravascular coagulation is characterized by:

a hypofibrinogenemia
b thrombocytosis   ✳
c negative D-dimer
d shortened thrombin time

DIC: ↑ PT, APTT, D-dimer ↓ fibrinogen, plts

333 A patient develops unexpected bleeding and the following test results were obtained:

MLS ONLY

PT and APTT: prolonged
fibrinogen: decreased
D-dimer: increased
platelets: decreased

What is the most probable cause of these results?

a familial afibrinogenemia
b primary fibrinolysis
c DIC
d liver disease

334 Patient results are as follows:

Test	Patient results	Reference range
PT	17.5 sec ↑	11-13 sec
APTT	56.7 sec ↑	25-35 sec
D-dimer	698 ng/mL ↑↑	<250 ng/mL
fibrinogen	123 mg/dL (1.23 g/L) ↓	200-400 mg/dL (2.0-4.0 g/L)
platelet count	$102 \times 10^3/\mu L$ (102×10^9/L) ↓	150-$450 \times 10^3/\mu L$ (150-450×10^9/L)

This workup suggests:

a blood clot
b hemorrhage
(c) DIC
d HUS

335 A patient develops severe unexpected bleeding following four transfusions. The following test results were obtained:

MLS ONLY

PT and APTT: prolonged
platelets: $50 \times 10^3/\mu L$ (50×10^9/L)
fibrinogen: 30 mg/dl (0.30 g/L)
D-dimer: increased

Given these results, which of the following blood products should be recommended to the physician for this patient?

a platelets
b Factor VIII
c cryoprecipitate
d fresh frozen plasma

336 The prothrombin time test requires that the patient's citrated plasma be combined with:

a platelet lipids
b thromboplastin
c Ca⁺⁺ and platelet lipids   ✳
(d) Ca⁺⁺ and thromboplastin (*tissue*)

337 In the APTT test, the patient's plasma is mixed with:

a ADP and calcium
b tissue thromboplastin and collagen
(c) phospholipid and calcium   ✳
d tissue thromboplastin and calcium

338 The APTT:

   a tests the extrinsic coagulation pathway
   b monitors Coumadin® therapy
   c requires tissue thromboplastin
   (d) monitors heparin therapy

339 Aliquots of plasma with a prolonged PT and prolonged APTT are mixed using various ratios of patient plasma and normal plasma. All samples are incubated at 37°C and tested at 10-, 30-, and 60-minute intervals. The PT and APTT results on all of the mixtures are corrected. These results would indicate the presence of:

Mixing studies -
both corrected = factor deficiency
✱ not corrected = inhibitor

   a circulating anticoagulant
   (b) factor deficiency
   c contaminated reagent
   d antibodies

340 A patient is taking 10 mg per day of Coumadin® (warfarin). The results of which of the following laboratory tests will be most impacted?

   (a) protein C level
   b antithrombin III level
   c Factor V Leiden mutation
   d Factor VIII level

341 A patient's thrombin time is 25.5 seconds, and the control is 11.5 seconds. The patient's plasma is mixed with an equal part of normal plasma. The thrombin time is rerun and is 28.0 seconds with a control of 11.5 seconds. These results indicate:
MLS ONLY

   a fibrinogen deficiency
   b thrombocyte antibodies present
   c Factor VII deficiency
   d circulating anticoagulant

↓ fibrinogen function
— not bother by heparin

342 A prolonged thrombin time and a normal reptilase-R time are characteristic of:

↓ fibrinogen, ↑FDP's, paraproteins,
heparin

   a dysfibrinogenemia   ✱ ✱
   b increased D-dimer
   c fibrin monomer-split product complexes
   (d) therapeutic heparinization

343 A 54-year-old man was admitted with pulmonary embolism and given streptokinase. Which of the following would be most useful in monitoring this therapy?
MLS ONLY

   a activated partial thromboplastin time
   b bleeding time
   c prothrombin time
   d thrombin time

344 The best test to determine if a sample is contaminated with heparin is:

   a fibrinogen
   (b) thrombin time   ✱
   c prothrombin time
   d stypven time

345 In a the Clauss fibrinogen method, the time to clot formation in plasma is measured after the addition of: ↓

   a calcium
   (b) thrombin   ✱
   c phospholipids
   d kaolin

346 If a patient presents with a prolonged APTT that <u>does not correct</u> upon mixing, the next
performed should be: *not factors*

    a Factor II
    ⓑ DRVVT
    c Factor VIII
    d platelet count

347 Excess D-dimer indicate that clots have been:

    a converted to fibrin monomers
    b released into circulation
    ⓒ formed and are being excessively lysed
    d stimulated to activate platelets

348 D-dimers are produced from:

    ⓐ cross-linked and stabilized fibrin clot
    b decreased fibrinogen and platelets
    c plasminogen converting to plasmin
    d generation of thrombin from endothelial cells

349 Which of the following laboratory procedures is most helpful in differentiating severe liver disease
MLS
ONLY and accompanying secondary fibrinolysis from disseminated intravascular coagulation?

    a presence of fibrin split products
    b increased APTT
    c Factor VIII activity
    d fibrinogen level

350 A bedside test that can be used to monitor heparin activity is the:

    ⓐ activated clotting time (ACT)
    b stypven time – *snake venom test for lupus*
    c reptilase time – *fibrinogen level on heparin patients*
    d partial thromboplastin time

351 Which of the following laboratory findings is associated with Factor XIII deficiency?

    a prolonged activated partial thromboplastin time
    ⓑ clot solubility in a 5 molar urea solution
    c prolonged thrombin time
    d prolonged prothrombin time

352 Heparin acts by:

    a precipitating fibrinogen
    b binding calcium
    c activating plasmin
    ⓓ inhibiting thrombin *and factor 10*

353 Low molecular weight heparin is monitored by a:

    ⓐ anti-Xa assay
    b̶ APTT – *not LMWH*
    c PT
    d anti-IIa assay

Hematology Laboratory Operations

354 In an automated cell counter, the WBC printed result is "+++". The next step is to: *exceeds upper reportable limit*

    a repeat after warming the sample to 37°C
    b make an appropriate dilution of the sample
    c recalibrate the machine from pooled samples
    d request a new sample immediately

355 A specimen run on an automatic cell counter has a platelet count of $19 \times 10^3/\mu L$ ($19 \times 10^9/L$). The first thing the technician should do is:

    a report the count after the batch run is completed
    b request a new specimen
    c review the stained blood smear
    d notify the laboratory manager

356 The electrical resistance method of cell counting requires:

    a equal-sized particles
    b a conductive liquid
    c 2 internal electrodes for current - *1 internal, 1 external*
    d three apertures for counting

357 An anemic patient has an RBC of $2.70 \times 10^6/\mu L$ ($2.7 \times 10^{12}/L$) and a hemoglobin of 13.5 g/dL
MLS ONLY (135 g/L) as determined by an electronic particle counter. Which of the following is the best explanation for these results? *rule of 3 not equal*

    a electrical interference
    b lipemia
    c high anticoagulant to blood ratio
    d a high coincidence rate

358 The following results were obtained on an electronic particle counter:
MLS ONLY

    WBC: $6.5 \times 10^3/\mu L$ ($6.5 \times 10^9/L$)
    RBC: $4.55 \times 10^6/\mu L$ ($4.55 \times 10^{12}/L$)
    Hgb: 18.0 g/dL (180 g/L)   *> rule of 3 not equal*
    Hct: 41.5%
    MCV: 90.1 μm^3 (90.1 fL)
    MCH: 39.6 pg
    MCHC: 43.4% - *high ↑*

    The first step in obtaining valid results is to:

    a perform a microhematocrit
    b correct the hemoglobin for lipemia
    c dilute the blood
    d replace the lysing agent

359 On an electronic particle counter, if the RBC is erroneously increased, how will other parameters be affected? ✳

    a increased MCHC
    b increased hemoglobin - *↑ RBC should not effect hgb*
    c decreased MCH
    d increased MCV

360 On setting up the electronic particle counter in the morning, one of the controls is slightly below the range for the MCV. Which of the following is indicated?

    a call for service
    b adjust the MCV up slightly
    c shut down the instrument
    d repeat the control

361 The following results were obtained on an electronic particle counter:

WBC: ++++ ✳ *dilution needed*
RBC: $2.01 \times 10^6/\mu L$ ($2.01 \times 10^{12}/L$)
Hgb: 7.7 g/dL (77 g/L)
Hct: 28.2%
MCV: 141 μm^3 (141 fL)
MCH: 38.5 pg
MCHC: 23.3%

What step should be taken before recycling the sample?

a clean the apertures
b warm the specimen
c replace the lysing agent
d dilute the specimen

362 In an electronic or laser particle cell counter, clumped platelets may interfere with which of the following parameters?
MLS ONLY

a white blood cell count
b red blood cell count
c hemoglobin
d hematocrit

363 Which of the following will not cause erroneous results when using a phase optical system for enumerating platelets?

a incipient clotting
b decreased hematocrit
c Howell-Jolly bodies
d leukocyte cytoplasmic fragments

364 The most common cause of error when using automated cell counters is:

a contamination of the diluent
b inadequate mixing of the sample prior to testing
c variation in voltage of the current supply
d a calibrating error

365 On an electronic cell counter, hemoglobin determinations may be falsely elevated due to the presence of:
MLS ONLY

✳✳ *Lipemia and ↑ bilirubin (icterus) = falsely ↑ hgb*

a lipemia or elevated bilirubin concentration – *(icterus)*
b a decreased WBC or lipemia
c an elevated bilirubin concentration or rouleaux
d rouleaux or lipemia

366 The calculated erythrocyte indices on an adult man are MCV = 89 fL, MCH = 29 pg and MCHC = 38%.
MLS ONLY The calculations have been rechecked; erythrocytes on the peripheral blood smear appear normocytic and normochromic with no abnormal forms. The next step is to:

80-100   26-32   32-36

a report the results
b examine another smear
c repeat the hemoglobin and hematocrit
d repeat the erythrocyte count and hematocrit

367 The following results were obtained on an electronic particle counter:

WBC:	$61.3 \times 10^3/\mu L$ ($61.3 \times 10^9/L$)
RBC:	$1.19 \times 10^6/\mu L$ ($1.19 \times 10^{12}/L$)
Hgb:	9.9 g/dL (99 g/L)
Hct:	21%
MCV:	125 μm³ (125 fL)
MCHC:	54.1%

What action should be taken to obtain accurate results?

  a dilute the specimen and recount   *cold agglutinins =*
  b warm the specimen and recount   *   ↓RBC, ↑MCV and MCHC
  c check the tube for clots
  d clean the aperture tubes and recount

368 A properly functioning electronic cell counter obtains the following results:

WBC:	$5.1 \times 10^3/\mu L$ ($5.1 \times 10^9/L$)
RBC:	$4.87 \times 10^6/\mu L$ ($4.87 \times 10^{12}/L$
Hgb:	16.1 g/dL (161 g/L)
Hct:	39.3%
MCV:	82.0 μm³ (82.0 fL)
MCH:	33.1 pg
MCHC:	41.3%

     *   *hgb x 3 doesn't match hematocrit*

What is the most likely cause of these results?

  a lipemia — *rule of 3 doesn't work*
  b cold agglutinins - *↑MCHC, rule of 3 out of wack*
  c increased WBC
  d rouleaux

369 Refer to the following illustration:

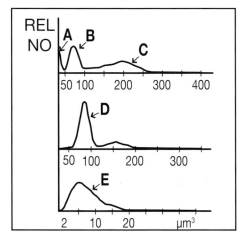

Which area in the automated cell counter histogram represents the RBC distribution curve?

  a A
  b B
  c C
  d D

370   Refer to the following illustration:

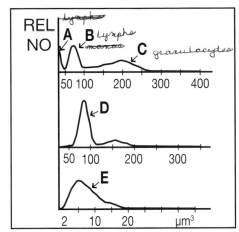

Which area of the automated cell counter histogram indicates the lymphocyte curve?

a A
b B
c C
d D

371   Refer to the following illustration:

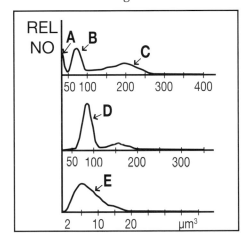

Which area of the automated cell counter histogram indicates the nonlymphocyte curve?

a B
b C
c D
d E

372   Hemoglobins are read on a photoelectric colorimeter in the laboratory. While reading the
MLS
ONLY   hemoglobins, a problem of drifting is encountered. To assess the problem, the **first** thing to do is:

a   recalibrate the instrument
b   check the filter
c   set up new hemoglobin samples
d   check the light source

373 The photo-optical method of endpoint detection is described as:

    a change in optical density as a result of a fibrin clot
    b measurement of tubidity of antigen-antibody formation (*nephelametry*)
    c decreased motion of a mechanical ball
    d color-producing chromophor

374 In laser flow cytometry, histograms combining the data from forward angle light scatter with
MLS ONLY the data from right-angle light scatter permit the operator to:

    a quantitate cell surface protein
    b determine absolute cell size
    c distinguish internal cell structures
    d differentiate cell populations from one another

375 In immunophenotyping by flow cytometry the emitting fluorescence intensity is proportional
MLS ONLY to the:

    a DNA content in the cell
    b amount of cell surface antigen
    c RNA content in the cell
    d size of the cell nucleus

376 The ideal capillary blood collection site on a newborn is:

    a tip of the thumb
    b ear lobe
    c plantar surface of the heel
    d the great toe

377 When evaluating a smear for a reticulocyte count, the technician observes that the red blood cells are overlapping throughout the entire slide. The most likely explanation is:

    a grease on the slide prevented even spreading
    b improper proportions of blood and stain were used
    c the slide was dried too quickly
    d the drop used for the slide preparation was too large

378 If a blood smear is dried too slowly, the red blood cells are often:

    a clumped
    b crenated   ✳
    c lysed
    d destroyed

379 A citrated blood specimen for coagulation studies is to be collected from a polycythemic patient. The anticoagulant should be:

    a the standard volume
    b reduced in volume – *plasma/citrate ratio wrong*
    c changed to EDTA
    d changed to oxalate

380 Blood collected in EDTA undergoes which of the following changes if kept at room temperature for 6-24 hours?

    a increased hematocrit and MCV   ✳
    b increased ESR and MCV
    c increased MCHC and MCV
    d decreased reticulocyte count and hematocrit

381　The specimen of choice for preparation of blood films for manual differential leukocyte counts is whole blood collected in:

　　(a) EDTA
　　b　oxalate
　　c　citrate
　　d　heparin

382　A platelet determination was performed on an automated instrument and a very low value was obtained. The platelets appeared adequate when estimated from the stained blood film. The best explanation for this discrepancy is:

　　(a) many platelets are abnormally large → *counted as ~~platelets~~ WBC's*
　　b　blood sample is hemolyzed
　　c　white cell fragments are present in the blood
　　d　red cell fragments are present in the blood

383　When platelets concentrate at the edges and feathered end of a blood smear, it is usually due to:

　　a　abnormal proteins
　　b　inadequate mixing of blood and anticoagulant
　　c　hemorrhage
　　(d) poorly made wedge smear

384　Platelet satellitosis is usually due to:

MLS ONLY
　　(a) abnormal proteins → *in vitro reaction to EDTA*
　　b　inadequate mixing of blood and anticoagulant
　　c　hemorrhage
　　d　poorly made wedge smear

385　On a smear made directly from a finger stick, no platelets were found in the counting area. The first thing to do is:

　　(a) examine the slide for clumping
　　b　obtain another smear
　　c　perform a total platelet count
　　d　request another finger stick

386　The anticoagulant of choice for routine coagulation procedures is:

　　a　sodium oxalate
　　(b) sodium citrate
　　c　heparin
　　d　sodium fluoride

387　A blue top tube is drawn for coagulation studies, the sample is a short draw results may be:

　　a　falsely shortened　　　　　*too much anticoagulant for the*
　　b　correct　　　　　　　　　　　　*plasma*
　　c　unable to be obtained
　　(d) falsely prolonged

388　The ISI in the INR represents the reagents:

　　a　activator
　　b　specificity
　　c　phospholipids
　　(d) sensitivity

389 Which of the following is the standard calibration method for hematology instrumentation
MLS
ONLY against which other methods must be verified?

    a latex particles of known dimension
    b stabilized red cell suspensions
    c stabilized 7 parameter reference controls
    d normal whole blood

390 Refer to the following illustration:
MLS
ONLY

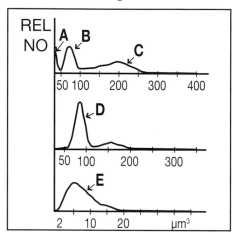

Which area of the automated cell counter histogram represents the platelet distribution curve?

    a A
    b B
    c C
    d E

391 Using automated coagulation instruments, duplication of normal tests is no longer
MLS
ONLY appropriate because:

    a the laboratory can document precision by collecting data to reflect precision performance
    b all technologists on all shifts can be taught quality control
    c it is difficult to have duplicates done in a blind fashion
    d one technologist can monitor quality control

392 When reviewing results on a Factor VIII the following results were obtained:
MLS
ONLY
    1:10 = 50%
    1:20 = 77%
    1:40 = 120%
    1:80 = 127%

This demonstrates the presence of a(n):

    a inhibitor
    b deficiency
    c clot
    d improper draw

393 The following CBC results were obtained from an automated cell counter on a patient sample with
lipemic plasma:

MLS
ONLY

WBC:	$7.2 \times 10^3/\mu L$ (7.2×10^9/L)
RBC:	$3.50 \times 10^6/\mu L$ (3.50×10^{12}/L)
Hgb:	13.8 g/dL (138 g/L)
Hct:	33.5%
MCV:	$92\ \mu m^3$ (92 fL)
MCH:	39.4 pg
MCHC:	41.0%

Which of the following tests would probably be in error?

  a WBC, RBC, MCV
  b RBC, Hct, MCV
  c RBC, Hgb, Hct
  d Hgb, MCH, MCHC

394 On Monday a patient's hemoglobin determination was 11.3 g/dL (113 g/L), and on Tuesday it
measured 11.8 g/dL (118 g/L). The standard deviation of the method used is ±0.2 g/dL (2 g/L).
Which of the following can be concluded about the hemoglobin values given?

  a one value probably resulted from laboratory error
  b there is poor precision; daily quality control charts should be checked
  c the second value is out of range and should be repeated
  d there is no significant change in the patient's hemoglobin concentration

1 d	59 d	117 a	175 d	233 d	291 d	349 c
2 b	60 a	118 b	176 c	234 b	292 a	350 a
3 a	61 d	119 b	177 d	235 c	293 d	351 b
4 b	62 d	120 a	178 a	236 a	294 a	352 d
5 b	63 b	121 c	179 b	237 a	295 b	353 a
6 d	64 d	122 d	180 b	238 d	296 c	354 b
7 c	65 a	123 b	181 d	239 c	297 a	355 c
8 d	66 a	124 b	182 b	240 a	298 a	356 b
9 a	67 d	125 c	183 d	241 d	299 a	357 b
10 d	68 d	126 d	184 a	242 d	300 d	358 b
11 d	69 b	127 b	185 d	243 b	301 c	359 c
12 d	70 c	128 b	186 d	244 a	302 d	360 d
13 d	71 c	129 c	187 d	245 b	303 d	361 d
14 b	72 a	130 c	188 c	246 a	304 c	362 a
15 d	73 c	131 c	189 d	247 b	305 c	363 b
16 d	74 a	132 a	190 c	248 d	306 c	364 b
17 a	75 b	133 d	191 c	249 c	307 d	365 a
18 b	76 b	134 d	192 a	250 a	308 c	366 c
19 c	77 b	135 c	193 a	251 c	309 d	367 b
20 a	78 a	136 c	194 d	252 b	310 a	368 a
21 a	79 a	137 a	195 c	253 d	311 b	369 c
22 c	80 d	138 d	196 d	254 c	312 a	370 b
23 b	81 a	139 d	197 d	255 c	313 b	371 b
24 b	82 d	140 a	198 b	256 a	314 a	372 d
25 b	83 c	141 b	199 d	257 c	315 d	373 a
26 b	84 a	142 a	200 a	258 d	316 b	374 d
27 b	85 c	143 b	201 a	259 c	317 c	375 b
28 b	86 b	144 c	202 d	260 b	318 d	376 c
29 c	87 a	145 d	203 b	261 b	319 d	377 d
30 d	88 d	146 b	204 b	262 d	320 a	378 b
31 d	89 c	147 c	205 a	263 c	321 a	379 b
32 b	90 b	148 c	206 d	264 c	322 b	380 a
33 c	91 d	149 b	207 b	265 a	323 b	381 a
34 c	92 c	150 d	208 a	266 b	324 c	382 a
35 b	93 d	151 a	209 b	267 a	325 b	383 d
36 b	94 d	152 b	210 d	268 c	326 a	384 a
37 d	95 a	153 b	211 a	269 b	327 c	385 a
38 a	96 d	154 a	212 c	270 d	328 c	386 b
39 d	97 c	155 b	213 c	271 c	329 c	387 d
40 a	98 a	156 c	214 a	272 d	330 b	388 d
41 b	99 b	157 c	215 c	273 b	331 c	389 d
42 c	100 a	158 b	216 a	274 d	332 a	390 d
43 a	101 c	159 a	217 c	275 d	333 c	391 a
44 d	102 d	160 b	218 c	276 d	334 c	392 a
45 a	103 d	161 b	219 b	277 a	335 c	393 d
46 b	104 d	162 d	220 a	278 b	336 d	394 d
47 a	105 a	163 d	221 b	279 a	337 c	
48 d	106 a	164 d	222 b	280 d	338 d	
49 d	107 d	165 c	223 a	281 d	339 b	
50 d	108 a	166 c	224 b	282 c	340 a	
51 c	109 c	167 c	225 c	283 a	341 d	
52 a	110 a	168 a	226 c	284 d	342 d	
53 c	111 b	169 b	227 d	285 d	343 d	
54 c	112 b	170 d	228 a	286 b	344 b	
55 c	113 c	171 b	229 d	287 a	345 b	
56 b	114 d	172 b	230 a	288 c	346 b	
57 c	115 b	173 d	231 b	289 a	347 c	
58 c	116 d	174 c	232 b	290 d	348 a	

Erythrocytes: Physiology

1   **d**   Morphological identifiable perinuclear halo.
[McKenzie 2002, pp108-109]

2   **b**   Correct order of heme synthesis.
MLS ONLY   [Harmening 2002, p103]

3   **a**   ⅔ iron in body bound to Hgb.
[Harmening 2002, p64]

4   **b**   Maintains in Fe^{++} form by way of reduced glutathione.
[Harmening 2002, p68]

5   **b**   Development time line of production of Hgb alpha chains.
[Harmening 2002, p66]

6   **d**   Development time line of production of Hgb beta chains.
[Harmening 2002, p66]

7   **c**   Development time line of production of Hgb gamma chains.
[Harmening 2002, p66]

8   **d**   Development time line of production of Hgb delta chains.
[Harmening 2002, p66]

9   **a**   Development time line of production of Hgb epsilon chains.
[Harmening 2002, p68]

10   **d**   Functional form of Fe (reduced).
[Harmening 2002, p68]

11   **d**   RBC morphology; disease state identification.
[Rodak 2007, p223]

12   **d**   Impaired DNA synthesis = macrocytes.
MLS ONLY   [Rodak 2007, p227]

13   **d**   Major site of destruction of senescent red blood cells.
[Rodak 2007, p90]

14   **b**   Normal degradation products of red blood cells.
[Rodak 2007, p90]

15   **d**   Formed with oxidization of Fe and formation of methemoglobin.
[Rodak 2007, p299]

16   **d**   RBC membrane defect (DAF) increases
MLS ONLY   susceptibility to complement mediated lysis.
[Rodak 2007, p302]

17   **a**   Primary functions of red blood cells.
[Rodak 2007, p77]

18   **b**   Erythropoietin action.
[Rodak 2007, p267]

19   **c**   May be referred to as hyperchromic because of decreased MCHC.
[McKenzie 2002, p175]

20   **a**   Hemochromatosis results in iron
MLS ONLY   deposited in tissues.
[Rodak 2007, p242]

Erythrocytes: Disease States

21   **a**   Iron loss with loss of blood.
MLS ONLY   [Rodak 2007, p476]

22   **c**   Positive DAT.
MLS ONLY   [Rodak 2007, p292]

23   **b**   Serum Fe levels low due to sequestration
MLS ONLY   in macrophages and hepatocytes.
[Rodak 2007, p137]

24   **b**   Erythropoietin production questionable
MLS ONLY   in chronic renal disease.
[Rodak 2007, p267]

25   **b**   Sickle cell disease, effect on lab results.
MLS ONLY   [Rodak 2007, p340]

26   **b**   Bone marrow, how affected by uremia.
MLS ONLY   [Rodak 2007, p68]

27   **b**   RBC membrane defects are common to PNH, HS, and HE.
[Rodak 2007, p287]

28   **b**   Iron studies—lab results.
MLS ONLY   [Rodak 2007, p237]

29   **c**   Iron studies: microcytic hypochromic anemia results in a decrease in serum and storage iron, but an increase in TIBC.
[Rodak 2007, p236]

30   **d**   Chronic blood loss frequently results in iron deficiency anemia.
[Rodak 2007, p236]

31   **d**   FEP-thalassemia.
MLS ONLY   [Rodak 2007, p368]

32   **b**   Mechanism of genetic abnormality in thalassemia reduces globin chain production.
[Rodak 2007, p356]

33   **c**   Thalassemia with elevated Hgb F and
MLS ONLY normal Hgb A_2 levels.
[Rodak 2007, p363]

34   **c**   Anemia related to uremia has normal-sized, normochromic cells; it is the number of RBCs that is decreased.
[Rodak 2007, p227]

35   **b**   Hemolytic anemia—laboratory results.
MLS ONLY [McKenzie 2002, p306]

36   **b**   G-6-PD deficiency.
[McKenzie 2002, p336]

37   **d**   G-6-PD deficiency—hemolytic stimulus.
[McKenzie 2002, p337]

38   **a**   G-6-PD deficiency—anti-malarial drugs.
[McKenzie 2002, p336]

39   **d**   Autoimmune hemolytic anemia: +DAT
MLS ONLY is characteristic.
[McKenzie 2002, p351]

40   **a**   Patients with pernicious anemia have fewer of all types of blood cells, but they are abnormally large.
[McKenzie 2002, pp274-275]

41   **b**   Anemia differentiation—vitamin B_{12} deficiency results in pernicious anemia (pancytopenia, macrocytosis).
[McKenzie 2002, p267]

42   **c**   Anemia differentiation—B_{12}/folate.
MLS ONLY [McKenzie 2002, p267]

43   **a**   Folate deficiency—peripheral smear will show abnormally large RBCs.
[Rodak 2007, pp251-252]

44   **d**   Pernicious anemia is a pancytopenia
MLS ONLY with low cell production.
[McKenzie 2002, p267]

45   **a**   Myelofibrosis is often accompanied by folate deficiency, which causes macrocytic anemia.
[McKenzie 2002, p272]

46   **b**   Megaloblastic anemia is caused by
MLS ONLY impaired DNA synthesis.
[Rodak 2007, p250]

47   **a**   Megaloblastic anemia laboratory results
MLS ONLY include low platelet and neutrophil counts.
[Rodak 2007, p250]

48   **d**   Iron studies in anemia of chronic disease show decreased serum iron and transferrin saturation; TIBC may be decreased as well.
[Rodak 2007, p238]

49   **d**   Morphology in Hgb C disease.
[Rodak 2007, p344]

50   **d**   Thalassemia cause.
[Rodak 2007, p356]

51   **c**   Thalassemia minor—laboratory results.
MLS ONLY [Rodak 2007, p360]

52   **a**   Hereditary spherocytosis—lab results.
[Rodak 2007, p291]

53   **c**   Polycythemia, in burn patient.
[Harmening 2002, p345]

54   **c**   Lead poisoning—basophilic stippling.
[Rodak 2007, p239]

55   **c**   Erythroleukemia: morphology.
MLS ONLY [Rodak 2007, p501]

56   **b**   Erythroleukemia: morphology.
MLS ONLY [Rodak 2007, p501]

57   **c**   Low M:E ratio is seen in
MLS ONLY erythroleukemia.
[Rodak 2007, p501]

58   **c**   RBC morphology in lead poisoning.
[Rodak 2007, p239]

59   **d**   Erythrocytosis: congenital heart defect.
MLS ONLY [Harmening 2002, p345]

60   **a**   Absolute reticulocyte count.
MLS ONLY [Harmening 2002, p571]

61   **d**   Polycythemia—diagnosis.
MLS ONLY [Rodak 2007, p476]

Erythrocytes: Laboratory Determinations

62 **d** In infectious mononucleosis, the leukocyte is usually increased due to an absolute lymphocytosis. The platelet count is often mildly decreased.
[McKenzie 2002, p406]

63 **b** When the shape or size of the red blood cells prevents rouleaux formation a decreased or low ESR is expected. This is observed with sickle cells, acanthocytes, and spherocytes.
[Harmening 2002, p576]

64 **d** Patients unable to synthesize normal amounts of hemoglobin show reduction in the MCH.
[Hillman 2005, p16]

65 **a** RDW-CV is a new parameter available from automated instruments.
[Hillman 2005, pp16-17]

66 **a** Tilting of the tube accelerates the fall of the red blood cells.
[Turgeon 2005, pp443-445]

67
MLS
ONLY **d** Red blood cell morphological features of malarial species.
[Turgeon 2005, p106]

68 **d** The absolute concentration of each type of cell in a WBC differential is important for determining an increase or decrease.
[McKenzie 2002, p88]

69 **b** Reticulocytes appear as polychromatophilic red blood cells on a Romanowsky-stained blood smear. These cells are usually larger than normal cells with a bluish tinge. The bluish tinge is caused by the presence of residual RNA in the cytoplasm.
[McKenzie 2002, p178]

70 **c** Recognize the laboratory findings in megaloblastic anemia.
[McKenzie 2002, pp266-267]

71 **c** Newborn infants have elevated reticulocyte counts.
[McKenzie 2002, Table A]

72 **a** Recognize spherocytes on a blood smear.
[McKenzie 2002, p175]

73 **c** Use knowledge of RBC indices to classify anemia.
[McKenzie 2002, pp182-183]

74 **a** Polychromatophilic red blood cells and basophilic stippling can be associated with accelerated heme synthesis.
[Turgeon 2005, p104]

75 **b** Hgb C crystals can be seen in patients with Hgb C disease, more often in individuals who have undergone splenectomy.
[Harmening 2002, pp176-177]

76 **b** Rouleaux and an increased sedimentation rate are caused by increased fibrinogen and/or with increased immunoglobulin.
[Harmening 2002, p576]

77 **b** The peripheral smear allows microscopic examination of the blood cells. The most characteristic finding in multiple myeloma is rouleaux formation of the red cells.
[Harmening 2002, p386]

78 **a** The National Polycythemia Vera Study group criteria for the diagnosis of polycythemia vera include increased red cell mass, increased platelet count, increased LAP score.
[Turgeon 2005, pp305-306]

79 **a** Increase in both myeloid and erythroid precursors.
[McKenzie 2002, p152]

80 **d** Patients who have suffered severe burns to more than 15% of their body generally show evidence of intravascular hemolysis. RBCs show changes including fragmentation, budding and microspherocytes formation.
[Harmening 2002, p221]

81 **a** RBC morphologic features of erythroleukemia include nuclear budding and fragmentation, cytoplasmic vacuoles, Howell-Jolly bodies, ringed sideroblasts and megaloblastic changes.
[McKenzie 2002, p565]

82 **d** Rouleaux is the stacking of red cells like coins and is caused by increased amounts of immunoglobulins in the blood causing the RBCs to adhere to each other.
[Harmening 2002, p386]

83 **c** In patients with cold agglutinins, the automated cell counters show an erroneously elevated MCV and an erroneously decreased red blood cell count due to clumping of the red cells.
[Harmening 2002, pp209-210]

Answers–Hematology

84 **a** Laboratory findings in iron deficiency
MLS ONLY anemia include decreased serum iron,
serum ferritin, % transferrin saturation
and increased TIBC, FEP, and serum soluble
transferrin receptor levels.
[Harmening 2002, pp104-106]

85 **c** Secondary hemochromatosis is
MLS ONLY associated with anemia with abnormally
high serum iron studies.
[McKenzie 2002, p211]

86 **b** A very high WBC count causes turbidity
in cyanmethemoglobin reagent-patient
specimen that will result in falsely elevated
hemoglobin values.
[McKenzie 2002, p133]

87 **a** Hgb A_2 is increased in beta thalassemia,
MLS ONLY but decreased in alpha thalassemia.
[McKenzie 2002, p244]

88 **d** Hgb C crystals can be seen in
patients with Hgb C disease, more
often in individuals who have
undergone splenectomy.
[Harmening 2002, pp175-177]

89 **c** The Kleihauer-Betke procedure is
commonly used as a screening test to
determine the amount of fetal blood that
has mixed with maternal blood.
[Turgeon 2005, p84]

90 **b** The solubility test is a rapid test for Hgb
S. This should not be used for screening
newborns, needs to be corrected in severe
anemia and is not specific for Hgb S as
there are other hemoglobins that will sickle.
The presence of Hgb S is confirmed by
hemoglobin electrophoresis.
[McKenzie 2002, p229]

91 **d** Hemoglobin concentration is calibrated
using commercially available HiCN solutions
of known content.
[Steine-Martin 1998, pp65-66]

92 **c** In delta-beta thalassemia, one or both
MLS ONLY of the gamma genes remain, resulting in
100% Hgb F.
[McKenzie 2002, p255]

93 **d** Hgb H does show increased oxygen
MLS ONLY affinity 10× that of Hgb A.
[McKenzie 2002, p247]

94 **d** In the Black and Swiss types of HPFH,
MLS ONLY both gamma and alpha chains are produced
in approximately equal amounts.
[McKenzie 2002, p257]

95 **a** Hgb H disease occurs when 3 of 4 alpha
MLS ONLY genes are deleted.
[McKenzie 2002, p246]

96 **d** The low hemoglobin can result in a
false-negative result.
[Turgeon 2005, p451]

97 **c** In beta-thalassemia major, reduced
synthesis of beta chains affects the
production of Hgb A. Hgb A_2 and Hgb F are
increased and Hgb A decreased.
[McKenzie 2002, pp250-251]

98 **a** Electrophoretic pattern for sickle trait
on cellulose acetate.
[McKenzie 2002, pp806-807]

99 **b** Hgb E trait has approximately 70% Hgb
MLS ONLY A and 30% Hgb E plus A_2.
[Harmening 2002, p177]

100 **a** Using RBC indices to classify anemia.
[McKenzie 2002, pp167-181]

101 **c** Calculating RBC indices.
[McKenzie 2002, pp167-169]

102 **d** Any turbidity in the
cyanmethemoglobin reagent-
patient specimen will result in falsely
elevated values.
[McKenzie 2002, p133]

103 **d** Autoagglutination of anticoagulated
blood can occur at room temperature in
patients with a cold autoagglutinin. The
MCV will be falsely elevated and the RBC
count falsely decreased, resulting in an
elevated MCHC. The blood sample should be
warmed to 37° and rerun.
[Harmening 2002, p210]

104 **d** Autoagglutination of anticoagulated
blood can occur at room temperature in
patients with a cold autoagglutinin. The
MCV will be falsely elevated and the RBC
count falsely decreased, resulting in an
elevated MCHC. The blood sample should be
warmed to 37° and rerun.
[Harmening 2002, p210]

105 **a** Autoagglutination of anticoagulated
blood can occur at room temperature in
patients with a cold autoagglutinin. The
MCV will be falsely elevated and the RBC
count falsely decreased, resulting in an
elevated MCHC. The blood sample should be
warmed to 37° and rerun.
[Harmening 2002, p210]

106 a LAP activity may be increased in polycythemia vera.
[Harmening 2002, p344]

107 d Calculation of RBC indices.
[Harmening 2002, pp573-574]

108 a Calculation of RBC indices.
[Harmening 2002, pp573-574]

109 c Calculation of RBC indices.
[Harmening 2002, pp573-574]

110 a Calculation of RBC indices.
[Harmening 2002, pp573-574]

111 b Calculation of RBC indices.
[Harmening 2002, pp573-574]

112 b Calculation of RBC indices.
[Harmening 2002, pp573-574]

113 c Calculation of RBC indices.
[Harmening 2002, pp573-574]

114 d Calculation of RBC indices.
[Harmening 2002, pp573-574]

115 b Calculation of RBC indices.
[Harmening 2002, pp573-574]

116 d Calculation of RBC indices.
[Harmening 2002, pp573-574]

117 a The principle screening test would be a peripheral smear and RBC indices. The confirmatory osmotic fragility is frequently a reference lab only test.
[McKenzie 2002, p318]

118 b The sucrose hemolysis test is still sometimes used for screening; however, the most accurate measurement is immunophenotyping.
[McKenzie 2002, pp325-327]

119 b Sideroblasts and siderocytes may be identified with Perl Prussian blue iron stain.
[McKenzie 2002, pp180, 126]

120 a Using a supravital stain, residual ribosomal RNA is precipitated within the reticulocytes.
[McKenzie 2002, p135]

121 c Using a supravital stain (new methylene blue), residual ribosomal RNA is precipitated within the reticulocytes.
[McKenzie 2002, p135]

122 d Prussian blue stain is used for assessing iron stores in bone marrow.
[McKenzie 2002, pp154-155]

123 b Prussian blue stain is used to differentiate siderotic granules (Pappenheimer bodies) from basophilic stippling.
[McKenzie 2002, pp154-155]

124 b Systemic lupus erythematosus (SLE) is an autoimmune disease. The ANA procedure is a screening tool for SLE.
[Turgeon 2005, p239]

125 c Iron deficiency anemia laboratory features include: decreased RBC, hemoglobin, MCV, MCH, MCHC, serum iron, serum ferritin % saturation, bone marrow iron stores; and increased RDW, TIBC, FEP and serum soluble transferrin receptor levels.
[Harmening 2002, p108]

Leukocytes: Physiology

126 d Morphology of Döhle bodies.
[CAP 1998, pp42-47]

127 b An increased amount of cytoplasmic basophilia in a blood cell indicates decreased cytoplasmic maturation.
[CAP 1998]

128 b Definition of left shift.
[CAP 1998, pp158-162]

129 c Definition of leukoerythroblastosis.
[Morris 2006, pp561-562]

130 c Lymphocyte function.
[Alberts 2008, p1539]

131 c The intermediate stage in the formation
MLS ONLY of the fibroblast is the peripheral blood monocyte.
[Alberts 2008, p1450]

132 a Secondary granule appearance in neutrophils.
[CAP 1998, pp16-17]

133 d Normal bone marrow differential.
[Morris 2006, pp24-26]

134 d Definition of absolute neutrophilic leukocytosis.
[Morris 2006, pp913-916]

135 c Definition of leukocytosis.
[Morris 2006, pp913-916]

136 c Definition of relative neutrophilic granulocytosis.
[Morris 2006, pp913-916]

137 a Definition of relative lymphocytosis.
[Morris 2006, pp1087-1089]

138 d TdT staining in lymphoblasts.
[Morris 2006, pp1042-1044]

139 d Definition of multipotent stem cell.
[Alberts 2008, p1450]

140 a Philadelphia chromosome composition.
[Morris 2006, pp1238-1246]

141 b Phagocytosis is performed by granulocytes.
[Alberts 2008, p1524]

142 a Glucocorticoid-induced neutrophilia.
MLS ONLY [Morris 2006, pp857-858]

143 b Immediate type hypersensitivity
MLS ONLY reaction, cell types involved in .
[Goldsby 2003, pp362-375]

144 c Hypersegmented neutrophils in pernicious anemia.
[CAP 1998, pp52-53; Morris 2006, p487]

Leukocytes: Disease States

145 d Differentiates anemia due to conditioned nutritional deficiency from those of bone marrow dysfunction.
[McPherson 2007, pp508-514]

146 b Demonstrates CGL as having predominant myeloid cell line.
[McPherson 2007, p559]

147 c Recall of FAB classification.
MLS ONLY [Lee 1999, pp2211-2212]

148 c Differentiates this from other myeloid leukemias or other red cell abnormities.
[McPherson 2007, p569]

149 b Recognizes multiple causes impacting granulocyte production.
[McPherson 2007, p548]

150 d Classic feature discriminates AGL from other types of erythroid/myeloid metaplasia.
[McPherson 2007, p566]

151 a Lab findings, increased WBC but with increased LAP; negative Philadelphia chromosome differentiates leukemoid response from leukemia.
[McPherson 2007, p547]

152 b Identifies predominant cell line impacted in viral response.
[McPherson 2007, p555]

153 b Delineates pathophysiology of initial B-cell proliferation in EBV infection.
[McPherson 2007, p555]

154 a T-cell activation follows during second week of IM in response to the EBV induced B-cell infection and activation.
[McPherson 2007, p555]

155 b Differentiates CMV as most common of viral diseases that lacks serological evidence of infection.
[McPherson 2007, p556]

156 c Differentiates diseases involving
MLS ONLY platelets from myelofibrosis with morphologically abnormal platelets.
[McPherson 2007, p561]

157 c Differentiates leukemia with classic granulocyte anomaly.
[McPherson 2007, p550]

158 b Delineates characteristics of
MLS ONLY Auer bodies.
[Williams 1972, p1393]

159 a Prognostic implications of
MLS ONLY Philadelphia chromosome.
[Lee 1999, p2351]

160 b Identifies classic cellular findings in CGL.
[McPherson 2007, p559]

161 b Demonstrates understanding of
MLS ONLY myeloid implication of skewed M:E ratio in cellular production.
[McPherson 2007, p547]

162 d Peripheral findings demonstrate
MLS ONLY condition as multiplasia, and exclude single cell-line diseases.
[McPherson 2007, p561]

163 d Results demonstrate a lymphoblastic
MLS ONLY cell line and ⅓ of cases of CGL in blast phase are consistent with ALL.
[McPherson 2007, pp559-560]

164 d >20% blasts in peripheral or marrow
MLS ONLY defines blast conversion. Lab results with % precursor and blasts identify progression of this patient from chronic to acute phase.
[McPherson 2007, p560]

165 **c** Leukopenia with immature granulocytes in all stages, including blast with markedly decreased LAP and Philadelphia chromosome, positively identify CML. Leukopenia is consistent with engorged marrow space.
[McPherson 2007, p559]

166 **c** Demonstrates the possible progression of multiple myeloma.
MLS ONLY
[Lee 1999, p2646]

167 **c** Demonstrates nature of basophils.
[McPherson 2007, p553]

168 **a** Lab findings are reflective of erythroid rather that myeloid metaplasia.
[McPherson 2007, p560]

169 **b** Demonstrates characteristics of Auer rods.
MLS ONLY
[McPherson 2007, pp566-567]

170 **d** >20% of myeloblasts without other immature stages differentiates AML from CML and myeloid metaplasia; erythroleukemia requires at least 50% erythroid precursors in marrow.
[McPherson 2007, p566]

171 **b** Recognizes myeloid predominance in AGL would increase normal (2:1 to 4:1) myeloid:erythroid ratio.
[Steine-Martin 1998, pp383-384]

172 **b** Findings differentiate PML from sideroblastic anemia, myelofibrosis and CGL.
MLS ONLY
[McPherson 2007, p567]

173 **d** Findings differentiate between CMML vs CGL, PML, and myelofibrosis.
[McPherson 2007, p563]

174 **c** Definition of 'hiatus' as opening or break demonstrates the absence of intermediate maturing cells.
[Steine-Martin 1998, p447]

175 **d** Classic discrimination between CGL vs other hematological conditions: sideroblastic anemia, PML, myelofibrosis.
[McPherson 2007, pp559-560]

176 **c** Demonstrates knowledge of disease progression into myeloid rather than erythroid forms.
MLS ONLY
[McPherson 2007, p569]

177 **d** Acute leukemia is characterized by a maturation defect, whereby immature hematopoietic progenitors cannot overcome a block in differentiation, also known as the leukemic hiatus.
[Morris 2006, pp1186-1187]

178 **a** Demonstrates difference between acute vs chronic leukemias; intermediate cell maturity seen in chronic myelogenous, but would not predominate in erythroleukemia.
[McPherson 2007, p569]

179 **b** Discriminates between conditions due to granulocytic precursor, which would exclude lymphocytic leukemia.
[McPherson 2007, pp559-562]

180 **b** Recognizes results reflect polycythemia vera's excessive proliferation of multiphasic cell lines (megakaryocytes, erythroid and myelocytoid).
[McPherson 2007, pp559-561]

181 **d** Recognizes red cell increase secondary to stimulation of excessive erythropoietin produced in kidney.
[McPherson 2007, p541]

182 **b** RBC production is inversely regulated by O_2 levels—O_2 would decrease in emphysema (hypoxia); therefore, RBC levels would compensate, ie, increase.
[McPherson 2007, p541]

183 **d** Discriminates between faulty function of platelets, which would inhibit clotting and other PCV characteristics.
[McPherson 2007, p560]

184 **a** Hypochromic, microcytic RBC is most commonly associated with iron deficiency, which would most likely result from repeated therapeutic phlebotomies.
[McPherson 2007, p560]

185 **d** Smear findings demonstrate drug impact: megaloblastic changes due to interference with DNA synthesis (oval macrocytes) as well as other toxic nuclear effects (Howell-Jolly; hypersegmentation).
[Steine-Martin 1998, p451]

186 **d** Differentiates morphologic features of IM.
[McPherson 2007, p556]

187 **d** Discriminates between reactive cell line and more homogenous malignant cell line.
[McPherson 2007, pp556-573]

188 **c**   T vs B origin in classification of
MLS
ONLY   lymphoid conditions.
[McPherson 2007, p571]

189 **d**   Differentiation between morphologic
MLS
ONLY   basis used by FAB vs WHO classification,
which focuses on cytogenetic and
molecular findings.
[McPherson 2007, p571]

190 **c**   Differentiates ALL from other
MLS
ONLY   acute nonlymphocytic leukemias and
Burkitt lymphoma.
[McPherson 2006, pp571; Wu 2006, p1697]

191 **c**   Characteristics of ALL; onset highest
1-5 years of age with peak at 2-3 years of
age; presents with lethargy, fever, bone pain,
with poor prognosis under 1 year of age.
[Lee 1999, pp2242-2246]

192 **a**   Recognizes ALL as possible progression
for ⅓ of CML cases.
[McPherson 2007, p560]

193 **a**   Recognizes ALL as most common
malignancy of children.
[McPherson 2007, p571]

194 **d**   Discrimination of CLL from other major
mature B cell neoplasms.
[McPherson 2007, p572]

195 **c**   Definition of hairy cell leukemia.
MLS
ONLY   [McKenzie 2002, p590]

196 **d**   Characteristics features of hairy cell
leukemia include all answers listed as well as
decreased resistance to infection.
[McPherson 2007, p574]

197 **d**   Recognition that Gaucher cell is from
lipid storage disease, not plasma cell variant.
[Steine-Martin 1998, pp505-506]

198 **b**   Differentiation of most common MM
MLS
ONLY   feature from others seen less frequently
(flame) or diagnostic of other disease
(Reed-Sternberg—Hodgkin lymphoma).
[Steine-Martin 1998, pp505-506]

199 **d**   Recognition of Waldenström as a
MLS
ONLY   lymphoplasmacytic lymphoma.
[McPherson 2007, pp573-574]

200 **a**   Identifies neoplastic cell line
MLS
ONLY   (lymphocytic) and defines origin in
mycosis fungoides.
[McPherson 2007, pp582, 585]

201 **a**   Identification of condition with
morphologic alteration in neutrophils,
representing giant fused lysosomes.
[McPherson 2007, p549]

202 **d**   Description of MH anomaly.
[McPherson 2007, pp549-551]

203 **b**   Morphologic alteration of neutrophils;
majority of nuclei are bilobed and rounded.
[McPherson 2007, pp549-551]

204 **b**   Morphologic alteration of neutrophils;
majority of nuclei are bilobed, rounded and
dumbbell-shaped.
[Steine-Martin 1998, pp364-365]

205 **a**   Giant granulocyte inclusions due to
fusion of lysosomes.
[McPherson 2007, pp549-551]

206 **d**   Morphologic alteration of neutrophils—
differentiated from Chédiak-Higashi; May-
Hegglin and Pelger-Huët anomalies.
[McPherson 2007, pp549-551]

207 **b**   Morphologic alteration of neutrophils—
differentiated from Chédiak-Higashi, CML
and Alder-Reilly anomalies.
[McPherson 2007, pp549-551]

208 **a**   Morphologic alteration of neutrophils—
primary feature is hyposegmentation.
[McPherson 2007, pp549-551]

209 **b**   Identification of cellular structure
where accumulation of partially degraded
mucopolysaccharides occurs.
[Lee 1999, p1892]

210 **d**   Discrimination of anomaly from others
involving nuclear hyposegmentation; large
granules in leukocytes; lipid storage disease.
[Steine-Martin 1998, pp364-368]

211 **a**   Differentiation of lipid storage disease
from other anomalies of leukocytes.
[Steine-Martin 1998, pp364-365]

212 **c**   Leukocyte function defect; CGD
MLS
ONLY   neutrophils, eos, monos and macrophages
fail to generate superoxide, hydrogen
peroxide and other oxygen radicals after
particle phagocytosis and thus have
decreased microbicidal activity.
[Lee 1999, p1896]

213 **c**   Primary characteristic distinguishing
May-Hegglin from other neutrophil and
lipid storage anomalies.
[McPherson 2007, pp549-551]

Leukocytes: Laboratory Determinations

214 **a** Effect of conventional chemotherapy on WBC count.
[McKenzie 2002, p494]

215 **c** Definition of absolute neutropenia.
[McKenzie 2002, inside cover]

216 **a** Definition of relative lymphocytosis.
[McKenzie 2002, inside cover]

217 **c** Correlation of gout with sodium urate crystals.
[McKenzie 2002, p646]

218 **c** Calculation of absolute from relative % and WBC.
[McKenzie 2002, inside cover]

219 **b** Calculation of absolute eosinophil count.
[McKenzie 2002, inside cover]

220 **a** Hemocytometer calculation .
[McKenzie 2002, p130]

221 **b** Hemocytometer calculation .
[McKenzie 2002, p130]

222 **b** Hemocytometer calculation .
[McKenzie 2002, p130]

223 **a** WBC correction for nRBC.
[McKenzie 2002, p815]

224 **b** WBC correction for nRBC.
[McKenzie 2002, p815]

225 **c** WBC correction for nRBC.
[McKenzie 2002, p815]

226 **c** WBC correction for nRBC.
[McKenzie 2002, p815]

227 **d** An elevation in the MCHC occurs in approximately 50% of individuals with hereditary spherocytosis. Elevation in the MCHC above the upper normal limit should prompt an investigation of the sample for autoantibodies that agglutinate RBC, or on older instruments when the hemoglobin concentration is artifactually elevated by lipemia.
[Morris 2006, pp729-733]

228 **a** An elevated hematocrit decreases the amount of plasma in whole blood, and causes an effective increase in the amount of citrate added to that plasma. Recalcification incompletely overcomes the additional citrate, and prolongations in clotting time tests can be expected, unless the amount of citrate is adjusted for the abnormal hematocrit.
[Marlar 2006, pp400-405]

229 **d** Morphology of a monocyte, although the RBC inclusions (Pappenheimer bodies) look more interesting.
[CAP 1998]

230 **a** Morphology of a myelocyte.
[CAP 1998]

231 **b** Morphology of a lymphocyte.
[CAP 1998]

232 **b** Morphology, recognition of
MLS
ONLY reactive lymphocytosis.
[CAP 1998]

233 **d** Morphological description of a monocyte.
[CAP 1998]

234 **b** Morphology of a basophil.
[CAP 1998]

235 **c** Morphology of a myelocyte.
[CAP 1998; Gulati 2007, p195]

236 **a** Correlation of sepsis with a leukemoid reaction.
[McKenzie 2002, p383]

237 **a** Morphology of reactive lymphocytes.
[CAP 1998]

238 **d** Morphology of Niemann-Pick cells.
MLS
ONLY [CAP 1998]

239 **c** Current T-cell markers.
MLS
ONLY [McKenzie 2002, p571]

240 **a** Association of pseudogout with calcium pyrophosphate crystals.
[CAP 1998]

241 **d** Association of traumatic arthritis with macrophages containing hemosiderin.
[CAP 1998]

242 **d** Myeloperoxidase as a marker of
MLS
ONLY the granulocytic lineage.
[McKenzie 2002, p550]

243 **b** Sudanophilia of myelocytes.
MLS
ONLY [McKenzie 2002, p550]

244 **a** Myeloperoxidase as a marker of
MLS ONLY the granulocytic lineage.
[CAP 1998]

245 **b** Lipid sudanophilia.
MLS ONLY [McKenzie 2002, p550]

246 **a** Cellular components identified by Sudan
MT ONLY black B.
[McKenzie 2002, p550]

247 **b** ID specific esterase substrate.
MLS ONLY [McKenzie 2002, p550]

248 **d** TRAP stain positivity in hairy
MLS ONLY cell leukemia.
[CAP 1998]

249 **c** Mixed staining results for AML
MLS ONLY monocytic subtypes.
[CAP 1998]

250 **a** Myeloperoxidase as a marker of primary
granules in granulocytes.
[CAP 1998]

251 **c** Hypogranular pseudo Pelger-Huët cells.
MLS ONLY [McKenzie 2002, pp534-535]

252 **b** APL morphology.
MLS ONLY [CAP 1998]

253 **d** AML monocytic subtypes
MLS ONLY staining results.
[CAP 1998]

254 **c** CLL lymphocytes express the pan B-cell
MLS ONLY markers as well as CD 5, which is normally
not expressed in normal B cells, but is on
the surface of normal T cells.
[Morris 2006, pp1350-1351]

255 **c** Hairy cell leukemia cells typically
MLS ONLY express the CD 11c subunit of the beta-2
integrin, classified as a myeloid marker.
[Morris 2006, p1351]

256 **a** In a flow cytometer, forward scatter
provides an estimate of cell volume or size.
[Morris 2006, pp28-29]

257 **c** In a flow cytometer, side scatter
provides an estimate of a cell complexity
or granularity.
[Morris 2006, pp28-29]

258 **d** CD138, or syndecan, is expressed on
MLS ONLY neoplastic plasma cells, and is useful in
the diagnosis of myeloma.
[Morris 2006, p1485]

259 **c** The t(8;14) typically found in
MLS ONLY Burkitt leukemia (ALL-L3), brings the
master cell cycle control factor *c-myc* on
chromosome 8 under the influence of
the strong immunoglobulin heavy chain
promoter on chromosome 14, driving
a leukemogenic process.
[Morris 2006, pp1429-1430]

260 **b** Older and newer tests designed to
MLS ONLY diagnose CGD are all based on redox
reactions carried out by the phagocyte
oxidase family of proteins. Deficiencies of,
or dysfunctional PHOX proteins cause CGD.
[Morris 2006, pp941-946]

261 **b** Aryl sulfatase b deficiency results
MLS ONLY in the accumulation of proteoglycans or
glycosaminoglycans in phagocytic cells
and urine.
[Stone 1998, pp207-25]

Platelets: Physiology

262 **d** vWF is a constituent of platelet
alpha granules, and is synthesized in
the megakaryocyte as it develops.
[McKenzie 2002, p665]

263 **c** Nuclear maturation and division
occurs first, and is largely complete before
cytoplasmic maturation begins.
[McKenzie 2002, pp660-661]

264 **c** Bone marrow and splenic macrophages
contain hemosiderin; histiocyte is
a collective term for macrophages.
[McKenzie 2002, pp104, 196]

265 **a** Megakaryocytes are the largest cell in
the bone marrow.
[McKenzie 2002, pp661,44,103,101]

266 **b** Average life span of platelets in
peripheral blood is 9.5 days.
[McKenzie 2002, p662]

267 **a** Aspirin interferes with prostaglandin
MLS ONLY metabolism in the platelet by inhibiting
cyclooxygenase, which participates in the
conversion of arachidonic acid to protein
G2; protein G2 is necessary to produce
thromboxane, which stimulates secretion
from the platelet granules.
[McKenzie 2002, pp667-668]

268 **c**   Capillary fragility and bleeding time tests evaluate vessel and platelet function; thromboplastin is not evaluated by routine testing procedures; prothrombin and fibrinogen are evaluated by PT, APTT & fibrinogen assays (fibrinogen only).
[McKenzie 2002, pp667, 785]

269 **b**   Aspirin interferes with prostaglandin metabolism in the platelet; see answer #267.
[McKenzie 2002, pp667,688]

270 **d**   Thrombocytes (platelets) participate in several aspects of hemostasis.
[McKenzie 2002, pp659,665]

271 **c**   The peripheral zone is associated with platelet adhesion and aggregation. The sol-gel zone provides a cytoskeletal system. The organelle zone contains alpha, dense, and lysosome granules. Membranes contain the dense tubular system.
[Rodak 2007, pp456-458]

Platelets: Disease States

272 **d**   May-Hegglin anomaly is characterized by decreased platelet counts; the other listed disorders do not necessarily present with low platelet counts.
[McKenzie 2002, pp394,717]

273 **b**   Acute ITP typically resolves within weeks and is more frequently seen in children; it is not gender-dependent; platelet destruction is increased.
[McKenzie 2002, pp713,714]

274 **d**   Thrombocytopenia is the most common cause of excessive or abnormal bleeding.
[McKenzie 2002, p710]

275 **d**   Neutrophilic leukemoid reaction is characterized by an increased WBC count, a left shift in the differential; and an increased LAP. Polycythemia vera is characterized by an increased WBC count, an increased LAP and an increased platelet count. Leukoerythroblastosis is characterized by nRBCs and immature WBCs on the differential.
[McKenzie 2002, pp490, 515]

276 **d**   Abnormalities in coagulation factors and DIC are ruled out by the normal PT/APTT and fibrinogen.
[McKenzie 2002, pp717, 748-750]

277 **a**   Patients with thrombotic thrombocytopenic purpura (TTP) present with platelet counts less than 20,000. Platelet thrombi are dispersed throughout the arterioles and capillaries subsequent to the accumulation of large vWF multimers made by endothelial cells and platelets. This is related to a deficiency of ADAMTS-13.
[Ciesla 2007, p248]

278 **b**   The pathogenesis of HIT is that antibodies are produced against heparin-platelet factor 4 complex. This complex binds to FC receptors causing platelet activation and the formation of platelet microparticles, thrombocytopenia and hypercoagulability.
[Ciesla 2007, p287]

279 **a**   Polycythemia vera is characterized by increased WBC, RBC, and platelet counts.
[McKenzie 2002, p519]

280 **d**   Definition of increased platelet count.
[McKenzie 2002, pp659, 718]

281 **d**   Congenital spherocytosis is characterized by an increased MCHC and an increased reticulocyte count; reactive thrombocytosis is not usually accompanied by abnormal platelets; myelofibrosis is characterized by abnormal RBC morphology and decreased platelets and reticulocytes.
[McKenzie 2002, pp317, 515, 718]

282 **c**   MM hemorrhage is typical of platelet disorders; remaining choices are typical of coagulation factor disorders.
[McKenzie 2002, p705]

283 **a**   Giant platelets, abnormal bleeding time, normal aggregation with ADP, decreased decreased platelet count are characteristic of Bernard-Soulier.
[McKenzie 2002, pp721-722]

284 **d**   Glanzmann disease is characterized by abnormal bleeding time, abnormal ADP aggregation, normal ristocetin aggregation and absence of clot retraction.
[McKenzie 2002, pp672, 721,722]

285 **d**   Cryoprecipitate is acceptable treatment for vWD, but DDAVP is preferred due to decreased risk of bloodborne pathogen transmission; DDAVP is most effective in type 1 vWD patients.
[McKenzie 2002, p736]

Platelets: Laboratory Determinations

286 b   There is no indication that any part of the procedure has been done incorrectly.
[McKenzie 2002, p132]

287 a   Manual chamber counts do not have a high degree of precision or reproducibility, and require a significant amount of time.
[McKenzie 2002, pp132, 816]

288 c   Standard calculation for hemacytometer cell count.
[McKenzie 2002, p131]

289 a   Platelet count matches estimate well (average of 17.8 platelets per oil immersion field × 20,000).
[McKenzie 2002, p144]

290 d   Platelet clumping is reduced by collecting sample in sodium citrate.
[McKenzie 2002, p143]

291 d   Platelet satellitism is reduced by collecting sample in sodium citrate.
[McKenzie 2002, p143]

292 a   An average of 5-10 megakaryocytes
MLS ONLY   are normally found in each 10× (low power field); 100× in this question refers to 10× objective and the 10× magnification of the oculars.
[McKenzie 2002, p152]

293 d   Glanzmann thrombasthenia is
MLS ONLY   characterized by abnormal aggregation to ADP, epinephrine and collagen, but normal aggregation with ristocetin.
[McKenzie 2002, pp722,723]

294 a   Bleeding time (BT) assesses platelet activity.
[McKenzie 2002, p785]

295 b   BT assesses platelet number and function; platelet count only assesses platelet number; PT and APTT do not assess platelet number or function.
[McKenzie 2002, pp785,724]

296 c   BT assesses both platelet number and function.
[McKenzie 2002, p785]

297 a   BT assesses platelet function; PT, TT and PTT do not assess platelet function.
[McKenzie 2002, p785]

298 a   Calcium is required for platelet aggregation.
[McKenzie 2002, pp669,671]

299 a   vWD is characterized by abnormal
MLS ONLY   platelet aggregation to ristocetin; normal platelet aggregation to epinephrine, ADP and collagen; and normal ADP amounts.
[McKenzie 2002, pp723,735]

300 d   Hemophilia A is a coagulation
MLS ONLY   protein abnormality; it has no platelet function abnormalities.
[McKenzie 2002, pp735,740]

301 c   Curve C shows primary platelet aggre-
MLS ONLY   gation, followed by a lack of secondary aggregation; curve A is typical of collagen aggregation; curve B of normal ADP/epi aggregation; curve D is not typical of ADP/epi aggregation.
[McKenzie 2002, pp787,788]

302 d   Thromboxane A_2 is necessary for normal
MLS ONLY   platelet aggregation.
[McKenzie 2002, pp667-670]

303 d   vWD shows abnormal aggregation
MLS ONLY   with ristocetin and normal with the other agonists listed.
[McKenzie 2002, pp723,735]

304 c   Glanzmann thrombasthenia is an
MLS ONLY   autosomal recessive disorder. Patients will have a prolonged bleeding time, normal platelet count and morphology and abnormal aggregation with all aggregating agents except ristocetin.
[Ciesla 2007, p251]

Hemostasis

305 c   Warfarin interferes with the carboxylation of vitamin K factors by interrupting the enzymatic phase of the reaction. Factors are inhibited according to their half life, VII having the shortest (4-5 hours) and II the longest (2-3 days).
[Rodak 2007, p533]

306 c   Vitamin K is present in green vegetables, fish, liver and tobacco and synthesized by bacteria in the intestine. Naturally occurring vitamin K is fat soluble. Warfarin is the most popular vitamin K antagonist. Heparin inhibits Factor Xa and thrombin.
[Rodak 2007, p532]

307   **d**   Factor VII (proconvertin) is a single-chain glycoprotein that is Vitamin K dependent and remains stable 4-5 hours in blood. Produced in the liver, it has the shortest half-life; therefore, it is the first factor affected when a Vitamin K antagonist such as warfarin is administered.
[Southern 1995, p470]

308   **c**   The extrinsic pathway is initiated by the release of tissue thromboplastin that has been expressed after damage to a vessel. Factor VII forms a complex with tissue thromboplastin and calcium. Factors II and VII are found in the common pathway, and Factor VIII is in the intrinsic pathway.
[Ciesla 2007, pp237-8]

309   **d**   Factor XII is a contact factor, which is activated to Factor XIIa. It is responsible for the activation of Factor XI to Factor XIa. Fibrinogen is converted to fibrin by the action of thrombin.
[Rodak 2007, p471]

310   **a**   Prothrombin is produced by the liver cells dependent on Vitamin K as a coenzyme for its functionality. It is released into the blood as a zymogen as a precursor for its active form thrombin.
[Rodak 2007, p467]

311   **b**   Factor V is called labile factor, because its activity diminishes quickly at room temperature. Factor II: prothrombin, VII: stable factors, X: Stuart-Prower.
[Rodak 2007, p469]

312   **a**   A clot is degraded by plasmin in the fibrinolytic system. Plasminogen is the zymogen produced when Factor XIIa and kallikrein are produced by contact activation.
[Rodak 2007, p477]

313   **b**   Patients with a deficiency of Factor XII tend to have thrombotic complications. They do not have bleeding problems most likely due to the lack of activation of fibrin lysis, also due to pathway activation of IX by VIIa/TF complex as well as the activation of Factor XI by thrombin.
[Rodak 2007, p471]

314   **a**   Patients with a deficiency of Factor XII tend to have thrombotic complications. They do not have bleeding problems most likely due to the lack of activation of fibrin lysis, also due to pathway activation of IX by VIIa/TF complex as well as the activation of Factor XI by thrombin.
[Rodak 2007, p471]

315   **d**   Factors V and VII are helpful in distinguishing between liver disease and Vitamin K deficiency. Factor VII is a Vitamin K dependent factor; however, Factor V is not and will not be decreased. Both factors will be decreased in liver disease.
[Rodak 2007, p590]

316   **b**   Liver disease affects all Vitamin K dependent factors (II, VII, IX, and X) which will be decreased. Factor VIII is an acute phase reactant that may be elevated in liver disease.
[Rodak 2007, p590]

317   **c**   A prolonged APTT with a normal PT denotes a problem with the intrinsic pathway, so Factors VIII, IX, XI would be looked at, these deficiencies would correct in a mixing study. A characteristic of prekallikrein deficiency is the correction of the PTT when incubated for 10 minutes with kaolin, Celite®, silica, or ellagic acid.
[Bick 1992, p121]

318   **d**   Warfarin is a Vitamin K antagonist; coagulation Factors II, VII, IX, X, Protein C, and S are reduced as nonfunctional molecules are produced. The rate of reduction is based on the half-life of the factors.
[Rodak 2007, p701]

319   **d**   Long-term antibiotic therapy disrupts normal flora, which provide a source of Vitamin K synthesis. This results in a Vitamin K deficiency.
[Ciesla 2007, p264]

320   **a**   All daughters of hemophiliac men are carriers of the disease; all sons are normal. The gene for Factor VIII lies on the X chromosome.
[Rodak 2007, p597]

321 **a**   Laboratory diagnosis of hemophilia
MLS ONLY reveals a normal PT and TT, abnormal
APTT and a decreased VIII. To distinguish
between vWD, additional testing of VIII
antigen, activity, and bleeding time should
be performed. Additional abnormalities will
help to diagnosis vWD.
[Rodak 2007, p596]

322 **b**   Laboratory diagnosis of hemophilia
MLS ONLY reveals a normal PT and TT, abnormal
APTT and a decreased VIII. To distinguish
between vWD, additional testing of VIII
antigen, activity, and bleeding time should
be performed. Additional abnormalities will
help to diagnosis vWD.
[Rodak 2007, p596]

323 **b**   Individuals with hemophilia B lack
MLS ONLY Factor IX clotting factor. Symptoms
mimic hemophilia A. Treatment includes
Factor IX concentrate.
[Ciesla 2007, p262]

324 **c**   Laboratory testing of hemophilia will
MLS ONLY result in a prolonged APTT, resulting from
a decreased Factor VIII. A patient with vWD
will also present with an abnormal platelet
screen (bleeding time or a PFA 100), and an
abnormal ristocetin cofactor assay. These
tests will both be normal in hemophilia.
[Rodak 2007, p596]

325 **b**   Factor XIII activity is <5% in congenital
or acquired disorders. In adults, bleeding is
slow and delayed. The PT, APTT, fibrinogen
and platelets will be normal.
[Rodak 2007, p693]

326 **a**   Patients suspected of a lupus
anticoagulant present with a prolonged
APTT. Laboratory assays to detect lupus
anticoagulants are the APTT, dilute Russel
viper venom test, and Kaolin clotting time.
In the presence of a LA, the mixing study
doesn't correct.
[Ciesla 2007, p287]

327 **c**   The dissolution of clots occurs several
MLS ONLY hours after the clot is formed, and the
key component is plasminogen. This is
converted to plasmin through TPA. This
substance is released through the activity
of endothelial damage and the production
of thrombin.
[Ciesla 2007, p272]

328 **c**   Protein C is inherited as an autosomal
MLS ONLY dominant trait. Venous thrombi and
pulmonary emboli occur in these patients.
[Bick 1992, p272]

329 **c**   AT inhibits the serum proteases
MLS ONLY thrombin and Factors IXa, Xa and XIa.
AT function is enhanced by heparin.
Factor VIII doesn't play a role in assaying AT.
[Rodak 2007, p608]

330 **b**   In a type I deficiency of protein S, there
MLS ONLY is a decreased activity assay. To determine
if the deficiency is a dysfunctional molecule
or a quantitative disorder, an ELISA assay
should be preformed to determine a
type II deficiency.
[Rodak 2007, p616]

331 **c**   A DNA test is available to confirm the
MLS ONLY specific point mutation of activated protein
C resistance is FVL.
[Ciesla 2007, p285]

332 **a**   The laboratory profile for a patient
with acute DIC is: increased PT, APTT,
D-dimer and a decrease in platelets and
hypofibrinogenemia.
[Ciesla 2007, p275]

333 **c**   The laboratory profile for a patient
MLS ONLY with acute DIC is: increased PT, APTT,
D-dimer and a decrease in platelets and
hypofibrinogenemia.
[Ciesla 2007, p275]

334 **c**   The laboratory profile for a DIC workup
includes increased PT, APTT and D-dimers,
with decreased fibrinogen and platelets.
[Ciesla 2007, p277]

335 **c**   FFP provides all the necessary clotting
MLS ONLY factors. However, fibrinogen is a concern,
and if the value is low and plasma volume
needs to be considered, cryoprecipitate will
provide this at a low volume.
[Rodak 2007, p624]

336 **d**   PT thromboplastin reagents are
prepared from recombinant or affinity
purified tissue factor suspended in
phospholipid mixed with a buffered 0.025M
solution of calcium chloride.
[Rodak 2007, p683]

337 **c**   The APTT reagent contains
phospholipid and a negatively-charged
particulate activator such as kaolin,
ellagic acid, or Celite®. Ionic calcium and
phospholipid are supplied as reagents.
[Rodak 2007, pp686-687]

338 **d**   The APTT is performed to monitor the effects of unfractionated heparin, to detect factor deficiencies, and the presence of inhibitors. The PT tests the extrinsic pathway and requires tissue thromboplastin. It is also used to monitor warfarin therapy.
[Rodak 2007, p686]

339 **b**   A mixing study, when corrected, indicates a factor deficiency. Lack of correction indicates an inhibitor. Some inhibitors may only become evident after the patient's plasma is allowed to interact with the normal plasma after incubation. In this case, correction occurred immediately, as well as after incubation, confirming a factor deficiency.
[Rodak 2007, p593]

340 **a**   Protein C is a vitamin K dependent protein; hence warfarin therapy will lower levels of this protein.
[Morris 2006, pp1983-1987]

341 **d**   Thrombin time is prolonged in
MLS ONLY dysfibrinogenemia, fibrinogen deficiency or elevated FDPs. No correction when mixed with normal plasma indicates the presence of an inhibitor.
[Ciesla 2007, pp591-592]

342 **d**   A prolonged thrombin time can indicate diminished or abnormal fibrinogen, the presence of FDPs, paraproteins, and heparin. Reptilase is insensitive to the effects of heparin, and sensitive to dysfibrinogenemia. Therefore, when the TT is prolonged and the reptilase test is normal, this confirms the presence of heparin.
[Rodak 2007, pp688-9]

343 **d**   In thrombolytic therapy, the thrombin
MLS ONLY time will be prolonged. It is reasonable to obtain a TT 4 hours post onset of therapy to document a systemic thrombolytic effect. The TT should be repeated after the streptokinase is stopped, and prior to heparin being started. The TT should be <2× prolonged.
[Bick 1992, p322]

344 **b**   A prolonged thrombin time may be considered evident of diminished or abnormal fibrinogen; however, the presence of AT activity, such as heparin, must be ruled out.
[Rodak 2007, p688]

345 **b**   In a Clauss fibrinogen, a standard amount of thrombin is added to diluted plasma, and the time required for clot formation is recorded.
[Arkin 2001, pp2-15]

346 **b**   If the initial APTT remains prolonged in
MLS ONLY a mix, a second assay should be performed. The lupus anticoagulant has multiple targets. The second test is the DRVVT, which triggers coagulation at Factor X.
[Rodak 2007, p688]

347 **c**   D-dimers are produced from crosslinked and stabilized fibrin clots. This clot is dissolved by plasma and d-dimers are released. Therefore, d-dimers suggest a breakdown of fibrin clots, and indicate that clots have been formed at the site of injury.
[Ciesla 2007, p273]

348 **a**   D-dimers are produced from crosslinked and stabilized fibrin clots. This clot is dissolved by plasma and d-dimers are released. Therefore, d-dimers suggest a breakdown of fibrin clots, and indicate that clots have been formed at the site of injury.
[Ciesla 2007, p273]

349 **c**   Severe liver disease shows a decrease in
MLS ONLY hepatic synthesis of Factors II, VII, IX and X, V, I, Xi and XII. The degree of decrease in each of these factors will be dependent on the degree of fibrinolysis and the degree of elevation of factors behaving as acute phase reactants, including Factor VIII.
[Bick 1992, p175]

350 **a**   The ACT monitors high-dose heparin therapy at clinics, bedside, cardiac catheterization or at a surgical suite. The Stypven time is a test using snake venom for testing for lupus. The reptilase time is used to distinguish between heparin contamination and a decreased fibrinogen level.
[Rodak 2007, p706]

351 **b**   Fibrin stabilizing factor is needed to polymerize a clot. Primary screening tests are normal in Factor XIII deficiency. A screening test is based on the solubility of a fibrin clot in 5M urea.
[Rodak 2007, p523]

352 **d**   Heparin acts by inhibiting thrombin and Factor Xa. Anticoagulants, such as sodium citrate, act by binding calcium to prevent a blood sample from clotting.
[Rodak 2007, p704]

Answers–Hematology

353 **a** The chromogenic anti-Xa assay is the only assay available to monitor LMWH; it may also be used to measure UFH. The APTT can not be used to monitor low-molecular-weight heparin therapy.
[Rodak 2007, p707]

Hematology Laboratory Operations

354 **b** "+++" is an indicator that the WBC count exceeds the upper reportable limit.
[McKenzie 2002, p849]

355 **c** Low platelet count values should be verified with a slide estimate.
[McKenzie 2002, p143]

356 **b** Coulter principle of particle counting.
[McKenzie 2002, pp816,817]

357 **b** MLS ONLY RBC × 3 should approximately equal the Hgb; this Hgb value is likely to be falsely high; common causes include lipemia.
[McKenzie 2002, pp133, 849, 850]

358 **b** MLS ONLY Falsely high Hgb indicated by no match with Hct (Hgb × 3 = Hct), and high MCHC.
[McKenzie 2002, pp133,849]

359 **c** Formulas for calculation of indices; falsely increased RBC should not affect Hgb.
[McKenzie 2002, p134]

360 **d** Repeat of one out-of-range control is the first appropriate course of action.
[McKenzie 2002, p847]

361 **d** "+++" indicates a WBC that is above the reportable range of the instrument; dilute the sample and rerun.
[McKenzie 2002, p849]

362 **a** MLS ONLY Clumped platelets in the WBC counting bath may be above the size threshold and be counted as WBCs.
[McKenzie 2002, p851]

363 **b** Howell-Jolly bodies and WBC fragments may be mistaken for platelets; clotting may affect platelet numbers; decreased Hct would have no effect on a phase platelet count.
[McKenzie 2002, p132]

364 **b** Problems with diluent contamination, voltage variation and calibration errors are not common and are detected by daily quality control.
[McKenzie 2002, pp41-42]

365 **a** MLS ONLY Lipemia and icterus are causes of falsely elevated Hgb values.
[McKenzie 2002, pp133,849]

366 **c** MLS ONLY Formula for MCHC calculation.
[McKenzie 2002, pp134,849]

367 **b** MLS ONLY Combination of decreased RBC, increased MCV and increased MCHC is likely to be due to cold agglutinins.
[McKenzie 2002, pp356,849]

368 **a** MLS ONLY Hgb × 3 does not match the Hct.
[McKenzie 2002, pp133, 849]

369 **d** Appearance of RBC histogram.
[McKenzie 2002, p818]

370 **b** Appearance of WBC histogram.
[McKenzie 2002, p819]

371 **b** Appearance of WBC histogram.
[McKenzie 2002, p819]

372 **d** MLS ONLY Variation in light source is a common cause of drift in reading of results, and should be checked first.
[Anderson 2007, pp88-89]

373 **a** Photo-optical endpoint is a change in optical density. Nephelometry is an immunometric method for measuring proteins. Chromogenic methods employs a color-producing substance called a chromophore. Immunologic assays are based on antigen-antibody reactions.
[Rodak 2007, p716]

374 **d** MLS ONLY Principle of flow cytometry and light scatter.
[McKenzie 2002, p421]

375 **b** MLS ONLY Principle of flow cytometry and immunophenotyping.
[McKenzie 2002, p422]

376 **c** The heel is the preferred site for drawing capillary blood from the newborn. The posterior curvature of the heel should never be used.
[Turgeon 2005, p22]

377 **d** Too large of a drop will produce a thick smear; slowly pushing the blood will affect the distribution of the cells.
[Turgeon 2005, p25]

378 **b** Prolonged drying of slides will produce erythrocyte distortion (crenated) on microscopic examination.
[Turgeon 2005, p25]

379 b   In polycythemia, the decrease in plasma volume relative to whole blood alters the 9 part blood to 1 part anticoagulant ratio, falsely prolonging results. Therefore, a tube with a reduced volume of anticoagulant is need when the Hct is > 55%.
[Rodak 2007, p553]

380 a   Tubes that remain at room temperature for >5 hours have unacceptable blood cell artifacts. This will affect the Hct and the MCV.
[Rodak 2007, p176]

381 a   High-quality blood smears can be made from the EDTA tube within 2-3 hours of collecting the specimen.
[Rodak 2007, p176]

382 a   Instruments count particles within defined size limits. The upper limit is to separate large platelets from erythrocytes. Large platelets may be counted as erythrocytes.
[Koepke 1991, p161]

383 d   Platelet clumping is expected if smears are made directly from the finger. Smears must be made promptly before any clotting begins. It is important to examine the edges for platelet clumping.
[Rodak 2007, p177]

384 a   Some patient's blood undergoes
MLS ONLY an in vitro phenomenon called platelet satellitosis, which is a result of EDTA-induced platelet clumping.
[Rodak 2007, p176]

385 a   Platelet clumping is expected if smears are made directly from the finger. Smears must be made promptly before any clotting begins. It is important to examine the edges for platelet clumping.
[Rodak 2007, p177]

386 b   Sodium citrate is the only anticoagulant used for hemostasis testing. Sodium citrate binds free calcium ions. EDTA inhibits the thrombin-mediated conversion of fibrinogen to fibrin and binds reagent calcium added to initiate clot based tests. Heparin inhibits IIa, Xa, XIIa, XIa and IXa.
[Rodak 2007, p553]

387 d   Falsely prolonged results will occur if there is too much anticoagulant for the plasma; this also occurs with an increased Hct. Conversely, if a tube is overdrawn, there may be too little anticoagulant, resulting in a clot.
[Ciesla 2007, p244]

388 d   The ISI represents the international sensitivity index. The most responsive reagents have an ISI of 1.
[Rodak 2007, p685]

389 d   Whole blood calibration using fresh
MLS ONLY whole blood specimens that have been assayed using reference methods is the preferred method of choice for validation.
[Koepke 1991, p51]

390 d   Ristocetin induces a monophasic
MLS ONLY aggregation tracing from a normal specimen. Patients with vWD produced a reduced or absent reaction.
[Rodak 2007, p680]

391 a   Precision describes the closeness of
MLS ONLY results obtained from repeated analysis of the same sample. Results that are both accurate and precise are desirable.
[Rodak 2007, p40]

392 a   If results from a factor assay do not
MLS ONLY lie in parallel with the reference curve, and more than 1 result falls within the known linear range, the presence of a coagulation inhibitor should be suspected.
[NCCLS 1997, p6]

393 d   Lipemia interferes with Hgb by falsely
MLS ONLY elevating the results and the associated parameter indices.
[Rodak 2007, p558]

394 d   The distribution of data around the mean is the standard deviation. Using a specific confidence interval of 95.5%, or 2 standard deviations, the results fall between ±0.2 (1SD) or ±0.4 (2SD).
[Rodak 2007, p41]

Answers–Hematology

Immunology

The following items have been identified generally as appropriate for both entry level medical laboratory scientists and medical laboratory technicians. Items that are appropriate for medical laboratory scientists **only** are marked with an "MLS ONLY."

Autoantibody Evaluation

1   Antinuclear antibody tests are performed to help diagnose:

   a acute leukemia
   b lupus erythematosus
   c hemolytic anemia
   d Crohn disease

2   In the anti-double-stranded DNA procedure, the antigen **most** commonly utilized is:
MLS ONLY

   a rat stomach tissue
   b mouse kidney tissue
   c *Crithidia luciliae*
   d *Toxoplasma gondii*

3   Refer to the following illustration:

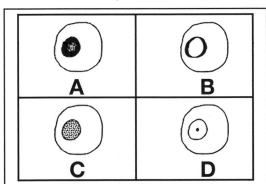

Which of the ANA patterns shown above would be associated with high titers of antibodies to the Sm antigen?

   a diagram A
   b diagram B-DNA
   c diagram C - SM
   d diagram D

4 Sera to be tested for IFA-ANA 6 days after drawing is best stored at:

    a room temperature
    b 5°C ± 2°C
    c −70°C in a constant temperature freezer
    d −20°C in a frost-free self-defrosting freezer

⑤ Antibodies directed at native DNA are **most** frequently associated with which pattern of fluorescence in the IFA-ANA test?

    a rim
    b diffuse
    c speckled
    d centromere

⑥ The technologist observes apparent homogenous staining of the nucleus of interphase cells while performing an IFA-ANA, as well as staining of the chromosomes in mitotic cells. This result is:

    a indicative of 2 antibodies, which should be separately reported after titration
    b expected for anti-DNA antibodies
    c inconsistent; the test should be reported with new reagent
    d expected for anti-centromere antibodies

7 The result of an anti-nuclear antibody test was a titer of 1:320 with a <u>peripheral pattern</u>. Which of the following sets of results best correlate with these results?

    a anti-dsDNA titer 1:80, and a high titer of antibodies to Sm
    b antimitochondrial antibody titer 1:160, and antibodies to RNP
    c anti-Scl-70, and antibodies to single-stranded DNA
    d high titers of anti-SS-A and anti-SS-B

⑧ Systemic lupus erythematosus patients often have which of the following test results?

    a high titers of DNA antibody
    b decreased serum immunoglobulin levels
    c high titers of anti-smooth muscle antibodies
    d high titers of antimitochondrial antibody

9 MLS ONLY Systemic lupus erythematosus patients with active disease often have which of the following test results?

    a high titers of antimicrosomal antibodies
    b high titers of anti-smooth muscle antibodies
    c marked decrease in serum CH_{50}
    d decreased serum immunoglobulin levels

10 MLS ONLY Which of the following is **decreased** in serum during the active stages of systemic lupus erythematosus?

    a anti-nuclear antibody
    b immune complexes
    c complement (C3)
    d anti-DNA

11 MLS ONLY A positive ANA with the pattern of anticentromere antibodies is **most** frequently seen in patients with:

    a rheumatoid arthritis
    b systemic lupus erythematosus
    c CREST syndrome
    d Sjögren syndrome

12 In the indirect fluorescent anti-nuclear antibody test, a homogenous pattern indicates
MLS
ONLY the presence of antibody to:

    a RNP
    b Sm
    c RNA
    d DNA

13 In the indirect fluorescent anti-nuclear antibody test, a speckled pattern may indicate the
MLS
ONLY presence of antibody to:

    a histone
    b Sm
    c RNA
    d DNA

14 A patient has the following test results:

ANA	ASO	Complement	RA
+, 1:320	50 Todd units	decreased	+

The above results could be seen in patients with:

    a rheumatic fever
  — **b** rheumatoid arthritis
    c lupus erythematosus – *autoantibody production in all systems*
    d glomerulonephritis

15 Autoantibodies in the absence of Sm are found in patients with:
MLS
ONLY
    a mixed connective tissue disease
    b systemic lupus erythematosus – *Sm*
    c Crohn disease – *centromere*
    d multiple myeloma – *monoclonal*

16 Which of the following is the most sensitive and appropriate method for the detection of
rheumatoid factor?

    a nephelometry
    b immunofixation electrophoresis   ✳
    c immunofluorescence
    d manual latex agglutination

17 Rheumatoid factor reacts with:

    a inert substances such as latex
    b Rh-positive erythrocytes   ✳
    c kinetoplasts of *Crithidia luciliae*
    d gamma globulin-coated particles   *RA testing*

18 A consistently and repeatedly negative IFA-ANA is:

    a strong evidence against untreated SLE
    b associated with active SLE
    c characteristic of SLE with renal involvement
  — **d** associated with lupus inhibitor

19 Positive rheumatoid factor is generally associated with:

    a hyperglobulinemia – *all autoimmune disorders*
    b anemia   ✳
    c decreased erythrocyte sedimentation rate
    d azotemia – ↑ *BUN*

20 The following results are from a rubella titer performed on acute and convalescent sera using a 2-fold serial dilution:

Date tested: 1/23/04
Acute serum titer: 1:8
Convalescent serum titer: 1:32

After evaluating the above results, the best interpretation is:

   a results are consistent with active infection with rubella
   b variation in the acute serum titers invalidates these results
   c test should be repeated by a different technologist
   d patient was not infected with rubella

21 Rheumatoid factors are immunoglobulins with specificity for allotypic determinants located on the:

   a Fc fragment of IgG
   b Fab fragment of IgG
   c J chain of IgM
   d secretory of component of IgA

22 Rheumatoid factor in a patient's serum may cause a false:

   a positive test for the detection of IgM class antibodies
   b negative test for the detection of IgM class antibodies
   c positive test for the detection of IgG class antibodies
   d negative test for the detection of IgG class antibodies

23 Rheumatoid factors are defined as:

   a antigens found in the sera of patients with rheumatoid arthritis
   b identical to the rheumatoid arthritis precipitin
   c autoantibodies with specificity for the Fc portion of the immunoglobulin (IgG) molecule
   d capable of forming circulating immune complexes only when IgM-type autoantibody is present

24 Tissue injury in systemic rheumatic disorders such as systemic lupus erythematosus is thought
MLS
ONLY to be caused by:

   a cytotoxic T cells
   b IgE activity
   c deposition of immune complexes
   d cytolytic antibodies

25 False-positive rheumatoid factor in agglutination and nephelometric methods can be due
MLS
ONLY to elevated levels of:

   a cryoglobulin
   b histidine-rich-glycoprotein
   c aspartame
   d C1q

26 An acute phase protein that binds to the membrane of certain microorganisms and activates
MLS
ONLY the complement system is:

   a C-reactive protein
   b tumor necrosis factor alpha
   c neutrophils
   d kinins

27 High titers of antimicrosomal antibodies are **most** often found in:

   a rheumatoid arthritis
   b systemic lupus erythematosus
   c chronic hepatitis
   d thyroid disease

28 Which of the following is an organ-specific autoimmune disease?

MLS ONLY

   a myasthenia gravis
   b rheumatoid arthritis
   c Addison disease
   d progressive systemic sclerosis

29 In chronic active hepatitis, high titers of which of the following antibodies are seen?

   a antimitochondrial
   b anti-smooth muscle
   c anti-DNA
   d anti-parietal cell

30 In primary biliary cirrhosis, which of the following antibodies is seen in high titers?

MLS ONLY

   a antimitochondrial
   b anti-smooth muscle
   c anti-DNA
   d anti-parietal cell

31 Anti-RNA antibodies are often present in individuals having an anti-nuclear antibody immunofluorescent pattern that is:

   a speckled
   b rim
   c diffuse
   d nucleolar

32 Anti-extractable nuclear antigens are **most** likely associated with which of the following anti-nuclear antibody immunofluorescent patterns?

   a speckled
   b rim
   c diffuse
   d nucleolar

33 In an anti-nuclear antibody indirect immunofluorescence test, a sample of patient serum shows a positive, speckled pattern. Which would be the **most** appropriate additional test to perform?

   a antimitochondrial antibody
   b immunoglobulin quantitation
   c screen for Sm and RNP antibodies
   d anti-DNA antibody using *C luciliae*

34 Anti-glomerular basement membrane antibody is **most** often associated with this condition:

MLS ONLY

   a systemic lupus erythematosus
   b celiac disease
   c chronic active hepatitis
   d Goodpasture disease

35 A 25-year-old woman is seen by a physician because of Raynaud phenomenon, myalgias, arthralgias and difficulty in swallowing. There is no evidence of renal disease. An ANA titer is 1:5120 with a speckled pattern with mitotic. Which of the following are also likely to be found in this patient?

MLS ONLY

   a high-level nDNA antibody and a low CH_{50} level
   b high-level Sm antibody
   c high-titer rheumatoid factor
   d high-level ribonucleoprotein (RNP) antibody

36 In pernicious anemia, which of the following antibodies is characteristically detected?
MLS ONLY

    a antimitochondrial

    b anti-smooth muscle

    c anti-DNA

    d anti-parietal cell

37 Anti-phospholipid antibodies associated with autoimmune disorders tend to have
MLS ONLY immunoglobulin (IgG) that belongs to which of the following subclasses?

    a IgG1 and IgG3

    b IgG2 and IgG4

    c IgG1 and IgG4

    d IgG2 and IgG3

38 The IIF staining pattern on ethanol-fixed leukocytes slides shows a perinuclear or nuclear staining
MLS ONLY pattern. This pattern is typically is due to:

    a C-ANCA

    b LKM

    c P-ANCA

    d GBM

39 The specificity of an immunoassay is determined by the:
MLS ONLY

    a label used on the antigen

    b method used to separate the bound from free antigen

    c antibody used in the assay

    d concentration of unlabeled antigen

40 In assessing the usefulness of a new laboratory test, sensitivity is defined as the percentage of:
MLS ONLY

    a positive specimens correctly identified

    b false-positive specimens

    c negative specimens correctly identified

    d false-negative specimens

41 In the indirect immunofluorescence method of antibody detection in patient serum, the labeled antibody is:

    a human anti-goat immunoglobulin

    b rheumatoid factor

    ⓒ goat anti-human immunoglobulin *w/ fleuorochrome*

    d complement

42 Which of the following describes an antigen-antibody reaction?

    ⓐ the reaction is reversible   ✳

    b the reaction is the same as a chemical reaction

    c a lattice is formed at prozone

    d a lattice is formed at postzone

43 The **most** common label in direct fluorescent antibody technique (DFA) is:

    a alkaline phosphatase

    b horseradish peroxidase

    ⓒ fluorescein isothiocyanate *→ green under UV*

    d calcofluor white

44 A substrate is first exposed to a patient's serum, then after washing, anti-human immunoglobulin labeled with a fluorochrome is added. The procedure described is:

    a fluorescent quenching

    b direct fluorescence   ✳ ✳

    ⓒ indirect fluorescence

    d fluorescence inhibition

45   Avidity may be defined as the:

   a degree of hemolysis
   b titer of an antigen
   c dilution of an antibody
   d strength of a reacting antibody ✳

46   In the interpretation of agglutination tests for febrile diseases, which of the following is of
      the greatest diagnostic importance?

   a anamnestic reactions caused by heterologous antigens
   b rise in titer of the patient's serum
   c history of previous vaccination
   d naturally occurring antibodies prevalent where the disease is endemic

47   Cholesterol is added to the antigen used in flocculation tests for syphilis to:

   a destroy tissue impurities present in the alcoholic beef heart extract
   b sensitize the sheep RBCs
   c decrease specificity of the antigen
   d increase sensitivity of the antigen

48   The strength of a visible reaction is known as:

   a prozone reaction
   b absorption
   c avidity - *reaction of an antibody with its antigen*
   d elution

49   Which of the following describes an antigen-antibody precipitation reaction of non-identity?

   a precipitin lines cross, forming double spurs
   b precipitin lines fuse, forming a single spur
   c no precipitin lines are formed
   d precipitin lines fuse, forming a single arc

50   Which test has the greatest sensitivity for antigen detection?

   a precipitin
   b agglutination
   c ELISA
   d complement fixation

51   Excess antigen in precipitation gel reactions will:

   a have no effect on the precipitate reaction
   b not dissolve precipitate after formation   ✳
   c enhance the precipitate reaction
   d dissolve the precipitate after formation

52   Soluble immune complexes are formed under the condition of:

   a antigen deficiency
   b antigen excess
   c antibody excess   ✳
   d complement

53   The visible serological reaction between soluble antigen and its specific antibody is:

   a sensitization
   b precipitation ✳ *soluble antigen + antibody*
   c agglutination
   d opsonization

54   The curve below was obtained by adding increasing amounts of a soluble antigen to fixed volumes of monospecific antiserum:

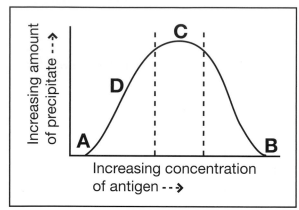

The area on the curve for equivalence precipitate is: *optimal antigen/antibody for maximum precipitation*

  a A
  b B
  c (C)
  d D

55   The curve below was obtained by adding increasing amounts of a soluble antigen to fixed volumes of monospecific antiserum:

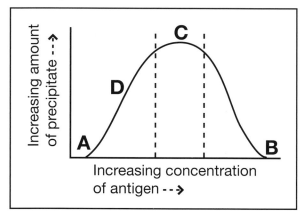

The area on the curve where no precipitate formed due to <u>antigen excess</u> is:

  a A
  (**b**) B
  c C
  d D

56   The curve below was obtained by adding increasing amounts of a soluble antigen to fixed volumes of monospecific antiserum:

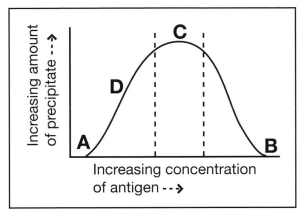

The area on the curve for prozone is:

   a A   *antibody excess → small complexes that do not visibly agglutinate*

   b B

   c C

   d D

57   The curve below was obtained by adding increasing amounts of a soluble antigen to fixed volumes of monospecific antiserum:

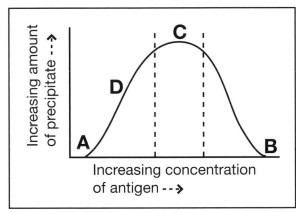

The area on the curve where soluble antigen-antibody complexes have begun to form is:

   a A

   b B

   c C

   d D

58   The curve below was obtained by adding increasing amounts of a soluble antigen to fixed volumes of monospecific antiserum:

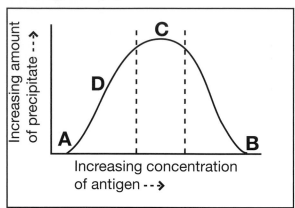

The area in which the addition of more antibody would result in the formation of additional precipitate is:

   a   A
   b   B
   c   C
   d   D

59   Refer to the following illustration:

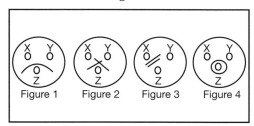

Which of the above figures demonstrates a reaction pattern of identity?

   a   Figure #1
   b   Figure #2
   c   Figure #3
   d   Figure #4

60   Refer to the following illustration:

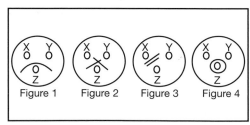

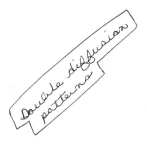

Which of the above figures demonstrates a reaction pattern of nonidentity?

   a   Figure #1
   b   Figure #2
   c   Figure #3
   d   Figure #4

61   Refer to the following illustration:

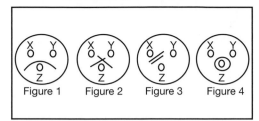

Which of the above figures demonstrates a reaction pattern showing 2 different antigenic molecular species?

a   Figure #1
b   Figure #2
ⓒ   Figure #3
d   Figure #4

62   Refer to the following illustration:
MLS
ONLY

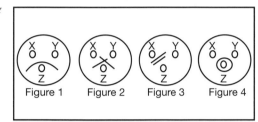

A nonspecific precipitin reaction is demonstrated in:

ⓐ   Figure #1
b   Figure #2
c   Figure #3
ⓓ   Figure #4

63   A series of 8 tubes are set-up with 0.79 mL of diluent in each. A serial dilution is performed by
MLS   adding 10 µL of serum to the first tube and then transferring 10 µL through each remaining tube.
ONLY   What is the serum dilution of tube 7?

a $1:2.431 \times 10^{11}$
b $1:2.621 \times 10^{11}$
c $1:1.920 \times 10^{13}$
d $1:2.097 \times 10^{13}$

64   The enzyme control tube in an ASO hemolytic assay exhibits no cell lysis. What is the **most** likely explanation for this?

a   incorrect pH of buffer
b   low ionic strength buffer
ⓒ   oxidation of the enzyme → should have complete hemolysis
d   reduction of the enzyme

65   The following pattern of agglutination was observed in an antibody titration:

Tube	1	2	3	4	5	6	7	8	9	10	11
	1+	2+	4+	4+	3+	3+	2+	1+	1+	0	0

This set of reactions **most** likely resulted from: *?.*

  a faulty pipetting technique
  b postzoning
  c prozoning (*antibody excess*)
  d the presence of a high-titer, low-avidity antibody

66   In a **positive** anti-streptolysin "O" enzyme inhibition test, the patient's:

  a streptolysin "O" enzyme in the patient serum neutralizes the anti-streptolysin "O" reagent, resulting in no hemolysis
  b red blood cells are hemolyzed by the streptolysin "O" enzyme in the reagent
  c anti-streptolysin "O" neutralizes the streptolysin "O" reagent, resulting in hemolysis
  d anti-streptolysin "O" inhibits the reagent streptolysin "O"'s, resulting in no hemolysis

an enzyme inhibition test
pt serum inhibits reagents hemolyzing effect
(antibody present)

Infectious Disease Serology

67   Blood is drawn from a patient for serological tests for a viral disease at the time of onset and again 4 weeks later. The results of the tests are considered diagnostic if the:

  a first antibody titer is 2× the second
  b first and second antibody titers are equal
  c first antibody is 4× the second
  d second antibody titer is at least 4× the first → *(antibody) four-fold between acute and convalescent*

68   Which of the following is **most** useful in establishing a diagnosis in the convalescence phase of a viral infection?

  a slide culture
  b serological techniques
  c shell vial
  d culture on McCoy media

69   The best method to detect infections due to rubella, Epstein-Barr and human immunodeficiency viruses is:

  a antigen detection by EIA
  b cell culture
  c antigen detection by Western blot
  d antibody detection by EIA → *sensitive, specific, can be automated*

70   Immunoassays are based on the principle of:

  a separation of bound and free analyte
  b antibody recognition of homologous antigen
  c protein binding to isotopes
  d production of antibodies against drugs

71   A DPT vaccination is an example of:

  a active humoral-mediated immunity - *vaccines stimulate antibody response*
  b passive humoral-mediated immunity
  c cell-mediated immunity
  d immediate hypersensitivity

72   Cells known to be actively phagocytic include:

    a neutrophils, monocytes, basophils
    b neutrophils, <u>eosinophils</u>, monocytes
    c monocytes, lymphocytes, neutrophils
    d lymphocytes, eosinophils, monocytes

Lymphocytes + basophils are not phagocytic

73   The presence of <u>HbsAg, anti-HBc</u> and often <u>HbeAg</u> is characteristic of:

    a early acute phase HBV hepatitis
    b early convalescent phase HBV hepatitis
    c recovery phase of acute HBV hepatitis
    d past HBV infection

early markers; Bs and Be disappear during convalescence

74   Refer to the following data:

MT ONLY

	HBsAg	anti-HBc IgM	anti-HAV IgM
patient #1	–	–	+
patient #2	+	+	–
patient #3	–	+	–

From the test results above, it can be concluded that patient #3 has:

    a recent acute hepatitis A
    b acute hepatitis B
    c acute hepatitis C (non-A/non-B hepatitis)
    d chronic hepatitis B

75   The disappearance of HBsAg and HBeAg, the persistence of anti-HBc, the appearance of anti-HBs, and often of anti-HBe indicate:

MLS ONLY

    a early acute HBV hepatitis
    b early convalescent phase HBV hepatitis
    c recovery phase of acute HBV hepatitis
    d carrier state of acute HBV hepatitis

76   An example of an organ specific disease with autoimmune antibodies is:

MLS ONLY

    a Wegener granulomatosus
    b rheumatoid arthritis
    c Hashimoto thyroiditis – *thyroid / others not organ specific*
    d systemic lupus erythematosus

77   When testing a patient for HIV antibody, which of the following is used to confirm a positive screening test?

    a radioimmunoassay
    b Western blot
    c immunofluorescence
    d ELISA

78   An example of a <u>live attenuated vaccine</u> used for human immunization is:

MLS ONLY

measles

    a rabies – *killed rabies virus*
    b tetanus – *toxoid*
    c hepatitis B – *recombinant subunit*
    d measles

79 A cold agglutinin titer end point is 1:16 after incubating overnight in the refrigerator and remains
MLS 1:16 after warming. The best course of action is to:
ONLY

  a report the titer as negative
  b report the titer as positive, 1:16
  c repeat the titer with a fresh sample
  d test for antibody specificity

80 What kind of antigen-antibody reaction would be expected if <u>soluble antigen</u> is added to homologous antibody?

  a precipitation
  b agglutination
  c complement fixation
  d hemagglutination

81 The Rapid Plasma Reagin test:

  a is useful in screening for syphilis – *tests for cardiolipids antibodies released by tissues damaged by syphillus, but also other diseases*
  b is useful in diagnosing syphilis
  c does not give false-positives
  d uses heated plasma

82 Flocculation tests for syphilis detect the presence of:

  a reagin antibody ✳
  b antigen
  c hemolysin
  d Forssman antigen

83 In the cold agglutinin test, the tubes containing the serum and erythrocytes are allowed to stand overnight in the refrigerator, and the results are read the next morning. If a disk of the erythrocytes floats up from the bottom of the tube with only the flick of finger, this is read as a:

  a 4+ reaction
  b 2+ reaction
  c 1+ reaction
  d negative reaction

84 <u>Flocculation</u> tests for syphilis use antigen composed of:

  a *Treponema pallidum*
  b reagin
  c cardiolipin and lecithin (*reagen antibody test*)
  d charcoal

85 The following cold agglutinin titer results are observed:

Tube #	1	2	3	4	5	6	7	8	9	10
dilution	1:1	1:2	1:4	1:8	1:16	1:32	1:64	1:128	1:256	1:512
4°C	+	+	+	+	+	+	+	+	0	0
37°C	0	0	0	0	0	0	0	0	0	0

✳

The best interpretation is:
  a positive, 1:128
  b negative
  c invalid because 37°C reading is negative
  d repeat the 4°C readings

86   A VDRL serum sample is heat inactivated, then placed in a refrigerator for overnight storage. Before being tested, the serum must be:

    a   kept colder than 10°C
    b   allowed to equilibrate to room temperature
    c   warmed to 37°C
    d   reheated to 56°C for 10 minutes *if longer than 4 hours*

87   Substances that are antigenic only when coupled to a protein carrier are:

    a   opsonins
    b   haptens– *antigenic only when coupled to a protein carrier*
    c   adjuvants
    d   allergens

88   A haptenic determinant will react with:
_{MLS ONLY}

    a   both T cells and antibody
    b   T cells but not antibody
    c   neither T cells nor antibody
    d   antibody but not T cells

89   A serological test for syphilis that depends upon the detection of cardiolipin-lecithin-cholesterol antigen is:

    a   FTA-ABS
    b   RPR
    c   MHA-TP
    d   TPI

90   The **most** important use of a nontreponemal antibody (NTA) test alone is in:
_{MLS ONLY}   *cannot be used for diagnosis; too many false positives*

    a   establishing the diagnosis of acute active syphilis
    b   establishing the diagnosis of chronic syphilis
    c   evaluating the success of therapy – *results in decreased titer*
    d   determining the prevalence of disease in the general population

91   The serological test for syphilis recommended for detecting antibody in cerebrospinal fluid is:

    a   nontreponemal antibody
    b   CSF-VDRL
    c   FTA-ABS
    d   MHA-TP

92   In the direct fluorescent antibody test for primary syphilis, spirochetes are detected by addition
_{MLS ONLY}   of labeled antibody to?

    a   *Treponema pallidum*
    b   cardiolipin
    c   human immunoglobulin
    d   nonpathogenic treponemes

93   In the FTA-ABS test, the presence of a beaded pattern of fluorescence along
_{MLS ONLY}   the treponeme indicates:

    a   positive identification of *Treponema pallidum*
    b   presumptive diagnosis of active syphilis
    c   presence of nontreponemal antibody (NTA)
    d   false-positive reaction

94   The FTA-ABS test for the serological diagnosis of syphilis is: *once positive for treponemal*
_{MLS ONLY}   *test → always positive*

    a   less sensitive and specific than the VDRL if properly performed
    b   likely to remain positive after adequate antibiotic therapy
    c   currently recommended for testing cerebrospinal fluid
    d   preferred over darkfield microscopy for diagnosing primary syphilis

95 A 16-year-old boy with infectious mononucleosis has a cold agglutinin titer of 1:2000. An
MLS ONLY important consideration of this antibody's clinical relevance is the:

    a thermal range
    b titer at 4°C
    c specificity
    d light chain type

96 What assay would confirm the immune status to hepatitis B virus?

    a HBsAg
    b anti-HBs *major antibody of immunity*
    c IgM anti-HBcAg
    d hepatitis C Ag

97 The following procedure has been routinely used for detection of hepatitis B surface antigen
(HBsAg) because of its high level of sensitivity:

    a hemagglutination
    b counterimmunoelectrophoresis
    c radial immunodiffusion
    d ELISA

98 In an indirect ELISA method designed to detect antibody to the rubella virus in patient serum,
the conjugate used should be:

    a anti-human IgG conjugated to an enzyme   ✳
    b anti-rubella antibody conjugated to an enzyme
    c rubella antigen conjugated to an enzyme
    d anti-rubella antibody conjugated to a substrate

99 A request is received in the laboratory for assistance in selecting the appropriate test(s) for
MLS ONLY detecting Lyme disease. Which of the following would be suggested?

    a Stool culture should be done to isolate the causative organism.
    b The organism is difficult to isolate, and antibody titers will provide the most help.
    c *Borrelia burgdorferi* is easily isolated from routine blood cultures.
    d This is an immunologic syndrome, and cultures are not indicated.

100 A bacterial protein used to bind human immunoglobulins is:
MLS ONLY
    a HAV antibody, IgA type
    b *Escherichia coli* protein C
    c staphylococcal protein A *– high affinity for Fc region of IgG*
    d HAV antibody, IgG type

101 Which of the following is the best indicator of an acute infection with the hepatitis A virus?

    a the presence of IgG antibodies to hepatitis A virus
    b the presence of IgM antibodies to hepatitis A virus *– IGM first indicator*
    c a sharp decline in the level of IgG antibodies to hepatitis A virus
    d a rise in both IgM and IgG levels of antibody to hepatitis A virus

102 Biological false-positive VDRL reactions are frequently encountered in patients with:

    a lupus erythematosus *– produce anti-cardiolipin*
    b acquired immune deficiency syndrome (AIDS)
    c gonorrhea
    d tertiary syphilis

103 Which serological marker of HBV (hepatitis B virus) infection indicates recovery and immunity?

  a viral DNA polymerase
  b HBe antigen
  c anti-HBs
  d HBsAg

104 The profile that matches the typical test profile for chronic active hepatitis due to hepatitis B virus is:
MLS ONLY

Profile	HBsAg	IgM anti-HBc	anti-HBc	anti-HBs
A	(+)	–	(+)	–
B	(+)	+	–	–
C	–	–	+	–
D	–	–	–	+

  a profile A
  b profile B
  c profile C
  d profile D

105 For diagnosis of late latent or tertiary syphilis, the **most** appropriate assay is:

  a RPR
  b VDRL
  c FTA-ABS
  d FTA-ABS IgM

106 A 26-year-old nurse developed fatigue, a low-grade fever, polyarthritis and urticaria. Two months earlier she had cared for a patient with hepatitis. Which of the following findings are likely to be observed in this nurse?

  a a negative hepatitis B surface antigen test
  b elevated AST and ALT levels
  c a positive rheumatoid factor
  d a positive Monospot™ test

107 The classic antibody response pattern following infection with hepatitis A is:

  a increase in IgM antibody; decrease in IgM antibody; increase in IgG antibody
  b detectable presence of IgG antibody only
  c detectable presence of IgM antibody only
  d decrease in IgM antibody; increase in IgG antibody of the IgG3 subtype

108 Refer to the following illustration of the hepatitis B virus:

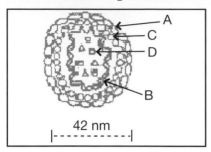

Select the corresponding lettered component indicated on the diagram for surface antigen.

(**a**) A
b B
c C
d D

109 Refer to the following illustration of the hepatitis B virus:

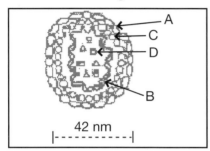

Select the corresponding lettered component indicated on the diagram for e antigen.

(soluble component in core)

a A
b B
c (C)
(**d**) D

110 Refer to the following illustration of the hepatitis B virus:

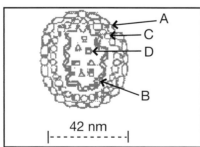

Select the corresponding lettered component indicated on the diagram for core antigen.

a A
(**b**) B
(**c**) C
d D

111 Refer to the following illustration of the hepatitis B virus:

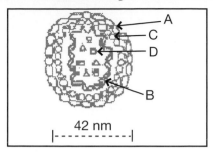

Select the corresponding lettered component indicated on the diagram for viral DNA.

  a A
  b B
  c C
  d D

112 The 20-nm spheres and filamentous structures of HBV are:

MLS ONLY

  a infectious
  b circulating aggregates of HBcAg
  c circulating aggregates of HBsAg
  d highly infectious when present in great abundance

113 The enzyme-linked immunosorbent assay (ELISA) technique for the detection of HBsAg:

  a requires radiolabeled Clq
  b is quantitated by degree of fluorescence
  c uses anti-HBs linked to horseradish peroxidase *(enzyme)*
  d uses beads coated with HBsAg

114 The antigen marker **most** closely associated with transmissibility of HBV infection is:

  a HBsAg
  b HBeAg ✱
  c HBcAg
  d HBV

115 Chronic carriers of HBV:

  a have chronic symptoms of hepatitis
  b continue to carry HBV
  c do not transmit infection
  d carry HBV but are not infectious

116 Hepatitis C differs from hepatitis A because it:

MLS ONLY

  a has a highly stable incubation period
  b is associated with a high incidence of icteric hepatitis
  c is associated with a high incidence of the chronic carrier state
  d is seldom implicated in cases of posttransfusion hepatitis

117 The initial immune response following <u>fetal</u> infection with rubella is the production of which class(es) of antibodies?

  a IgG – Mom's
  b IgA – breast milk from Mom
  c IgM
  d both IgG and IgA

118 A maternal serum rubella titer that is equal to or greater than 1:8 indicates:

   a probable immunity to rubella – *titer* ≥ 1:8
   b evidence of acute rubella infection – *2 fold rise between 2 pt samples*
   c susceptibility to rubella infection – *neg antibody result*
   d absence of acute rubella

119 A false-negative cold agglutinin test may result if:
   MLS ONLY

   a the specimen is centrifuged at room temperature
   b the cold agglutinin demonstrates anti-I specificity
   c the specimen is refrigerated prior to serum separation
   d adult human O red cells are used in the assay

120 Which of the following is a treponemal test?

   a RST
   b RPR
   c FTA-ABS
   d VDRL

121 The air temperature throughout the serology laboratory is 20°C. How will this affect VDRL and RPR test results? *temperature range: 23°-29°*

   a no effect—the acceptable test range is 20°-24°C   ✳
   b weaken reactions so that false negatives occur
   c strengthen reactions so that positive titers appear elevated
   d increase the number of false positives from spontaneous clumping

122 Which laboratory technique is **most** frequently used to diagnose and follow the course of therapy of a patient with secondary syphilis?

   a flocculation   ✳
   b precipitation
   c complement fixation
   d indirect immunofluorescence

123 A patient suspected of having toxoplasmosis has a specific IgG antibody titer of 1:64 upon initial testing. The titer of a second serum sample from the patient, taken 3 weeks later, was 1:256. These results are indicative of:
   MLS ONLY

   a past infection
   b present infection
   c allergic response
   d recent vaccination

124 The **most** commonly used serological indicator of recent streptococcal infection is the antibody to:

   a streptolysin O
   b hyaluronidase
   c NADase
   d DNA

Protein Analysis

125 Antibodies composed of IgG immunoglobulin:

   a occur during the primary response to antigen
   b are larger molecules than IgM antibodies
   c can cross the placenta from mother to fetus
   d can be detected in saline crossmatches

126 Measurement of serum levels of which of the following immunoglobulins can serve as a screening test for multiple allergies?

    (a) IgA
    (b) IgE – *allergies* ✱
    c IgG
    d IgM

127 Cells that are precursors of plasma cells and also produce immunoglobulins are:

    a macrophages
    (b) B lymphocytes
    c T lymphocytes
    d monocytes

128 IgM antibodies are frequently hemolytic because of:

    a their dimeric structure
  –b the molecule's 5 antigen binding sites
    c their sedimentation coefficient of 7-15 S
  –(d) their efficient ability to fix complement → *causes hemolysis*

129 To which of the following classes do the antibodies that cause hemolytic disease of the newborn belong?

    a IgA
    b IgE
    (c) IgG
    d IgD

130 It is important to note that when an infant is born, levels of specific antibody of the following class are used to indicate neonatal infection:

    a IgA
    b IgG
    (c) IgM
    d IgD

131 The immunoglobulin classes **most** commonly found on the surface of circulating B lymphocytes
MLS ONLY in the peripheral blood of normal persons are:

    a IgM, IgA
    b IgM, IgG
    (c) IgM, IgD – *B cell receptor*
    d IgM, IgE

132 Antibodies are produced by:

    a killer cells
    b marrow stem cells
    c mast cells
    (d) B cells

133 Antibody class and antibody subclass are determined by major physiochemical differences and antigenic variation found primarily in the:

    (a) constant region of heavy chain ✱ *Fc area*
    b constant region of light chain
    (c) variable regions of heavy and light chains
    d constant regions of heavy and light chains

134 The ratio of kappa to lambda light chain producing cells in normal individuals is:

MLS ONLY

   a 1:1
   (b) 2:1
   c 3:1
   d 4:1

135 Which of the following immunoglobulin classes is associated with a secretory component (transport piece)?

   (a) IgA – *secretory* ✳
   b IgD   *(tears, saliva)*
   c IgE
   d IgG

136 The immunoglobulin class typically found to be present in saliva, tears and other secretions is:

   a IgG
   (b) IgA
   c IgM
   d IgD

137 Treatment of IgG with papain results in how many fragments from each immunoglobulin molecule?

   a 2   ✳
   (b) 3
   c 4
   d 5

138 The immunoglobulin class associated with immediate hypersensitivity or atopic reactions is:

   a IgA
   b IgM
   c IgD
   (d) IgE

139 Which of the following immunoglobulins is the **most** efficient at agglutination?

   a IgG
   b IgA
   (c) IgM
   d IgE

140 Polyclonal B cell activation:

MLS ONLY

   a inhibits antibody production
   b requires the participation of T helper cells
   c results from the activation of suppressor T cells
   (d) can induce autoantibody production

141 Antibodies to which of the following immunoglobulins is known to have produced anaphylactic reactions following blood transfusion?

MLS ONLY

   (a) IgA
   b IgD
   c IgE
   d IgG

142 The key structural difference that distinguishes immunoglobulin subclasses is the:

   a number of domains
   b stereometry of the hypervariable region
   (c) the sequence of the constant regions   ✳
   d covalent linkage of the light chains

143 Immunoglobulin idiotypic diversity is best explained by the theory of:

MLS ONLY

   a somatic mutation
   b germ line recombination
   c antigen induction
   d clonal selection

144 Which of the following are true statements about selective IgA deficiency?

MLS ONLY

   a associated with a decreased incidence of allergic manifestations
   b high concentration of secretory component in the saliva
   c associated with an increased incidence of autoimmune diseases
   d found in approximately 1 out of every 50 persons

145 Which class of immunoglobulin is thought to function as an antigenic receptor site on the surface of immature B lymphocytes?

MLS ONLY

   a IgD
   b IgE
   c IgA
   d IgG

146 The IgM molecule is a:

   a dimer
   b trimer
   c tetramer
   d pentamer

147 Which of the following immunoglobulins is present in the highest concentration in normal human serum?

   a IgM
   b IgG
   c IgA
   d IgE

148 Which of the following statements about immunoglobulins is true?

   a immunoglobulins are produced by T lymphocytes
   b IgA class is determined by the gamma heavy chain
   c IgA class exists as serum and secretory molecules
   d there are only 2 subclasses of IgG

149 Membrane-bound immunoglobulin molecules:

MLS ONLY

   a have an additional amino-terminal sequence of about 40 residues
   b are not anchored in a transmembrane configuration
   c are anchored by a hydrophobic sequence of about 26 residues
   d are anchored by a hydrophilic region

150 The area of the immunoglobulin molecule referred to as the hinge region is located between which domains?

MLS ONLY

   a V_H and V_L
   b C_{H1} and C_{H2}
   c C_{H2} and C_{H3}
   d C_{H3} and V_L

151 Antibody idiotype is dictated by the:

   a constant region of heavy chain
   b constant region of light chain
   c variable regions of heavy and light chains
   d constant regions of heavy and light chains

152 Antibody allotype is determined by the:

idiotype versus allotype

   a constant region of heavy chain
   b constant region of light chain
   c variable regions of heavy and light chains
   (d) constant regions of heavy and light chains

153 Which IgG subclass is **most** efficient at crossing the placenta?

IgG
Subclass function

   (a) IgG1
   b IgG2
   c IgG3
   d IgG4

154 The J-chain is associated with which of the following immunoglobulins?

Immunoglobulin structure

   (a) IgA
   b IgG
   c IgE
   d IgD

155 The assembly of the complement "membrane attack unit" is initiated with the binding of:

MLS ONLY

   a C1
   b C3
   c C4
   (d) C5

156 Macrophages are characterized by:

MLS ONLY

   (a) surface receptors for C3b complement
   b surface CD3 expression
   c in vitro synthesis of immunoglobulin
   d large amounts of rough endoplasmic reticulum

157 Macrophage phagocytosis of bacteria is enhanced by which of the following:

   (a) opsonin–
   b antigen
   c hapten–
   d secretory piece

158 Which of the following is **most** likely to activate the alternative pathway of complement activation?

   a lipopolysaccharides
   b glycoproteins   *
   (c) haptens
   d IgG complexed with antigen

159 Which of the following is the larger residual split portion of C3?

   a C3a – *small; anaphylatoxin*
   (b) C3b – *larger; opsonin; lands on target surface and becomes part of C5*
   c C4
   d C1q

160 Which of the following activities is associated with C3b?

   (a) opsonization
   b anaphylaxis
   c vasoconstriction
   d chemotaxis

161 After a penicillin injection, a patient rapidly develops respiratory distress, vomiting and hives. This reaction is primarily mediated by:

    a IgG
    b IgA
    c IgM
    (d) IgE

162 Which of the following is the "recognition unit" in the classical complement pathway?

    (a) C1q – *recognition unit*
    b C3a
    c C4
    d C5 – *membrane*

163 In immunofixation electrophoresis:

    a the antibody reacts with the antigen and then the complex is electrophoresed
    b the antigen is electrophoresed into an antibody containing gel   *
    (c) the antigen is electrophoresed and then monospecific antisera is reacted with it
    d the antigen is electrophoresed, transferred to nitrocellulose and then antibody reacts with it and an EIA is performed

164 Which of the following is the "membrane attack complex" of complement activation?

    a C1
    b C3
    c C4, C2, C3   *C5-9 Membrane attack unit*
    (d) C5b, C6, C7, C8, C9

165 Which of the following releases histamine and other mediators from basophils?

    (a) C3a, C4a, and C5a all release histamine
    b properdin factor B
    c C1q
    d C4

166 The complement component C3:
MLS ONLY

    a is increased (in plasma levels) when complement activation occurs
    (b) can be measured by immunoprecipitin assays *(RID)*
    c causes the conversion of C4 to C4a + C4b
    d is not involved in the alternate complement pathway

167 The serum hemolytic complement level (CH_{50}):
MLS ONLY

    (a) is a measure of total complement activity
    b provides the same information as a serum factor B level
    c is detectable when any component of the classical system is congenitally absent
    d can be calculated from the serum concentrations of the individual components

168 A single, reliable screening test for detecting neonatal infection in the absence of clinical signs is:

    a serum immunoelectrophoresis
    b differential leukocyte count
    c CD4 cell counts
    (d) quantitative serum IgM determination

169 Bence Jones proteins are:

    a immunoglobulin catabolic fragments in the urine
    (b) monoclonal light chains   *
    c whole immunoglobulins in the urine
    d Fab fragments of a monoclonal protein

170 A patient's serum IgA as measured by radial immunodiffusion (RID) was 40 mg/dL. Another
laboratory reported IgA absent. A possible explanation for this discrepancy is that the:

   a rabbit antiserum was used in the RID plates and rabbit antisera should not be utilized in RID
assays

   b IgA has an Fc deletion that cause complex formation in vivo

   c IgA antiserum has kappa specificity

   d patient serum has antibodies against a protein in the antiserum in the agarose of the RID
utilized by the first lab

171 Goat anti-human IgG heavy chain specific alkaline phosphatase conjugate is a:

   a monoclonal reagent that reacts with gamma heavy chains

   b monoclonal reagent that reacts with light chains

   c polyclonal reagent that reacts with gamma heavy chains

   d polyclonal reagent that reacts with light chains

172 Humoral antibodies are produced by which cells?

   a macrophages

   b T lymphocytes

   c B lymphocytes

   d neutrophils

173 Initiation of the activation mechanism of the alternative complement pathway differs from that
of the classical pathway in that:

   a antigen-antibody complexes containing IgM or IgG are required

   b endotoxin alone cannot initiate activation

   c C1 component of complement is involved

   d antigen-antibody complexes containing IgA or IgE may initiate activation

174 Which of the following is cleaved as a result of activation of the classical complement pathway?

   a properdin factor B

   b C1q

   c C4

   d C3b

175 The component associated only with the alternative pathway of complement activation is:

   a C4

   b C1q

   c properdin factor B

   d C3a

176 Which of the following complement components is a strong chemotactic factor as well as a
strong anaphylatoxin?

   a C3a

   b C3b

   c C5a

   d C4a

177 The C3b component of complement:

   a is undetectable in pathological sera

   b is a component of the C3 cleaving enzyme of the classical pathway

   c is cleaved by C3 inactivator into C3c and C3d; acts as control

   d is not part of the alternative pathway

178 Components of the complement system **most** likely to coat a cell are:
MLS
ONLY
   a C1 and C2
   b C3 and C4
   c C6 and C7
   d C8 and C9

179 The serological test that can be modified to selectively detect only specific IgM antibody in
MLS
ONLY untreated serum is:

   a Ouchterlony
   b enzyme immunoassay
   c hemagglutination inhibition
   d passive hemagglutination

180 A patient's serum is being analyzed in a sandwich assay. This patient has received mouse monoclonal
MLS
ONLY antibody therapy, and shows a false positive reaction in the sandwich assay, which is due to:

   a the mouse antibody in the patient's serum reacting to the antigen
   b the presence of human anti-mouse antibody activity
   c antibody to a mouse virus
   d production of a monoclonal gammopathy of unknown significance after the antibody
       treatment

181 A monoclonal spike of IgG, Bence Jones proteinuria, and bone pain are usually associated with:
MLS
ONLY
   a Burkitt lymphoma
   b Bruton disease
   c severe combined immunodeficiency disease
   d multiple myeloma

182 The hyperviscosity syndrome is **most** likely to be seen in monoclonal disease of which of
MLS
ONLY the following immunoglobulin classes?
                              Waldenstrom macroglobulinemia
   a IgA
   b IgM
   c IgG
   d IgD

183 Patients suffering from Waldenström macroglobulinemia demonstrate excessively increased
MLS
ONLY concentrations of which of the following?

   a IgG
   b IgA
   c IgM
   d IgD

184 Which of the following is the **most** common humoral immune deficiency disease?
MLS
ONLY
   a Bruton agammaglobulinemia
   b IgG deficiency
   c selective IgA deficiency
   d Wiskott-Aldrich syndrome

185 Which of the following is a true statement about Bruton agammaglobulinemia?
MLS
ONLY
   a it is found ~~only in females~~ *in males (X-linked)*
   b there are normal numbers of circulating B cells (*pre-B cell stage problem*)
   c there are decreased to absent concentrations of immunoglobulins
   d the disease presents with pyogenic infections ~~1 week~~ after birth
                              2-6 months

186 Immunodeficiency with thrombocytopenia and eczema is often referred to as:

MLS ONLY

   a DiGeorge syndrome
   b Bruton agammaglobulinemia
   c ataxia telangiectasia
   (d) Wiskott-Aldrich syndrome (X-linked)

187 The autosomal recessive form of severe combined immunodeficiency disease is also referred to as:

MLS ONLY

   a Bruton agammaglobulinemia
   (b) Swiss-type lymphopenic agammaglobulinemia - autosomal recessive
   c DiGeorge syndrome
   d Wiskott-Aldrich syndrome

188 In hybridoma technology, the desirable fused cell is the:

MLS ONLY

   a myeloma-myeloma hybrid
   (b) myeloma-lymphocyte hybrid   tumor   spleen
   c lymphocyte-lymphocyte hybrid
   d lymphocyte-granulocyte hybrid

189 Potent chemotactic activity is associated with which of the following components of the complement system:
                          chemotaxin =
   a C1q
   (b) C5a
   c C3b
   d IgG

190 Hereditary angioedema is characterized by:

   a decreased activity of C3   ✳
   (b) decreased activity of C1 esterase inhibitor
   c increased activity of C1 esterase inhibitor
   d increased activity of C2

191 Which of the following has been associated with patients who have homozygous C3 deficiency?
                                              (worst to have)
   a undetectable hemolytic complement activity in the serum
   b systemic lupus erythematosus
   c no detectable disease
   (d) a lifelong history of life-threatening infections

192 Hereditary deficiency of early complement components (C1, C4 and C2) is associated with:

   a pneumococcal septicemia
   b small bowel obstruction
   (c) lupus erythematosus like syndrome   ✳
   d gonococcemia

193 Hereditary deficiency of late complement components (C5, C6, C7 or C8) can be associated with which of the following conditions?

   a pneumococcal septicemia
   b small bowel obstruction
   c systemic lupus erythematosus   ✳
   (d) a systemic gonococcal infection if exposed

194 For several months a 31-year-old woman has had migratory polyarthritis and a skin rash. Upon admission to the hospital, the following laboratory data were obtained:

	Patient	Reference range
leukocyte count:	$4.7 \times 10^3/\mu L$	$5.0\text{-}10.0 \times 10^3/\mu L$
differential:	normal	
serum hemolytic complement:	<22 U	80-150 U
ANA:	positive in a homogenous pattern	
rheumatoid factor test:	negative	
urinalysis:	protein 1+, occasional RBCs	

This patient's test results are consistent with:

a dermatomyositis
b C1INH deficiency
c systemic lupus erythematosus (C3 deficiency)
d mixed connective tissue disease

195 Infantile X-linked agammaglobulinemia is referred to as:

a Bruton agammaglobulinemia
b DiGeorge syndrome
c Swiss-type agammaglobulinemia
d ataxia telangiectasia

196 Combined immunodeficiency disease with loss of muscle coordination is referred to as:

a DiGeorge syndrome
b Bruton agammaglobulinemia
c ataxia telangiectasia
d Wiskott-Aldrich syndrome

197 In skin tests, a wheal and flare development is indicative of: *edema erythema*

a immediate hypersensitivity
b delayed hypersensitivity
c anergy
d Arthus reaction

198 Which immunologic mechanism is usually involved in bronchial asthma?

a immediate hypersensitivity
b antibody mediated cytotoxicity   ✳
c immune complex
d delayed hypersensitivity

199 Antihistamines like Benadryl®:

a depress IgE production
b block antigen binding to surface IgE   ✳
c bind histamine
d block H_1 histamine receptors

200 Which of the following is used to detect allergen specific IgE?

a RIST
b IEP
c RAST
d CRP

201 A child has severe hay fever. A total IgE measurement was performed by the Ouchterlony immunodiffusion method. No lines of precipitation appeared on the immunodiffusion plate. The **most** likely explanation is:

    a IgE antibodies are not produced in children who have hay fever
    b hay fever is mediated by the cellular system ✳
    c IgE is in too low a concentration to be detected by this method
    d IgA is the antibody commonly produced in people with hay fever

Cellular Immunity and Histocompatibility Techniques

202 Which test is used to evaluate the cellular immune system in a patient?

    a skin test for commonly encountered antigens (hypersensitivity)
    b determination of isohemagglutinin titer
    c immunoelectrophoresis of serum
    d measurement of anti-HBsAg after immunization

203 T cells are incapable of:

    a collaborating with B cells in antibody responses
    b secretion of immunoglobulins
    c secretion of cytokines
    d producing positive skin tests

204 T lymphocytes are incapable of functioning as:

    a cytotoxic cells
    b helper cells
    c phagocytic cells
    d regulatory cells

205 Nonspecific killing of tumor cells is carried out by:

    a cytotoxic T cells
    b helper T cells
    c natural killer cells
    d antibody and complement

206 Tumor markers found in the circulation are **most** frequently measured by:

    a immunoassays
    b thin-layer chromatography ✳
    c high-pressure liquid chromatography
    d colorimetry

207 A patient with a B-cell deficiency will **most** likely exhibit:

    a decreased phagocytosis
    b increased bacterial infections
    c decreased complement levels
    d increased complement levels

208 A patient with a T-cell deficiency will **most** likely exhibit:

    a increased immune complex formation
    b increased parasitic infections
    c decreased IgE-mediated responses
    d decreased complement levels

209 Which of the following is an important cellular mediator of immune complex tissue injury?

    a mast cell
    b neutrophil — *deposet of immune complexes → neutrophils → lysosomal enzymes*
    c basophil
    d eosinophil

210 Which of the following mediators is released during T-cell activation?

    a immunoglobulins
    b thymosin
    c serotonin
    d cytokines

211 The HLA antibodies used in histocompatibility typing have been obtained from which of the following?

    a multiparous women
    b nonidentical siblings
    c sheep blood
    d rabbit serum

212 Which of the following terms describes a graft between genetically unidentical individuals belonging to the same species?

    a autograft — *same individual*
    b isograft — ~~genetic~~ *genetically identical individuals*
    c allograft — *genetically unidentical individuals*
    d xenograft — *different species*

213 Incompatibility by which of the following procedures is an absolute contraindication to allotransplantation?

    a MLC (mixed lymphocyte culture)
    b HLA typing
    c Rh typing
    d ABO grouping

214 Which is a recognized theory of the origin of autoimmunity?

    a enhanced regulatory T-cell function
    b diminished helper T-cell activity
    c production of antibodies that cross-react with tissue components
    d deficient B-cell activation

215 C3b and Fc receptors are present on:

    a B lymphocytes
    b monocytes
    c B lymphocytes and monocytes
    d neither B lymphocytes and monocytes

216 T lymphocytes that possess the CD8 surface marker mediate which of the following T-cell functions? *(suppressor)*

    a delayed type hypersensitivity
    b regulatory
    c cytotoxic
    d helper

217 Delayed hypersensitivity may be induced by:

    a contact sensitivity to inorganic chemicals
    b transfusion reaction
    c anaphylactic reaction
    d bacterial septicemia

※ contact dermatitis = delayed hypersensetivity

218 The **most** rapid immediate hypersensitivity reaction is associated with:

    a transfusion
    b anaphylaxis
    c contact dermatitis
    d serum sickness

219 The normal controls for a quantitative B lymphocyte assay should have a value of what percentage of total lymphocytes counted?

MLS ONLY

    a 21% – *B cells (20%)*
    b 48%
    c 76% – *T cells (80%)*
    d 89%

220 An immunofluorescence test using reagent antibody directed against the CD3 surface marker would identify which of the following cell types in a sample of human peripheral blood?

    a all mature T lymphocytes
    b T helper lymphocytes only
    c cytotoxic T lymphocytes only
    d T regulatory cells only

221 Refer to the following results for peripheral blood samples:

MLS ONLY

	% **T lymphocytes**
patient #1:	85%
patient #2:	23%
patient #3:	51%
patient #4:	82%
normal control:	44%

The data above indicates:

    a patient #1 has an abnormally high T lymphocyte count
    b patient #2 has a normal T lymphocyte count
    c patients #1 and #3 have normal T lymphocyte counts
    d the normal control is too low and another sample should be selected

222 Refer to the following flow cytometric data.

MLS ONLY

absolute WBC:	8,930
total lymphocytes:	30%
B lymphocytes:	40%
T lymphocytes:	58%

WBC × Lymphocyte total % × B cell %
8,930 × .40 = 3,572
6,930 × .30 = 2,679 × .40 =

Calculate the absolute count for B lymphocytes.

    a 1,072
    b 2,679
    c 3,572
    d 6,251

223 A concentrate of lymphocytes can be prepared from peripheral blood by:

MLS
ONLY
   a density gradient centrifugation
   b ultracentrifugation
   c zone electrophoresis
   d freeze fractionation

224 In flow cytometry, labeled cells:

   a scatter the light and absorb fluorescence
   b absorb fluorescence and emit electronic impulses
   c scatter the light and emit fluorescence
   d absorb both fluorescence and light

225 A marked decrease in the CD4 lymphocytes and decrease in the CD4/CD8 ratio:

   a is diagnostic for bacterial septicemia
   b may be seen in **most** hereditary immunodeficiency disorders
   c is associated with a viral induced immunodeficiency (HIV)
   d is only seen in patients with advanced disseminated cancer

226 Refer to the following data from a peripheral blood sample:

MLS
ONLY

total WBC:	$10.0 \times 10^3/\mu L$
Differential:	
neutrophils:	68%
lymphocytes:	25% (40% T cells)
monocytes:	4%
eosinophils:	2%
basophils:	1%

$10,000 \times 25\% \times .40 = 1,000$

The expected total number of T cells is:

   a 200
   b 1,000
   c 2,000
   d 2,500

227 A peripheral blood total leukocyte count is $10.0 \times 10^3/\mu L$. The differential reveals 55% neutrophils,
MLS
ONLY
2% eosinophils, 40% lymphocytes and 3% monocytes. Assuming a lymphocyte recovery of
85%-95%, what is the expected number of T cells in a normal individual?

   a 750/μL
   b 2,500/μL
   c 4,000/μL
   d 8,000/μL

228 In laser flow cytometry, applying a voltage potential to sample droplets as they stream past the
MLS
ONLY
light beam and using charged deflector plates results in:

   a an emission of red fluorescence from cells labeled with fluorescein isothiocyanate
   b an emission of green fluorescence from cells labeled with rhodamine
   c a 90° light scatter related to cell size
   d the separation of cells into subpopulations based on their charge

229 What is the immunologic method utilized in the flow cytometer?

   a latex agglutination
   b enzyme linked immunoassay
   c immunofluorescence
   d radioimmunoassay

230 Given the following data:

WBC:	$5.0 \times 10^3/\mu L$
lymphs:	15%
CD4:	8%

$5,000 \times .15 \times .08 =$

Calculate the absolute CD4:

  a   40
  b   60
  c   400
  d   750

231 Given this hematologic data:

WBC:	$5.0 \times 10^3/\mu L$
lymphs:	15%
CD4:	8%

Which of the following is the correct interpretation?

  a   CD4% and absolute CD4 normal
  b   consistent with an intact immune system
  c   consistent with a viral infection such as HIV
  d   technical error

232 Bone marrow transplant donors and their recipients must be matched for which antigen system(s)?

MLS ONLY

  a   ABO-Rh
  b   HLA
  c   CD4/CD8
  d   Pl^{a1}

233 A 28-year-old man is seen by a physician because of several months of intermittent low back pain. The patient's symptoms are suggestive of ankylosing spondylitis. Which of the following laboratory studies would support this diagnosis?

MLS ONLY

  a   a decreased synovial fluid CH_{50} level
  b   low serum CH_{50} level
  c   positive HLA-B27 antigen test
  d   rheumatoid factor in the synovial fluid

234 Cells from a patient with <u>hairy cell leukemia</u> have immunologic and functional features of:

MLS ONLY

  a   mast cells and B lymphocytes
  b   B lymphocytes and T lymphocytes
  c   granulocytes and monocytes
  d   B lymphocytes and monocytes

235 Which T-cell malignancy may retain "helper" activity with regard to immunoglobulin synthesis by B cells?

MLS ONLY

  a   Hodgkin lymphoma
  b   acute lymphocytic leukemia (ALL)
  c   Sézary syndrome
  d   chronic lymphocytic leukemia (CLL)

236 A patient's abnormal lymphocytes are positive for CD2 antigen, lack C3 receptors, and are negative for surface immunoglobulin. This can be classified as a disorder of:

  a   T cells $CD_2 + CD_3$
  b   B cells → surface immunoglobulin
  c   monocytes
  d   natural killer cells

237 HLA typing of a family yields the following results:

	Locus A	Locus B
father	(8, 12)	(17, 22)
mother	(7, 12)	(13, 27)

On the basis of these genotypes, predict the possibility of ankylosing spondylitis in this percentage of their children.

   a   25% of their children
   b   50% of their children
   c   75% of their children
   d   100%

238 HLA-B8 antigen has been associated with which of the following pairs of diseases?

   a   ankylosing spondylitis and myasthenia gravis
   b   celiac disease and ankylosing spondylitis
   c   myasthenia gravis and celiac disease
   d   Reiter disease and multiple sclerosis

239 Which of the following is an important marker for the presence of immature B cells in patients with acute lymphocytic leukemia (ALL)?

   a   terminal deoxynucleotidyl transferase (TdT) — *differentiates ALL from mature B-cell leukemias*
   b   adenosine deaminase
   c   glucose-6-phosphate dehydrogenase
   d   purine nucleoside phosphorylase

1	b	59	a	117	c	175	c	233	c
2	c	60	b	118	a	176	c	234	d
3	c	61	c	119	c	177	c	235	c
4	b	62	d	120	c	178	b	236	a
5	a	63	d	121	b	179	b	237	b
6	b	64	c	122	a	180	b	238	c
7	a	65	c	123	b	181	d	239	a
8	a	66	d	124	a	182	b		
9	c	67	d	125	c	183	c		
10	c	68	b	126	b	184	c		
11	c	69	d	127	b	185	c		
12	d	70	b	128	d	186	d		
13	b	71	a	129	c	187	b		
14	c	72	b	130	b	188	b		
15	a	73	a	131	c	189	b		
16	a	74	b	132	d	190	b		
17	d	75	c	133	a	191	d		
18	a	76	c	134	b	192	c		
19	a	77	b	135	a	193	d		
20	a	78	d	136	b	194	c		
21	a	79	d	137	b	195	a		
22	a	80	a	138	d	196	c		
23	c	81	a	139	c	197	a		
24	c	82	a	140	d	198	a		
25	d	83	a	141	a	199	d		
26	a	84	c	142	c	200	c		
27	d	85	a	143	b	201	c		
28	c	86	d	144	c	202	a		
29	b	87	b	145	a	203	b		
30	a	88	d	146	d	204	c		
31	d	89	b	147	b	205	c		
32	a	90	c	148	c	206	a		
33	c	91	b	149	c	207	b		
34	d	92	a	150	b	208	b		
35	d	93	d	151	c	209	b		
36	d	94	b	152	d	210	d		
37	b	95	a	153	a	211	a		
38	c	96	b	154	a	212	c		
39	c	97	d	155	d	213	d		
40	a	98	a	156	a	214	c		
41	c	99	b	157	a	215	c		
42	a	100	c	158	c	216	c		
43	c	101	b	159	b	217	a		
44	c	102	a	160	a	218	b		
45	d	103	c	161	d	219	a		
46	b	104	a	162	a	220	a		
47	d	105	c	163	c	221	d		
48	c	106	b	164	d	222	a		
49	a	107	a	165	a	223	a		
50	c	108	a	166	b	224	c		
51	d	109	d	167	a	225	c		
52	b	110	c	168	d	226	b		
53	b	111	b	169	b	227	b		
54	c	112	c	170	d	228	d		
55	b	113	c	171	c	229	c		
56	a	114	b	172	c	230	b		
57	d	115	b	173	d	231	c		
58	b	116	c	174	c	232	b		

Autoantibody Evaluation

1 b ANA detects circulating antibodies to nuclear antigens in systemic rheumatic diseases.
[Detrick 2006, p995]

2 **c** The Crithidia substrate has giant
MLS
ONLY mitochondrion containing native DNA that is free from contaminating histone antigens.
[Detrick 2006, p1028]

3 c Sm is characteristic of a speckled pattern.
[Detrick 2006, p996]

4 b Storage at 4°C is sufficient for samples analyzed up to a week after collection. For longer periods (months or years) –20 °C is preferable.
[Rose 2002, p926]

5 a Antigen target in the homogeneous pattern is DNA.
[Detrick 2006, p996]

6 b Homogeneous pattern may indicate the presence of anti-DNA antibodies for both single- or double-stranded DNA.
[Rose 2002, p923]

7 a Peripheral pattern reacts with the antigenic determinants of doublestrandedness of DNA.
[Miller 1991, pp314-315]

8 a Anti-DNA antibodies are prototypic autoantibodies found in the sera of SLE patients.
[Detrick 2006, p1027]

9 **c** CH50 is a good screening test for
MLS
ONLY complement deficiencies in the classical pathway. In SLE patients the classical pathway is critical for immune complex clearance.
[Rose 2002, p914]

10 **c** C3 becomes depleted due to
MLS
ONLY the autoantibody called C3-nephritic factor (C3NeF).
[Benjamin 2000, p273]

11 **c** A centromere is the specialized area
MLS
ONLY of chromosome constriction during metaphase. Autoantibodies to centromere antigens are found in 22% of patients with progressive systemic sclerosis (PSS, or diffuse scleroderma) and in 90% of patients with the subset of scleroderma known as the CREST syndrome (calcinosis, Raynaud, esophageal dysfunction, sclerodactyly, and telangiectasia).
[Detrick 2006, pp996-997]

12 **d** The homogeneous/rim ANA pattern
MLS
ONLY can be caused by: antibodies to double and single-stranded DNA (seen in SLE in high titers and in lower titers in other rheumatic diseases).
[Detrick 2006, p996]

13 **b** Sm antigen is a non-histone nuclear
MLS
ONLY protein composed of several polypeptides of differing molecular weights. Sm causes a speckled pattern.
[Detrick 2006, p996]

14 **c** Systemic lupus is characterized by an
MLS
ONLY association of autoantibody production; generalized multisystem.
[Detrick 2006, p1027]

15 **a** Systemic lupus erythematosus patients
MLS
ONLY usually have Sm antibodies; patients with Crohn disease have centromere antibodies; patients with multiple myeloma have an increase in monoclonal antibodies.
[Rose 2002, p951]

16 a Nephelometry and latex agglutination are used to detect rheumatoid factor. The sensitivity of detection of immune complexes containing rheumatoid factor has been increased by nephelometry over the sensitivity of manual latex agglutination methods.
[Detrick 2006, p1035]

17 d Source for latex agglutination of RF is gamma globulin pools from humans, rabbits, or cattle.
[Detrick 2006, p1034]

18 **a** Small percentage of normal healthy individuals and individuals with disorders not classified as autoimmune may have positive ANA. But positive ANA occurs most commonly in patients with systemic rheumatic diseases.
[Miller 1991, p340]

19 **a** Hypergammaglobulinemia such as a polyclonal increase is associated with autoimmune disorders. Hypergammaglobulinemia such as a monoclonal increase is associated with such disease states as multiple myeloma, lymphomas, etc.
[Miller 1991, p98]

20 **a** In a rubella infection, a titer of 1:8 or greater indicates protective antibodies. An acute infection would indicate a rise in titer between 2 serum samples collected 2 or more weeks apart.
[Miller 1991, pp314-315]

21 **a** Antigen detected is located on the Fc portion of the IgG molecule.
[Detrick 2006, p1034]

22 **a** IgM RF is the species most commonly measured in clinical assays.
[Detrick 2006, p1033]

23 **c** Rheumatoid factor is an autoantibody to the Fc portion of the immunoglobulin molecule.
[Rose 2002, p923]

24 **c** Large soluble complexes often accumulate along the basement membrane in the kidney. Impaired ability to process and clear immune complexes in SLE.
MLS ONLY
[Benjamin 2000, p273]

25 **d** C1q like RF will bind and cross link IgG; Cryoglobulin—false negative.
MLS ONLY
[Rose 2002, p964]

26 **a** Kinins act on smooth muscle; neutrophils are phagocytic cells; and TNF released by activated macrophages.
MLS ONLY
[Benjamin 2000, pp24-25]

27 **d** TPO (thyroid peroxidase) is the microsomal antigen of the thyroid epithelial cell. TPO antibodies are positive for about 90% of patients with chronic thyroiditis.
[Detrick 2006, p1065]

28 **c** Addison disease has antibodies circulating to adrenal antigens.
MLS ONLY
[Detrick 2006, p1065]

29 **b** Chronic Active Hepatitis (CAH) has at least 2 subsets, the classic or type I, which is associated with a positive ANA test and positive smooth muscle antibodies. The condition is associated with an attack on the hepatocytes.
[Folds 1999, p161]

30 **a** PBC is characterized by the presence of antimitochondrial antibodies.
MLS ONLY
[Detrick 2006, p1084]

31 **d** Nucleolar pattern is characteristic of staining of the nucleolus seen as 1 or 2 large dots within each nucleus and is produced most frequently in the presence of antibody to nucleolar RNA.
[Miller 1991, p341]

32 **a** Rnp/Sm extractable nuclear antigens show coarse nuclear speckles.
[Detrick 2006, p996]

33 **c** Rnp/Sm extractable nuclear antigens show coarse nuclear speckles.
[Detrick 2006, p996]

34 **d** Goodpasture syndrome is an autoimmune disease mediated by circulating autoantibodies with specificity to the GBM and the alveolar basement membrane.
MLS ONLY
[Detrick 2006, pp1110-1111]

35 **d** Coarse nuclear speckles are seen in Raynaud syndrome. Autoantibodies, eg, anti-nRNP, are associated with certain symptoms such as Raynaud phenomenon.
MLS ONLY
[Rose 2002, p936]

36 **d** Parietal cell antibodies are found in 90% of the cases with pernicious anemia. The other autoantibodies are not organ specific.
MLS ONLY
[Detrick 2006, pp1066-1067]

37 **b** IgG2 and IgG4 are associated with autoimmune disorders; IgG1 and IgG3 are dominant in infections.
MLS ONLY
[Rose 2002, p974]

38 **c** C-ANCA shows a granular cytoplasmic
MLS
ONLY
staining, and P-ANCA shows a perinuclear
or nuclear staining pattern.
[Detrick 2006, p1056]

39 **c** Specificity refers to the ability of an
MLS
ONLY
individual antibody combining site to react
with only 1 antigenic determinant or the
ability of a population of antibody molecules
to react with only 1 antigen.
[O'Gorman 2008, p43]

40 **a** The ratio of the true positives
MLS
ONLY
to the sum of true positives plus the
false negatives.
[O'Gorman 2008, p43]

41 **c** Fluorochrome is a labeled anti-
human immunoglobulin for indirect
immunofluorescent assays.
[Miller 1991, p62]

42 **a** Antigen-antibody binding is governed
by the law of mass action: free reactants are
in equilibrium with bound reactants.
[Stevens 1996, p113]

43 **c** Fluorescein isothiocyanate fluoresces
a visible green color when excited by UV.
[Benjamin 2000, p102]

44 **c** First react the target with an unlabeled
antibody, then follow with a fluorescent dye.
[Benjamin 2000, p103]

45 **d** Describes the overall interaction of
an antibody with its antigen.
[Detrick 2006, p10]

46 **b** A rising titer of antibody during the
progression and resolution of an illness is an
indication of infection with an organism.
[Gorbach 2003]

47 **d** VDRL antigen contains 0.9% cholesterol.
[Larsen 1998]

48 **c** Describes the overall interaction of
an antibody with its antigen.
[Detrick 2006, p10]

49 **a** Non-identity: each antigen forms
an independent precipitin line with
the corresponding antibody at an
equivalence point.
[Benjamin 2000, pp96-97]

50 **c** ELISA is a solid phase immunoassay
that uses anti-immunoglobulins that are
labeled with an enzyme that can be detected
by the appearance of color on the addition of
a substrate.
[Benjamin 2000, p101]

51 **d** Precipitation does not occur due to lack
of free antibody.
[Rose 2002, p7]

52 **b** As more antigen is added, the reaction
moves to antigen excess. Precipitation does
not occur due to lack of free antibody. Upon
the addition of antigen to a fixed quantity of
antibody, immune complexes start forming
immediately.
[Rose 2002, p7]

53 **b** Precipitation takes place when
antibodies and soluble antigens are mixed.
[Benjamin 2000, p94]

54 **c** The proportion of antigen to antibody is
optimal for maximal precipitation.
[Benjamin 2000, p95]

55 **b** Excess of antigen results in soluble
complexes.
[Benjamin 2000, pp94-95]

56 **a** "*Prozone*—suboptimal precipitation
occurs in the region of antibody excess.
Prozone effect—Occasionally, it is observed
that when the concentration of antibody
is high (ie, lower dilutions), there is no
agglutination and then, as the sample is
diluted, agglutination occurs. The lack of
agglutination at high concentrations of
antibodies is called the *prozone effect*. Lack
of agglutination in the prozone is due to
antibody excess resulting in very small
complexes that do not clump to form visible
agglutination."
[Benjamin 2000, pp94-95]

57 **d** Zone of antigen excess is depicted on
the figure as D.
[Benjamin 2000, pp94-95]

58 **b** In the figure, B is the zone of
antibody excess.
[Benjamin 2000, pp94-95]

59 **a** Continuous coalescing precipitin lines
form when the 2 antigens are identical.
[Benjamin 2000, pp96-97]

Answers–Immunology

60 **b** Two nonrelated antigens form independent precipitin lines that cross over each other.
[Benjamin 2000, pp96-97]

61 **c** Identity arc indicates that the 2 antigens are identical in figure #1. Figure #2, partial identity, shares a determinant that is part of antigen #1.
[Benjamin 2000, pp96-97]

62 **d** Identity arc indicates that the 2 antigens
MLS ONLY are identical in figure #1. Figure #2, partial identity, shares a determinant that is part of antigen #1.
[Benjamin 2000, pp96-97]

63 **d** A dilution involves the solute, the
MLS ONLY material being diluted and the diluent. 1/dilution= (amount of solute)/(total volume). In the problem, the 8th tube is diluted.
[Stevens 1996, pp7-8]

64 **c** There should be complete hemolysis in the streptolysin O control tube.
[Miller 1991, p192]

65 **c** Prozone—suboptimal precipitation occurs in the region of antibody excess.
[Benjamin 2000, pp94-95]

66 **d** ASO is an enzyme inhibition test. In the ASO test, a serum results in inhibition of the reagent's enzymatic ability to lyse human red blood cells.
[Miller 1991, pp190-191]

Infectious Disease Serology

67 **d** A 4-fold or greater increase in antibody titer from 2 serum specimens taken from a patient during the acute and convalescent phases of an infection are considered to be diagnostic.
[Mahon 2006, p238]

68 **b** Cell culture methods are best used during the acute phase of a viral infection, when the viral titer is high. Serological techniques, which detect antibody to the virus, would be better in detecting viral infection during the convalescence phase, when the patient is recovering and the number of viral particles has decreased.
[Mahon 2006, pp831-834]

69 **d** Serological tests are commonly used to detect antibodies in infections with viruses that are difficult to culture, such as rubella, HIV, and EBV. EIA is a common serological method because it is sensitive, specific, and can be automated.
[Stevens 2003, p325]

70 **b** "Immunoassay" is a general term for an assay involving binding of an antibody to a specific antigen.
[Mahon 2006, p103]

71 **a** Vaccines stimulate the host to produce antibodies against a specific antigen to prevent disease.
[Kindt 2007, pp477-478]

72 **b** Lymphocytes and basophils are not phagocytic.
[Kindt 2007, pp34-37]

73 **a** The markers listed appear early during hepatitis B infection; HBsAg and HBeAg disappear prior to convalescence and recovery.
[Stevens 2003, pp327-328]

74 **b** IgM anti-HBc may be the only marker
MLS ONLY present during the "window period" between disappearance of HBsAg and the appearance of anti-HBs in late acute hepatitis B.
[Stevens 2003, pp327-328]

75 **c** Anti-HBs and anti-HBe are associated
MLS ONLY with recovery and development of immunity in hepatitis B, while HBsAg and HBeAg are antigens from HBV that are present during the infectious stages of disease.
[Stevens 2003, pp327-328]

76 **c** In Hashimoto disease, the auto-
MLS ONLY antibodies produced are specifically directed against the thyroid gland, whereas in the other diseases, they are not organ-specific.
[Mahon 2006, p139]

77 **b** Western blot has been the traditional confirmatory test for HIV antibody because it is very specific.
[Stevens 2003, pp357-358]

78 **d** To prevent measles, a vaccine consisting
MLS ONLY of live, weakened measles (rubeola) virus is used. The vaccine for rabies consists of killed rabies virus; the vaccine for tetanus is a toxoid; and the vaccine for hepatitis B is made up of a recombinant subunit.
[Goldsby 2003, p482]

79 **d**   Because the antibody is still reactive
MLS
ONLY
upon warming, a test for antibody specificity
can help distinguish pathological from
harmless autoantibodies.
[Rudman 2005, pp494-495]

80 **a**   By definition, precipitation involves
combination of antigen and soluble antibody
to form insoluble complexes that fall out
of solution.
[Stevens 2003, p129]

81 **a**   The RPR is the most widely used
nontreponemal test to screen for syphilis
because it is rapid and inexpensive. It uses
unheated serum to test for antibodies to
cardiolipin, a lipid released during tissue
damage in syphilis patients, but also present
in other diseases with tissue damage.
[Stevens 2003, pp298-299]

82 **a**   Flocculation is the aggregation of fine
particles to form small clumps. This reaction
occurs in nontreponemal tests for syphilis
when reagin antibody reacts with the fine
cardiolipin antigen particles.
[Stevens 2003, pp298-299]

83 **a**   When 1 solid agglutinate is present,
the reaction is classified as 4+.
[Blaney 2009, p161]

84 **c**   Flocculation tests for syphilis are
nontreponemal tests that detect antibody
specific for cardiolipin antigen. When this
antibody, called reagin, combines with the
fine cardiolipin particles, small clumps are
formed in a reaction called flocculation.
[Stevens 2003, p298]

85 **a**   A cold agglutinin titer is read as the last
dilution showing agglutination at 4°C.
[Miller 1991, p364]

86 **d**   To avoid reactivation of complement,
standard practice is to reheat the specimen
for 10 minutes at 56°C if more than 4
hours has elapsed since the specimen was
first inactivated.
[Miller 1991, p29]

87 **b**   This is the definition of a hapten.
[Stevens 2003, p47]

88 **d**   In the immune response to a
MLS
ONLY
hapten-carrier complex, the hapten
portion of the molecule binds to B cells,
while the carrier portion binds to T cells,
and the B cell is stimulated to produce
hapten-specific antibody.
[Abbus 2007, pp225-226]

89 **b**   Nontreponemal tests for syphilis, such
as the RPR, detect antibody to cardiolipin
antigen complexed with lecithin and
cholesterol.
[Stevens 2003, p298]

90 **c**   Because of the high rate of false-positive
MLS
ONLY
results, nontreponemal tests cannot be used
alone to establish a diagnosis of syphilis, but
once the patient is known to have syphilis,
they can be used to monitor therapy, since
successful therapy will result in a decrease in
the nontreponemal antibody titer.
[Stevens 2003, p298]

91 **b**   The VDRL test is the only serological
test recommended for testing of spinal
fluid because of the low incidence of
false positives.
[Stevens 2003, p299]

92 **a**   Direct detection of *T pallidum* organisms
MLS
ONLY
in lesions from patients with primary
or secondary syphilis can be performed
by dark-field microscopy or fluorescent
antibody testing. In direct testing, labeled
antibody that is specific for *T pallidum* binds
directly to the spirochetes.
[Stevens 2003, pp297-298]

93 **d**   Serum from patients with lupus
MLS
ONLY
erythematosus may produce a false-positive
result in the FTA-ABS test, which appears
as a beaded pattern of fluorescence.
[Miller 1991, p213]

94 **b**   Once a patient shows reactivity in a
MLS
ONLY
treponemal test, such as the FTA-ABS,
that patient will remain positive for life,
regardless of whether or not they have
received therapy.
[Stevens 2003, pp299-300]

Answers–Immunology

95 **a**   It is important to determine the thermal
MLS
ONLY range of reactivity, because cold antibodies
are most likely to cause disease if they react
with red blood cells at temperatures from
30°C to 32°C.
[Rudman 2005, pp494-495]

96 **b**   Antibody to the surface antigen of
hepatitis B virus (anti-HBs) is the major
protective antibody in hepatitis B and
provides evidence of immunity against
this infection.
[Turgeon 2009, p283]

97 **d**   Of all the methods listed, ELISA is
the most sensitive and the only one that
is used for detection of HBsAg in the
clinical laboratory.
[Stevens 2003, p328]

98 **a**   In an indirect ELISA, patient antibody
to an antigen (eg, rubella antigen) is
detected by addition of an enzyme-labeled
antibody to human immunoglobulin, which,
in turn, binds to the patient's IgG.
[Stevens 2003, p161]

99 **b**   It is difficult to isolate *Borrelia*
MLS
ONLY *burgdorferi* from skin, blood, or other clinical
samples; therefore, laboratory detection of
Lyme disease is based on serological assays
such as EIA, IFA, and Western blot.
[Stevens 2003, pp304-306]

100 **c**   Protein A, found in the cell walls of
MLS
ONLY *Staphylococcus aureus* bacteria, has a high
affinity for the Fc region of IgG, and can be
used to bind IgG in some laboratory assays.
[Kindt 2007, pp162-164]

101 **b**   IgM is the first antibody to be produced
during an immune response, and levels
decline within 6-12 months; it is therefore
an indicator of a current infection.
[Stevens 2003, p326]

102 **a**   Patients with the autoimmune disease,
lupus erythematosus, frequently produce
antibody against cardiolipin, the same
antibody that is used to screen for syphilis
by the VDRL test.
[Stevens 2003, p218]

103 **c**   Antibody to the surface antigen
of hepatitis B virus (anti-HBs) appears
after the acute stage of infection during
convalescence and is a marker of recovery
and immunity, while the other markers
listed are components of the virus itself.
[Turgeon 2009, p283]

104 **a**   HBsAg is an indicator of active
MLS
ONLY infection, either acute or chronic. While
IgM anti-HBc is present in acute infection,
it disappears after this stage, while IgG
antibody to the core antigen persists for
life. Anti-HBs is an indicator of immunity,
and this has not been achieved in chronic
active hepatitis.
[Stevens 2003, pp327-328]

105 **c**   Treponemal tests, such as the FTA-
ABS, remain positive throughout the
course of syphilis (except for IgM, which
is only positive in the early stages),
while nontreponemal tests are generally
nonreactive in the late stages of disease.
[Turgeon 2009, p220]

106 **b**   The nurse's history and symptoms
suggest that she has hepatitis. The liver
enzymes, alanine aminotransferase (ALT)
and aspartate aminotransferase (AST) are
elevated in hepatitis as general indicators of
liver inflammation.
[Stevens 2003, p326]

107 **a**   The immune response to HAV follows
the classic pattern for an antibody response,
with IgM appearing first, followed by a
decline in IgM and appearance of IgG.
[Mahon 2006, p118]

108 **a**   Hepatitis B surface antigen (HBsAg) is
located in the outer envelope of the virus.
[Nester 2001, p610]

109 **d**   Hepatitis Be antigen (HBeAg) is a
soluble component in the core of the
hepatitis B virus.
[Nester 2001, p610]

110 **c**   The hepatitis B core antigen (HBc) is a
protein in the nucleocapsid of HBV.
[Nester 2001, p610]

111 **b**   Double-stranded DNA is present in the
core of the virus.
[Nester 2001, p610]

112 **c**   These structures, which consist entirely
MLS
ONLY of HBsAg, circulate in the serum but are
not infectious since they lack the other viral
components.
[Turgeon 2009, p282]

113 **c**   The ELISA for HBsAg is a sandwich
technique in which HBsAg in patient serum
binds to anti-HBs on a solid phase; the
HBsAg is then detected by the addition of an
anti-HBs labeled with an enzyme.
[Stevens 2003, p328]

114 b   HBeAg is present in patient serum during periods of active HBV replication, and is therefore a marker of high infectivity.
[Stevens 2003, p327]

115 b   Some patients who become infected with HBV do not develop immunity and become long-term carriers of the virus who can transmit the infection to others.
[Turgeon 2009, pp284-285]

116 c   About 85% of persons infected with
MLS
ONLY   HCV will develop a chronic infection, while hepatitis A does not progress to a chronic state.
[Stevens 2003, pp326, 329]

117 c   IgM is the first immunoglobulin to be produced during an immune response, and is produced by infants with congenital infections. IgG in the blood of a newborn infant is primarily of maternal origin, since it can cross the placenta, while IgA would be acquired through mother's breast milk.
[Turgeon 2009, p302]

118 a   In serological assays for rubella, a titer of 1:8 or greater indicates presence of protective antibodies. An acute infection would be indicated by a rise in antibody titer between 2 serum samples collected 2 or more weeks apart, while susceptibility to rubella would be indicated by a negative antibody result.
[Turgeon 2009, pp301-302]

119 c   Prior to collecting serum for the cold
MLS
ONLY   agglutinin test, blood must be warmed; refrigeration would result in the binding of the patient's cold agglutinin antibodies to his/her own red blood cells prior to the collection of serum, resulting in depletion of these antibodies from the serum, and a false-negative result when that serum is incubated with the human type O red blood cells used in the test.
[Miller 1991, pp363-364]

120 c   The only treponemal test listed is the FTA-ABS (fluorescent treponemal antibody absorbed test), while the others are all nontreponemal tests that detect antibody to cardiolipin.
[Stevens 2003, pp298-299]

121 b   It is recommended that the VDRL and RPR tests be performed at a temperature range between 23°C and 29°C; optimal agglutination does not occur at temperatures below that range, resulting in false negative tests.
[Turgeon 2009, pp219-222]

122 a   Nontreponemal tests are used to screen for syphilis and monitor syphilis patients during therapy. These tests, the VDRL and RPR, are based on the principle of flocculation, created by the clumping of the fine cardiolipin particles used in the tests, after binding to patient's antibody.
[Stevens 2003, p298]

123 b   A 4-fold or greater increase in antibody
MLS
ONLY   titer between 2 serum samples taken from the same patient over time indicates a current infection.
[Stevens 2003, p373]

124 a   Patients with recent streptococcal infections produce antibodies to several enzymes produced by Streptococcal bacteria. The antibodies detected most commonly in the laboratory are those directed against streptolysin O or DNase B.
[Stevens 2003, p316]

Protein Analysis

125 c   Biological functions of immunoglobulins; IgG crosses the placenta.
[Stevens 2003, p64]

126 b   Biological functions of immunoglobulins; IgE is the antibody involved in multiple allergies.
[Stevens 2003, p67]

127 b   Biological functions of lymphocytes; B cells make antibody, become plasma cells.
[Stevens 2003, p31]

128 d   Biological functions of immunoglobulins; IgM binds complement well and is hemolytic.
[Stevens 2003, p65]

129 c   Biological functions of immunoglobulins; IgG antibody crosses the placenta and is involved in hemolytic disease of the newborn.
[Stevens 2003, p201]

130 b/c   Babies' IgG comes from their mother, but if they have elevated IgM, an in utero, or neonatal infection is indicated.
[Stevens 2003, p64]

131 c   IgM and IgD are the classes of
MLS
ONLY   immunoglobulin that are found on most circulating B cells. They are in effect the B-cell receptor.
[Stevens 2003, p31]

Answers–Immunology

132 **d** The function of B cells is to produce antibodies.
[Stevens 2003, p29]

133 **a** The area on the immunoglobulin molecule that is the antigen-specific region is the Fab region (this is the amino terminal end). *Fab* stands for *fragment antigen binding*, and indicates a fragment after papain cleavage. The biological function of the immunoglobulin, ie, whether it goes to the placenta, whether it binds complement, and what effector cells it binds, resides in the Fc region, on the carboxy terminal end. The *Fc* stands for *fragment crystallizable*, and indicates the part of the immunoglobulin molecule after papain cleavage that has structural identity, and thus can be crystallized.
[Stevens 2003, ch5 p.61]

134 **b** The immunoglobulin molecule is
MLS ONLY made up of one or more units (# of units depending on heavy chain type) composed of 2 heavy chains and 2 light chains. The light chains can be either the kappa or lambda type. About 65% of the human immunoglobulin molecules have kappa chains and 35% have lambda chains.
[Turgeon 2009, p20]

135 **a** A secretory IgA molecule is composed of 2 units of 2 heavy chains and 2 light chains. These chains are joined by the J chain, and are protected from the harsher environment where there are secreted by an additional chain called the secretory piece.
[Stevens 2003, ch5]

136 **b** Immunoglobulin A (IgA) is the most abundant immunoglobulin in saliva, tears, and other mucosal secretions and plays an important role in mucosal immunity.
[Stevens 2003, p66]

137 **b** The area on the immunoglobulin molecule that is the antigen-specific region is the Fab region (called the amino terminal end). *Fab* stands for *fragment antigen binding*, and indicates a fragment after papain cleavage. The biological function of the immunoglobulin, ie, whether it goes to the placenta, whether it binds complement, and what effector cells it binds, resides in the Fc region, on the carboxy terminal end. The *Fc* stands for *fragment crystallizable*, and indicates the part of the immunoglobulin molecule after papain cleavage that has structural identity, and thus can be crystallized.
[Stevens 2003, p61]

138 **d** Immunoglobulin function; IgE is the immunoglobulin involved with allergy.
[Stevens 2003, p68]

139 **c** Immunoglobulin function; IgM best at agglutination.
[Stevens 2003, p65]

140 **d** Autoimmunity, theories of how
MLS ONLY it develops.
[Stevens 2003, p213]

141 **a** Immunoglobulin deficiency, patients
MLS ONLY with IgA deficiency can have an anaphylactic reaction during transfusions.
[Stevens 2003, p251]

142 **c** Immunoglobulin subclasses differ from each other in their Fc regions; this is the reason that the different classes have different biological function. The Fc region is the region that is crystallizable after papain cleavage. It varies in sequence in the different classes of immunoglobulin.
[Stevens 2003, pp61-62]

143 **b** The diversity sequence of the variable
MLS ONLY region, which is expressed as many idiotypic differences, is what allows so many different antigens to be bound by antibody. This huge diversity in the variable region develops due to VDJ recombinant events for the heavy chain and VJ recombinant events for the light chain.
[Stevens 2003, p69]

144 **c** Immunoglobulin deficiency, IgA
MLS ONLY deficiency is related to autoimmune diseases.
[Stevens 2003, ch16 p251]

145 a The main function of IgD is in B cell
MLS
ONLY development; it is the class of surface
immunoglobulin on immature B cells.
[Stevens 2003, p31]

146 d Immunoglobulin structure; IgM is
a pentamer.
[Stevens 2003, p65]

147 b IgG highest in concentration in
normal sera.
[Stevens 2003, p64]

148 c Immunoglobulin structure; IgA is in
serum and secretions.
[Stevens 2003, p66]

149 c IgD and surface IgM are anchored in the
MLS
ONLY B cell membrane; in order to be anchored
in the membrane, they must contain a
hydrophobic region. The hydrophobic region
is about 26 residues long.
[Stevens 2003, p64]

150 b Immunoglobulin structure, hinge is
MLS
ONLY between CH1 and CH2.
[Stevens 2003, p62]

151 c Immunoglobulin structure, idiotype is
in variable regions of heavy and light chains.
[Stevens 2003, p62]

152 d Immunoglobulin allotype is in constant
regions of heavy and light chains.
[Stevens 2003, p62]

153 a Immunoglobulin IgG subclass function,
IgG1 goes through placenta best.
[Stevens 2003, p63]

154 a Immunoglobulin structure, J chain
associated with IgA.
[Stevens 2003, p66]

155 d Complement, the membrane attack unit
MLS
ONLY begins with C5.
[Stevens 2003, p96]

156 a Macrophages have surface receptors
MLS
ONLY for C3b.
[Stevens 2003, p96]

157 a Macrophage phagocytosis enhanced
by opsonins.
[Stevens 2003, p13]

158 c Haptens initiate the alternative pathway
of complement.
[Stevens 2003, p97]

159 b C3 breaks down to a small C3a, which
floats away and is an anaphylatoxin, and the
larger C3b, which lands on the target surface
and becomes part of C5 convertase, is also a
powerful opsonin.
[Stevens 2003, p94]

160 a C3 breaks down to a small C3a, which
floats away and is an anaphylatoxin, and the
larger C3b, which lands on the target surface
and becomes part of C5 convertase, is also a
powerful opsonin.
[Stevens 2003, p96]

161 d Biological functions of
immunoglobulins, IgE mediates
immediate type hypersensitivity seen in
penicillin allergy.
[Stevens 2003, p68]

162 a Complement C1q is the recognition
piece.
[Stevens 2003, p94]

163 c In immunoelectrophoresis, first the
serum is separated in an agarose gel by
electrophoresis, then in a trough that is cut
parallel to the plane of the electrophoresis,
antiserum is placed. The antibody diffuses
toward the serum proteins and arcs of
antibody antigen precipitation occur.
[Stevens 2003, p95]

164 d Complement, C5 - C9, is the membrane
attack unit.
[Stevens 2003, p6]

165 a C3a, C4a and C5a are anaphylatoxins
and cause release of histamine from
basophils and mast cells.
[Stevens 2003, ch7]

166 b Complement, C3 can be measured
MLS
ONLY by RID.
[Stevens 2003, ch7]

167 a Complement, definition of the
MLS
ONLY CH50 reaction.
[Stevens 2003, ch7]

168 d Babies' IgG comes from their mother,
but if they have elevated IgM, an in utero, or
neonatal infection is indicated.
[Stevens 2003, ch5]

169 b Definition of Bence Jones protein.
[Stevens 2003, ch15]

170 **d** An radioimmunodiffusion assay
MLS measures the precipitin reaction of an
ONLY antibody with an antigen. Normally the
antibody in the gel reacts with an antigen
diffusing from a well. If, however, the
patient has an antibody to a protein in the
antiserum, then the ring of precipitation
that is measured can be the patient's
immunoglobulin diffusing out of the well,
and reacting with a serum antigen.
[Stevens 2003]

171 **c** A gamma-specific antibody would react
MLS only to the gamma heavy chain, not to the
ONLY light chains or it would react with all classes
of antibody. Monoclonal antibodies will
usually say monoclonal in their name, and
these are usually of mouse origin. Although
rat monoclonal and rabbit monoclonal
antibodies have been made, these are rarely
used.
[Stevens 2003, p11]

172 **c** B cells make humoral antibodies.
[Stevens 2003, p31]

173 **d** IgA and IgE do not initiate the classical
pathway of complement but can initiate
the alternative pathway.
[Stevens 2003, ch7]

174 **c** Classical complement pathway:
C1 is activated by binding 2 Fcs of
immunoglobulin, then C4 is split to C4a
and C4b; C4b binds, and next C2 is bound
and cleaved; this forms C3 convertase, so
C3 binds and is cleaved; C3b stays bound;
C3a floats away; C5 next is split and C5b
binds and C5a floats away. C6, C7, C8, and
C9 bind sequentially and cause a hole in
the membrane.
[Stevens 2003, ch7]

175 **c** Classical complement pathway
(see answer 174); alternative pathway: C3+
Factor B→ iC3B + Factor D and Mg++→
C3Bb or C3bBb; this is stabilized by
properdin to make C3bBbC3bP, which is a C5
convertase, and C5 is split to C5a and C5b,
and next C6, C7, C8 and C9 are activated
and form a hole in the cell.
[Stevens 2003, ch7]

176 **c** C5a is both chemotactic and
MLS an anaphylatoxin.
ONLY
[Stevens 2003, ch7]

177 **c** C3 is a very powerful amplifying step
MLS of the classical and alterative pathways and
ONLY also forms a powerful opsinogen. Thus it
must be subject to controls, and one such
control is that it can be broken down to C3c
and C3d.
[Stevens 2003, ch7]

178 **b** Conversion of C4 to C4a + C4b is an
MLS amplifying step with 30 molecules of C4
ONLY for every molecule of C1; C3 conversion
is a large amplifying step with about
200 molecules converted for every C3
convertase. These extra molecules can bind
to the cell surface.
[Stevens 2003, ch7]

179 **b** Indirect labeled assays can be designed
MLS to utilize class specific anti-human
ONLY immunoglobulin, that is IgM specific.
[Stevens 2003, p11]

180 **b** Patients that have received mouse
MLS monoclonal antibody therapy may have a
ONLY false-postive when tested with a sandwich
assay due to the mouse monoclonal IgM
utilized in the assay to test for a hepatitis
B surface antigen.
[Abbott 2008]

181 **d** Multiple myeloma shows a monoclonal
MLS IgG spike in serum protein electrophoresis
ONLY and light chains in the urine called Bence
Jones protein. In addition, the tumor cells
can grow in the bone forming round lesions
that are very painful.
[Stevens 2003, p15]

182 **b** Waldenström macroglobulinemia
MLS is a monoclonal gammopathy in which
ONLY the tumor cells are making IgM. The
uncontrolled secretion of such a high
molecule weight compound causes a severe
increase in viscosity.
[Stevens 2003, p15]

183 **c** Waldenström macroglobulinemia
MLS is a monoclonal gammopathy in which
ONLY the tumor cells are making IgM. The
uncontrolled secretion of such a high
molecule weight compound causes a severe
increase in viscosity.
[Stevens 2003, p15]

184 **c** Selective IgA deficiency is the most
MLS common immunodeficiency.
ONLY
[Stevens 2003, p15]

185 **c** Bruton agammaglobulinemia is an
MLS
ONLY X-linked disease (therefore, usually found
in males) in which there is a decreased
immunoglobulin concentration, which
becomes apparent at 2-6 months of age, ie,
after the infant's maternally-transferred
immunoglobulin has decreased due
to its biological half-life. Problem is in
differentiation at the pre-B cell stage.
[Stevens 2003, p15]

186 **d** Wiskott-Aldrich syndrome is
MLS
ONLY an X-linked recessive defect that
exhibits immunodeficiency, eczema
and thrombocytopenia.
[Stevens 2003, p15]

187 **b** Swiss-type agammaglobulinemia is a
MLS
ONLY type of severe combined immunodeficiency
disease (SCID) that is autosomal recessive.
[Stevens 2003, p15]

188 **b** Monoclonal antibodies are produced
MLS
ONLY by cells that are a fused hybrid of a mouse
spleen cell with a mouse myeloma cell. The
spleen cell confers the antibody specificity,
and the tumor cells give it the ability to
keep reproducing.
[Stevens 2003, pp70-72]

189 **b** C5a is a chemotaxin for neutrophils,
basophils, mast cells and monocytes.
[Stevens 2003, p102]

190 **b** C1 esterase inhibitor is associated with
hereditary angioedema.
[Stevens 2003, p104]

191 **d** C3 deficiency is the worst deficiency
to have; it causes a lifelong history of
life-threatening infections.
[Stevens 2003, p104]

192 **c** C1, C4, C2 deficiencies are associated
with a lupus erythematosus-like syndrome.
[Stevens 2003, p104]

193 **d** C5, C6, C7, C8 deficiencies associated
with a worse *Neisseria* infection if
the patient is exposed due to less
pathogen clearance.
[Stevens 2003, ch7 p104]

194 **c** C2 deficiency is associated with a lupus
like syndrome.
[Stevens 2003, p104]

195 **a** X-linked infantile agammaglobulinemia
MLS
ONLY is Bruton agammaglobulinemia; DiGeorge
syndrome is a T-cell deficiency; Swiss-type
is a SCID; ataxia has additional muscular
coordination problems.
[Stevens 2003, p251]

196 **c** X-linked infantile agammaglobulinemia
MLS
ONLY is Bruton agammaglobulinemia; DiGeorge
syndrome is a T-cell deficiency; Swiss-type
is a SCID; ataxia has additional muscular
coordination problems.
[Stevens 2003, p255]

197 **a** Immediate hypersensitivity is tested by
MLS
ONLY skin tests with edema and erythema, which
also can be called wheal and flare.
[Stevens 2003, p198]

198 **a** Immediate hypersensitivity is involved
in bronchial asthma.
[Stevens 2003, p197]

199 **d** Antihistamines block histamine binding
to histamine receptors.
[Stevens 2003, p197]

200 **c** RAST tests for allergen specific IgE.
MLS
ONLY [Stevens 2003, p199]

201 **c** IgE is in too low a concentration
for precipitation; therefore it cannot be
detected by this method.
[Stevens 2003, p133]

Cellular Immunity and Histocompatibility Techniques

202 **a** Skin tests are used to determine
whether the delayed type hypersensitivity
response mediated by T cells is functioning
properly. All other tests listed evaluate
humoral antibody responses.
[Stevens 2003, pp256-257]

203 **b** While T cells help B cells in the process
of antibody production, they are not capable
of secreting immunoglobulins themselves.
Immunoglobulins are produced only by
B cells and plasma cells.
[Turgeon 2009, p55]

204 **c** Phagocytosis is mediated by
macrophages and neutrophils, not
by lymphocytes.
[Turgeon 2009, p31]

205 **c** Natural killer cells do not specifically
bind to tumor antigens, as do T lymphocytes
and antibodies, and can kill tumor cells
without having had prior exposure to them.
[Stevens 2003, pp35-36]

206 **a**   Immunoassays that employ monoclonal antibody reagents are commonly used to quantify circulating tumor antigens because they are highly sensitive and specific.
[Bishop 2005, p609]

207 **b**   Antibodies are important in defense against bacterial infections. Patients with B-cell deficiencies are unable to produce adequate amounts of antibodies, and therefore exhibit increased bacterial infections. Also, B cells are not phagocytic and do not produce complement.
[Stevens 2003, p249]

208 **b**   T cells and cell-mediated immunity are important in defense against intracellular pathogens such as viruses, fungi, and parasites. Patients with T-cell deficiencies will therefore exhibit increased parasitic infections.
[Stevens 2003, p249]

209 **b**   The tissue damage resulting from type III hypersensitivity is caused by the deposition of immune complexes, which recruit neutrophils to the tissues. The neutrophils release their lysosomal enzymes, resulting in inflammation and damage to the surrounding tissues.
[Mahon 2006, pp95-96]

210 **d**   While B cells are involved in humoral immunity through the production of antibodies, T cells mediate their responses through the release of soluble proteins called cytokines.
[Turgeon 2009, p63]

211 **a**   Multiparous women, or those having
MLS
ONLY
multiple children, frequently produce antibodies to fetal HLA antigens, which are of paternal origin. The serum from these women has therefore been used as a source for the HLA antibodies that are employed in the complement-dependent cytotoxicity test to type HLA antigens.
[Mahon 2006, p279]

212 **c**   By definition, an allograft is a graft between genetically unidentical individuals of the same species. An isograft is between genetically identical individuals, a xenograft is between individuals of different species, and an autograft is transplanted from 1 location to another in the same individual.
[Turgeon 2009, p432]

213 **d**   ABO incompatibility results in
MLS
ONLY
hyperacute rejection. This reaction is mediated by anti-A or anti-B antibodies that naturally occur in individuals who lack the corresponding A or B antigen.
[Stevens 2003, p265]

214 **c**   The theory of molecular mimicry states
MLS
ONLY
that antibodies produced against foreign antigens, such as certain microorganisms, can cross-react with self antigens to produce autoimmunity. All the other answers are incorrect because they would result in a decreased immune response.
[Turgeon 2009, pp367-368]

215 **c**   Receptors for the C3b component
MLS
ONLY
of complement and for the Fc portion of immunoglobulin are found both on B cells and on monocytes, and are thought to play a role in the clearance of immune complexes.
[Turgeon 2009, p34]

216 **c**   Cytotoxic T cells, which are capable of destroying targets such as tumor cells and virus-infected cells, bear the CD8 surface marker, while the other cell types listed are positive for the CD4 surface marker.
[Stevens 2003, p34]

217 **a**   Contact dermatitis is a delayed type hypersensitivity reaction due to T-cell responses to environmental chemicals or metals. The other conditions are examples of other types of hypersensitivity.
[Mahon 2006, pp.96-98]

218 **b**   Anaphylactic, or type I hypersensitivity, occurs very rapidly, usually within 30 minutes after antigen exposure. While transfusion reactions and serum sickness are also examples of immediate hypersensitivity, they generally do not occur as rapidly. Contact dermatitis is a delayed hypersensitivity reaction, manifesting between 24 and 72 hours after antigen exposure.
[Mahon 2006, pp89-91]

219 **a**   Normal peripheral blood should contain
MLS
ONLY
approximately 80% T lymphocytes and 20% B lymphocytes.
[Turgeon 2009, p52]

220 **a**   CD3 is a marker used to identify T lymphocytes. It is present on the surface of all mature T-cells, regardless of T-cell subset.
[Mahon 2006, p26]

221 **d** About 70%-85% of peripheral blood
MLS ONLY lymphocytes should be T cells. The value for the normal control is therefore too low, and the test should be repeated with a fresh control sample before patient results can be interpreted.
[Turgeon 2009, p55]

222 **a** The absolute number of B lymphocytes
MLS ONLY would be calculated by multiplying the absolute white blood cell count by the percentage of total lymphocytes to get the total leukocyte count; then multiplying the total leukocyte count by the percentage of B lymphocytes. $8,930 \times 0.30 \times 0.40 = 1,072$.
[Turgeon 2009, p65]

223 **a** Lymphocytes can be obtained by
MLS ONLY density gradient centrifugation with Ficoll-Hypaque. Following centrifugation, the lymphocytes can be found in the layer of mononuclear cells that overlays the layer of Ficoll-Hypaque.
[Stevens 2003, p37]

224 **c** In flow cytometry, a laser beam hits cells as they pass through the instrument in single file. The amount of light scatter is measured from each cell at 2 different angles, and is used to identify the cell type on the basis of size and granularity. Cells are also identified on their ability to emit fluorescence after they have been incubated with fluorescent-labeled monoclonal antibodies that bind to specific surface markers.
[Stevens 2003, p38]

225 **c** A decrease in the number of T helper (CD4+) cells and a decrease in the ratio of CD4+:CD8+ cells is a characteristic finding of HIV infection and AIDS.
[Stevens 2003, p354]

226 **b** The total number of T cells is calculated
MLS ONLY by multiplying the total WBC ($10 \times 10^3/\mu$L) by the percent of lymphocytes (25%, or 0.25) and the percent of T cells (40%, or 0.40). The answer for this calculation is 1×10^3 or 1,000.
[Turgeon 2009, p65]

227 **b** A normal individual would have
MLS ONLY approximately 63%-84% T cells. With the values given in this example, the absolute T cell number would range from 2.52×10^3 (2,520; calculated by multiplying the total leukocyte count (10×10^3) by the % of lymphocytes (40% or 0.40), and by the lower limit of the % of T cells (63%) to 3.36×10^3 (3,360; calculated by multiplying the total leukocyte count (10×10^3) by the % of lymphocytes (40% or 0.40), and by the upper limit of the % of T cells (84%). With a % recovery of 85%-95%, values would range between 2,142 ($2,520 \times 0.85$) and 3,192 ($3,360 \times 0.95$).
[Turgeon 2009, p61, 65]

228 **d** Laser flow cytometry is the underlying
MLS ONLY principle of cell sorting into subpopulations.
[Turgeon 2009, p174]

229 **c** Flow cytometry uses fluorescent-labeled monoclonal antibodies to identify cells of interest by binding to specific components within or on the surface of the cells.
[Turgeon 2009, p173]

230 **b** The total number of lymphocytes can be calculated by multiplying the WBC (5×10^3, or 5,000) by the % of lymphocytes (15% or 0.15) to get 750. This number is then multiplied by the % of CD4+ cells (8% or 0.08) to get an absolute CD4 cell count of 60.
[Stevens 2003, pp354-355]

231 **c** The patient's percent of CD4+ cells (8%) is well below the normal range of 50%-60%, and the patient's absolute number of CD4+ cells ($5,000 \times 0.15 \times 0.08 = 60$) is also far below the normal range of 500-1,300 cells/μL peripheral blood. These findings are consistent with AIDS, which is caused by HIV.
[Stevens 2003, pp354-355]

232 **b** Mis-matches in HLA antigens between
MLS ONLY a donor and recipient of a bone marrow transplant can lead to graft-vs-host disease, in which T lymphocytes in the bone marrow graft mount an immune response against the foreign histocompatibility antigens of the immunocompromised recipient.
[Stevens 2003, pp266, 270]

233 **c** More than 95% of patients with
MLS ONLY ankylosing spondylitis are positive for theHLA-B27 antigen; therefore, a positive result for this test would support the diagnosis.
[Mahon 2006, p181]

234 **d** Hairy cell leukemia cells have surface
MLS ONLY markers such as CD19 and CD20, which
are characteristic of B cells, and other
markers, such as CD11c, which are found
on monocytes. They also stain positive for
tartrate resistant acid phosphatase, which is
found in osteoclasts and macrophages.
[McKenzie 2004, p591]

235 **c** Sézary cells are cells that have the helper
MLS ONLY T cell phenotype (CD3+, CD4+).
[McKenzie 2004, p592]

236 **a** CD2 and CD3 are T-cell markers, while
surface immunoglobulin is a B-cell marker.
[Stevens 2003, pp29, 30]

237 **b** HLA-B27 is associated with ankylosing
MLS ONLY spondylitis. There is a 50% chance that
the mother will transmit her B27 allele to
her children.
[Mahon 2006, pp172, 181]

238 **c** Individuals who are HLA-B8+ have a
MLS ONLY 5× greater risk than HLA B8– persons of
developing myasthenia gravis, and a 9×
greater risk of developing celiac disease over
a lifetime.
[Turgeon 2009, p429]

239 **a** TdT is an enzyme that adds nucleotides
MLS ONLY onto the 3′ end of a DNA molecule. It is
present in immature T cells and B cells, and
is used to differentiate ALL from mature
B-cell malignancies.
[McKenzie 2004, p491]

Microbiology

The following items have been identified generally as appropriate for both entry level medical laboratory scientists and medical laboratory technicians. Items that are appropriate for medical laboratory scientists **only** are marked with an "MLS ONLY."

Preanalytical and Susceptibility Testing

1. Proper media for culture of a urethral discharge from a man include:
       (PEA – isolates staph / inhibits gram negs, particularly proteus)
   a sheep blood and phenylethyl alcohol agars
   b eosin-methylene blue and sheep blood agars   *chocolate*
   c thioglycollate broth and chocolate agar
   d chocolate and modified Thayer-Martin agars
       (chocolate for Neisseria)

2. A sheep blood agar plate inoculated with 0.001 mL of urine grows 70 colonies of *Staphylococcus aureus*. How many colony forming units per mL of urine should be reported?

   a   70
   b   700
   c 7,000
   d 70,000

3. The lowest concentration of antibiotic that inhibits growth of a test organism is the:

   a minimum inhibitory concentration
   b serum inhibitory concentration
   c minimum bactericidal titer
   d maximum inhibitory titer

4. Which of the following clean catch urine culture colony counts indicates the patient likely has a urinary tract infection?

   a 10^1 CFU/mL
   b 10^3 CFU/mL ✳
   c 10^5 CFU/mL
   d no growth

5   The steam autoclave method of sterilization:

    ⓐ uses 15 lbs of pressure for 15 minutes   *121°C for 15 minutes*
    b utilizes dry heat for 20 minutes   *with 15 lbs pressure*
    c produces a maximum temperature of 100°C
    d requires a source of ethylene oxide

6   The expected colony count in a <u>suprapubic</u> urine from a healthy individual is:

    ⓐ   0 CFU/mL
    b   100 CFU/mL
    c   1,000 CFU/mL
    d 100,000 CFU/mL

7   An aspirate of a deep wound was plated on blood agar plates and incubated aerobically and anaerobically. At 24 hours there was growth on both plates. This indicates that the organism is a(n):

    a nonfermenter
    b obligate anaerobe
    c aerobe
    ⓓ facultative anaerobe

8̸   The proper blood-to-broth ratio for blood cultures to reduce the antibacterial effect of serum in
MLS ONLY   adults is:

    a 1:2
    b 1:3
    c 1:10
    d 1:30

⑨   A penicillin-resistant *Neisseria gonorrhoeae* produces:

    a alpha-hemolysin
    ⓑ beta-lactamase
    c enterotoxin
    d coagulase

⑩   Which selective medium is used for the isolation of gram-positive microorganisms?

    ⓐ Columbia CNA with 5% sheep blood
    b trypticase soy agar with 5% sheep blood – *enriched media*
    c eosin methylene blue – *inhibits gram pos*
    d modified Thayer-Martin – *chocolate with antibiotics to isolate Neisseria*
       vanco → gram positives   colistin → gram ⊖
       nystatin → yeast   enterics

11   The **most** sensitive <u>substrate</u> for the detection of beta-lactamases is:

    a penicillin
    b ampicillin
    c cefoxitin
    ⓓ nitrocefin

~~12~~
MLS
ONLY
A *Staphylococcus aureus* isolate has an MIC of 4 µg/mL to oxacillin. There is uncertainty as to whether this represents an oxacillin (heteroresistant) resistant strain or a hyperproducer of beta-lactamase.

Strain	Oxacillin	Amoxicillin-clavulanic acid
strain A	susceptible	susceptible
strain B	susceptible	resistant
strain C	resistant	susceptible
strain D	resistant	resistant

Based on the above results for oxacillin and amoxicillin-clavulanic acid, which strain is **heteroresistant**?

a strain A
b strain B
c strain C
d strain D   *→ aminoglycoside resistance*

(13) An *Enterococcus* isolated from multiple blood cultures in a patient endocarditis should be:

   ~~a~~ screened for high level aminoglycoside resistance *Enterococcus: treated w/*
   b checked for tolerance   *aminoglycoside + penicillin*
   c assayed for serum antimicrobial activity   *together   (cellwall agent*
  – **d** tested for beta-lactamase production

(14) In the Kirby-Bauer disc diffusion susceptibility test, which variable is critical when testing *Pseudomonas* species for antibiotic susceptibility to aminoglycosides?

   a incubation temperature
   b duration of incubation
   ⓒ cation content of media *(calcium, mg) ↑ -too small zone; ↓ -too large zone*
   d depth of agar

(15) The procedure that assures the **most** accurate detection of mecA-mediated oxacillin resistance in routine broth microdilution susceptibility testing against *S aureus* is:

   a addition of 4% NaCl   *(2% NaCl, 37° incubation for 24 hours)*
   b incubation at 30°C
   c incubation for 48 hours
   ⓓ use of cefoxitin for testing *→ > 4 µg/mL = oxacillin resistant*

16 When performing a stool culture, a colony type typical of an enteric pathogen is subcultured on a blood agar plate. The resulting pure culture is screened with several tests to obtain the following results:

TSI:	acid butt, alkaline slant, no gas, no H_2S
phenylalanine deaminase:	negative
motility:	positive
serological typing:	*Shigella flexneri* (*Shigella* subgroup B)

The serological typing is verified with new kit and controls. The best course of action would be to:

   a report the organism as *Shigella flexneri* without further testing
 –ⓑ verify reactivity of motility medium with positive and negative controls
   c verify reactivity of the TSI slants with positive and negative controls for H_2S production
   d verify reactivity of phenylalanine deaminase with positive and negative controls

17   Susceptibility testing performed on quality control organisms using a new media lot number yielded zone sizes that were too large for all antibiotics tested. The testing was repeated using media from a previously used lot number, and all zone sizes were acceptable. Which of the following best explains the unacceptable zone sizes?

     a   the antibiotic disks were not stored with the proper desiccant
     b   the depth of the media was too thick
     c   the depth of the media was too thin
     d   the antibiotic disks were not properly applied to the media

18   Three sets of blood cultures were obtained from an adult patient with fever and suspected endocarditis. The aerobic bottle of one set had growth of *Staphylococcus epidermidis* at 5 days of incubation. This indicates that:

     a   there was low-grade bacteremia
     b   the organism is **most** likely a contaminant
     c   the patient has a line infection
     d   the blood culture bottles are defective

19   In order to isolate *Campylobacter coli/jejuni,* the fecal specimen should be:
         microaerophellic / 42°

     a   inoculated onto selective plating media and incubated in reduced oxygen with added CO_2 at 42°C
     b   stored in tryptic soy broth before plating to ensure growth of the organism
     c   inoculated onto selective plating media and incubated at both 35°C and at room temperature
     d   incubated at 35°C for 2 hours in Cary-Blair media before inoculating onto selective plating media

20   An expectorated sputum is sent to the laboratory for culture from a patient with respiratory distress. The Gram stain of the specimen shows many squamous epithelial cells (>25/lpf) and rare neutrophils. The microscopic appearance of the organisms present include:

        moderate gram-positive cocci in chains and diplococci
        moderate gram-negative diplococci
        moderate palisading gram-positive bacilli all in moderate amounts

   This Gram stain is **most** indicative of:

     a   a pneumococcal pneumonia
     b   an anaerobic infection
     c   an *Haemophilus* pneumonia
     d   oropharyngeal flora

21   Which type of microscope would be **most** useful in examining viruses and the structure of microbial cells?

     a   electron – *viruses cannot be seen using light source; too small*
     b   phase-contrast
     c   dark-field
     d   bright-field

22   After satisfactory performance of daily disk diffusion susceptibility quality control is documented, the frequency of quality control can be reduced to:

     a   twice a week
     b   every week
     c   every other week
     d   every month

23   In disk diffusion susceptibility testing, as an antimicrobial agent diffuses away from the disk, the concentration of antibiotic is:

    a increased
    b decreased
    c unchanged
    d inoculum dependent

24   The **most** common cause for failure of a GasPak™ anaerobic jar to establish an adequate environment for anaerobic incubation is:

    a the failure of the oxidation-reduction potential indicator system due to deterioration of methylene blue
    b the failure of the packet to generate adequate H_2 and/or CO_2
    c condensation of water on the inner surface of the jar
    d catalysts that have become inactivated after repeated use

2 most common causes: ① defective jar seal ② inactivated catalyst pellets

25   (MLS ONLY) Which of the following is the **most** appropriate method for collecting a urine specimen from a patient with an indwelling catheter?

    a remove the catheter, cut the tip, and submit it for culture
    b disconnect the catheter from the bag, and collect urine from the terminal end of the catheter
    c collect urine directly from the bag
    d aspirate urine aseptically from the catheter tubing

26   Which one of the following specimen requests is acceptable?

    a feces submitted for anaerobic culture
    b Foley catheter tip submitted for aerobic culture *– contaminated with colonizing organisms*
    c rectal swab submitted for direct smear for gonococci
    d urine for culture of acid-fast bacilli *– renal tuberculosis*

27   Which of the following groups of specimens would be acceptable for anaerobic culture?

    a vaginal, eye
    b ear, leg tissue
    c pleural fluid, brain abscess
    d urine, sputum

28   A liquid fecal specimen from a three-month-old infant is submitted for microbiological examination. In addition to culture on routine media for *Salmonella* and *Shigella*, this specimen should be routinely:

    a examined for the presence of *Entamoeba hartmanni* *– non-pathogenic parasite*
    b examined for the presence of *Campylobacter* sp *– most common pathogen for diarrhea*
    c screened for the detection of enterotoxigenic *Escherichia coli*
    d placed in thioglycollate broth to detect *Clostridium botulinum*

29   Cerebrospinal fluid from a febrile 25-year-old man with possible meningitis is rushed to the laboratory for a stat Gram stain and culture. While performing the Gram stain, the technologist accidentally spills **most** of the specimen. The smear shows many neutrophils and no microorganisms. Since there is only enough CSF to inoculate one plate, the technologist should use a:

    a blood agar plate
    b chopped meat glucose *(Clostridium)*
    c chocolate agar plate *– doesn't inhibit growth; provides factors for Neisseria and Haemophilus*
    d Thayer-Martin plate *(Neisseria)*

30. A diabetic foot swab from a 82-year-old woman with recurrent infections is submitted for culture. The Gram stain reveals:

    > many neutrophils, no squamous epithelial cells
    > many gram-negative bacilli
    > many gram-positive cocci in chains

    The physician requests that all pathogens be worked up. In addition to the sheep blood and MacConkey agar plates routinely used for wound cultures, the technologist might also process a(n):

    a CNA agar plate – *gram pos*
    b chocolate agar plate
    c XLD agar plate – *enterics*
    d chopped meat glucose – *clostridium* *clostridium*

31. Which of the following is the **most** appropriate specimen source and primary media battery?

    a endocervical-chocolate, Martin Lewis
    b sputum-sheep blood, Thayer-Martin, KV-laked blood (*blood + Mac*)
    c CSF-Columbia CNA, MacConkey (*blood + choc*)
    d urine-sheep blood, chocolate, Columbia CNA (*blood + Mac*)

32. Which of the following is the **most** appropriate organism and media combination?

    a *Legionella* species—Regan Lowe (*Bordetella*)
    b *Clostridium difficile*—phenylethyl alcohol (PEA) – *gram ⊕*
    c *Campylobacter* species—charcoal yeast extract
    d *Yersinia enterocolitica*—cefsulodin-irgasan-novobiocin (CIN) – *Yersinia*

33. A Gram stain from a swab of a hand wound reveals:

    > moderate neutrophils
    > no squamous epithelial cells
    > – moderate gram-positive cocci in chains
    > – moderate large gram-negative bacilli

    Select the appropriate media that will selectively isolate each organism.
    (aerobic)   *(Neisseria)*
    a KV-laked agar, Thayer-Martin
    b sheep blood, MacConkey
    c Columbia CNA, chocolate
    d Columbia CNA, MacConkey
        (gram +)   *(gram –)*

34. Upon review of a sputum Gram stain, the technician notes that the nuclei of all of the neutrophils present in the smear are staining dark blue. The best explanation for this finding is:

    a the slide was inadequately decolorized with acetone/alcohol
    b the sputum smear was prepared too thin
    c the cellular components have stained as expected
    d the iodine was omitted from the staining procedure

35. When performing a Kovac indole test, the substrate must contain:

    a indole
    b tryptophan
    c ornithine
    d paradimethylaminobenzaldehyde

36. The ONPG test allows organisms to be classified as a lactose fermenter by testing for which of the following?

    a permease
    b beta-galactosidase
    c beta-lactamase
    d phosphatase

37 Sodium bicarbonate and sodium citrate are components of which of the following?

a JEMBEC system
b MTM agar
c NYC medium
d ML agar

38 Chocolate agar base containing vancomycin, colistin, anisomycin, and trimethoprim is also known as:

a EMB agar
b modified Thayer-Martin agar
c Columbia CNA agar
d Martin Lewis agar

39 A medium that aids in the presumptive identification of organisms based on their appearance on the medium is called:

a enriched
b selective
c differential
d specialized

40 SPS is used as an anticoagulant for blood cultures because it:

a inactivates penicillin and cephalosporins
b prevents clumping of red cells
c inactivates neutrophils and components of serum complement
d facilitates growth of anaerobes

41 When evaluating a new susceptibility testing system, if the new system characterizes a susceptible isolate as resistant, this is termed a:

a very major error
b major error
c minor error
d acceptable error

42 Which of the following methods is inadequate for the detection of vancomycin-<u>intermediate</u> *S aureus*?

a broth macrodilution
b agar dilution
c gradient diffusion
d disk diffusion

43 In a disk diffusion susceptibility test, which of the following can result if disks are placed on the inoculated media and left at room temperature for an hour before incubation?

— **a** the antibiotic would not diffuse into the medium, resulting in no zone
— **b** zones of smaller diameter would result
—**c** zones of larger diameter would result
+ **d** there would be no effect on the final zone diameter

* delay of >15 minutes will cause excess prediffusion → larger zones

44 Which of the following factors would make an organism appear to be more resistant on a disk diffusion susceptibility test?

a too little agar in the plate
— **b** too many organisms in the inoculum
c the presence of 0.5% NaCl in the medium
d a medium with a pH of 7.4

(45) First-generation cephalosporins can be adequately represented by:

*
    a cefotetan
    b ceftriaxone   *cephalothin → cefotetan + cefoxitin → ceftriaxone*   (1st) (2nd)
    c cephalothin
    d cefoxitin

(46) An antibiotic that inhibits cell wall synthesis is:

*
    a chloramphenicol – *protein*
    b penicillin – *cell wall*
    c sulfamethoxazole – *folic acid*
    d colistin – *↑ cell wall permability permeability*

(47) Which one of the following organisms does not require susceptibility testing to the antimicrobial indicated when isolated from a clinically significant source?

*
    a *Staphylococcus aureus*-clindamycin
    b *Proteus mirabilis*-gentamicin   *no resistance to penicillin*
    c *Streptococcus pyogenes*-penicillin   *by strep*
    d *Escherichia coli*-levofloxacin

(48) Which of the following antibiotics would routinely be tested and reported for isolates of *Pseudomonas aeruginosa*?

*
    a penicillin
    b erythromycin   *Pseudomonas = gent*
    c clindamycin
    d gentamicin

49 Which of the following must be incubated in a microaerophilic environment for optimal recovery of the organism?

    a *Campylobacter jejuni*
    b *Escherichia coli* – FA
    c *Pseudomonas aeruginosa* – *aerobe*
    d *Proteus mirabilis* – FA

50   Diagnosis of typhoid fever can be confirmed best by culture of :
MLS
ONLY
    a stool
    b urine
    c blood
    d bone marrow

51   *Vibrio parahaemolyticus* can be isolated best from feces on:

    a eosin methylene blue (EMB) agar – *gram neg enterics*
    b Hektoen enteric (HE) agar – *Salmonella/Shigella*
    c Salmonella Shigella (SS) agar –
    d thiosulfate citrate bile salts (TCBS) agar – *Vibrio sp.*

(52) Which of the following media can be used to culture *Campylobacter jejuni*?

    a Skirrow medium – *campy*
    b CIN agar – *Yersinia*
    c anaerobic CNA agar – *gram ⊕*
    d bismuth sulfite – *Salmonella*

(53) Tests for beta-lactamase production in *Haemophilus influenzae*:

*
    a are not commercially available   *20 – 40% beta-lactamase producers*
    b include tests that measure a change to an alkaline pH   *perform cephalosporin test*
    c should be performed on all blood and CSF isolates
    d are not valid for any other bacterial species

54 Media used to support growth of *Legionella pneumophila* should contain which of the following additives?

   a X and V factors
   b hemin and Vitamin K
   c charcoal and yeast extract *— specific for Legionella*
   d dextrose and laked blood

55 The best medium for culture of *Bordetella pertussis* is:

   a Regan-Lowe agar
   b cystine blood agar
   c Martin Lewis agar
   d Ashdown agar

56 The best medium for culture of *Francisella tularensis* is:

   a Bordet-Gengou medium *- Bord*
   b cystine glucose blood agar : *cystine required for Francisella growth*
   c Loeffler medium *- C. diphtheriae*
   d charcoal selective medium

57
MLS
ONLY
The **most** rapid method for detection of *Francisella tularensis* is:

   a serological slide agglutination utilizing specific antiserum
   b dye stained clinical specimens
   c fluorescent antibody staining techniques on clinical specimens
   d polymerase chain reaction

58 When processing throat swabs for a group A *Streptococcus* culture, the medium of choice is:

   a sheep blood agar *- clear cut hemolysis*
   b rabbit blood agar
   c human blood agar
   d horse blood agar

59 The ability to detect oxacillin-resistant *Staphylococcus aureus* may be enhanced by:

   a shortening incubation of standard susceptibility plates
   b incubating susceptibility plates at 39°-41°C
   c using Mueller-Hinton broth with 2% NaCl
   d adjusting inoculum to 0.1 McFarland before inoculating susceptibility plates

60 The optimal wound specimen for culture of anaerobic organisms should be:

   a a swab of lesion obtained before administration of antibiotics
   b a swab of lesion obtained after administration of antibiotics
   c a syringe filled with pus, obtained before administration of antibiotics
   d a syringe filled with pus, obtained after administration of antibiotics

61 A 21-year-old patient presents with pharyngitis. A throat swab is collected and submitted for anaerobic culture. This specimen should be:

   a set up immediately
   b rejected as unacceptable
   c inoculated into thioglycollate broth
   d sent to a reference laboratory

62
MLS
ONLY
Anaerobic susceptibility testing is helpful in the management of patients with:

   a synovial infections
   b rectal abscesses
   c streptococcal pharyngitis
   d pilonidal sinuses

63 An antibiotic used to suppress or kill contaminating fungi in media is:

   a penicillin
   b cycloheximide– *added to media*
   c streptomycin
   d amphotericin B

64 Production of beta-lactamase is <u>inducible</u> in which of the following:
   (causes when exposed)

   a *Haemophilus influenzae*
   b *Staphylococcus aureus*
   c *Corynebacterium diphtheriae*
   d *Streptococcus pyogenes*

65 A sputum specimen is received for culture and Gram stain. The Gram stained smear from this specimen is seen in the image (total magnification 100×):

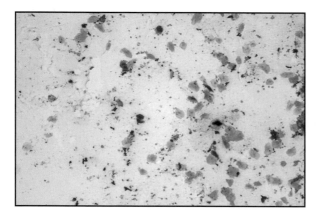

The technologist's best course of action would be to:

   a inoculate appropriate media and incubate anaerobically
   b inoculate appropriate media and incubate aerobically
   c call the physician and notify him of this "life-threatening" situation
   d call the patient care area and request a new specimen

66 A technologist is reading a Gram stain from a CSF and observes many neutrophils and lancet-shaped gram-positive diplococci. Which set of chemistry and hematology CSF results would **most** likely be seen in someone with this type of infection?

CSF results	WBC	Glucose	Protein
A	increased	increased	increased
B	decreased	decreased	decreased
C	increased	decreased	increased
D	decreased	increased	decreased

   a result A
   b result B
   c result C
   d result D

67 Refer to the following illustration:

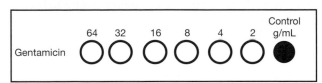

Gentamicin   64   32   16   8   4   2   Control g/mL

Examine the broth microdilution susceptibility test shown above and determine the MIC for gentamicin.   *well showing no growth*

   a   >64 µg/mL
   b   32 µg/mL
   c   16 µg/mL
   d   <2 µg/mL

68 Which of the following tests is used to monitor bactericidal activity during antimicrobic therapy in cases of endocarditis?
MLS ONLY

   a Elek
   b tolerance
   c Sherris synergism
   d Schlichter

69 Quality control results for disk diffusion susceptibility tests yield the following results: aminoglycoside zones too small and penicillin zones too large. This is **most** likely due to the:
MLS ONLY

   a inoculum being too heavy
   b inoculum being too light
   c pH of Mueller-Hinton agar being too low
   d calcium and magnesium concentration in the agar being too high

70 When using a control strain of *Staphylococcus aureus*, the technologist notices that the zone around the oxacillin disk is too small. Which of the following is the **most** likely explanation?

   a inoculation of the plates 10 minutes after preparing the inoculum
   b incubation of the Mueller-Hinton plates at 35°C
   c use of a 0.25 McFarland standard to prepare inoculum
   d use of outdated oxacillin disks

71 In the disk diffusion method of determining antibiotic susceptibility, the size of the inhibition zone used to indicate susceptibility has been determined by:
MLS ONLY

   a testing 30 strains of 1 genus of bacteria
   b correlating the zone size with minimum inhibitory concentrations
   c correlating the zone size with minimum bactericidal concentrations
   d correlating the zone size with the antibiotic content of the disk

72 Which of the following organisms may be mistaken for *Neisseria gonorrhoeae* in Gram stained smears of uterine cervix exudates?

   a *Lactobacillus* species - *gram⊖ rod*
   b *Streptococcus agalactiae* - *gram⊕*
   c *Pseudomonas aeruginosa*
   d *Moraxella osloensis* - *gram⊖ coccobacillus*

73   A 73-year-old man diagnosed as having pneumococcal meningitis is not responding to his
      penicillin therapy. Which of the following tests should be performed on the isolate to best
      determine this organism's susceptibility to penicillin?

    a beta-lactamase
    b oxacillin disk diffusion
    c penicillin disk diffusion
    d Schlichter test

74   *Salmonella enteritidis* is isolated from multiple blood cultures in a patient with fever. Susceptibility
MLS   results are as follows: ampicillin-susceptible, ceftriaxone-susceptible, ciprofloxacin-susceptible,
ONLY trimethoprim/sulfamethoxazole-resistant. What is the next best step?

    a report all of the susceptibility testing results with no changes
    b perform a beta-lactamase test on the isolate before reporting the ampicillin as susceptible
    c test the isolate against nalidixic acid and if resistant report the ciprofloxacin as resistant
    d report gentamicin since the trimethoprim/sulfamethoxazole is resistant

75   Which of the following antimicrobials would be inappropriate to report on an *E coli* isolated from
      a wound culture?

    a gentamicin
    b ampicillin
    c cefazolin
    d nitrofurantoin – *URINARY TRACT INFECTIONS ONLY!*

76   The susceptibility results below are reported on an *Enterococcus faecalis* isolated from peritoneal
      fluid.

        ampicillin: susceptible
        vancomycin: resistant
        clindamycin: susceptible
        levofloxacin: resistant
        linezolid: susceptible

The physician calls questioning the results. Which of the following should have been done before
the report was released?

    a the clindamycin result should have been removed from the report since it is inactive against
       Enterococcus
    b the ampicillin result should have been changed to resistant since the isolate is vancomycin
       resistant
    c the linezolid result should have been removed from the report since it is inactive against
       Enterococcus
    d ciprofloxacin should have been added to the report since levofloxacin was resistant

~~Enterococcus~~
ENTEROCOCCUS → not treatable with
               CLINDAMYCIN
               CEPHALASPORINS
               SULFAS

77 A D test is performed on an isolate of *Staphylococcus aureus* to determine inducible clindamycin resistance:

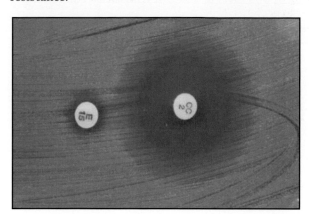

Double disk test:
E = erythromycin
CC = Clindamycin

formation of D-shaped zone by erythromycin shows resistance to clindamycin.

Based on the result seen in the image how should the erythromycin and clindamycin be reported?

  a erythromycin: resistant; clindamycin: resistant
  b erythromycin: resistant; clindamycin: susceptible   *negative D test*
  c erythromycin: susceptible; clindamycin: resistant
  d erythromycin: susceptible; clindamycin: susceptible

78 Which of the following combinations is useful for confirming the presence of extended spectrum beta-lactamases in *E coli*?

  a ampicillin + cefepime
  b cefoxitin + penicillin
  c ceftazidime + clavulanic acid *— used to test extended spectrum BL; used in conjunction with drug*
  d cefpodoxime + cefotaxime

79
Enzymatic drug modification is a mechanism of resistance for which antimicrobial?

  a levofloxacin
  b sulfamethoxazole
  c vancomycin
  d gentamicin

80 Which of the following is the **most** important variable in the recovery of organisms in patients with bacteremia?

  a subculture of all bottles at day 5 of incubation
  b the volume of blood cultured
  c use of chlorhexadine for skin antisepsis
  d collection of multiple blood culture sets from a single venipuncture

81   A 24-year-old man presents with pain on urination and urethral discharge. A Gram stain of the discharge is seen in the image:

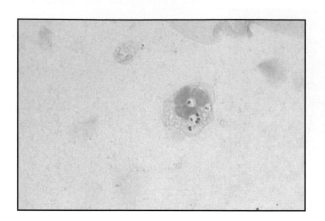
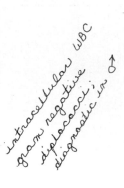

intracellular WBC
gram negative
diplococci;
diagnostic in ♂

What is the **most** likely identification of this organism?

a   *Acinetobacter baumannii*
b   *Neisseria gonorrhoeae*
c   *Haemophilus ducreyi*
d   *Escherichia coli*

82   A 10-year-old child with cystic fibrosis presents with cough and shortness of breath. Her sputum Gram stain is seen in the image:

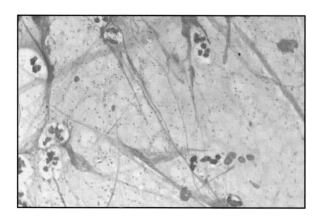
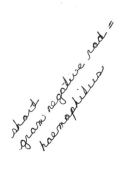

short
gram negative rod =
haemophilus

Based on the Gram stain what would be the best medium and incubation condition to optimize recovery of the organism seen?

a   MacConkey agar incubated in CO_2
b   Tinsdale agar incubated in ambient air
c   chocolate agar incubated in CO_2
d   CNA agar incubated in ambient air

83   The image depicts a Gram stain (final magnification 1,000×) of a knee fluid from a patient who has recently undergone knee replacement surgery:

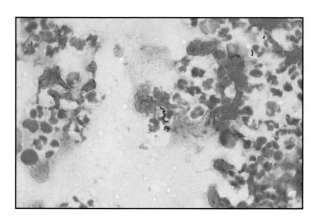
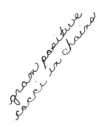

gram positive cocci in chains

The best interpretation of this Gram stain is:

a gram-positive cocci suggestive of *Staphylococcus*
b gram-positive bacilli suggestive of *Corynebacterium*
c gram-positive bacilli suggestive of *Listeria*
d gram-positive cocci suggestive of *Streptococcus*

84   A vaginal/rectal swab is collected from a pregnant patient to screen for group B *Streptococcus* colonization. What is the best medium to use for specimen inoculation?

a blood agar
b LIM broth — *for Group B strep*
c CNA agar
d thioglycollate broth

85   A pregnant patient is screened at 36 weeks gestation for group B *Streptococcus* (GBS). A vaginal
swab is collected and cultured in Todd-Hewitt broth with 8 µg gentamicin/mL and 15 µg nalidixic acid/mL. The broth is subcultured onto sheep blood agar after 24 hours of incubation. No GBS are seen on the subculture and the results are reported as negative. The patient later goes on to deliver an infant with early onset GBS disease. What is the **most** likely reason for the negative GBS culture?

a the patient was screened to early since screening after 38 weeks is recommended
b a vaginal swab was collected instead of a vaginal/rectal swab
c the Todd-Hewitt broth used was inhibitory to the organism
d the selective broth was incubated only 24 hours before subculture

86   Susceptibility testing is performed on a *Staphylococcus aureus* isolate from a blood culture with the following results:

oxacillin:	resistant
cefazolin:	susceptible
clindamycin:	susceptible
erythromycin:	susceptible
trimethoprim/sulfamethoxazole:	susceptible
vancomycin:	susceptible

What should the technologist do next?

a ceftriaxone should be reported instead of cefazolin
b clindamycin should be tested for inducible resistance prior to reporting
c the trimethoprim/sulfamethoxazole result should be removed since all *S aureus* are resistant
d the cefazolin result should be changed to resistant since the oxacillin result is resistant

87   To quality control the autoclave, a vial of *Bacillus stearothermophilus* is autoclaved and should then be:

     a inoculated to blood agar
     b incubated at 37°C
     c inoculated to chocolate agar
     d incubated at 56°C

88   In a quality control procedure on a new batch of Mueller-Hinton plates using a stock culture of *Staphylococcus aureus* (ATCC 25923), all the disk zone sizes are too small. The **most** likely reason for this is that the:

     a Mueller-Hinton plates were poured too thin
     b potency of the antibiotic disks is too high
     c bacterial suspension was not diluted to the proper concentration
     d disks should have been set up on mannitol salt

89   Which one of the following combinations of organisms would be appropriate as controls to test the functions listed?

     a beta-hemolysis-negative *Escherichia coli* and *Streptococcus pyogenes*
     b catalase-negative *Staphylococcus aureus* and *Staphylococcus epidermidis*
     c H$_2$S production-negative *Proteus mirabilis* and *Staphylococcus epidermidis*
     d indole-negative *Escherichia coli* and *Proteus mirabilis*

(margin note: all positive)

Aerobic Gram-Positive Cocci

90   A urine Gram stain shows gram-positive cocci in clusters. The organism tested catalase positive. To **speciate** this organism from culture, the technician should perform a coagulase test and a/an:

     a polymyxin B susceptibility
     b novobiocin susceptibility
     c oxidase
     d beta-lactamase

91   The Gram stain from a blood culture shows gram-positive cocci in chains. No growth occurs on blood agar plates incubated both aerobically and anaerobically. Additional testing should be done to detect the presence of:

     a *Staphylococcus saprophyticus*
     b *Aerococcus urinae*
     c *Abiotrophia defectiva* — *nutritionally defective streptococci*
     d *Streptococcus pneumoniae*

92   Viridans streptococci can be differentiated from *Streptococcus pneumoniae* by:

     a alpha hemolysis
     b morphology
     c catalase reaction
     d bile solubility

93   A reliable test for distinguishing *Staphylococcus aureus* from other staphylococci is:

     a oxidase
     b coagulase
     c catalase
     d optochin susceptibility

94   The optochin (ethylhydrocupreine hydrochloride) disk is used for the identification of:

   a *Haemophilus influenzae*
   b group A beta-hemolytic streptococci
   c *Streptococcus pneumoniae* - OPTOCHIN SENSITIVE
   d alpha-hemolytic streptococci

95   In the optochin (ethylhydrocupreine hydrochloride) susceptibility test, if there is a zone of inhibition of 19-30 mm surrounding the disk following overnight incubation at 37°C, the colony **most** likely consists of:

   a staphylococci
   b streptococci
   c pneumococci (S. pneumoniae)
   d intestinal bacilli

96   Which 2 diseases are usually preceded by infection with beta-hemolytic streptococci?

   a rheumatic fever, undulant fever
   b glomerulonephritis, rheumatic fever
   c rheumatic fever, tularemia
   d glomerulonephritis, undulant fever

97   The enterotoxin produced by certain strains of hemolytic, coagulase positive *Staphylococcus aureus*:

   a is destroyed by boiling for 15-30 minutes
   b is identical to the dermonecrotic toxin
   c causes one type of bacterial food poisoning – enterotoxin same
   d is highly antigenic

98   A gamma-hemolytic *Streptococcus* that blackens bile esculin agar but does not grow in 6.5% NaCl broth is **most** likely:

   a group B *Streptococcus* - beta
   b *Enterococcus* ⊕ BEA/ ⊕ NaCl
   c group D *Streptococcus* ⊕BEA/⊖NaCl
   d *Streptococcus pneumoniae* -alpha

99   Gram stain examination from a blood culture bottle shows dark blue, spherical organisms in clusters. Growth on sheep blood agar shows small, round, pale yellow colonies. Further tests should include:

   a catalase production and coagulase test
   b bacitracin susceptibility and serological typing
   c oxidase and deoxyribonuclease reactions
   d Voges-Proskauer and methyl red reactions gram ⊖

100   Gram-positive cocci in chains are seen on a Gram stain from a blood culture. The organism grows as a beta-hemolytic colony. Further tests that could be performed include:

   a bile esculin, PYR, bacitracin, and hippurate
   b catalase and coagulase
   c oxidase and deoxyribonuclease
   d Voges-Proskauer and methyl red

101   "Nutritionally deficient" streptococci are:

   a enterococci
   b group D nonenterococci
   c cell wall-deficient streptococci
   d in the genera *Granulicatella* and *Abiotrophia* ✻✻

102 After 24 hours a blood culture from a newborn grows catalase-negative, gram-positive cocci. The
     bacterial colonies are small, translucent and beta-hemolytic on a blood agar plate. Biochemical
     test results of a pure culture are:

     bacitracin: resistant
     CAMP reaction: positive
     bile esculin: not hydrolyzed
     6.5% NaCl broth: no growth

     Assuming that all controls react properly and reactions are verified, the next step would be to:

     (a) perform a *Streptococcus* group typing
     b report the organism as *Streptococcus pneumoniae*
     c report the organism as *Staphylococcus aureus*
     d report the organism as *Staphylococcus epidermidis*

103 A beta-hemolytic streptococcus that has been isolated from an ear culture grows up to the edge of
     a 0.04 unit bacitracin disk. Which of the following tests would help to determine if the organism
     is *Enterococcus*?

     (a) growth in 6.5% NaCl broth
     b growth in the presence of penicillin
     c optochin susceptibility
     d fermentation of 10% lactose

104 The organism **most** commonly associated with neonatal purulent meningitis is:

     a *Neisseria meningitidis*   *all can cause meningitis*
     b *Streptococcus pneumoniae*
     (c) group B streptococci – *neonatal*
     d *Haemophilus influenzae*

105 An important cause of acute exudative pharyngitis is:

     a *Staphylococcus aureus* (beta-hemolytic)
     b *Streptococcus pneumoniae*
     c *Streptococcus agalactiae*
     (d) *Streptococcus pyogenes*

106 Of the following bacteria, the **most** frequent cause of prosthetic heart valve infections occurring
     within 2-3 months after surgery is:

     a *Streptococcus pneumoniae*
     b *Streptococcus pyogenes*
     c *Staphylococcus aureus*
     (d) *Staphylococcus epidermidis*

107 Which of the 2 different antimicrobial agents listed below are commonly used and may result in
MLS synergistic action in the treatment of endocarditis caused by *Enterococcus faecalis*?
ONLY
     a an aminoglycoside and a macrolide
     (b) a penicillin derivative and an aminoglycoside
     c a cell membrane active agent and nalidixic acid
     d a macrolide and a penicillin derivative

108 A catheterized urine is inoculated onto blood and MacConkey agar using a 0.01 mL loop. After 48 hours, 68 colonies of a small translucent nonhemolytic organism grew on blood agar but not MacConkey. Testing reveals small gram-positive, catalase-negative cocci. The preliminary report and follow-up testing would be:

   a growth of 680 colonies/mL of gram-positive cocci, optochin and bacitracin susceptibility tests to follow

   b growth of 6,800 colonies/mL of a *Staphylococcus* species, coagulase test to follow

   ⓒ growth of 6,800 colonies/mL of a *Streptococcus* species, esculin hydrolysis and NaCl growth test to follow

   d growth of 6,800 colonies/mL of a *Streptococcus* species, no further testing

109 Children who have infections with beta-hemolytic streptococci can develop:

   a acute pyelonephritis

   ⓑ acute glomerulonephritis

   c chronic glomerulonephritis

   d nephrosis

110 A gram-positive coccus isolated from a blood culture has the following characteristics:

optochin susceptibility:	negative
bacitracin (0.04 U) susceptibility:	negative
bile esculin hydrolysis:	negative *BE⊖*
hippurate hydrolysis:	positive
catalase:	negative *(strep)*

This organism is **most** likely:

   a *Staphylococcus aureus*

   b *Streptococcus pneumoniae*

   c *Streptococcus pyogenes*

   ⓓ *Streptococcus agalactiae*

Strep agalactiae: catalase ⊖
optochin and bacitracin R⊖
BEA ⊖
hippurate ⊕

111 A beta-hemolytic streptococci that is bacitracin-sensitive and <u>CAMP-negative</u> is:

   a group B

   ⓑ group A

   c beta-hemolytic, not group A, B, or D

   d beta-hemolytic, group D

Group A: bacitracin S
CAMP negative

112 A beta-hemolytic *Streptococcus* that is bacitracin-resistant and <u>CAMP-positive</u> is:

   a group A or B

   b group A

   ⓒ group B

   d beta-hemolytic, group D

113 Group B, beta-hemolytic streptococci may be distinguished from other hemolytic streptococci by which of the following procedures?

   ⓐ latex antigen typing

   b growth in 6.5% NaCl broth

   c growth on bile esculin medium

   d bacitracin susceptibility

114 It is important to differentiate between *Enterococcus* and group D streptococci because:

   a viridans streptococci are often confused with enterococci

   b several enterococci cause severe puerperal sepsis

   c group D streptococci are avirulent

   ⓓ enterococci often show more antibiotic resistance than group D streptococci

115 *Streptococcus pneumoniae* can be differentiated best from the viridans group of streptococci by:

   a Gram stain
   b the type of hemolysis
   c colonial morphology
   d bile solubility

*[handwritten: * Strep pneumo: bile solubility ⊕ / Strep viridans: ⊖]*

116 Characteristically, enterococci are:

   a unable to grow in 6.5% NaCl
   b relatively resistant to penicillin
   c sodium hippurate positive
   d bile esculin negative

[handwritten: Enterococci: NaCl ⊕ / BEA ⊕ / hippurate ⊖]

117 A beta-hemolytic, catalase-positive, gram-positive coccus is coagulase negative by the slide coagulase test. Which of the following is the **most** appropriate action in identification of this organism?

   a report a coagulase-negative *Staphylococcus*
   b report a coagulase-negative *Staphylococcus aureus*
   c reconfirm the hemolytic reaction on a fresh 24-hour culture
   d do a tube coagulase test to confirm the slide test

118 Which of the following would best differentiate *Streptococcus agalactiae* from *Streptococcus pyogenes* ?

   a ability to grow in sodium azide broth
   b a positive bile-esculin reaction
   c hydrolysis of sodium hippurate
   d beta-hemolysis on sheep blood agar

119 The **most** critical distinction between *Staphylococcus aureus* and other *Staphylococcus* is:

   a phosphatase reaction
   b DNA production
   c coagulase production
   d hemolysis

120 Which of the following organisms is, to date, considered universally susceptible to penicillin:

   a *Haemophilus influenzae*
   b *Neisseria gonorrhoeae*
   c *Streptococcus pyogenes*
   d *Corynebacterium diphtheriae*

121 A beta-hemolytic gram-positive coccus was isolated from the cerebrospinal fluid of a 2-day-old infant with signs of meningitis. The isolate grew on sheep blood agar under aerobic conditions and was resistant to a bacitracin disc. Which of the following should be performed for the identification of the organism?

   a oxidase production
   b catalase formation
   c latex antigen typing
   d esculin hydrolysis

122 How many hours after eating contaminated food do initial symptoms of staphylococcal food poisoning typically occur?

   a 2-6 hours
   b 12-18 hours
   c 24-48 hours
   d 72 hours to a week

123 During the past month, *Staphylococcus epidermidis* has been isolated from blood cultures at 2-3 times the rate from the previous year. The **most** logical explanation for the increase in these isolates is that:

    a the blood culture media are contaminated with this organism
    b the hospital ventilation system is contaminated with *Staphylococcus epidermidis*
    c there has been a break in proper skin preparation before drawing blood for culture
    d a relatively virulent isolate is being spread from patient to patient

124 An outbreak of *Staphylococcus aureus* has occurred in a hospital nursery. In order to establish the epidemiological source of the outbreak, the **most** commonly used typing method is:
MLS ONLY

    a pulsed-field gel electrophoresis
    b serological typing
    c coagulase testing
    d catalase testing

125 A yellow colony from a wound culture tested catalase-positive and coagulase-negative. The *staph*   *CNS* organism stained as gram-positive cocci in clusters. Which of the following tests would differentiate between a coagulase-negative *Staphylococcus* and *Micrococcus*?

    a novobiocin susceptibility   *FURAZOLIDONE:*
    b leucine aminopeptidase production   *CNS: S*
    c furazolidone (100 µg/disk) susceptibility   *Micrococcus. R*   ***
    d bile esculin

126 A light yellow colony from a skin lesion grew aerobically and tested as catalase positive and coagulase negative. The organism gram stained as positive cocci in clusters. The organism was *MLS ONLY* modified oxidase positive, bacitracin (0.04U) susceptible and resistant to lysostaphin. What is the identification of this organism?

    a *Staphylococcus aureus*
    b *Micrococcus luteus*
    c *Staphylococcus epidermidis*
    d *Peptostreptococcus anaerobius*

127 An isolate of an unknown beta-hemolytic *Streptococcus* is streaked perpendicular to a streak of beta-lysin-producing *Staphylococcus aureus*. After incubation a zone of arrowhead hemolysis is noted at the interface of the 2 streaks. What is the name of the test and the presumptive identification of the unknown *Streptococcus*?

    a hippurate hydrolysis and *S agalactiae*
    b CAMP test and *S pyogenes*
    c hippurate hydrolysis and *S pyogenes*
    d CAMP test and *S agalactiae*

128 Which of the following may be used as a positive quality control organism for the bile esculin test?

    a *Staphylococcus epidermidis*
    b *Staphylococcus aureus*   *all negative*
    c *Streptococcus pyogenes*
    d *Enterococcus faecalis*

Gram-Negative Bacilli

129 Infection of the urinary tract is **most** frequently associated with:

    a *Staphylococcus aureus*
    (b) *Escherichia coli*
    c *Enterococcus faecalis*
    d *Serratia marcescens*

130 MacConkey media for screening suspected cases of hemorrhagic *E coli* O157:H7 must contain: *⊖ for sorbitol / all other E. Coli's ⊕*

    a indole
    b citrate
    (c) sorbitol
    d lactose

131 Members of the family *Enterobacteriaceae* share which one of the following characteristics?

    a produce cytochrome oxidase
    b ferment lactose
    c produce beta-hemolysis
    (d) reduce nitrate to nitrite

132 Which one of the following genera is among the least biochemically reactive members of the *Enterobacteriaceae*?

    a *Proteus*
    (b) *Pseudomonas*
    c *Citrobacter*
    (d) *Shigella* - Lactose⊖, gas⊖, VP⊖, urea⊖, lysine⊖, citrate⊖, non-motile

133 Which one of the following gram-negative bacilli ferments glucose?

    a *Alcaligenes faecalis*
    b *Pseudomonas cepacia* ⎬ non-fermenters
    c *Acinetobacter lwoffii*
    (d) *Yersinia enterocolitica*

134 A sputum culture from an alcoholic seen in the ER grows gray, <u>mucoid, stringy colonies</u> on sheep blood agar. The isolate grows readily on MacConkey agar and forms mucoid, dark pink colonies. The colonies yield the following test results:

ONPG:	+
indole:	−
glucose:	+
oxidase:	−
citrate:	+
VP:	+

The organism is **most** likely:

    a *Edwardsiella tarda*
    (b) *Klebsiella pneumoniae*
    c *Escherichia coli*
    d *Proteus vulgaris*

135 An organism was inoculated to a TSI tube and gave the following reactions:
    K/A
    alkaline slant/acid butt, H_2S, gas produced

This organism **most** likely is:

    a *Klebsiella pneumoniae* A/A
    b *Shigella dysenteriae*
    (c) *Salmonella typhimurium*
    d *Escherichia coli* A/A

136 An isolate from a stool culture gives the following growth characteristics and biochemical reactions:

MacConkey agar: colorless colonies NLF
Hektoen agar: yellow-orange colonies
TSI: acid slant/acid butt, no gas, no H_2S A/A/
urea: positive

These screening reactions are consistent with which of the following enteric pathogens?

a *Yersinia enterocolitica* – yellow colonies on Hektoen
b *Shigella sonnei* – colorless colonies on Mac + Hektoen
c *Vibrio parahaemolyticus* – needs 1% NaCl
d *Campylobacter jejuni*

137 A TSI tube inoculated with an organism gave the following reactions:

alkaline slant, acid butt, no H_2S, no gas produced   K/A, no H_2S, no gas

This organism is **most** likely:

a *Yersinia enterocolitica* A/A
b *Salmonella typhi*
c *Salmonella enteritidis*
d *Shigella dysenteriae*

138 An organism gave the following reactions:

TSI: acid slant/acid butt; no H_2S gas produced   A/A, no H_2S
indole: positive   +
motility: positive   – –
citrate: negative
lysine decarboxylase: positive
urea: negative
VP: negative

This organism **most** likely is:

a *Klebsiella pneumoniae* – non-motile
b *Shigella dysenteriae* – non-motile
c *Escherichia coli*
d *Enterobacteria cloacae* – indole neg

139 Which of the following organisms can grow in the small bowel and cause diarrhea in children, traveler's diarrhea, or a severe cholera-like syndrome through the production of enterotoxins?

a *Yersinia enterocolitica*
b *Escherichia coli* – enterotoxins   ✱
c *Salmonella typhi*
d *Shigella dysenteriae*

140 One of the enterotoxins produced by enterotoxigenic *Escherichia coli* in traveler's diarrhea is
MLS
ONLY   similar to a toxin produced by:

a *Clostridium perfringens*
b *Clostridium difficile*
c *Vibrio cholerae*
d *Yersinia enterocolitica*

141 *Shigella* species characteristically are:

a urease positive
b nonmotile
c oxidase positive
d lactose fermenters

142 A gram-negative bacillus has been isolated from feces, and the confirmed biochemical reactions fit those of *Shigella*. The organism does not agglutinate in *Shigella* antisera. What should be done next?

    a test the organism with a new lot of antisera
    b test with Vi antigen
    c repeat the biochemical tests
    d boil the organism and retest with the antisera

143 Biochemical reactions of an organism are consistent with *Shigella*. A suspension is tested in antiserum without resulting agglutination. However, after 15 minutes of boiling, agglutination occurs in group D antisera. The *Shigella* species is:

    a *dysenteriae* - Group A
    b *flexneri*
    c *boydii*
    d *sonnei* - Group D

144 >100,000 CFU/mL of a gram-negative bacilli were isolated on MacConkey from a urine specimen. Biochemical results are as follows:

    glucose: acid, gas produced
    indole: negative
    urea: positive
    TDA: positive
    H₂S: positive

The organism is **most** likely:

    a *Morganella morganii* - no H₂S
    b *Proteus mirabilis* -- indole ⊖
    c *Proteus vulgaris* -- indole ⊕
    d *Providencia stuartii* - no H₂S

145 A urine culture had the following culture results:

    sheep blood: swarming
    Columbia CNA: no growth
    MacConkey: 1. >100,000 CFU/mL nonlactose-fermenter
                     2. >100,000 CFU/mL nonlactose-fermenter with red pigment

The isolates from MacConkey agar had the following biochemical reactions:

Test	Isolate 1	Isolate 2
TSI	alk/acid	alk/acid
urea	positive	negative
TDA	positive	negative
H₂S	positive	negative

The organisms are **most** likely:

    a *Proteus vulgaris* and *Enterobacter cloacae*
    b *Proteus mirabilis* and *Serratia marcescens* - red pigment
    c *Morganella morganii* and *Klebsiella pneumoniae*
H₂S⊕   **d** *Providencia stuartii* and *Serratia liquefaciens*
swarming

146 An 8-year-old girl was admitted to the hospital with a three-day history of fever, abdominal pain, diarrhea, and vomiting. A stool culture grew many lactose-negative colonies that yielded the following test results:

oxidase:	negative
TSI:	acid slant/acid butt
indole:	negative
urease:	positive
ornithine decarboxylase:	positive
sucrose:	positive
H_2S:	negative
motility at 25°C:	positive

The **most** probable identification of this organism is:

a *Escherichia coli*
b *Providencia stuartii*
c *Yersinia enterocolitica*
d *Edwardsiella tarda*

147 Which of the following sets of tests best differentiates *Salmonella* and *Citrobacter* species?

a KCN, malonate, beta-galactosidase, lysine decarboxylase
b dulcitol, citrate, indole, H_2S production
c lactose, adonitol, KCN, motility
d lysine decarboxylase, lactose, sucrose, malonate, indole

148 A fecal specimen, inoculated to xylose lysine deoxycholate (XLD) and Hektoen enteric (HE) produced colonies with black centers. Additional testing results are as follows:

Biochemical screen	Result	Serological test	Result
glucose	positive	polyvalent	no agglutination
H_2S	positive	group A	no agglutination
lysine decarboxylase	positive	group B_l	no agglutination
urea	negative	group C	no agglutination
ONPG	negative	group D	no agglutination
indole	positive	group V_i	no agglutination

The **most** probable identification is:

a *Salmonella enterica*
b *Edwardsiella tarda*
c *Proteus mirabilis*
d *Shigella sonnei*

149 A 10-year-old boy was admitted to the emergency room with lower right quadrant pain and tenderness. The following laboratory results were obtained:

	Patient value	Normal range
% segmented neutrophils	75%	16%-60%
WBC count	$200 \times 10^3/\mu L$ ($200 \times 10^9/L$)	$13.0 \times 10^3/\mu L$ ($13.0 \times 10^9/L$)

The admitting diagnosis was appendicitis. During surgery the appendix appeared normal; an enlarged node was removed and cultured. Small gram-negative bacilli were isolated from the room temperature plate. The organism **most** likely is:

a *Prevotella melaninogenica*
b *Shigella sonnei*
c *Listeria monocytogenes*
d *Yersinia enterocolitica*

150 A 25-year-old man who had recently worked as a steward on a transoceanic grain ship presented to the emergency room with high fever, diarrhea and prostration. Axillary lymph nodes were hemorrhagic and enlarged. A Wayson stain of the aspirate showed bacilli that were bipolar, resembling safety pins. The **most** likely identification of this organism is:

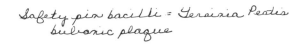

Safety pin bacilli = Yersinia Pestis
bubonic plague

   a *Brucella melitensis*
   b *Streptobacillus moniliformis*
   c *Spirillum minus*
   (d) *Yersinia pestis*

151 Biochemical reactions of an organism are consistent with *Salmonella*. A suspension is tested in polyvalent antiserum A through G and Vi antiserum. There is agglutination in the Vi antiserum only. What should be done next?
(MLS ONLY)

   a boil suspension of the organism for 10 minutes to inactivate the Vi antigen
   b test organism with individual antisera for agglutination
   c report "no *Salmonella* isolated"
   d repeat biochemical identification of the organism

152 A clean catch urine sample from a nursing home patient is cultured using a .001 mL loop. It grows 67 colonies of a lactose fermenter that has the following biochemical reactions:

TSI:	acid/acid	*A/A*	*67,000*
oxidase:	negative		
motility:	positive		
indole:	negative	*—*	*+ +*
citrate:	positive		
VP:	positive		
lysine decarboxylase:	negative		
ornithine decarboxylase:	positive		
urea:	negative		

What should the microbiologist report?

   a   670 CFU/mL *Serratia marsecens* sp
   b 6,700 CFU/mL *Providencia stuartii*
   (c) 67,000 CFU/mL *Enterobacter cloacae* *- + +*
   d 67,000 CFU/mL *Klebsiella oxytoca* *- nonmotile*

(153) *Plesiomonas shigelloides* is a relatively new member of the family *Enterobacteriaceae*. What characteristic separates it from other members of the *Enterobacteriaceae*?

   (a) it is oxidase positive
   b it ferments glucose
   c it produces pyocyanin
   d it requires 10% CO_2 for growth

✳✳

154 A 64-year-old male with lymphoma has a positive blood culture at 18 hours incubation. The
MLS organism is a nonlactose fermenting gram-negative bacillus on MacConkey agar. Further testing
ONLY gives the following reactions:

oxidase:	negative
TSI:	alkaline/acid, no hydrogen sulfide
motility:	positive
indole:	positive
citrate:	positive
ornithine decarboxylase:	negative
urea:	positive
phenylalanine deaminase:	positive
VP:	negative

NLF gram ⊖ rod
K/A, no H₂S
motile
+　 - +
urea +

The genus is:

a　*Morganella*
b　*Proteus*
ⓒ　*Providencia* - *no H₂S, phenylalanine deaminase⊕*
d　*Serratia*

155　The stock cultures needed for quality control testing of motility are:

a　*Salmonella typhimurium/Escherichia coli*
b　*Escherichia coli/Pseudomonas aeruginosa*
c　*Serratia marcescens/Escherichia coli*
ⓓ　*Klebsiella pneumoniae/Escherichia coli*
　　　⊖　　　　　　　　　⊕

156　The stock cultures needed for quality control testing of oxidase production are:

a　*Escherichia coli/Klebsiella pneumoniae*
b　*Salmonella typhimurium/Escherichia coli*
　　　⊖　　　　　　　　　⊕
ⓒ　*Escherichia coli/Pseudomonas aeruginosa*
d　*Proteus mirabilis/Escherichia coli*

157　The stock cultures needed for quality control testing of deamination activity are:

a　*Escherichia coli/Klebsiella pneumoniae*
b　*Salmonella typhimurium/Escherichia coli*　　*Proteus mirabilis = phenylalanine*
c　*Escherichia coli/Pseudomonas aeruginosa*　　　　　　*deaminase ⊕*
ⓓ　*Proteus mirabilis/Escherichia coli*
　　　⊕　　　　　　　　⊖

158　The stock cultures needed for quality control testing of deoxyribonuclease (DNase) production are:

a　*Salmonella typhimurium/Escherichia coli*
b　*Escherichia coli/Pseudomonas aeruginosa*　　*Serratia marcescens = DNase ⊕*
c　*Proteus mirabilis/Escherichia coli*
d　*Serratia marcescens/Escherichia coli*
　　　⊕　　　　　　　　⊖

159　Quality control of the spot indole test requires the use of ATCC cultures of:

a　*Pseudomonas aeruginosa/Proteus mirabilis*
b　*Salmonella typhi/Shigella sonnei*　　　　✱✱
c　*Escherichia coli/Proteus vulgaris*
d　*Escherichia coli/Enterobacter cloacae*
　　　⊕　　　　　　　　⊖

160　An organism that exhibits the satellite phenomenon around colonies of staphylococci is:

ⓐ　*Haemophilus influenzae* - *needs X and V factors*　　✱✱　*X = sheep blood*
b　*Neisseria meningitidis*　　　　　　　　　　　　　　　*V = staph*
c　*Neisseria gonorrhoeae*
d　*Klebsiella pneumoniae*

161 An organism isolated from the surface of a skin burn is found to produce a diffusible green pigment on a blood agar plate. Further studies of the organism would **most** likely show the organism to be: *pyocyanin pigment*

   a *Staphylococcus aureus*
   b *Serratia marcescens*
   c *Flavobacterium meningosepticum*
   d *Pseudomonas aeruginosa*

162 A nonfermenting gram-negative bacillus is isolated from a wound. The nitrate and oxidase are strongly positive. The growth on sheep blood agar has a grape-like odor. The organism is:

   a *Burkholderia cepacia*
   b *Moraxella lacunata*
   c *Chryseobacterium (Flavobacterium) meningosepticum*
   d *Pseudomonas aeruginosa* + oxidase

163 A small, gram-negative bacillus is isolated from an eye culture. It grows only on chocolate agar and is oxidase-variable. The **most** likely organism is:

   a *Acinetobacter lwoffii*
   b *Haemophilus influenzae*
   c *Stenotrophomonas maltophilia*
   d *Pseudomonas aeruginosa*

164 *MLS ONLY* A blood culture bottle with macroscopic signs of growth is Gram stained and the technician notes small, curved gram-negative bacilli resembling "gull wings." It is subcultured to blood and chocolate agar, and incubated aerobically and anaerobically. After 24 hours, no growth is apparent. The next step should be to:

   a subculture the bottle, and incubate in microaerophilic conditions
   b assume the organism is nonviable, and ask for repeat specimen *gull wings = campy*
   c utilize a pyridoxal disk to detect *Aeromonas*
   d subculture the bottle to a medium containing X and V factors

165 The optimal incubator temperature for isolation of the *Campylobacter jejuni/coli* group is: *other colon bacteria inhibited at high temp*

   a 4°C
   b 20°C
   c 25°C
   d 42°C

166 *MLS ONLY* A patient with a nosocomial pneumonia has a sputum Gram stain that shows many neutrophils and numerous small gram-negative coccobacilli. The organism grew in 24 hours as a mucoid, hemolytic colony on blood agar and a colorless colony on a MacConkey agar. The organism had the following characteristics:

oxidase:	negative
catalase:	positive
nitrate:	negative
ONPG:	negative
ornithine decarboxylase:	negative
lysine decarboxylase:	negative

The organism is:

   a *Stenotrophomonas maltophilia*
   b *Alcaligenes faecalis*
   c *Moraxella lacunata*
   d *Acinetobacter baumannii*

167 A gastroenterologist submits a gastric biopsy from a patient with a peptic ulcer. To obtain presumptive evidence of *Helicobacter pylori*, a portion of the specimen should be added to which media?

   a urea broth
   b tetrathionate
   c selenite
   d tryptophan

168 A 4-year-old boy is admitted to the hospital with suspected meningitis. He has not had **most** of the childhood vaccines. The suspected pathogen is:

   a *Listeria monocytogenes*
   b *Haemophilus influenzae*
   c *Streptococcus agalactiae*
   d *Neisseria meningitidis*

169 *Acinetobacter lwoffii* differs from *Neisseria gonorrhoeae* in that the former:
MLS ONLY

   a exhibits a gram-negative staining reaction
   b will grow on MacConkey and EMB media
   c is indophenol oxidase-positive
   d produces hydrogen sulfide on a TSI slant

170 A 4-year-old is admitted with symptoms of meningitis, and a Gram stain of the cerebrospinal fluid reveals small, pleomorphic, gram-negative coccobacilli. After 24 hours incubation at 35°C, small, moist, gray colonies, which are oxidase variable, are found on the chocolate agar plate only. Which of the following biochemical data would be consistent with this isolate?

   a CTA dextrose: positive
      CTA maltose: positive
      ONPG: negative
   b sodium hippurate hydrolysis: positive
      A disc: negative
      CAMP test: positive   *Haemophillus influenzae*
   c X factor: no growth
      V factor: no growth
      XV factor: growth
      horse blood: no hemolysis
   d catalase: positive
      esculin hydrolysis: positive
      methyl red: positive
      "umbrella" motility at room temperature

171 A Gram stain of a touch prep from a gastric biopsy shows gram-negative bacilli that are slender and curved. The **most** likely pathogen is:

   a *Burkholderia cepacia* – respiratory
   b *Corynebacterium urealyticum*
   c *Helicobacter pylori* – gram ⊖ curved bacilli
   d *Pasteurella multocida*

172 A cerebrospinal fluid has been inoculated onto sheep blood and chocolate agar plates and into a tube of trypticase soy broth. All media were incubated in an atmosphere of 5% CO$_2$. Which of the following organisms would usually be isolated by this procedure?

   a *Francisella tularensis* – requires special media
   b *Haemophilus influenzae*
   c *Bordetella pertussis* – requires special media
   d *Bacteroides fragilis* – an aerobe

173 If present, a characteristic that is helpful in separating *Pseudomonas aeruginosa* from other members of the *Pseudomonas* family is:

   a a positive test for cytochrome oxidase
   b oxidative metabolism in the OF test
   c production of fluorescein pigment
   d growth at 42°C

P. aeruginosa grows at 42°; other pseudomonas sp. do NOT

174 A *Campylobacter* species isolated from a stool culture gives the following biochemical reactions:

MLS ONLY

nalidixic acid:	susceptible
cephalothin:	resistant
hippurate hydrolysis:	positive
oxidase:	positive
catalase:	positive

This biochemical profile is consistent with:

   a *Campylobacter fetus*
   b *Campylobacter jejuni*
   c *Campylobacter coli*
   d *Campylobacter laridis*

175 Which one of the following results is typical of *Campylobacter jejuni*:

   a optimal growth at 42°C
   b oxidase ~~negative~~ *positive*
   c catalase ~~negative~~ *positive*
   d ~~non~~motile

176 Optimum growth of *Campylobacter jejuni* is obtained on suitable media incubated at 42°C in an atmosphere containing:

   a 6% O_2, 10%-15% CO_2, 85%-90% nitrogen
   b 10% H_2, 5% CO_2, 85% nitrogen
   c 10% H_2, 10% CO_2, 80% nitrogen
   d 25% O_2, 5% CO_2, 70% nitrogen

177 The porphyrin test was devised to detect strains of *Haemophilus* capable of:

MLS ONLY

   a ampicillin degradation
   b capsule production
   c synthesis of hemin
   d chloramphenicol resistance

178 *Haemophilus influenzae* is **most** likely considered normal indigenous flora in the:

   a oropharynx
   b female genital tract
   c large intestine
   d small intestine

179 *Haemophilus influenzae* becomes resistant to ampicillin when the organism produces a(n):

   a capsule of polysaccharide material
   b affinity for the beta-lactam ring of the ampicillin
   c porphobilinogen
   d beta-lactamase enzyme

180 An isolate on chocolate agar from a patient with epiglottitis was suggestive of *Haemophilus* species. Additional testing showed that the isolate required NAD for growth and was nonhemolytic. The organism is **most** likely *Haemophilus*:

   a *haemolyticus* – *hemolytic*
   b *ducreyi* – *doesn't cause epiglottitis*
   c *influenzae* – *needs hemin*
   (d) *parainfluenzae* – *needs NAD but not hemin (X factor)*

181 Which of the following specimens is considered to be the **most** sensitive for the recovery of *Brucella* in cases of chronic infection?

   a blood *Brucella → bone marrow best recovery*
   b urine
   (c) bone marrow
   d lymph node

182 A genus that is found in soil and water and causes infections in immunocompromised patients has the following characteristics:
MLS ONLY

sheep blood agar:	violet pigment
MacConkey agar:	growth
42°C incubation:	growth
oxidase:	positive
OF glucose:	fermenter
indole:	negative

The genus is:

   a *Campylobacter*
   b *Chromobacterium*
   c *Aeromonas*
   d *Serratia*

183 Which one of the following results is typical of *Campylobacter fetus* subspecies *fetus*?
MLS ONLY

   a optimal growth at 42°C
   b oxidase negative
   c growth at 37°C
   d catalase negative

184 Multiple blood cultures from a patient with endocarditis grew a facultatively anaerobic, pleomorphic gram-negative bacilli with the following characteristics:
MLS ONLY

hemolysis:	negative
MacConkey agar:	no growth
sheep blood agar:	growth in 5%-10% CO_2
chocolate agar:	growth in 5%-10% CO_2
catalase:	negative
V factor:	not required
X factor:	not required
oxidase:	negative
nitrate:	positive, reduced to nitrites
indole:	negative

The **most** likely identification is:

   a *Brucella abortus*
   b *Actinobacillus actinomycetemcomitans*
   c *Haemophilus aphrophilus*
   d *Cardiobacterium hominis*

185   A gram-negative bacillus with bipolar staining was isolated from a wound infection caused by a bite from a pet cat. The following characteristic reactions were seen:

     oxidase: positive
     glucose OF: fermentative
     catalase: positive
     motility: negative
     MacConkey agar: no growth

Which of the following is the **most** likely organism?

    a   *Pseudomonas aeruginosa*
    b   *Pasteurella multocida* – animal bites; AtF no growth on MacConkey
    c   *Aeromonas hydrophila* – water infections
    d   *Vibrio cholerae* – cholera; motile

186   A culture from an infected dog bite on a small boy's finger yielded a small, gram-negative coccobacillus that was smooth, raised and beta-hemolytic on blood agar. The isolate grew on MacConkey agar, forming colorless colonies. The organism was motile, catalase positive, oxidase positive, reduced nitrate, and was urease positive within 4 hours. No carbohydrates were fermented. The **most** likely identification of this isolate is:

    a   *Brucella canis*
    b   *Yersinia pestis*
    c   *Francisella tularensis*
    d   *Bordetella bronchiseptica*

187   While swimming in a lake near his home, a young boy cut his foot, and an infection developed. The culture grew a nonfastidious gram-negative, <u>oxidase positive</u>, <u>beta-hemolytic</u>, <u>motile</u> bacilli that produced deoxyribonuclease. The **most** likely identification is:

    a   *Enterobacter cloacae* – oxidase ⊖
    b   *Serratia marcescens* – oxidase ⊖
    c   *Aeromonas hydrophila* – water infections
    d   *Escherichia coli* – oxidase ⊖

188   An aerobic, gram-negative coccobacillus was isolated on Bordet-Gengou agar from a nasopharyngeal swab 48 hours after culture from a 6-month-old infant with suspected pertussis. The organism exhibited the following characteristics:

     MacConkey agar: no growth
     urea: negative at 4 hours, positive at 24 hours
     oxidase: negative
     catalase: positive

The **most** probable identification of this isolate is:

    a   *Moraxella lacunata*
    b   *Pasteurella ureae*
    c   *Bordetella pertussis*
    d   *Bordetella parapertussis*

189   Which of the following characteristics best differentiates *Bordetella bronchiseptica* from *Alcaligenes* species?

    a   flagellar pattern
    b   growth at 24°C
    c   oxidase activity
    d   rapid hydrolysis of urea

190 Serum samples collected from a patient with pneumonia demonstrate a rising antibody titer to *Legionella*. A bronchoalveolar lavage (BAL) specimen from this patient had a positive antigen test for *Legionella* but no organisms were recovered on buffered charcoal yeast extract medium after 2 days of incubation. The best explanation is that the:

   a antibody titer represents an earlier infection
   b positive antigen test is a false positive
   c specimen was cultured on the wrong media
   (d) culture was not incubated long enough

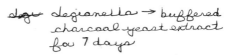

~~dogu~~ legionella → buffered charcoal yeast extract for 7 days

191 Which characteristic best differentiates *Acinetobacter* species from *Moraxella* species?

oxidase ⊖   *oxidase ⊕*

   (a) production of indophenol oxidase
   b growth on MacConkey agar- *both*
   c motility - *both*
   d susceptibility to penicillin- *both*

(192) An organism has been identified as a member of the fluorescent group of *Pseudomonas*. Which of the following sets of tests should be used to determine the species of the organism?

   (a) growth at 42°C, pyocyanin production, gelatinase production   ✳✳
   b pyocyanin production, gelatinase production, OF glucose
   c growth at 37°C, pyocyanin production, OF glucose
   d gelatinase production, growth at 52°C, H_2S

193 Appropriate culture requirements for a specimen from a patient suspected of having tularemia include:

   Francisella

   (a) a media with cysteine such as buffered charcoal yeast extract agar - *needs cysteine*
   b colistin nalidixic acid agar
   c Mueller-Hinton agar with 5% sheep blood agar
   d Regan-Lowe media

194 A child was bitten on the arm by her sibling and the resulting wound grew a slender gram-negative
_{MLS ONLY} bacilli that has the following characteristics:

   growth on SBA: colonies that "pit" the agar
   colonies odor: like bleach
   catalase: negative
   oxidase: positive
   TSI: no growth

The identification of this organism is:

   a *Moraxella catarrhalis*
   b *Eikenella corrodens*
   c *Kingella kingae*
   d *Legionella pneumophila*

195 Characteristics of the genus *Capnocytophaga* include:
_{MLS ONLY}

   a grows in ambient air
   b colonies are large and spreading after 2-4 days
   c considered "nonfermenter"
   d gram-positive bacillus

196 A laboratory aid receives a bronchoscopy sample with the request for culture of *Legionella*. The assistant asks a microbiologist for direction on plating protocol. The correct response from the microbiologist is:

   a culture on thiosulfate citrate bile salt media
   b incubate the culture media anaerobically
   c reject the specimen and request a sputum sample
   (d) culture on buffered charcoal yeast extract agar with antibiotics

197 A community hospital microbiology laboratory is processing significant numbers of stool cultures because of an outbreak of diarrhea following heavy rains and flooding in the county. A media that should be incorporated in the plating protocol is:

    a colistin nalidixic acid for *Listeria*
    b MacConkey agar with sorbitol for *Campylobacter*
    c mannitol salt agar for *Enterococcus* species
    (d) thiosulfate citrate bile salts sucrose for *Vibrio* species

198 A college student attended a beach party where raw oysters and other shellfish were consumed.
MLS ONLY The next day, he had symptoms of septicemia. The blood cultures grew gram-negative bacilli with the following characteristics:

    oxidase: positive
    MacConkey agar: pink colonies
    O/129 (150 µg): susceptible

    The **most** likely organism is:

    a *Aeromonas hydrophila*
    b *Pseudomonas putida*
    c *Serratia marcescens*
    d *Vibrio vulnificus*

199 Differentiating tests that will separate *Burkholderia* from *Stenotrophomonas* include:

    a Gram stain reaction
    b growth on MacConkey agar
    c glucose fermentation
    (d) oxidase

200 A 17-year-old female with cystic fibrosis is diagnosed with pneumonia. A sputum sample grew
MLS ONLY gram-negative bacilli with yellow, smooth colonies that have the following biochemical reactions:

    oxidase: positive
    TSI: alk/alk
    glucose: oxidized
    fluorescence: negative
    lysine decarboxylase: positive

    The **most** likely organism is:

    a *Burkholderia cepacia*
    b *Klebsiella pneumoniae*
    c *Shewanella putrefaciens*
    d *Stenotrophomonas maltophilia*

201 Characteristics of the HACEK group of bacteria include:
MLS ONLY
    a association with urinary tract infections
    b Gram stain of pleomorphic gram-positive bacilli
    c requirement of 5%-10% CO_2 for growth
    d requirement of 42°C for growth

202 The laboratory receives a blood culture from a veterinarian who has been ill for many weeks with fevers in the afternoon and evenings, arthritis, and fatigue. The blood culture is positive after 5 days, and the organism has the following characteristics:

    Gram stain: small, gram-negative coccobacilli
    sheep blood agar: growth after 48 hours with <u>small, smooth, raised colonies</u>

    What should the microbiologist do next?

    a consider the growth contamination and perform another gram stain
    b perform biochemical identification for HACEK organisms
    c perform identification and susceptibility testing using an automated system
    (d) take extra safety precautions for possible *Brucella*

Aerobic Gram-Negative Cocci

203   The primary isolation of *Neisseria gonorrhoeae* requires:

    a   anaerobic conditions
    b   starch media
    c   carbon dioxide- *requires ↑ CO_2*
    d   blood agar

204   Assuming the agent isolated from a patient's spinal fluid produces a positive oxidase test, the **most** likely diagnosis is:

    a   tuberculous meningitis
    b   meningococcal meningitis → *oxidase ⊕*
    c   viral meningitis
    d   pneumococcal meningitis

205   The following results were obtained from a culture of unknown origin:

Gram stain:	gram-negative diplococci
indophenol oxidase:	positive
glucose:	positive
maltose:	negative
sucrose:	negative

carbohydrate panel   *N. gonorrhea*

    The **most** likely source of the specimen would be the:

    a   respiratory tract
    b   blood
    c   genitourinary tract
    d   cerebrospinal fluid

206   An urethral swab obtained from a man with an urethral exudate was plated directly on chocolate agar and modified Thayer-Martin agar, and a Gram stain was made. The Gram stain showed gram-negative diplococci. The culture plates were incubated at 35°C, but had no growth at 48 hours. The **most** likely failure for organism growth is that the:

    a   wrong media were used
    b   Gram stain was misread
    c   organism only grows at room temperature
    d   organism requires CO_2 for growth

207   A Gram stain performed on a sputum specimen revealed gram-negative diplococci within PMNs. Oxidase testing is positive and <u>carbohydrate degradation tests are inert</u>. The organism is:

    a   *Neisseria lactamica*   *Neisseria → carbohydrates*
    b   *Moraxella catarrhalis*
    c   *Neisseria meningitidis*
    d   *Neisseria sicca*

208   Coagglutination is associated with:

    COAGGULTINATION = N. gonorrhoeae

    a   *Chlamydia trachomatis*
    b   *Neisseria gonorrhoeae*
    c   *Streptococcus pneumoniae*
    d   *Klebsiella pneumoniae*

209   Clinical resistance to penicillin correlates **most** frequently with beta-lactamase production in:

    a   *Neisseria gonorrhoeae* → *beta lactamase production*
    b   *Neisseria meningitidis*
    c   *Streptococcus agalactiae*
    d   *Streptococcus pyogenes*

210 All species of the genus *Neisseria* have the enzyme to oxidize:

    a naphthylamine   ✱✱
    b dimethylaminobenzaldehyde
    c glucopyranoside
    d tetramethyl-phenylenediamine – *all oxidase* ⊕

211 The diagnosis of *Neisseria gonorrhoeae* in females is best made from:

    a clinical history
    b an endocervical culture
    c a Gram stain of cervical secretions – *too many non-pathogenic Neisseria*
    d examination for clue cells

212 A vaginal smear is submitted for a Gram stain for *Neisseria gonorrhoeae*. The technologist finds the
(MLS ONLY) following results on the Gram stain:

    many white blood cells
    few epithelial cells
    many gram-positive bacilli
    few gram-negative diplococci
    few gram-positive cocci in chains

The technologist should:

    a report out smear positive for gonorrhea
    b report out smear negative for gonorrhea
    c request a new specimen due to number of white blood cells
    d not read or report a Gram stain on a vaginal specimen

213 Which of the following is the **most** reliable test to differentiate *Neisseria lactamica* from
Neisseria meningitidis?   *maltose + lactose*
    maltose + glucose
    a acid from maltose
    b growth on modified Thayer-Martin agar
    c lactose degradation
    d nitrite reduction to nitrogen gas

214 Definitive identification of *Neisseria gonorrhoeae* is made with the:

    a Gram stain
    b oxidase test
    c degradation of amino acids
    d hydrolysis of carbohydrates

215 A gram-negative diplococcus that grows on modified Thayer-Martin medium can be further
confirmed as *Neisseria gonorrhoeae* if it is: *glucose* ⊕ / *oxidase* ⊕
    a oxidase positive, glucose positive, and maltose positive
    b oxidase positive and glucose positive, maltose negative
    c oxidase positive and maltose positive, glucose negative
    d glucose positive, oxidase negative and maltose negative

216 An organism previously thought to be nonpathogenic, *Moraxella catarrhalis*, is now known to be
associated with opportunistic respiratory infection and nosocomial transmission. Characteristic
identification criteria include:

    a oxidase negative   ✱✱
    b carbohydrates negative (asaccharolytic)
    c beta-lactamase negative
    d gram-negative bacilli

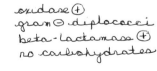
oxidase ⊕
gram ⊖ *diplococci*
beta-lactamase ⊕
no carbohydrates

217 An autopsy performed on an 8-year-old child revealed Waterhouse-Friderichsen syndrome. Blood and throat cultures taken just prior to death were positive for which organism? *↓ most severe complication of N. meningitidis (hemorrhage of adrenal glands)*

   a *Neisseria gonorrhoeae*
   b *Neisseria meningitidis*
   c *Haemophilus influenzae*
   d *Klebsiella pneumoniae*

218 An aspirated specimen of purulent material was obtained from a brain abscess. After 24 hours incubation, pinpoint colonies grew on sheep blood and small, yellowish colonies grew on chocolate. Gram stain of the organism showed gram-negative cocci. Results of carbohydrate degradation studies were as follows:

      glucose: acid
      maltose: acid
      sucrose: acid
      lactose: negative

Additional testing revealed that the organism was oxidase positive and beta-galactosidase negative. The organism is **most** likely *Neisseria*:

   a *meningitidis*
   b *sicca* — *glucose, maltose and sucrose*   ※ ※
   c *lactamica*
   d *gonorrhoeae*

Aerobic or Facultative Gram-Positive Bacilli

219 A Gram stain of organisms on <u>Loeffler agar</u> showed pleomorphic gram-positive bacilli. The organism should be subcultured to: *C. Diphtheriae*

   a blood
   b chocolate
   c MacConkey
   d potassium tellurite

220 Which organism commonly causes food poisoning by consumption of foods containing excessive populations of organisms or preformed enterotoxin?

   a *Salmonella enteritidis*
   b *Shigella sonnei*
   c *Bacillus cereus*
   d *Escherichia coli*

221 An organism recovered from a sputum has the following characteristics:

culture:	growth at 7 days on Lowenstein-Jensen agar, incubated under aerobic conditions with CO_2 at 35°C
Gram stain:	delicate branching gram-positive bacilli ※
acid-fast stain:	branching, filamentous, "partially" acid-fast bacterium

These results are consistent with which of the following genera?

   a *Nocardia*
   b *Mycobacterium*
   c *Actinomyces*
   d *Streptomyces*

222 The best procedure to differentiate *Listeria monocytogenes* from *Corynebacterium* species is:

    a catalase
    b motility at 25°C
    c motility at 35°C
    d Gram stain

223 Establishing the pathogenicity of a microorganism isolated from a child's throat and identified as *Corynebacterium diphtheria* would depend upon:

    a the morphological appearance as revealed by Gram stain
    b the type of hemolysis on blood agar
    c a positive toxigenicity test (PCR test)
    d the appearance of growth on Tinsdale tellurite agar

224 Which feature distinguishes *Erysipelothrix rhusiopathiae* from other clinically significant non-spore-forming, gram-positive, facultatively anaerobic bacilli?

    a "tumbling" motility – Listeria
    b beta-hemolysis
    c more pronounced motility at 25°C than 37°C – Listeria
    d H_2S production ✶ERYSIPELOTHRIX RHUSIOPATHIAE – only gram ⊕ rod that produces H_2S on TSI agar

✶✶

225 *Listeria* can be confused with some streptococci because of its hemolysis and because it is:

    a nonmotile
    b catalase negative   ✶✶   Listeria = beta-hemolytic esculin ⊕
    c oxidase positive
    d esculin positive

226 Fluid from a cutaneous black lesion was submitted for routine bacterial culture. After 18 hours of incubation at 35°C there was no growth on MacConkey agar, but 3+ growth on sheep blood agar. The colonies were nonhemolytic, nonmotile, 4-5 mm in diameter and off-white with a ground glass appearance. Each colony had an irregular edge with comma-shaped outgrowths that stood up like "beaten egg whites" when gently lifted with an inoculating needle. A Gram stain of a typical colony showed large, gram-positive rectangular bacilli. The organism is **most** likely:

    a *Clostridium perfringens*   box car
    b *Aeromonas hydrophila*   "medusa head"
    c *Bacillus anthracis*
    d *Mycobacterium marinum*

227 A branching gram-positive, partially acid-fast organism is isolated from a bronchial washing on a 63-year-old woman receiving chemotherapy. The organism does **not** hydrolyze casein, tyrosine or xanthine. The **most** likely identification is:

    a *Actinomadura madurae*
    b *Nocardia caviae*
    c *Streptomyces somaliensis*
    d *Nocardia asteroides* – doesn't use casein

Anaerobes

228 The characteristic that is **most** commonly associated with the presence of strict anaerobic bacteria and can be taken as presumptive evidence of their presence in a clinical specimen is the:

 a presence of a single bacterial species
 b production of gas in a thioglycollate broth culture
 c growth on a blood agar plate incubated in an anaerobic jar
 d presence of a foul, putrid odor from tissue specimens and cultures

anaerobes = SMELL
polymicrobic

229 Gram stain of a thigh wound showed many gram-positive spore-forming bacilli. The specimen was placed on brain heart infusion blood agar and incubated aerobically at 35°C for 3 days. At the end of that time, the plates showed no growth. The **most** likely explanation is that some of the specimen should have been incubated:

 a on chocolate agar
 b for 5 days
 c under 5% CO_2
 d anaerobically

230 An aspirate of a deep wound was plated on blood agar plates aerobically and anaerobically. At 24 hours there was growth on the anaerobic plate only. The next step in the evaluation of this culture is to:

 a reincubate for another 24 hours
 b begin organism identification
 c issue the final report
 d set up a Bauer-Kirby sensitivity

231 Anaerobic infections differ from aerobic infections in which of the following?

 a they usually respond favorably with aminoglycoside therapy
 b they usually arise from exogenous sources
 c they are usually polymicrobic
 d Gram stains of specimens are less helpful in diagnosis

232 The following growth results were observed on media inoculated with a foot abscess aspirate and incubated in 3%-5% CO_2.

MLS ONLY

SBA:	2+ large gray colonies
PEA:	no growth
chocolate:	3+ large gray colonies
MacConkey:	3+ lactose fermenters
trypticase soy broth:	gram-negative bacilli and gram-positive bacilli

Biochemicals were set up on the colonies from the MacConkey agar plate. What should the microbiologist do next?

 a set up biochemicals on the colonies from SBA
 b send out final report to the physician after biochemicals are interpreted
 c subculture TSB to SBA aerobic and SBA anaerobic
 d test colonies on chocolate agar with hemin and NAD

233 Which of the following pairs of organisms usually grow on kanamycin, vancomycin, laked blood agar?

 a *Bacteroides* and *Prevotella*
 b *Mobiluncus* and *Gardnerella*
 c *Porphyromonas* and *Enterococcus*
 d *Veillonella* and *Capnocytophaga*

234 Acceptable specimens for culture of anaerobic bacteria that cause disease include:

 a abscesses
 b gingival swabs
 c skin swabs   *> too much normal flora*
 d vaginal swabs

235 *Propionibacterium acnes* is **most** often associated with:

    a normal oral flora
    b post-antibiotic diarrhea   ✳ ✳
    c tooth decay
    d blood culture contamination — *normal skin flora*

236 The etiologic agent of botulism is:

    a highly motile
    b non-spore-forming
    c *Clostridium perfringens*
    d an exotoxin producer

237 A strict anaerobe that produces terminal spores is:

    a *Clostridium tetani*
    b *Corynebacterium diphtheriae*
    c *Bacillus anthracis*
    d *Propionibacterium acnes*

238 An anaerobic, spore-forming, nonmotile, gram-positive bacillus isolated from a foot wound is **most** likely;

    a *Actinomyces israelii* – *no spores*
    b *Clostridium perfringens*
    c *Bacillus subtilis* – *aerobic*
    d *Eubacterium lentum* – *no spores*

239 The lab has been using a latex agglutination assay to detect *Clostridium difficile* in stools, which
MLS ONLY
    identifies a nontoxin cell wall antigen. The lab is considering adoption of an EIA method that detects *Clostridium difficile* toxin A. Which of the following would provide the best comparison?

    a latex agglutination vs culture on cycloserine cefoxitin-egg-fructose agar
    b latex agglutination vs EIA vs cell culture cytotoxin assay
    c EIA vs culture on cycloserine cefoxitin-egg-fructose agar
    d EIA vs cell culture cytotoxin assay

240 The reverse CAMP test, lecithinase production, <u>double zone hemolysis,</u> and Gram stain morphology are all useful criteria in the identification of:

    a *Clostridium perfringens*
    b *Streptococcus agalactiae*
    c *Propionibacterium acnes*
    d *Bacillus anthracis*

241 Which one of the following anaerobes is inhibited by sodium polyanethol sulfonate (SPS)?
MLS ONLY

    a *Bacteroides fragilis*
    b *Propionibacterium acnes*
    c *Peptostreptococcus anaerobius*
    d *Veillonella parvula*

242 At the present time *Clostridium difficile* toxin can be detected by:
MLS ONLY

    a fluorescent staining
    b EIA
    c latex agglutination
    d high-pressure liquid chromatography

243 An anaerobic gram-positive bacilli with subterminal spores was isolated from a peritoneal abscess. The **most** likely identification of this organism is:

    a *Bacillus cereus* – *not anaerobic*
    b *Clostridium septicum* – *subterminal spores*
    c *Eubacterium lentum* ⎱ *non - spore producers*
    d *Bifidobacterium dentium*

244 The **most** meaningful laboratory procedure in confirming the diagnosis of clinical botulism is:

  a demonstration of toxin in the patient's serum, *feces, vomit or gastric contents*
  b recovery of *Clostridium botulinum* from suspected food   ✳ ✳
  c recovery of *Clostridium botulinum* from the patient's stool
  d Gram stain of suspected food for gram-positive, sporulating bacilli

245 A stool sample is sent to the laboratory for culture to rule out *Clostridium difficile*. What media should the microbiologist use and what is the appearance of the organisms on this media?

  a BBE: colonies turn black   ✳
  b *Brucella* agar: red pigmented colonies
  c CCFA: yellow, ground glass colonies – LF
  d CNA: double zone hemolytic colonies

246 A Gram stain of a necrotic wound specimen showed large gram-positive bacilli. There was 3+ growth on anaerobic media only, with colonies producing a double zone of hemolysis. To identify the organism, the microbiologist should:

  a determine if the organism ferments glucose
  b perform the oxidase test
  c set up egg yolk agar plate - *lecithinase* ⊕
  d test for bile tolerance

247 A patient has a suspected diagnosis of subacute bacterial endocarditis. His blood cultures grow
MLS ONLY non-spore-forming pleomorphic gram-positive bacilli only in the anaerobic bottle. What test(s) will give a presumptive identification of this microorganism?

  a beta-hemolysis and oxidase
  b catalase and spot indole
  c esculin hydrolysis
  d hydrolysis of gelatin

248 The Gram stain of drainage from a pulmonary sinus tract shows many WBCs and 3+ branching
MLS ONLY gram-positive bacilli. Colonies grow only on anaerobic media after 3 days incubation. They are yellow-tan and have a molar tooth appearance. The **most** likely genus is:

  a *Actinomyces*
  b *Bacteroides*
  c *Fusobacterium*
  d *Nocardia*

249 Which organism is the **most** common anaerobic bacteria isolated from infectious processes of
MLS ONLY soft tissue and anaerobic bacteremia?

  a *Bacteroides fragilis*
  b *Fusobacterium nucleatum*
  c *Porphyromonas asaccharolytica*
  d *Clostridium perfringens*

250 Which of the following genera include anaerobic gram-negative nonsporulating bacilli?

  a *Brucella* → *aerobic*, GNR
  b *Pasteurella*
  c *Actinomyces* - *anaerobe*, GPR
  d *Bacteroides* - *anaerobic* GNR *no spores*

251 An organism from a peritoneal abscess is isolated on kanamycin-vancomycin laked blood agar and
MLS ONLY grows black colonies on BBE agar. It is nonpigmented, catalase positive, and indole negative. The genus of this organism is:

  a *Acidominococcus*
  b *Bacteroides*
  c *Porphyromonas*
  d *Prevotella*

252 Which of the following sets of organisms may exhibit a brick red fluorescence?

MLS
ONLY
    a *Porphyromonas asaccharolytica* and *Clostridium ramosum*
    b *Clostridium difficile* and *Fusobacterium* sp
    c *Veillonella parvula* and *Prevotella melaninogenica*
    d *Fusobacterium* sp and *Veillonella parvula*

253 A 1-2 mm translucent, nonpigmented colony, isolated from an anaerobic culture of a lung abscess

MLS
ONLY
after 72 hours, was found to fluoresce brick-red under ultraviolet light. A Gram stain of the organism revealed a coccobacillus that had the following characteristics:

growth in bile:	inhibited
vancomycin:	resistant
kanamycin:	resistant
colistin:	susceptible
catalase:	negative
esculin hydrolysis:	negative
indole:	negative

The identification of this isolate is:

    a *Bacteroides ovatus*
    b *Prevotella oralis*
    c *Prevotella melaninogenica*
    d *Porphyromonas asaccharolytica*

254 A thin, gram-negative bacillus with tapered ends isolated from an empyema specimen grew

MLS
ONLY
only on anaerobic sheep blood agar. It was found to be indole positive, lipase negative, and was inhibited by 20% bile. The **most** probable identification of this isolate would be:

    a *Bacteroides distasonis*
    b *Prevotella melaninogenica*
    c *Fusobacterium nucleatum*
    d *Clostridium septicum*

255 Which one of the following anaerobes would be negative for indole?

MLS
ONLY
    a *Bacteroides fragilis*
    b *Fusobacterium nucleatum*
    c *Porphyromonas asaccharolytica*
    d *Proteus mirabilis*

256 The presence of 20% bile in agar will allow growth of:

MLS
ONLY
    a *Fusobacterium necrophorum*
    b *Bacteroides ovatus*
    c *Prevotella melaninogenica*
    d *Porphyromonas gingivalis*

257 A control strain of *Clostridium* should be used an anaerobe jar to assure:
    obligate anaerobe
    a that plate media is working
    b that an anaerobic environment is achieved
    c that the jar is filled with a sufficient number of plates
    d that the indicator strip is checked

258 Which one of the following organisms could be used as the positive quality control test for

MLS
ONLY
lecithinase on egg yolk agar?

    a *Bacteroides fragilis*
    b *Fusobacterium necrophorum*
    c *Clostridium perfringens*
    d *Clostridium sporogenes*

Fungi

259 The major features by which molds are routinely identified are:

    a macroscopic characteristics and microscopic morphology
    b biochemical reactions and microscopic morphology
    c macroscopic characteristics and selective media
    d specialized sexual reproductive structures

260 A sputum specimen from a patient with a known *Klebsiella pneumoniae* infection is received in the laboratory for fungus culture. The proper procedure for handling this specimen is to:

    a reject the current specimen and request a repeat culture when the bacterial organism is no longer present
    b incubate culture tubes at room temperature in order to inhibit the bacterial organism
    c include media that have cycloheximide and chloramphenicol added to inhibit bacterial organisms and saprophytic fungi
    d perform a direct PAS stain; if no fungal organisms are seen, reject the specimen

261 Many fungal infections are transmitted to man via inhalation of infectious structures. Which of the following is usually contracted in this manner?

    a *Sporothrix schenckii*
    b *Trichophyton rubrum*
    c *Malassezia furfur*
    d *Histoplasma capsulatum* — *most frequently transmitted by inhalation*

262 A smear of skin tissue reveals fluorescent septate hyphae. The smear was prepared using:

    a acridine orange
    b calcofluor white — *fungi (binds to cellulose + chitin in cell walls)*
    c auramine rhodamine
    d periodic acid-Schiff

263 Antifungal susceptibility tests for yeasts are:
MLS ONLY

    a performed routinely
    b highly reproducible
    c not clinically relevant
    d more useful in identifying resistant strains

264 In preparing an India ink slide, the technician should ensure that the:
MLS ONLY

    a CSF is unspun
    b sputum is well mixed
    c proper amount of reagent is added
    d slide is properly dried first

265 An organism that demonstrates budding yeast cells with wide capsules in an India ink preparation of spinal fluid is probably:

    a *Cryptococcus neoformans* — *capsules*
    b *Histoplasma capsulatum*
    c *Blastomyces dermatitidis*
    d *Candida albicans*

266 The formation of germ tubes presumptively identifies:

    a *Candida tropicalis*
    b *Candida parapsilosis*
    c *Candida glabrata*
    d *Candida albicans*

267 An HIV-positive patient began to show signs of meningitis. A spinal fluid was collected and cultured for bacteria and fungus. A budding, encapsulated yeast was recovered. Which organism is consistent with this information?

   a *Cryptococcus neoformans* – *polysaccharide capsule* *used birdseed agar – forms brown colonies*
   b *Aspergillus fumigatus*
   c *Microsporum audouinii*
   d *Sporothrix schenckii*

268 *MLS ONLY* Staib medium (birdseed agar) is useful in the identification of which of the following?

   a *Candida albicans*
   b *Candida glabrata*
   c *Saccharomyces cerevisiae*
   d *Cryptococcus neoformans*

269 Gram stain examination of a CSF specimen indicates the presence of yeast-like cells with gram-positive granular inclusions. Which of the following techniques should be used next to assist in the identification of this organism?

   a 10% KOH – *nail decomposer*
   b lactophenol cotton blue
   c India ink – *fungi stain / shows C. Neoformans' capsule*
   d periodic acid-Schiff

270 *MLS ONLY* The one characteristic by which an unknown *Cryptococcus* species can be identified as *Cryptococcus neoformans* is:

   a appearance of yellow colonies
   b positive urease test
   c presence of a capsule
   d positive phenol oxidase test

271 *MLS ONLY* A urine culture from a patient with a urinary tract infection yields a yeast with the following characteristics:

   failure to produce germ tubes
   hyphae not formed on cornmeal agar
   urease-negative
   assimilates trehalose

   The **most** likely identification is:

   a *Saccharomyces cerevisiae*
   b *Cryptococcus laurentii*
   c *Candida pseudotropicalis*
   d *Candida glabrata*

272 A yeast isolate from a CSF specimen produced the following results:

   India ink: no encapsulated yeast cells – *not C. Neoformans*
   cryptococcal antigen: negative
   urea: negative
   germ tube: negative – *not C. albicans*

   What should the technologist do next to identify this organism?

   a inoculate bird seed agar
   b ascospore stain
   c cycloheximide susceptibility
   d carbohydrate assimilation

273 The recovery of some *Cryptococcus* species may be compromised if the isolation media contains:

    (a) cycloheximide – *fungi inhibitor*
    b gentamicin
    c chloramphenicol
    d penicillin

274 A neonatal blood culture collected through a catheter grows a small yeast. Microscopically, the yeast appear round at one end, with a budlike structure on a broad base at the other end. Growth is enhanced around olive oil-saturated discs. The organism isolated is:

    a *Candida tropicalis*
    b *Malassezia furfur*
    c *Candida lipolytica*
    d *Malassezia pachydermatis*

275 Two blood cultures are positive for yeast from a patient with an intravenous catheter. One culture grew *Candida albicans*, while the other grew *Candida krusei*. Which medium should the technologist use to subculture the blood bottles to in order to verify that the cultures are pure?

    a Sabouraud dextrose agar
    b potato dextrose agar
    c cornmeal agar
    d chromogenic agar

276 Quality control testing of CHROMagar™ *Candida* medium shows very weakly colored colonies after incubation at 25°C, ambient atmosphere for 48 hours. The technologist should:

    a repeat the quality control tests to verify results
    b repeat the quality control tests but incubate at 35°C
    c repeat the quality control tests using new subcultures of the quality control organisms
    d discard this lot of CHROMagar™ and repeat the quality control tests on a new lot number

277 The morphological characteristics of a yeast grown in rabbit plasma are shown in the image:

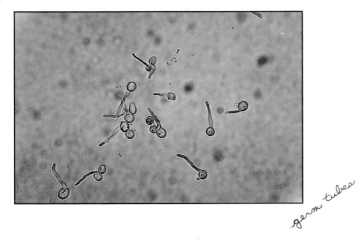

germ tubes

The **most** likely identification of this yeast is:
    a *Candida tropicalis*
    b *Candida krusei*
    (c) *Candida albicans*
    d *Candida glabrata*

278 The **most** sensitive test for the initial diagnosis of cryptococcal disease is:

    a India ink
    b Gram stain
    (c) cryptococcal antigen
    d Giemsa stain

279 Which of the following statements concerning the germ tube test is true?

    a using a heavy inoculum enhances the rapid production of germ tubes
    b germ tubes should be read after 2 hours incubation at 25°C *37° C.*
    c *Candida albicans* and *Candida tropicalis* can be used as positive and negative controls, respectively
    d serum will be stable for 1 year if stored at 4°C prior to use

280 Which of the following procedures should be performed to confirm that an unknown mold is one of the pathogenic dimorphic fungi:

    a animal inoculation
    b culture conversion to yeast form
    c demonstration of sexual and asexual reproduction
    d serological studies

dimorphic fungi:
RT: mold
37° (body temp): yeast
e.g., COCCIDIOIDES IMMITUS
C. ALBICANS SPOROTHRIX SCHENCKII
HISTOPLASMA CAPSULATUM

281 Lab workers should always work under a biological safety hood when working with cultures of:

    a *Streptococcus pyogenes*
    b *Staphylococcus aureus*
    c *Candida albicans*
    d *Coccidioides immitis* — *arthroconidia highly infectious when inhaled*
    causes valley fever (SW US) lung disease

282 *(MLS ONLY)* Structures important in the microscopic identification of *Coccidioides immitis* are:

    a irregular staining, barrel-shaped arthrospores
    b tuberculate, thick-walled macroconidia
    c thick-walled sporangia containing sporangiospores
    d small pyriform microconidia

283 *(MLS ONLY)* Which of the following is the **most** useful morphological feature in identifying the mycelial phase of *Histoplasma capsulatum*?

    a arthrospores every other cell
    b 2-5 µm microspores
    c 8-14 µm tuberculate macroconidia
    d 5-7 µm nonseptate macroconidia

284 *(MLS ONLY)* A mold grown at 25°C exhibited delicate septate hyaline hyphae and many conidiophores extending at right angles from the hyphae. Oval, 2-5 µm conidia were formed at the end of the conidiophores giving a flowerlike appearance. In some areas "sleeves" of spores could be found along the hyphae as well. A 37°C culture of this organism produced small, cigar-shaped yeast cells. This organism is **most** likely:

    a *Histoplasma capsulatum*
    b *Sporothrix schenckii*
    c *Blastomyces dermatitidis*
    d *Acremonium falciforme*

285 Which of the following is a <u>dimorphic fungus</u>? *See # 280*

    a *Sporothrix schenckii*
    b *Candida albicans*
    c *Cryptococcus neoformans*
    d *Aspergillus fumigatus*

286 A fungal isolate from the sputum of a patient with a pulmonary infection is suspected to be
MLS
ONLY *Histoplasma capsulatum.* Tuberculate macroconidia were seen on the hyphae of the mold phase,
which was isolated at room temperature on Sabouraud dextrose agar containing chloramphenicol
and cycloheximide (SDA-CC). A parallel set of cultures incubated at 35°C showed bacterial growth
on SDA, but no growth on SDA-CC. Which of the following is the appropriate course of action?

   a repeat subculture of the mold phase to tubes of moist SDA-CC, incubate at 35°C
   b subculture the mold phase to tubes of moist BHI-blood media, incubate at 25°C
   c subculture the mold phase to moist BHI-blood media, incubate at 35°C
   d perform animal inoculation studies

287 Skin scrapings obtained from the edge of a crusty wrist lesion were found to contain thick-walled,
MLS
ONLY spherical yeast cells (8-15 μm in diameter) that had single buds with a wide base of attachment.
Microscopic examination of the room temperature isolate from this specimen would probably
reveal the presence of:

   a "rosette-like" clusters of pear-shaped conidia at the tips of delicate conidiophores
   b thick-walled, round to pear-shaped tuberculate macroconidia
   c numerous conidia along the length of hyphae in a "sleevelike" arrangement
   d round or pear-shaped small conidia attached to conidiophores of irregular lengths

288 Examination of a fungal culture from a bronchial washing reveals white, cottony aerial mycelium.
MLS
ONLY A tease preparation in lactophenol cotton blue shows the structures shown in the image:

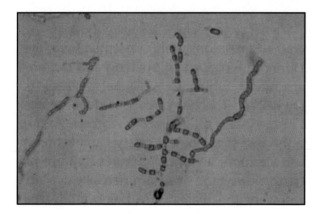

The **most** rapid test for definitive identification is:
   a nucleic acid probe
   b animal inoculation
   c exoantigen test
   d slide culture

289 *Penicillium* species is isolated from a bone marrow culture of a patient that travelled to southeast
MLS
ONLY Asia. After 7 days the isolate produces a red pigment that diffuses into the medium. The
technologist should:

   a prepare a slide culture
   b repeat the tease preparation
   c transfer a colony to BHI at 35°C
   d perform a nucleic acid probe

290 The microscopic structures that are **most** useful in the identification of dermatophytes are:

MLS ONLY

   a septate and branching hyphae
   b racquet and pectinate hyphae
   c chlamydospores and microconidia
   d macroconidia and microconidia

291 Which of the following is **most** often used to prepare a slide from a plate culture of a dermatophyte for microscopic observation?

   (a) lactophenol cotton blue
   b potassium hydroxide
   c iodine solution
   d Gram stain

DERMATOPHYTE : pathogenic fungus of the skin

TRICOPHYTON

292 A specimen of hair that fluoresced under a Wood lamp was obtained from a child with low-grade scaling lesions of the scalp. Cultures revealed a fungus with mycelium and very few macroconidia or microconidia. This fungus is **most** likely:

MLS ONLY

   a *Microsporum gypseum*
   b *Microsporum audouinii*
   c *Trichophyton tonsurans*
   d *Epidermophyton floccosum*

293 Which of the following is the best aid in the identification of *Epidermophyton floccosum* macroconidia?

MLS ONLY

   a parallel side walls with at least 10 cells
   b spindle-shaped spore with thin walls
   c spindle-shaped spore, thick walls and distinct terminal knob with echinulations
   d smooth walls, club-shaped

294 Culture of a strand of hair, that fluoresced yellow-green when examined with a Wood lamp, produced a slow-growing, flat gray colony with a salmon-pink reverse. Microscopic examination demonstrated racquet hyphae, pectinate bodies, chlamydospores, and a few abortive or bizarre-shaped macroconidia. The **most** probable identification of this isolate is:

MLS ONLY

   a *Epidermophyton floccosum*
   b *Microsporum canis*
   c *Microsporum audouinii*
   d *Trichophyton rubrum*

295 On day 3 of a fungal culture, grayish cottony growth is observed that is filling the container. The **most** likely mold isolated is a:

   a dermatophyte
   b dimorphic mold
   (c) zygomycete - *grow rapidly; fill container with cottony growth*
   d dematiaceous mold

296 The appropriate specimen for the diagnosis of mucormycosis is:

hyphae grow in and around blood vessels

   a nasal swab
   b sputum
   c sinus washing
   (d) eschar biopsy

297 *Penicillium* can best be separated from *Aspergillus* by:

MLS ONLY

   a color of the colonies
   b optimum growth temperature
   c presence of rhizoids
   d arrangement of the conidia on the conidiophore

298 A fungus superficially resembles *Penicillium* species but may be differentiated because its phialides
MLS are long and tapering and bend away from the central axis. The **most** probable identification is:
ONLY

    a *Exophiala*
    b *Acremonium*
    c *Cladosporium*
    d *Paecilomyces*

299 An isolate from a cornea infection had the following culture results:
MLS
ONLY

    Sabouraud dextrose: white & cottony at 2 days, rose color at 6 days
    slide culture: slender sickle shape macroconidia

The **most** likely organism is :

    a *Acremonium*
    b *Aspergillus*
    c *Fusarium*
    d *Geotrichum*

300 In the USA, the **most** common organism causing eumycotic mycetoma is:
MLS
ONLY

    a *Pseudallescheria boydii*
    b *Nocardia brasiliensis*
    c *Blastomyces dermatitidis*
    d *Aspergillus fumigatus*

301 Crust from a cauliflower-like lesion on the hand exhibited brown spherical bodies 6-12 μm in
MLS diameter when examined microscopically. After 3 weeks of incubation at room temperature, a
ONLY slow-growing black mold grew on Sabouraud dextrose agar. Microscopic examination revealed
Cladosporium, *Phialophora* and *Fonsecaea* types of sporulation. The probable identification of this
organism is:

    a *Fonsecaea pedrosoi*
    b *Pseudallescheria boydii*
    c *Phialophora verrucosa*
    d *Cladosporium carrionii*

302 Pus from a draining fistula on a foot was submitted for culture. Gross examination of the
MLS specimen revealed the presence of a small (0.8 mm in diameter), yellowish, oval granule. Direct
ONLY microscopic examination of the crushed granule showed hyphae 3-4 μm in diameter and the
presence of chlamydospores at the periphery. After 2 days a cottony, white mold was seen
that turned gray with a gray to black reverse after a few days. When viewed microscopically,
moderately large hyaline septate hyphae with long or short conidiophores, each with a single
pear-shaped conidium, 5-7 × 8-10 μm, were seen. The **most** likely identification is:

    a *Exophiala jeanselmei*
    b *Fonsecaea pedrosoi*
    c *Pseudallescheria boydii*
    d *Cladosporium carrionii*

303 In processing clinical specimens and fungal isolates, laboratory workers may contract systemic
fungal infections through:

    a inhalation – *aerosal spray*
    b ingestion
    c skin contact
    d insect vector

Mycobacteria – *waxy cell wall*

304   A sputum specimen received at 8 AM for an AFB smear reveals acid-fast bacilli. An additional sputum is submitted that afternoon. This specimen was concentrated by the NALC-sodium hydroxide method and inoculated on 2 Lowenstein-Jensen slants and held for 8 weeks at 35°C in 5%-10% CO_2. No growth occurs. The best explanation is that:

     a   the hypochlorite technique was not used
     b   an improper specimen was submitted for culture – *early morning specimen optimal*
     c   improper media was used for culture
     d   cultures were held for an insufficient period of time

305   The preferred carbon source for mycobacteria is:

     a   glycerol
     b   glucose
     c   fatty acids
     d   casein hydrolysate

         ✷✷ *MYCOBACTERIA = waxy cell wall*
                                  AFB stain
                                    glycerol carbohydrate source
                                    slow grower (12 weeks)

306   A first morning sputum is received for culture of mycobacteria. It is digested and concentrated by the N-acetyl-L-cysteine alkali method. Two Lowenstein-Jensen slants are incubated in the dark at 35°C with 5%-10% CO_2. The smears reveal acid-fast bacilli, and after 7 days no growth appears on the slants. The best explanation is:

     a   improper specimen submitted
     b   incorrect concentration procedure
     c   exposure to CO_2 prevents growth
     d   cultures held for insufficient length of time – *up to 12 weeks*

307   A first morning sputum specimen is received for acid-fast culture. The specimen is centrifuged, and the sediment is inoculated on 2 Lowenstein-Jensen slants, which are incubated at 35°C in 5%-10% CO_2. After 1 week, the slants show abundant growth over the entire surface. Stains reveal gram-negative bacilli. To avoid this problem:

     a   utilize a medium that inhibits bacterial growth
     b   add sodium hypochlorite to the sediment before inoculation
     c   incubate the tubes at room temperature to retard bacterial growth
     d   decontaminate the specimen with sodium hydroxide ($NaOH$)

308   A first morning sputum is received for culture of acid-fast bacilli. It is digested and concentrated by the N-acetyl-L-cysteine alkali method. Two Sabouraud dextrose slants are incubated in the dark at 35°C with 5%-10% CO_2. The smears reveal acid-fast bacilli, but the slants show no growth after 8 weeks. The explanation is:

     a   improper media used
     b   incorrect concentration procedure used
     c   improper specimen submitted
     d   exposure to CO_2 prevents growth

309   In reviewing the number of *Mycobacterium* isolates for the current year, it was noted that there
MLS ONLY   were 76% fewer isolates than the previous year (115 vs 28). The technologist in charge of the area has documented that the quality control of media, reagents and stains has been acceptable and there has been no gross contamination of the cultures noted. The **most** appropriate course of action to pursue would be:

     a   stop use of commercial media and produce in-house
     b   change to different formulations of egg and agar based media
     c   change over to the Bactec™ system for isolation of *Mycobacterium*
     d   review the digestion and decontamination procedure

310 Which of the following combinations of media provides an egg base, agar base, and a selective egg or agar base media?

    a Lowenstein-Jensen, American Thoracic Society (ATS), Middlebrook 7H11 *(egg base) (agar base)*

    b Lowenstein-Jensen, Middlebrook 7H11, Lowenstein-Jensen Gruft— *selective egg base*

    c Middlebrook 7H10, Petragnani, Lowenstein-Jensen

    d Middlebrook 7H10, Middlebrook 7H11, Mitchison 7H11

311 Which of the following reagents should be used as a mucolytic, alkaline reagent for digestion and decontamination of a sputum for mycobacterial culture?

    a N-acetyl-L-cystine and NaOH - *digestion decontamination*

    b NaOH alone

    c zephiran-trisodium phosphate

    d oxalic acid

312 The function of N-acetyl-L-cysteine in the reagent for acid-fast digestion-decontamination procedure is to:

    a inhibit growth of normal respiratory flora

    b inhibit growth of fungi

    c neutralize the sodium hydroxide

    d liquefy the mucus

313 When staining acid-fast bacilli with Truant auramine-rhodamine stain, potassium permanganate is used as a:

    a decolorizing agent

    b quenching agent— *reduces background fluorescence of cellular debris*

    c mordant

    d dye

314 Middlebrook 7H10 and 7H11 media must be refrigerated in the dark, and incubated in the dark as well. If these conditions are not met, the media may prove toxic for mycobacteria because:

    a carbon dioxide will be released

    b growth factors will be broken down

    c light destroys the ammonium sulfate

    d formaldehyde may be produced → *agar based media*

315 The method used for processing specimens for mycobacterial culture contaminated with *Pseudomonas* is:

    a N-acetyl-L-cystine and NaOH

    b NaOH

    c zephiran-trisodium phosphate

    d oxalic acid *for Pseudomonas contaminated specimens*

316 An AFB broth culture is positive for acid-fast bacilli at 1 week while the agar slant shows no growth. The **most** likely explanation for this is:

    a the organism is a contaminant

    b AFB grow more rapidly in liquid media

    c PANTA was added to the broth

    d the agar slant was incubated in 5% CO_2

317 A bronchial washing is processed for acid-fast bacilli. Which of the following precautions should be taken in order to prevent infection of laboratory personnel?

    a add an equal amount of NALC to the specimen
    b process all specimens under ultraviolet light
    c centrifuge specimen only after the addition of preservative
    (d) process all specimens in a biological safety hood

318 Tubercle bacilli are specifically stained by:

    a crystal violet
    b 1% acid fuchsin   ✶✶
    c methylene blue
    d carbol fuchsin (KINYOUN)

319 The species of mycobacteria that will give a positive niacin test is *Mycobacterium*:
MLS ONLY

    a *leprae*
    b *kansasii*
    c *fortuitum*
    d *tuberculosis*

320 A digested and decontaminated sputum is inoculated into a Bactec™ 12B bottle and incubated in air at 37°C. On day 14, a positive growth index is obtained, and the auramine-rhodamine stain is positive. Broth from the initial bottle is inoculated into one Bactec™ 12B bottle, and one Bactec™ 12B bottle with NAP. After reincubation, the inoculated growth bottle shows an increase in growth index, while the bottle containing NAP shows no increase. The organism cultured from the sputum is **most** likely *Mycobacterium*:
MLS ONLY

    a *marinum*
    b *kansasii*
    c *tuberculosis*
    d *avium-intracellulare*

321 On a culture suspected to be *Mycobacterium tuberculosis*, the **most** important test to perform is:
MLS ONLY

    a catalase production
    b tellurite reduction
    c Tween® 80 hydrolysis
    d niacin production

322 A positive niacin test is **most** characteristic of *Mycobacterium*:
MLS ONLY

    a *chelonae*
    b *marinum*
    c *tuberculosis*
    d *xenopi*

323 Characteristics necessary for the definitive identification of *Mycobacterium tuberculosis* are:
MLS ONLY

    a buff color, slow growth at 37°C, niacin production-positive, nitrate reduction-negative
    b rough colony, slow growth at 37°C, nonpigmented
    c rough, nonpigmented colony, cording positive, niacin production-negative, catalase-negative at pH 7/68°C
    d rough, nonpigmented colony, slow growth at 37°C, niacin production-positive, nitrate reduction-positive

324 A 2-week-old culture of a urine specimen produced a few colonies of acid-fast bacilli, which were
**MLS
ONLY** rough and nonpigmented. The niacin test was weakly positive and the nitrate test was positive.
Which of the following is the **most** appropriate action when a presumptive identification has
been requested as soon as possible?

  a report the organism as presumptive *Mycobacterium tuberculosis*

  b wait a few days and repeat the niacin test; report presumptive *Mycobacterium tuberculosis* if the
     test is more strongly positive

  c subculture the organism and set up the routine battery of biochemicals; notify the physician
     that results will not be available for 3 weeks

  d set up a thiophene-2-carboxylic acid hydrazide (T^2H); if the organism is sensitive, report
     Mycobacterium bovis

325 The disease-producing capacity of *Mycobacterium tuberculosis* depends primarily upon:

  a production of exotoxin

  b production of endotoxin

  (**c**) capacity to withstand intracellular digestion by macrophages ✶✶ *remains dormant for*
  d lack of susceptibility to the myeloperoxidase system   *many years*

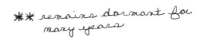

326 Which species of *Mycobacterium* includes a BCG strain used for vaccination against tuberculosis?

  a *tuberculosis*

  (**b**) *bovis* – *weakened (live attenuated)*

  c *kansasii*

  d *fortuitum/chelonae* complex

327 AFB smear positive respiratory specimens may be reliably identified as *Mycobacterium tuberculosis*
the same day the smear was read by:

  a cording seen on the AFB smear

  (**b**) nucleic acid amplification (*PCR*)

  c QuantiFERON®-TB test

  d DNA probes

328 A physician calls the laboratory to verify a result of *Mycobacterium tuberculosis*, stating that the
**MLS
ONLY** clinical history of the patient is not compatible with tuberculosis. On review of the patient's
culture, the smear was negative and the culture became positive at 5 weeks in the broth culture
only. Additionally, it was determined that another patient's specimen that was processed the same
day was 4+ AFB on smear and the culture was positive at 10 days for *Mycobacterium tuberculosis*.
The lab should:

  a include a positive control when processing specimens

  b perform molecular fingerprinting on both isolates

  c repeat the nucleic acid probe

  d set up susceptibility tests

(**329**) Which of the following is considered a primary drug for the treatment of
Mycobacterium tuberculosis?

  (**a**) rifampin

  b kanamycin

  c rifabutin

  d ethionamide

330 An unusual number of *Mycobacterium gordonae* have been isolated. The **most** likely source is:
**MLS
ONLY**

  a an outbreak of infections due to *Mycobacterium gordonae*

  b contamination by water organisms

  c contamination of commercial Lowenstein-Jensen tubes

  d contamination of the specimen collection containers

331 When grown in the dark, yellow to orange pigmentation of the colonies is usually demonstrated by:
   a *Mycobacterium tuberculosis*
   b *Mycobacterium kansasii*
   c *Mycobacterium fortuitum*
   d *Mycobacterium scrofulaceum*

332 The mycobacteria that produce a deep yellow or orange pigment both in the dark and light are:

   a photochromogens
   b scotochromogens
   c nonchromogens
   d rapid growers

333 Mycobacteria that produce pigment only after exposure to light are classified as:

   a photochromogens
   b scotochromogens
   c rapid growers
   d nonchromogens

334 In a suspected case of Hansen disease (leprosy), a presumptive diagnosis is established by:

   a isolation of organisms on Lowenstein-Jensen medium
   b detection of weakly acid-fast bacilli in infected tissue
   c isolation of organisms in a cell culture
   d detection of niacin production by the isolated bacterium

335 The best medium for culture of *Mycobacterium tuberculosis* is:

   a Bordet-Gengou agar
   b Loeffler medium
   c Lowenstein-Jensen medium (*egg base*)
   d cystine blood agar

336 A 27-year-old scuba diver has an abrasion on his left thigh. A culture of this wound grew an
acid-fast organism at 30°C. This isolate **most** likely is:

   a *Mycobacterium chelonae*
   b *Mycobacterium marinum*
   c *Mycobacterium tuberculosis*
   d *Mycobacterium xenopi*

337 A nonchromogen that grows best at 42°C and is highly resistant to antibiotics is:
   a *Mycobacterium chelonae*
   b *Mycobacterium marinum*
   c *Mycobacterium tuberculosis*
   d *Mycobacterium xenopi*

338 Photochromogens produce pigment when:

   a kept in the dark at 22°C
   b exposed to light for 1 hour
   c grown in the presence of CO_2
   d incubated with x-ray film

339 An acid-fast bacillus recovered from an induced sputum had the following characteristics:

MLS
ONLY

pigmentation:	yellow in the dark, turning a deeper yellow-orange after 2 weeks of light exposure
nitrate reduction:	negative
Tween® hydrolysis:	positive at 5-10 days
urease:	negative

Based on this information, the organism is **most** likely *Mycobacterium*:

a *scrofulaceum*
b *gordonae*
c *szulgai*
d *flavescens*

340 Which of the following characteristics best distinguishes *Mycobacterium scrofulaceum* from *Mycobacterium gordonae*?

MLS
ONLY

a iron uptake
b Tween® hydrolysis
c good growth at 25°C
d niacin production

341 Differentiation of *Mycobacterium avium* from *Mycobacterium intracellulare* can be accomplished by:

a nitrate reduction test
b Tween® hydrolysis test
c resistance to 10 μg thiophene-2-carboxylic acid hydrazide (TCH)
(d) DNA probe

342 Which one of the following species of *Mycobacterium* does **not** usually fluoresce on fluorochrome stain?

(a) *Mycobacterium fortuitum* - rapid grower ✳
b *Mycobacterium tuberculosis*
c *Mycobacterium ulcerans*
d *Mycobacterium bovis*

343 A mycobacterial isolate that causes multiple skin nodules, grows at 30°C and requires hemin for growth is *Mycobacterium*:

MLS
ONLY

a *marinum*
b *genavense*
c *haemophilum*
d *xenopi*

344 AFB smears of a lymph node biopsy from a child are positive. At the end of 8 weeks, the AFB cultures are no growth. To enhance the possibility of recovery of the causative organism, the technologist should:

MLS
ONLY

a incubate the cultures an additional 4 weeks
b add mycobactin J to the media
c transfer the cultures to a 30°C incubator
d subculture the liquid culture to chocolate agar

345 The nitrate test for mycobacteria can be performed with a reagent impregnated paper strip or by the use of standard reagents. In order to quality control the test properly, which of the following should be used for a positive control?

MLS
ONLY

a *Mycobacterium bovis*
b *Mycobacterium gordonae*
c *Mycobacterium tuberculosis*
d *Mycobacterium intracellulare*

Viruses and Other Microorganisms

346 Virus transport medium containing penicillin, gentamicin and amphotericin is used to collect and transport specimens for virus culture because this medium:

    a enables rapid viral growth during the transport time
    (b) inhibits bacterial and fungal growth
    c destroys nonpathogenic viruses
    d inhibits complement-fixing antibodies

347 Which of the following indicates the presence of a viral infection in tissue smears or biopsies?

    a cytopathic effect
    (b) intranuclear inclusions
    c cell lysis
    d mononuclear inflammatory cells

348 Respiratory syncytial virus is best isolated using a(n):

    (a) nasopharyngeal aspirate
    b cough plate   *RSV infects respiratory epithelium*
    c expectorated sputum   *cells*
    d throat swab

349 A urine specimen was submitted for isolation of cytomegalovirus (CMV). The urine was inoculated
MLS ONLY into human fibroblast tissue culture tubes. After 72 hours, no cytopathic effect was observed in the culture tubes. The **most** appropriate course of action is to:

    a incubate the culture tubes for 2-3 weeks longer
    b request a fecal specimen as urine is inappropriate
    c repeat the test using monkey kidney cell culture tubes
    d request CMV serology as CMV cannot be isolated

350 The genus of virus associated with anogenital warts, cervical dysplasia and neoplasia is:
         (cancer)
    (a) herpes simplex virus
    (b) papillomavirus
    c cytomegalovirus
    d coxsackievirus

351 Encephalitis is **most** commonly associated with which of the following viruses?

    a Epstein-Barr
    (b) herpes simplex ✳✳
    c coxsackie B
    d varicella zoster

352 Colds and other acute respiratory diseases are **most** often associated with:

    a Epstein-Barr virus
    (b) adenovirus
    c coxsackie B
    d reovirus

353 The Epstein-Barr virus is associated with which of the following?
MLS ONLY   *(mono)*
    a chickenpox
    b Hodgkin lymphoma
    (c) Burkitt lymphoma
    d smallpox

354 Which organism fails to grow on artificial media or in cell cultures?
MLS ONLY
    a *Chlamydia trachomatis*
    b *Neisseria gonorrhoeae*
    (c) *Treponema pallidum* – *syphillus*
    d herpes simplex virus

355 Darkfield microscopy is can be used to visualize:

MLS ONLY
 a *Pseudomonas aeruginosa*
 b *Streptococcus pneumoniae*
 c *Treponema pallidum*
 d *Legionella pneumophila*

356 A Wright stain on a conjunctival smear from a neonate shows granular cytoplasmic perinuclear
MLS ONLY inclusions. This is **most** indicative of:

 a *Chlamydia trachomatis*
 b herpes simplex virus
 c cytomegalovirus
 d varicella-zoster virus

357 Iodine staining of a McCoy cell monolayer culture of a cervical swab reveals a large brown
MLS ONLY intracytoplasmic inclusion. What is the **most** likely infecting organism?

 a cytomegalovirus
 b *Ehrlichia chaffeensis*
 c *Chlamydia trachomatis*
 d *Rickettsia prowazekii*

358 Which compound, detected by Lugol iodine, is used in the nonimmunologic detection of
MLS ONLY *Chlamydia trachomatis* in cell culture?

 a DNA
 b RNA
 c glycogen
 d DNA polymerase

359 Microorganisms resembling L-forms have been isolated from the blood of patients treated with
MLS ONLY antibiotics that:

 a complex with flagellar protein
 b interfere with cell membrane function
 c inhibit protein synthesis
 d interfere with cell wall synthesis

360 Relapsing fever in humans is caused by:

 a *Borrelia recurrentis* ✳
 b *Brucella abortus*
 c *Leptospira interrogans*
 d *Spirillum minus*

361 Psittacosis is transmissible to man via contact with: *CHLAMYDOPHILA PSITTACI*
 inhalation from parrots

 a insects
 b birds (*parrots*)
 c cattle
 d dogs

362 Chlamydial infections have been implicated in:

 a urethritis and conjunctivitis
 b gastroenteritis and urethritis
 c neonatal pneumonia and gastroenteritis
 d neonatal meningitis and conjunctivitis

363 Mycoplasmas differ from bacteria in that they:

 a do not cause disease in humans
 b cannot grow in artificial inanimate media
 c lack cell walls - *cannot be gram stained*
 d are not serologically antigenic

364 A jaundiced 7-year-old boy, with a history of playing in a pond in a rat-infested area, has a urine
MLS
ONLY specimen submitted for a direct darkfield examination. Several spiral organisms are seen. Which of
the following organisms would **most** likely be responsible for the patient's condition?

   a *Spirillum minus*
   b *Streptobacillus moniliformis*
   c *Listeria monocytogenes*
   d *Leptospira interrogans*

365 A jaundiced 7-year-old boy, with a history of playing in a pond in a rat-infested area, has a urine
MLS
ONLY specimen submitted for a direct dark-field examination. No organisms are seen in the specimen.
Which medium should be inoculated in an attempt to isolate the suspected organism?

   a blood cysteine dextrose
   b PPLO agar
   c Fletcher semisolid
   d chopped meat glucose

366 Which of the following is a growth requirement for the isolation of *Leptospira*?
MLS
ONLY
   a an atmosphere of 10% CO_2
   b an incubation temperature of 4°C
   c 4-5 day incubation
   d medium containing 10% serum plus fatty acids

367 Blood cultures from a case of suspected leptospiremia should be drawn:
MLS
ONLY
   a between 10 PM and 2 AM
   b in the first 7-10 days of infection
   c during febrile periods, late in the course of the disease
   d after the first 10 days of illness

368 What material should be used to prepare slides for direct smear examination for virus detection by
MLS
ONLY special stains or FA technique?

   a vesicular fluid
   b leukocytes from the edge of the lesion
   c the top portion of the vesicle
   d epithelial cells from the base of the lesion

369 A 29-year-old man is seen for recurrence of a purulent urethral discharge 10 days after the successful
MLS
ONLY treatment of culture proven gonorrhea. The **most** likely etiology of his urethritis is:

   a *Mycoplasma hominis*
   b *Chlamydia trachomatis*
   c *Trichomonas vaginalis*
   d *Neisseria gonorrhoeae*

370 *Ureaplasma urealyticum* are difficult to grow in the laboratory on routine media because of their
MLS
ONLY requirement for:

   a sterols
   b horse blood
   c ferric pyrophosphate
   d surfactant such as Tween® 80

371 A cell culture line used for the recovery of *Chlamydia trachomatis* from clinical specimens is:

   a HeLa 229   ** also buffalo green monkey kidney cells
   b Hep-2
   c BHK-21
   ⓓ McCoy cells

372 *Rickettsiae* infecting man multiply preferentially within which of the following cells?
MLS
ONLY
   a reticuloendothelial
   b hepatic
   c renal tubule
   d endothelial

Parasites

373 Artifacts found in a stool specimen that can be confused with ova or cysts are:

   a partially digested meat fibers
   b degenerated cells from the gastrointestinal mucosa
   c dried chemical crystals
   (d) pollen grains

374 Polyvinyl alcohol used in the preparation of permanently stained smears of fecal material:
MLS
ONLY
   a concentrates eggs
   b dissolves artifacts
   c serves as an adhesive
   d enhances stain penetration

375 The method of choice to detect *Acanthamoeba* sp from corneal ulcer scrapings is:
MLS
ONLY
   a Novy, MacNeal and Nicolle (NNN) medium
   b culture on McCoy cells
   c direct exam
   d blood agar flooded with a 24-hour growth of *E coli*

376 Primary amoebic encephalitis may be caused by:
MLS
ONLY
   a *Entamoeba coli*
   b *Dientamoeba fragilis*
   c *Endolimax nana*
   d *Naegleria fowleri*

377 A formed stool is received in the laboratory at 3 AM for ova and parasite exam. The night shift
MLS
ONLY technologist is certain that the workload will prevent examination of the specimen until 6 AM
when the next shift arrives. The technologist should:

   a request that a new specimen be collected after 6 AM
   b perform a zinc sulfate floatation procedure for eggs and hold the remaining specimen at room
      temperature
   c examine a direct prep for trophozoites and freeze the remaining specimen
   d preserve the specimen in formalin until it can be examined

378 A batch of trichrome-stained slides for ova and parasite examination contains numerous minute
MLS
ONLY crystals, which totally obscure the microscopic field. Which of the following measures is the **most**
appropriate remedial action?

   a change the Schaudinn fixative, remove coverslips and restain
   b change the acid alcohol and restain
   c remove coverslips and remount using fresh Permount™ or similar medium
   d change the iodine alcohol solution to obtain a strong tea-colored solution, restain

379 The advantage of thick blood smears for malarial parasites is to:
MLS
ONLY
   a improve staining of the organisms
   b improve detection of the organisms
   c remove RBC artifacts
   d remove platelets

380 Multifocal brain lesion in AIDS patients is commonly caused by:

   (a) *Toxoplasma gondii* brain lesions in AIDS patients
   b *Pneumocystis jiroveci*   **✳✳**
   c *Cryptosporidium parvum*
   d *Giardia lamblia*

381 A 44-year-old man was admitted to the hospital following a 2-week history of low-grade fever,
MYS
ONLY malaise and anorexia. Examination of a Giemsa stain revealed many intraerythrocytic parasites.
Further history revealed frequent camping trips near Martha's Vineyard and Nantucket Island,
but no travel outside the continental United States. This parasite could easily be confused with:

a *Trypanosoma cruzi*
b *Trypanosoma rhodesiense/gambiense*
c *Plasmodium falciparum*
d *Leishmania donovani*

382 A patient is suspected of having amebic dysentery. Upon microscopic examination of a fresh fecal
specimen for ova and parasites, the following data were obtained:

> a trophozoite of 25 μm
> progressive, unidirectional crawl
> evenly distributed peripheral chromatin
> finely granular cytoplasm

This information probably indicates:

a *Entamoeba coli* – *irregular chromatin; sluggish motility*
b *Entamoeba histolytica* – *large troph; progressive crawl; uniform chromatin*
c *Endolimax nana* – *small*
d *Iodamoeba bütschlii* – *no chromatin*

383 Refer to the following image:

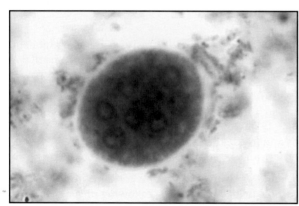

Entamoeba coli
non-pathogenic

Trophozoites of the cyst shown above are likely to:

a contain red blood cells
b have clear, pointed pseudopodia
c contain few, if any, vacuoles
d have slow, undefined motility

384 Refer to the following image:

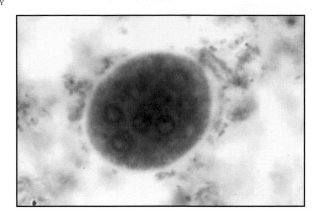

Upon finding the above in a fecal concentrate, the technologist should:

a telephone the report of this pathogen to the physician immediately
b review the fecal concentration carefully for the presence of other microorganisms that may be pathogenic
c look for motile trophozoites
d request a new specimen because of the presence of excessive pollen grains

385 Refer to the following image:

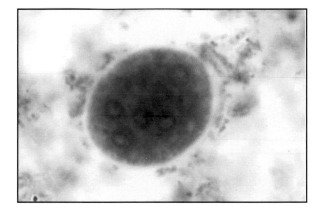

E. Coli - more than 4 nuclei
larger than E. histolytica

An inexperienced parasitology student may confuse the above organism with:

a *Entamoeba histolytica*
b *Dientamoeba fragilis* - *flagellate*
c *Giardia lamblia*
d *Trichomonas vaginalis*

386 Refer to the following image:

MLS
ONLY

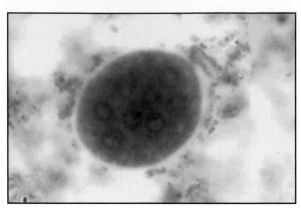

E. Coli

This structure depicts a:

a cyst of a nonpathogenic amoeba
b trophozoite of a nonpathogenic amoeba
c cyst of a pathogenic amoeba
d trophozoite of a pathogenic amoeba

387 Refer to the following image:

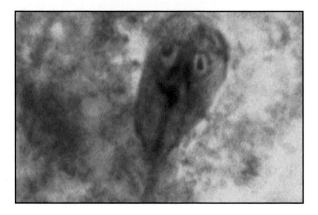

The organism depicted is a(n):

a amoeba
b flagellate
c filaria
d sporozoan

388 Refer to the following image:

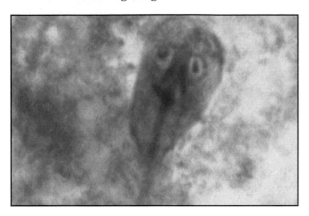

A 24-year-old woman, who just returned from vacationing in Russia, became ill with steatorrheal diarrhea. The above organism was found in her stool. The patient **most** likely is suffering from:

a giardiasis *– consumption of contaminated water*
b amebiasis
c ascariasis
d balantidiasis

389 A liquid stool specimen is collected at 10:00 PM and brought to the laboratory for culture and ova and parasite examination. It is refrigerated until 10:10 AM the next day, when the physician requests that the technologist look for amoebic trophozoites. The best course of action would be to:

a request a fresh specimen
b perform a concentration on the original specimen
c perform a trichrome stain on the original specimen
d perform a saline wet mount on the original specimen

390 Protozoan cysts are found in a wet mount of sediment from ethyl-acetate concentrated material. The cysts are without peripheral chromatin on the nuclear membrane. Each cyst has 4 nuclei, and each nucleus has a large karyosome, which appears as a refractive dot. These oval cysts are **most** likely:

a *Endolimax nana*
b *Chilomastix mesnili*
c *Entamoeba histolytica*
d *Entamoeba hartmanni*

391 The term "internal autoinfection" is generally used in referring to infections with:

a *Ascaris lumbricoides*
b *Necator americanus*
c *Trichuris trichiura*
d *Strongyloides stercoralis*

392 The best method to demonstrate the ova of *Enterobius vermicularis* is:
(PINWORM) ✳

a acid-ether concentration
b cellophane tape preparation
c formalin-ether concentration
d zinc sulfate flotation

393 Proper collection of a sample for recovery of *Enterobius vermicularis* includes collecting:

a a 24-hour urine collection
b a first morning stool collection with proper preservative
c a scotch tape preparation from the perianal region
d peripheral blood from a finger

394 A fibrous skin nodule is removed from the back of a patient from Central America. A microfilaria
MLS
ONLY   seen upon microscopic exam of the nodule is:

    a *Wuchereria bancrofti*
    b *Brugia malayi*
    c *Onchocerca volvulus*
    d *Loa loa*

395 Refer to the following image:

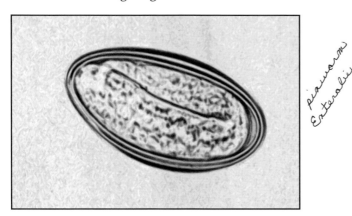

pinworm
Enterobius vermicularis

  The egg depicted above is **most** likely to be found in children suffering from:

    a diarrhea
    b constipation
    c perianal itching
    d stomach pain

396 Refer to the following illustration:

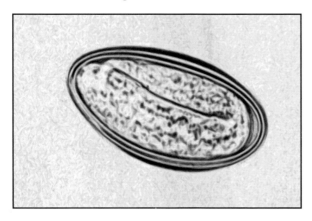

  The specimen of choice for finding the above parasite is:

    a stool
    b duodenal washing
    c rectal swab
    d scotch tape preparation

397 The examination of human feces is no help in the detection of:
MLS
ONLY

    a *Strongyloides stercoralis*
    b *Entamoeba histolytica*
    c *Echinococcus granulosus*
    d *Ancylostoma duodenale*

398 The causative agent of cysticercosis is:
cysts embed in tissue

   (a) *Taenia solium*
   b *Taenia saginata*
   c *Ascaris lumbricoides*
   d *Trichuris trichiura*

399 Organisms that can be easily identified to the species level from the ova in fecal specimens include:

   a *Metagonimus yokogawai, Heterophyes heterophyes*
   b *Taenia solium, Taenia saginata*
   c *Necator americanus, Ancylostoma duodenale*   ✳✳
   (d) *Paragonimus westermani, Hymenolepis nana* – *only ones DX by ova in feces*

400 The scolex of *Taenia saginata* has:

   (a) 4 suckers - *no hooks*
   b no suckers and 14 hooklets
   c 24 hooklets
   d 26-28 sucking discs

401 When stool examination is negative, the preferred specimen for the diagnosis of paragonimiasis is:
MLS ONLY

   a bile drainage
   b duodenal aspirate
   c sputum
   d rectal biopsy

402 A stool specimen for ova and parasite examination contained numerous rhabditiform larvae. Which factor does **not** aid in the identification of larvae?

   a larva tail morphology –
   (b) type of water vegetation consumed
   c length of the buccal cavity ·   *Factors in larvae identification!!!*
   d appearance of the genital primordium –

1	d	59	c	117	d	175	a	233	a	291	a	349	a
2	d	60	c	118	c	176	a	234	a	292	b	350	b
3	a	61	b	119	c	177	c	235	d	293	d	351	b
4	b	62	a	120	c	178	a	236	d	294	c	352	b
5	a	63	b	121	c	179	d	237	a	295	c	353	c
6	a	64	b	122	a	180	d	238	b	296	d	354	c
7	d	65	d	123	c	181	c	239	b	297	d	355	c
8	c	66	c	124	a	182	b	240	a	298	d	356	a
9	b	67	d	125	c	183	c	241	c	299	c	357	c
10	a	68	d	126	b	184	c	242	b	300	a	358	c
11	d	69	c	127	d	185	b	243	b	301	a	359	d
12	d	70	d	128	d	186	d	244	a	302	c	360	a
13	a	71	b	129	b	187	c	245	c	303	a	361	b
14	c	72	d	130	c	188	d	246	c	304	b	362	a
15	d	73	b	131	d	189	d	247	b	305	a	363	c
16	b	74	c	132	d	190	d	248	a	306	d	364	d
17	c	75	d	133	d	191	a	249	a	307	d	365	c
18	b	76	a	134	b	192	a	250	d	308	a	366	d
19	a	77	b	135	c	193	a	251	b	309	d	367	b
20	d	78	c	136	a	194	b	252	c	310	b	368	d
21	a	79	d	137	d	195	b	253	c	311	a	369	b
22	b	80	b	138	c	196	d	254	c	312	d	370	a
23	b	81	b	139	b	197	d	255	a	313	b	371	a
24	d	82	c	140	c	198	d	256	b	314	d	372	d
25	d	83	d	141	b	199	d	257	b	315	d	373	d
26	d	84	b	142	d	200	a	258	c	316	b	374	c
27	c	85	b	143	d	201	c	259	a	317	d	375	d
28	b	86	d	144	b	202	d	260	c	318	d	376	d
29	c	87	d	145	b	203	c	261	d	319	d	377	d
30	a	88	c	146	c	204	b	262	b	320	c	378	d
31	a	89	d	147	a	205	c	263	d	321	d	379	b
32	d	90	b	148	b	206	d	264	c	322	c	380	a
33	d	91	c	149	d	207	b	265	a	323	d	381	c
34	a	92	d	150	d	208	b	266	d	324	b	382	b
35	b	93	b	151	a	209	a	267	a	325	c	383	d
36	b	94	c	152	c	210	d	268	d	326	b	384	b
37	a	95	c	153	a	211	b	269	c	327	b	385	a
38	d	96	b	154	c	212	d	270	d	328	b	386	a
39	c	97	c	155	d	213	c	271	d	329	a	387	b
40	c	98	c	156	c	214	d	272	d	330	b	388	a
41	b	99	a	157	d	215	b	273	a	331	d	389	a
42	d	100	a	158	d	216	b	274	b	332	b	390	a
43	c	101	d	159	d	217	b	275	d	333	a	391	d
44	b	102	a	160	a	218	b	276	b	334	b	392	b
45	c	103	a	161	d	219	d	277	c	335	c	393	c
46	b	104	c	162	d	220	c	278	c	336	b	394	c
47	c	105	d	163	b	221	a	279	c	337	d	395	c
48	d	106	d	164	a	222	b	280	b	338	b	396	d
49	a	107	b	165	d	223	c	281	d	339	b	397	c
50	d	108	c	166	d	224	d	282	a	340	b	398	a
51	d	109	b	167	a	225	d	283	c	341	d	399	d
52	a	110	d	168	b	226	c	284	b	342	a	400	a
53	c	111	b	169	b	227	d	285	a	343	c	401	c
54	c	112	c	170	c	228	d	286	c	344	a	402	b
55	a	113	a	171	c	229	d	287	d	345	c		
56	b	114	d	172	b	230	b	288	a	346	b		
57	d	115	d	173	d	231	c	289	c	347	b		
58	a	116	b	174	b	232	c	290	d	348	a		

Preanalytical and Susceptibility Testing

1   **d**   Chocolate agar and chocolate agar-based selective media should be used for recovery of *Neisseria gonorrhoeae* from urethral discharge. Chocolate agar provides the nutrients required by *N gonorrhoeae* and selective media contains antimicrobial agents that inhibits other organisms and permits recovery of pathogenic *Neisseria*.
[Murray 2007, p591]

2   **d**   When 0.001 mL of urine is plated, the growth of one colony is equivalent to 1000 CFU/mL. Thus 70 colonies is 70,000 CFU/mL.
[Isenberg 1992, p1.17.7]

3   **a**   The MIC is a basic laboratory measurement of the activity of an antibiotic against an organism. It is the lowest concentration of antibiotic that inhibits visible growth of the organism. It does not represent the concentration of antibiotic that is lethal to the organism.
[Murray 2007, pp1103-1104]

4   **b**   Patients with infection often have at least 100,000 bacteria/mL of urine in the bladder. However one third of young women with symptomatic cystitis have less than 100,000 bacteria/mL of urine. The Infectious Disease Society of America consensus definition of cystitis is greater than or equal to 1,000 CFU/mL of a uropathogen.
[Mandell 2005, p885]

5   **a**   The traditional gravity displacement steam sterilization cycle is 121°C for 15 minutes at 15 pounds per square inch. Ethylene oxide is an alternative sterilization method.
[Isenberg 1992, pp11.9.8-11.9.9.]

6   **a**   Urine in the bladder is normally sterile. Suprapubic aspiration removes urine directly from the bladder and yields a specimen free of urethral contamination.
[Mandell 2005, p885]

7   **d**   Facultative anaerobes are organisms that can grow under both aerobic and anaerobic conditions.
[Koneman 2005, p195]

8   **c**   Human blood contains substances that
MLS ONLY   may inhibit microbial growth. Diluting blood in culture broth reduces the concentration of these substances as well as any antibiotics that may be present. The recommended blood broth ratio is 1:5-1:10. Dilutions less than this may cause the blood to clot trapping organisms in the clot. Greater dilutions may increase the time to detection.
[Baron 2005, pp11-12]

9   **b**   Antimicrobial resistance in *Neisseria gonorrhoeae* is widespread. The production of beta-lactamase (penicillinase) breaks open the beta lactam ring of penicillin, destroying its activity. Thus, *N gonorrhoeae* that produce beta lactamase are resistant to penicillin.
[Murray 2007, p597]

10   **a**   Columbia CNA agar contains colistin and nalidixic acid, which inhibit most gram-negative organisms. Eosin methylene blue is selective and inhibits gram-positive organisms and modified Thayer Martin is selective and inhibits gram-positive organisms, gram-negative bacilli and yeast.
[Murray 2007, p265]

11   **d**   The chromogenic cephalosporin test using nitrocefin is the most sensitive and specific test for detection of beta lactamase. Acidimetric tests employing penicillin are less expensive, but not as sensitive, as the nitrocefin assay.
[Koneman 2005, pp996, 1001]

12   **d**   A *Staphylococcus aureus* isolate with an
MLS ONLY   MIC of 4 µg/mL is resistant to oxacillin. As per the Clinical and Laboratory Standards Institute (CLSI) recommendations a heteroresistant strain would be defined as a methicillin (oxacillin) resistant *S aureus* (MRSA/ORSA). An MRSA/ORSA isolate would be reported as resistant to all beta lactam agents, beta lactam/beta lactamase inhibitor combinations, such as amoxicillin-clavulanic acid, and carbapenems.
[Murray 2007, p1182]

13 **a** Systemic enterococcal infections, such as endocarditis, are commonly treated with a cell-wall-active agent and an aminoglycoside. These agents act synergistically to kill the organism. If the organism is resistant to one or both, there is no synergy, and the combination will fail. It is important to detect aminoglycoside and beta-lactam resistance in these cases. Enterococci have intrinsic moderate level resistance to aminoglycosides. Acquired resistance corresponds to very high MICs (greater than 500 μg/mL) for gentamicin and is termed high level resistance.
[Murray 2007, p1178]

14 **c** Variations in the concentrations of divalent cations primarily calcium and magnesium affect the results of aminoglycoside, tetracycline and colistin tests with *P aeruginosa* isolates. A cation concentration that is too high results in smaller zone sizes, and a concentration that is too low increases zone sizes.
[Murray 2007, p1120]

15 **d** Cefoxitin is used as a surrogate for mecA-mediated oxacillin resistance in *S aureus*. *S aureus* with cefoxitin MICs >4 μg/mL are considered oxacillin resistant. The Clinical Laboratory Standards Institute (CLSI) recommends addition of 2% NaCl, incubation at 35±2°C, and incubation for 24 hours when performing susceptibility testing of *S aureus* against oxacillin.
[CLSI 2008, p167]

16 **b** All of the biochemical and serological reactions listed are consistent with an identification of *Shigella flexneri*, with the exception of motility. All *Shigella* are nonmotile.
[Murray 2007, p638]

17 **c** All Mueller-Hinton agar used for disk diffusion susceptibility testing should be poured to a depth of 4mm. If the depth of the media is <4mm, this may be associated with excessively large zones and false-positive susceptibility results. Agar that is >4mm in depth may cause excessively small zone sizes.
[Murray 2007, p1120]

18 **b** Coagulase-negative staphylococci are commonly associated with contaminated blood cultures; however, they are also increasing as a cause of true bacteremia. Significant bacteremia in a patient with endocarditis is usually continuous and low grade. In most cases, all blood cultures drawn will yield positive results. The facts that only 1 bottle of 1 set was positive, and that the bottle did not become positive until day 5 of incubation, indicate that this isolate is most likely a contaminant.
[Mandell 2005, p985]

19 **a** *Campylobacter coli/jejuni* require a microaerophilic atmosphere for optimal recovery. The use of selective media is recommended for recovery from fecal specimens. Selective media for *Campylobacter* contains antibiotics to inhibit the growth of enteric gram-negative flora. Unlike other enteric pathogens, *C coli/jejuni* grow well at 42°C.
[Murray 2007, p905]

20 **d** Sputum specimen quality is assessed to determine if the specimen is representative of the site of infection. The presence of white blood cells is an indicator of infection, and presence of squamous epithelial cells is an indicator of oropharyngeal contamination. In this specimen, >25 epithelial cells per low power field is an indicator of poor specimen quality, and the bacteria present are representative of oropharyngeal flora.
[Koneman 2005, pp15-17]

21 **a** Due to the small size of viruses, they are not visible using light microscopy. Electron microscopy is used to visualize viruses and the internal structure of microorganisms.
[Koneman 2005, p1330]

22 **b** Daily disk diffusion quality control can be converted to weekly testing when 30 days of consecutive testing demonstrates no more than 3 antibiotic/organism combinations outside of the acceptable limits.
[CLSI 2006, p24]

23 **b** The amount of antibiotic used in disk diffusion susceptibility testing is standardized and constant. Once the disk is placed on the inoculated plate and makes contact with the agar, the antibiotic in the disk begins to diffuse out. As it diffuses into the media, the concentration of antibiotic gets lower the further it diffuses from the disk.
[Murray 2007, pp1120-1121]

24   **d**   The 2 most common causes of failure of the GasPak™ system is a defective gasket in the jar lid that allows escape of gas from inside the jar and inactivated catalyst pellets.
[Koneman 2005, pp895-897]

25   **d**   Indwelling catheters are closed
MLS ONLY systems, and should not be disconnected for specimen collection. Urine samples should not be collected from catheter bags, and Foley catheter tips are unsuitable for culture because they are contaminated with colonizing organisms. Urine from indwelling catheters should be collected by aseptically puncturing the tubing (collection port).
[Koneman 2005, p85]

26   **d**   Urine is an appropriate specimen for the detection of renal tuberculosis. Since feces contain anaerobic organisms as part of the indigenous flora, it is an unacceptable specimen for anaerobic culture. Foley catheter tips are also not acceptable for culture, because they are contaminated with colonizing organisms. Gram stain smears of rectal swabs for *N gonorrhoeae* should also not be performed, since the presence of organisms with similar morphologies may lead to overinterpretation of smears.
[Murray 2007, pp287, 543, 590]

27   **c**   Materials collected from sites not harboring indigenous flora (sterile body fluids, abscess exudate and tissue) should be cultured for anaerobic bacteria. However, since anaerobes normally inhabit the skin and mucus membranes as part of the indigenous flora, specimens such as urine, sputum, and vaginal, eye and ear swabs are not acceptable for culture.
[Koneman 2005, pp890-91]

28   **b**   *Campylobacter* continues to be the most common enteric pathogen isolated from patients with diarrhea. Routinely fecal specimens should be cultured for *Salmonella*, *Shigella* and *Campylobacter*. Fecal specimens are not routinely cultured for enterotoxigenic *E coli* or *C botulinum*. *E hartmanni* is a nonpathogenic parasite and does not cause diarrhea.
[Murray 2007, pp655, 902]

29   **c**   Enriched media such as chocolate agar has no inhibitory effects on bacterial growth and contains additional nutrients that support the growth of fastidious organisms such as *H influenzae* and *Neisseria*.
[Koneman 2005, p27]

30   **a**   CNA agar is a selective medium commonly used in the isolation of gram-positive aerobic and anaerobic organisms. Since the Gram stain indicates a mixture of gram-positive and gram-negative organisms, use of CNA will aid in the recovery of the gram-positive cocci in culture.
[Murray 2007, p370]

31   **a**   Chocolate agar and chocolate agar-based selective media (Martin Lewis) are routinely used for the recovery of *Neisseria gonorrhoeae* from genital specimens. Sputum and urine specimens are routinely processed using a general purpose media (blood agar) and a selective agar (EMB or MacConkey). In addition chocolate agar is routinely included to enhance recovery of fastidious organisms such as *H influenzae*. CSF is routinely processed using blood and chocolate agars.
[Murray 2007, pp370, 591]

32   **d**   CIN agar is a selective and differential medium for the isolation and differentiation of *Y enterocolitica*. This medium contains sodium desoxycholate, crystal violet, cefsulodin, irgason (triclosan), and novobiocin as selective agents, and mannitol as the carbohydrate.
[Murray 2007, p369]

33   **d**   Columbia CNA agar is a selective medium used for the isolation of gram-positive organisms. The medium contains colistin and nalidixic acid, which inhibits gram-negative organisms. MacConkey agar is a selective and differential medium used for the isolation of gram-negative organisms. The medium contains bile and crystal violet, which inhibits gram-positive organisms.
[Murray 2007, pp370, 374]

34   **a**   Problems with analysis of Gram staining generally result from errors including interpretation of the slide (smear prepared too thick), excessive heat fixing, and improper decolorization. Inadequate decolorization with acetone/alcohol results in a smear in which host cells (neutrophils and squamous cells), as well as bacteria, all appear blue.
[Murray 2007, p363]

35   **b**   The indole test is used for determining an organism's ability to produce indole from deamination of tryptophan by tryptophanase.
[Murray 2007, p357]

Answers–Microbiology

36 **b** Through the action of the enzyme beta-galactosidase, ONPG cleaves into galactose and o-nitrophenol (a yellow compound).
[Koneman 2005, p1451]

37 **a** The JEMBEC system is a transport and
MLS ONLY inoculation medium used for direct plating of specimens for *N gonorrhoeae*. Chocolate-based selective medium is inoculated with the specimen. This is placed in an impermeable plastic bag with a bicarbonate-sodium citrate pellet that absorbs moisture to generate a carbon dioxide-rich environment.
[Koneman 2005, p590]

38 **d** Martin Lewis agar is a modification of
MLS ONLY the modified Thayer Martin formulation, and contains a higher concentration of vancomycin and anisomycin instead of nystatin. These modifications provide better inhibition of gram-positive organisms and *Candida*.
[Murray 2007, p374]

39 **c** Differential media contain compounds, often carbohydrates, that provide a presumptive identification based on colony color or a precipitate around the colony. Examples include MacConkey, Hektoen and xylose lysine desoxycholate agar.
[Murray 2007, pp264-265]

40 **c** Most commercially available
MLS ONLY blood culture media contain sodium polyanetholsulfonate (SPS) in concentrations between 0.025 and 0.05%. SPS has anticoagulant activity, and inactivates neutrophils as well as some antibiotics including gentamicin and polymyxin. It also precipitates components of serum complement.
[Koneman 2005, p102]

41 **b** When evaluating susceptibility testing
MLS ONLY systems the following conventions are used: a *very major error* occurs when the system characterizes a resistant isolate as susceptible; a *major error* occurs when the system characterizes a susceptible isolate as resistant; and a *minor error* occurs when the system characterizes a susceptible or resistant isolate as intermediate, or an intermediate isolates as susceptible or resistant.
[Koneman 2005, pp968-69]

42 **d** The disk diffusion procedure will not differentiate *S aureus* strains with reduced susceptibility to vancomycin (MICs 4-8 µg/mL) from susceptible stains even when incubated for 24 hours.
[CLSI 2008, p50]

43 **c** A delay of more than 15 minutes between placing the disks on an inoculated plate and incubation permits excess prediffusion of the antimicrobial agent from the disk. This would result in a larger than expected zone diameter.
[Murray 2007, p1121]

44 **b** To ensure the reproducibility of disk diffusion testing, the inoculum must be standardized. If the inoculum is too dense (too many organisms), zone sizes would be smaller than expected and appear falsely resistant.
[Murray 2007, p1121]

45 **c** Cephalothin is a first-generation cephalosporin, cefotetan and cefoxitin are second-generation cephalosporins, and ceftriaxone is a third generation cephalosporin.
[CLSI 2008, p172]

46 **b** Penicillin inhibits penicillin binding proteins that are essential to peptidoglycan (cell wall) synthesis. Chloramphenicol inhibits protein synthesis, colistin increases cell membrane permeability, and sulfamethoxazole inhibits folate metabolism.
[Murray 2007, p1039]

47 **c** Susceptibility testing should be performed when the susceptibility of the organism cannot reliably be predicted and resistance is known or suspected. Susceptibility testing of penicillins for treatment of *S pyogenes* does not need to be performed routinely since resistance has not been documented.
[Murray 2007, p1102]

48 **d** Aminoglycoside antibiotics such as gentamicin are active against *Pseudomonas* and routinely tested and reported on these isolates. Penicillin, erythromycin, and clindamycin are not active against *Pseudomonas*.
[Murray 2007, p1046]

49 **a** Most *Campylobacter* species grow best under lower oxygen tension in an atmosphere of 5% oxygen, 10% carbon dioxide and 85% nitrogen. *E coli* and *Proteus mirabilis* are facultative anaerobes and *Pseudomonas aeruginosa* is an aerobe.
[Koneman 2005, p195]

50 **d** The sensitivity of blood culture is only
MLS
ONLY
50%-70%. Stool cultures are positive in <50% of patients and urine cultures are positive even less frequently. Bone marrow has a sensitivity of up to 90%. Higher colony counts are present in bone marrow and counts are not decreased by up to 5 days of antimicrobial therapy prior to specimen collection.
[Mandell 2005, p2645]

51 **d** TCBS is a highly selective and differential medium for the recovery of most *Vibrio* species including *V parahaemolyticus*. Hektoen and Salmonella-Shigella agars are selective and differential for the isolation and differentiation of enteric pathogens such as *Salmonella* and *Shigella*. EMB is a selective and differential medium for gram-negative enteric bacilli.
[Murray 2007, p379]

52 **a** Skirrow medium is an enriched selective blood agar medium used for the isolation of *Campylobacter* from specimens with mixed flora. CIN and bismuth sulfite agars are selective and differential for *Yersinia enterocolitica* and *Salmonella*, respectively. CNA agar is selective for gram-positive organisms.
[Murray 2007, p378]

53 **c** As many as 20%-40% of *H influenzae* produce beta-lactamases. Detection of these enzymes should be performed on any isolate considered to be a pathogen using the chromogenic cephalosporin (nitrocefin) test.
[Koneman 2005, p1002]

54 **c** Buffered charcoal yeast extract medium is a specialized enrichment medium for the isolation of *Legionella*. The nutritive base includes yeast extract. Charcoal is added to the medium as a detoxifying agent.
[Murray 2007, p368]

55 **a** Regan-Lowe agar is an enriched and selective medium for the isolation of *B pertussis*. Cephalexin is added to inhibit nasopharyngeal flora. It provides better isolation of *B pertussis* than Bordet-Gengou medium.
[Murray 2007, p784]

56 **b** *Francisella tularensis* is fastidious and not readily recovered in culture. Cysteine blood glucose agar is an enriched medium with beef heart infusion, peptones, glucose and rabbit blood. It also includes cystine, which is required by *F tularensis* for growth.
[Murray 2007, p371]

57 **d** Methods for rapid diagnosis of
MLS
ONLY
Francisella tularensis include fluorescent antibody staining of smears and tissues, antigen detection in urine detection of lipopolysaccharide using specific monoclonal antibodies and PCR. Only PCR has gained widespread use. PCR is appealing because smears and cultures are usually negative, and organism isolation may be hazardous. Serological diagnosis may take weeks to confirm.
[Mandell 2005, pp2681-2682]

58 **a** Sheep blood agar is preferred because clear-cut patterns of hemolysis are obtained.
[Mandell 2005, p2366]

59 **c** For optimum detection of oxacillin-resistant *S aureus*, a suspension with a turbidity equivalent to a 0.5 McFarland standard should be inoculated into a cation-adjusted Mueller-Hinton broth with 2% NaCl. Plates should be incubated at 35 ± 2°C for 24 hours. Temperatures above 35°C may not detect oxacillin resistance.
[CLSI 2008, p110]

60 **c** The use of swabs for collection of specimens for anaerobic culture is discouraged. Aspiration with a needle and syringe is recommended. Whenever possible cultures should be obtained before the administration of antibiotics to optimize organism recovery.
[Koneman 2005, pp12-13]

61 **b** Many anaerobic bacteria are commensal flora in the oropharynx. Anaerobic bacteria do not cause pharyngitis. The most common cause of pharyngitis is *Streptococcus pyogenes*. Other causes include *Arcanobacterium haemolyticum*, *Corynebacterium diphtheriae*, *Neisseria gonorrhoeae* and viruses.
[Koneman 2005, p72]

Answers—Microbiology

62
MLS
ONLY
a There is evidence that antimicrobial resistance among anaerobic organisms is significant, and that inappropriate therapy correlates with poor patient outcomes. Susceptibility testing is useful when anaerobes are isolated from normally sterile sites such as synovial fluid. Rectal abscesses and pilonidal sinuses are polymicrobial in nature, and often resolved by surgical management.
[Murray 2007, p1141]

63 **b** Cyclohexamide, which inhibits protein synthesis, is the common agent used in Mycosel® or mycobiotic agar to inhibit faster-growing saprophytic fungi. Penicillin and streptomycin do not inhibit fungi. Amphotericin B is not routinely used as an additive in fungal media.
[Murray 2007, p1691]

64 **b** Some bacteria such as *Enterococcus* sp, *H influenzae* and *Neisseria gonorrhoeae* continually produce beta-lactamase. *S aureus* produces beta-lactamase only after exposure to an inducing agent (such as penicillin). *C diphtheriae* and *S pyogenes* do not produce beta-lactamase.
[Murray 2007, p1184]

65 **d** There are several sputum-screening systems for assessing the quality of respiratory specimens. In general, neutrophils are a positive indicator of quality, and squamous epithelial cells are a negative indicator of quality, suggesting oropharyngeal contamination. This specimen contains an abundance of squamous cells (>10/low power field), and would be unacceptable for culture.
[Murray 2007, p316]

66 **c** The classic CSF alterations associated with bacterial meningitis are a high WBC count with a neutrophil predominance as well as a low CSF glucose and a high CSF protein.
[Koneman 2005, p92]

67 **d** When reading a broth microdilution susceptibility test, growth in each well is determined by comparison with the growth control well and indicated by turbidity. The well with the lowest concentration of antibiotic displaying no growth is read as the minimum inhibitory concentration (MIC).
[Murray 2007, p1117]

68
MLS
ONLY
d The serum bactericidal, or Schlichter, test can be used to assess the activity of patient's serum when they are receiving long-term therapy for endocarditis or osteomyelitis. High titers of antibacterial activity in the serum suggest adequate dosing, a nontolerant isolate or normal elimination of the antibiotic.
[Murray 2007, p1188]

69
MLS
ONLY
c Mueller-Hinton agar used for disk diffusion susceptibility testing is standardized at pH 7.2-7.4. Penicillins function better in an acidic environment, so zone sizes would become larger if the media pH is too low. Aminoglycosides, on the other hand, are less effective in an acidic environment, so zone sizes would become smaller if the pH of the media is too low. Plates should not be incubated in a carbon dioxide atmosphere, which lowers the pH of the media.
[Koneman 2005, p997]

70 **d** Deterioration of the antimicrobial agent in the disk will cause the zone sizes to be too small (falsely resistant). Standardization of the inoculum turbidity to less than a 0.5 McFarland standard would result in an inoculum that is too light and resulting zone sizes that are too large. Incubation of the plates at 35°C and inoculating plates within 10 minutes of preparation would not have an adverse effect on zone sizes.
[Koneman 2005, p997]

71
MLS
ONLY
b The zone size observed has no meaning in and of itself. Interpretive standards are derived from a correlation between zone sizes and minimum inhibitory concentrations. Usually a large number of organisms from a given species or group (eg, *Enterobacteriaceae*) are tested.
[Koneman 2005, p987]

72 **d** *Moraxella osloensis* is a gram-negative coccobacillus that is often plump and occurs in pairs and demonstrates a morphology similar to *Neisseria*. The presence of this organism in endocervical specimens contaminated with vaginal secretions can lead to over interpretation of smears for *N gonorrhoeae*.
[Murray 2007, p590]

73   **b**   With the exception of the oxacillin disk screening test, disk diffusion is not recommended for testing *S pneumoniae* against beta-lactam agents. *S pneumoniae* does not produce beta-lactamase, so beta-lactamase testing would not be useful. The Schlichter test is not a method for determining an organism's susceptibility to a given agent.
[Murray 2007, p1129]

74   **c**   Extraintestinal isolates of *Salmonella*
MLS ONLY should be tested for resistance to nalidixic acid in addition to fluoroquinolones. Fluoroquinolones susceptible stains of *Salmonella* that are resistant to nalidixic acid may be associated with clinical failure or delayed response to therapy. In the case where ciprofloxacin is susceptible and nalidixic acid is resistant the nalidixic acid result should be used for reporting.
[CLSI 2008, p101]

75   **d**   Certain antimicrobials, such as nitrofurantoin and norfloxacin, are used only or primarily to treat urinary tract infections. These agents should not be reported for pathogens recovered from other sites of infection.
[CLSI 2008, p18]

76   **a**   Enterococcus species may appear active in vitro to clindamycin, cephalosporins and trimethoprim/sulfamethoxazole but are not effective clinically and should not be reported as susceptible.
[CLSI 2008, p116]

77   **b**   The image displays a negative D test result. There is no flattening of the zone of inhibition around the clindamycin disk adjacent to the erythromycin disk. Thus, there is no inducible clindamycin resistance, and the isolate is reported as clindamycin-susceptible, while the erythromycin is reported as resistant.
[CLSI 2008, pp164-65]

78   **c**   Extended spectrum beta lactamases (ESBL) are inhibited by clavulanic acid. Confirmatory tests of the presence of ESBL are based on the enhanced activity of a beta-lactam antibiotic, usually cefotaxime or ceftazidime, when it is tested with clavulanic acid compared to the activity of the beta-lactam tested alone.
[Murray 2003, p1185]

79   **d**   Aminoglycoside modifying enzymes
MLS ONLY modify aminoglycosides, such as gentamicin, resulting in poor binding to the bacterial ribosome. Resistance to levofloxacin, vancomycin and sulfamethoxazole is a result of nonenzymatic alteration of the antimicrobial target causing reduced antibiotic binding or activity.
[Murray 2007, pp1077-1078]

80   **b**   The volume of blood collected is the single most important variable in the recovery of organisms in patients with bloodstream infections. Since many cases of adult bacteremia are of low magnitude, there is a direct relationship between the yield of blood culture (positivity) and volume of blood collected. The collection of multiple blood culture sets from a single venipuncture is an unacceptable practice due to the potential for contamination. The practice of terminal subculture of blood culture bottles at 5 days is no longer recommended. The use of chlorhexadine for skin antisepsis does not affect organism recovery, but aids in decreasing blood culture contamination.
[Baron 2005, pp3-4]

81   **b**   Gonococcal urethritis in adult males is often diagnosed by the observation of gram-negative diplococci within or closely associated with neutrophils in smears prepared from urethral discharge. The Gram stain in males has a sensitivity of 90%-95% and a specificity of 95%-100% for diagnosing gonorrhea in symptomatic males.
[Murray 2007, p590]

82   **c**   The Gram stain demonstrates numerous neutrophils and small, pleomorphic gram-negative bacilli suggestive of *Haemophilus*. *H influenzae* is an important cause of lower respiratory tract infections in patient with pre-existing lung disease such as cystic fibrosis. *Haemophilus* are fastidious, and require the use of an enriched medium such as chocolate agar and incubation at 35°-37°C in a moist environment supplemented with 5%-10% CO_2.
[Murray 2007, pp626-627]

83   **d**   The Gram stain depicts gram-positive cocci arranged in chains. Members of the genus *Streptococcus* characteristically grow in pairs and chains, and tend to chain more in fluid. Staphylococci are also gram-positive cocci that can appear singly, in pairs, short chains or, more typically, clusters.
[Koneman 2005, pp643, 709]

84 **b** Detection of group B *Streptococcus* (GBS) in the genital and gastrointestinal tracts of pregnant women can identify infants at risk for GBS infection. The CDC currently recommends the collection of vaginal and rectal swabs or a single swab inserted first into the vagina and then the rectum at 35-37 weeks gestation. The swab(s) should be inoculated into a selective broth medium such as LIM broth (Todd-Hewitt broth with colistin and nalidixic acid). The use of vaginal/rectal swabs and selective broth medium greatly increases the recovery of GBS.
[Murray 2007, p408]

85 **b** Group B *Streptococcus* (GBS) colonizes both the genital and gastrointestinal tracts of pregnant women. Collection of a vaginal and rectal specimen is recommended by the CDC to maximize GBS detection in this population. Patients should be screened at 35-37 weeks gestation. In addition selective broth culture is recommended (Todd-Hewitt broth with antibiotics) although other selective media are also available. When selective broth culture is used it should be incubated for 18-24 hours prior to subculture onto blood agar.
[Murray 2007, p408]

MLS ONLY

86 **d** Oxacillin resistant staphylococci are resistant to all beta-lactam agents, beta-lactam/beta-lactamase inhibitor combinations and carbapenems. Results for these antibiotics should be reported as resistant or should not be reported.
[CLSI 2008, p110]

87 **d** *Bacillus stearothermophilus* is commonly used as an indicator organism for the appropriate functioning of autoclaves. Unlike most *Bacillus* species, *B stearothermophilus* grows at 56°C.
[Isenburg 1992, p12.3.4]

88 **c** Quality control zone sizes that are too small could indicate that the organism inoculum is too high, plates were poured too thick, or that the potency of the antibiotic disks is too low.
[Murray 2007, p1169]

89 **d** Of the combinations listed, the use of *E coli* and *Proteus mirabilis* will produce a positive and negative result for indole, respectively. The remainder of the organisms are all positive for the test described.
[Murray 2007, pp652-653]

Aerobic Gram-Positive Cocci

90 **b** The organism in this urine culture is a *Staphylococcus* species. Coagulase will differentiate *S aureus* from coagulase-negative staphylococci (CNS) and novobiocin susceptibility will differentiate *S saprophyticus* from other CNS. *S saprophyticus* is a common cause of urinary tract infections in young females.
[Koneman 2005, p684]

91 **c** Nutritionally deficient streptococci such as *Abiotrophia* do not grow on sheep blood agar without the addition of cysteine or proximity to *S aureus* colonies.
[Mahon 2006, p406]

92 **d** Bile solubility testing of alpha-hemolytic streptococci differentiates *S pneumoniae* (soluble) from other alpha-hemolytic streptococci, such as viridans streptococci (insoluble).
[Murray 2007, p423]

93 **b** Coagulase is the biochemical test used to distinguish *S aureus* (positive) from coagulase-negative staphylococci (negative).
[Koneman 2005, p645]

94 **c** Optochin susceptibility is used to differentiate *S pneumoniae*, which are susceptible, from other alpha-hemolytic streptococci, which are resistant.
[Murray 2007, p423]

95 **c** Optochin susceptibility is used to differentiate *S pneumoniae*, which are susceptible, from other alpha-hemolytic streptococci, which are resistant.
[Murray 2007, p423]

96 **b** Noninfectious sequelae associated with infection with *Streptococcus pyogenes* are glomerulonephritis and rheumatic fever.
[Koneman 2005, p680]

97 **c** *Staphylococcus aureus* produces an enterotoxin that is associated with short-incubation food poisoning.
[Mahon 2006, p372]

98 **c** Group D streptococci and *Enterococcus* produce a positive bile esculin test; however, of these 2, only *Enterococcus* grows in the presence of 6.5% NaCl.
[Mahon 2006, p400]

99   **a**   The Gram stain and culture growth describe a *Staphylococcus* species. Catalase production confirms that the organism belonged to the genus *Staphylococcus* and coagulase is used to differentiate *S aureus* from coagulase-negative staphylococci.
[Mahon 2006, p375, 383]

100   **a**   Bile esculin, PYR, bacitracin and hippurate are biochemicals/tests used in the presumptive or definitive identification of beta-hemolytic streptococci such as *S pyogenes*, *S agalactiae* and *Enterococcus*.
[Mahon 2006, p387]

101   **d**   Organisms that used to be categorized as nutritionally variant or deficient streptococci have been reclassified into the genera *Abiotrophia* and *Granulicatella*.
[Murray 2007, p443]

102   **a**   The colony description and biochemical results presented describe *Streptococcus agalactiae*. The identification of this organism is confirmed by streptococcus antigen typing.
[Mahon 2006, p385]

103   **a**   Of the biochemicals listed, only growth in 6.5% NaCl will aid in the identification of *Enterococcus*, which has the ability to grow in the presence of high salt concentrations.
[Mahon 2006, p387]

104   **c**   All of the organisms listed are potential causes of meningitis. Group B *Streptococcus* is associated with neonatal meningitis and meningitis in the elderly.
[Koneman 2005, p684]

105   **d**   *Streptococcus pyogenes* is the cause of exudative pharyngitis, commonly called strep throat.
[Koneman 2005, p679]

106   **d**   *Staphylococcus epidermidis* is the most common cause of prosthetic valve endocarditis.
[Koneman 2005, p639]

107   **b**   *Enterococcus* species are relatively
MLS ONLY   resistant to beta-lactam agents and aminoglycosides. Combination therapy with a beta-lactam agent or vancomycin and an aminoglycoside provide a synergistic combination to effectively treat enterococcal infections.
[Murray 2007, p437]

108   **c**   The number of colonies isolated is multiplied by 100 when a 0.01 mL loop is used for inoculation. Gram-positive, catalase negative cocci are indicative of streptococci.
[Koneman 2005, p726]

109   **b**   Noninfectious sequelae associated with infection with *Streptococcus pyogenes* are glomerulonephritis and rheumatic fever.
[Koneman 2005, p680]

110   **d**   *Streptococcus agalactiae* is catalase and bile esculin hydrolysis negative and bacitracin and optochin resistant. *Streptococcus agalactiae* hydrolyzes hippurate.
[Mahon 2006, p387]

111   **b**   Group A streptococci (*Streptococcus pyogenes*) are susceptible to bacitracin and CAMP test negative.
[Mahon 2006, pp386-387]

112   **c**   Group B streptococci (*Streptococcus agalactiae*) are resistant to bacitracin and CAMP test positive.
[Mahon 2006, pp386-387]

113   **a**   Growth in 6.5% NaCl, growth in bile esculin medium and susceptibility are not used in the routine identification of *Streptococcus agalactiae*. Polysaccharide typing for group B antigen is routinely used for identification of *S agalactiae*.
[Koneman 2005, p719]

114   **d**   *Enterococcus* species are more resistant to antimicrobial therapy than group D streptococci such as *S bovis*.
[Murray 2007, p437]

115   **d**   Bile solubility testing of alpha-hemolytic streptococci differentiates *S pneumoniae* (soluble) from other alpha-hemolytic streptococci such as viridans streptococci (insoluble).
[Murray 2007, p423]

116   **b**   Enterococci are bile esculin-positive, hippurate-negative and have the ability to grow in 6.5% NaCl. Enterococci are relatively resistant to penicillin and require combination therapy to treat serious infections.
[Murray 2007, p437]

117 d *Staphylococcus aureus* are usually beta-hemolytic. Some strains may not produce bound coagulase detected by the slide coagulase test. A tube coagulase is performed to detect free coagulase and should be performed on colonies with typical *S aureus* morphology that are slide coagulase-negative.
[Mahon 2006, pp374-375]

118 c Of the biochemicals listed only hydrolysis of sodium hippurate will differentiate *Streptococcus agalactiae* (positive) from *S pyogenes* (negative).
[Mahon 2006, p387]

119 c Coagulase production is the primary biochemical used to differentiate *S aureus* from other coagulase-negative staphylococci.
[Mahon 2006, p375]

120 c *Haemophilus influenzae* and *Neisseria gonorrhoeae* do not have predictable susceptibility to penicillin. *Corynebacterium diphtheriae* is not universally susceptible to penicillin. To date, no penicillin resistance has been demonstrated in *Streptococcus pyogenes*.
[Mahon 2006, p397]

121 c The most likely organism isolated from this specimen is *Streptococcus agalactiae*. Polysaccharide antigen typing will confirm the identification of *S agalactiae* and differentiate it from other beta-hemolytic streptococci.
[Koneman 2005, p719]

122 a *Staphylococcus aureus* produces an enterotoxin that is associated with food poisoning. Symptoms typically appear within 2-6 hours.
[Murray 2007, p393]

123 c Appropriate skin antisepsis is the most important factor in preventing contaminated blood cultures. *Staphylococcus epidermidis* is a common blood culture contaminant because it is a common inhabitant of the skin.
[Koneman 2005, p100]

124 a The most commonly used method
MLS ONLY to determine the relatedness of 2 or more bacterial strains is pulsed-field gel electrophoresis.
[Murray 2007, p402]

125 c *Micrococcus* and *Staphylococcus* can be differentiated by susceptibility to furazolidone (100 µg/disk). *Staphylococcus* is susceptible and *Micrococcus* is resistant.
[Koneman 2005, p645]

126 b *Micrococcus* is modified oxidase positive,
MLS ONLY bacitracin (0.04U) susceptible and resistant to lysostaphin.
[Mahon 2006, p368]

127 d The question describes the CAMP test, which is positive for *Streptococcus agalactiae*.
[Mahon 2006, p390]

128 d *Enterococcus* is positive for the bile esculin test while *Streptococcus pyogenes* and staphylococci are negative.
[Isenburg 1992, p1.20.19.IV.A]

Gram-Negative Bacilli

129 b >80% of uncomplicated UTIs are caused by *E coli*.
[Koneman 2005, p507]

130 c Sorbitol replaces lactose in MacConkey. *E coli* O157:H7 does not ferment sorbitol, whereas other species of *E coli* are positive for fermentation of sorbitol. This makes the media a good screen for O157:H7.
[Koneman 2005, p248]

131 d Members of *Enterobacteriaceae* are oxidase negative, ferment glucose, and reduce nitrate to nitrite.
[Koneman 2005, p213]

132 d *Shigella* is lactose negative, most species do not produce gas, are VP, urea, lysine decarboxylase and citrate negative, and they are nonmotile.
[Koneman 2005, p249]

133 d *Alcaligenes*, *Pseudomonas* and *Acinetobacter* are all nonfermenters; *Yersinia* is a member of the *Enterobacteriaceae* and, by definition, ferments glucose.
[Mahon 2006, p503]

134 b *Klebsiella* is the only distractor that is VP positive, and the other biochemical reactions are typical for *K pneumoniae*.
[Mahon 2006, pp530-537]

135 c *Salmonella* is the only distractor that produces H_2S. Also, *Klebsiella* and *E coli* produce acid/acid reactions in TSI.
[Mahon 2006, pp530-537]

136 a   *Shigella* has colorless colonies on both MacConkey and Hektoen agars. *Yersinia* is lactose negative, but Hektoen agar (has both lactose and sucrose) produces yellow colonies from the fermentation of sucrose. *V parahaemolyticus* needs at least 1% NaCl to grow and *Campylobacter* does not grow on MacConkey or Hektoen agars.
[Mahon 2006, pp550-551]

137 d   *Salmonella* produce H$_2$S in TSI and *Yersinia* produces an acid slant and acid butt. *Shigella* fits this biochemical profile.
[Mahon 2006, pp530-537]

138 c   These biochemicals are characteristic for *E coli*. *Klebsiella pneumoniae* is indole negative and nonmotile. *Shigella dysenteriae* is nonmotile and *Enterobacter cloacae* is indole negative.
[Koneman 2005, pp217, 234; Mahon 2006, pp530-537]

139 b   *E coli* can produces several different types of toxins that result in different gastroenteritis manifestations.
[Mahon 2006, pp508-512]

140 c   The toxin produced by enterotoxigenic *E coli* is similar in action and amino acid sequence to cholera toxin.
[Mahon 2006, p509]
MLS ONLY

141 b   The biochemical characteristic that best fits *Shigella* is that it is nonmotile. *Shigella* are urease negative and oxidase negative. *Shigella* are lactose nonfermenters.
[Mahon 2006, p536]

142 d   Some *Shigella* produce capsular antigen that mask the cell wall and boiling removes the capsule.
[Mahon 2006, p539]

143 d   Boiling removed the capsule so that the antiserum could react with cell wall antigen. Group D *Shigella* is *S sonnei*.
[Mahon 2006, p539]

144 b   *Morganella* and *Providencia* do not produce H$_2$S; the indole reaction differentiates *P mirabilis* and *P vulgaris*.
[Mahon 2006, p534]

145 b   *Serratia* can produce a red pigment; *Proteus mirabilis* swarms, is TDA positive and produces H$_2$S.
[Mahon 2006, pp515, 534-536]

146 c   *Edwardsiella* produces H$_2$S; *E coli* is indole positive; *Providencia* has a TSI reaction of alkaline/acid. *Yersinia* typically shows motility at 25°C and not 35°C.
[Mahon 2006, p523]
MLS ONLY

147 a   *Salmonella* are positive for lysine decarboxylase and most are negative for KCN, malonate, and ONPG. *Citrobacter* are negative for lysine decarboxylase and positive for growth in KCN.
[Mahon 2006, pp530-535]
MLS ONLY

148 b   *Shigella* is H$_2$S negative, while *Salmonella*, *Edwardsiella* and *Proteus* are H$_2$S positive. *Proteus mirabilis* is indole negative, so a lack of agglutination with *Salmonella* antisera indicates the presence of *Edwardsiella*.
[Mahon 2006, p534]
MLS ONLY

149 d   The history of the patient suggests an appendicitis-like syndrome, which is consistent with *Yersinia enterocolitica*. Also, *Y enterocolitica* grows better at 25°C.
[Mahon 2006, p523]
MLS ONLY

150 d   *Yersinia pestis* is classically described as having a "safety pin" appearance on Wayson stain. This patient's presentation is classic for bubonic plague.
[Murray 2007, pp617, 675-676, 798-799; Mahon 2006, p523]

151 a   If the Vi antigen is present, it will not permit agglutination of the polyvalent antisera. The Vi antigen is heat labile, so boiling will remove it and appropriate agglutination can take place.
[Mahon 2006, p539]
MLS ONLY

152 c   The correct quantitation on a urine sample is obtained by counting the colonies and multiplying them by the dilution factor, which in this case is 1000 because a .001 µL loop was used for culture. The biochemicals are characteristic of *Enterobacter cloacae*.
[Mahon 2006, pp532; Koneman 2005, pp85-86]

153 a   Enterobacteriaceae ferment glucose and are oxidase negative. *Plesiomonas* was a member of the Vibrio family in part because it is oxidase positive. However, it was moved to the Enterobacteriaceae family despite its positive oxidase reaction.
[Mahon 2006, pp552-555]

154 c   These are typical biochemical reactions for *Providencia*. Key reactions that separate it from most other enteric organisms are lack of hydrogen sulfide production and phenylalanine deaminase positivity. Citrate and ornithine reactions differentiate *Providencia* and *Morganella*.
[Mahon 2006, p517]
MLS ONLY

155 d   Of the organisms listed only *Klebsiella pneumoniae* is nonmotile.
[Murray 2007, p653]

156 c   Of the organisms listed only *Pseudomonas aeruginosa* is oxidase positive.
[Isenburg 1992, 1.19.32`]

157 d   Of the organisms listed only *Proteus mirabilis* is phenylalanine deaminase positive.
[Murray 2007, pp653-654]

158 d   Of the organisms listed only *Serratia marcescens* is DNase positive.
[Murray 2007, pp653-654]

159 d   Quality control of indole requires both a positive and a negative control. *E coli* and *E cloacae* respectively produce a positive and negative reaction with indole.
[Murray 2007, pp652-653]

160 a   *Haemophilus influenzae* requires X and V factors. Sheep blood agar supplies X factor, and the staphylococci produce V factor, so colonies grow around staph colonies.
[Koneman 2005, p464]

161 d   *Pseudomonas aeruginosa* produces the blue-green pigment, pyocyanin.
[Mahon 2006, p568]

162 d   *Pseudomonas aeruginosa* often has a sweet odor that smells like grapes.
[Mahon 2006, p568]

163 b   Growth only on chocolate agar is typical for *Haemophilus influenzae*, which is a gram-negative coccobacillus that causes upper respiratory infections.
[Koneman 2005, p432]

164 a   *Campylobacter* are gram-negative,
MLS ONLY   curved bacilli that require microaerophilic conditions for growth.
[Mahon 2006, pp558-559]

165 d   *Campylobacter jejuni/coli* grow better at 42°C than 37°C and other organisms in the colon are inhibited at this high temperature.
[Mahon 2006, pp558-559]

166 d   *Alcaligenes* and *Moraxella* are oxidase
MLS ONLY   positive; *Stenotrophomonas* is a gram-negative bacillus and is lysine and ONPG positive; *Acinetobacter baumannii* is nitrate and ONPG negative, and it is a gram-negative coccobacillus.
[Murray 2007, pp740, 753; Koneman 2005, p357]

167 a   *Helicobacter pylori* produces large amounts of extracellular urease and is positive for urea within 2 hours.
[Koneman 2005, p559]

168 b   *Haemophilus influenzae* was previously the most common cause of bacterial meningitis in young children. However, the *Haemophilus influenzae* type B vaccine has been in use for several years, resulting in a low incidence of *H influenzae* causing meningitis. This patient has not had most childhood vaccinations, so he is susceptible to *H influenzae*.
[Mahon 2006, pp465, 982]

169 b   Both organisms are gram-negative.
MLS ONLY   *Neisseria gonorrhoeae* is fastidious and does not grow on MacConkey or EMB agar, but *Acinetobacter* does. *Neisseria* is oxidase positive and *Acinetobacter* is oxidase negative.
[Mahon 2006, p570]

170 c   These are classic gram stain, growth and biochemicals for *Haemophilus influenzae*.
[Koneman 2005, p432]

171 c   *Helicobacter pylori* is known to cause gastritis and is a gram-negative, curved bacillus.
[Mahon 2006, pp559, 567, 967-968]

172 b   *Haemophilus influenzae* is recovered on chocolate agar. *Francisella* and *Bordetella pertussis* are fastidious and require special media for growth. *Bacteroides* is an anaerobe that will not grow aerobically.
[Murray 2007, pp639-642]

173 d   *Pseudomonas aeruginosa* grows at 42°C, but this temperature is inhibitory for other *Pseudomonas* species.
[Koneman 2005, p355]

174 b   *Campylobacter jejuni* and *C coli* are closely
MLS ONLY   related and both are pathogens. The test that differentiates the two is hippurate hydrolysis.
[Koneman 2005, pp398-399]

175 a   *Campylobacter jejuni* will grow at 37°C, but prefers 42°C. It is oxidase and catalase positive and motile.
[Koneman 2005, p399]

176 a   *Campylobacter* is microaerophilic, and requires a decreased oxygen and increased carbon dioxide atmosphere for growth.
[Koneman 2005, pp395-396]

177 c   The porphyrin test is an alternative
MLS ONLY   method for detecting heme-producing species of *Haemophilus*. It detects whether or not the organism converts the substrate delta-amino levulinic acid into porphyrins or porphobilinogen, which are intermediates in synthesis of Factor X.
[Mahon 2006, p469]

178 a   *Haemophilus influenzae* is indigenous flora of the upper respiratory tract.
[Mahon 2006, p464]

179 d   The beta-lactamase enzyme produced by *Haemophilus influenzae* inactivates the antibiotics that have a beta-lactam ring in their structure, such as penicillins and cephalosporins.
[Mahon 2006, p470]

180 d   *Haemophilus parainfluenzae* requires NAD for growth but not hemin. This distinguishes it from *H influenzae*. *H haemolyticus* is hemolytic, and *H ducreyi* does not cause epiglotittis.
[Mahon 2006, p471]

181 c   Bone marrow is considered the most sensitive specimen for the recovery of *Brucella*.
[Koneman 2005, p488]

182 b   The violet pigment on sheep blood
MLS ONLY   agar is a characteristic for the genus *Chromobacterium*. *Serratia* is oxidase negative, and *Campylobacter* does not produce a pigment and does not grow on MacConkey agar.
[Mahon 2006, pp579-580; Koneman 2005, p416]

183 c   Most *Campylobacter* grow at 42°C, except
MLS ONLY   *C fetus*. *C fetus* grows best at 37°C and is catalase and oxidase positive.
[Mahon 2006, p560]

184 c   Biochemicals and growth characteristics
MLS ONLY   are indicative of *Haemophilus aphrophilus*. *Brucella* and *Cardiobacterium* are oxidase positive, and *Actinobacillus* are catalase positive.
[Murray 2007, pp626-627]

185 b   *Pasteurella multocida* does not grow on MacConkey agar, and is associated with wounds resulting from dog and cat bites. *Vibrio cholerae* is motile and *Pseudomonas* and *Aeromonas* grow on MacConkey.
[Mahon 2006, pp477, 479]

186 d   *Bordetella bronchiseptica* are normal flora
MLS ONLY   in the respiratory tract of various animals. A key reaction is that it is rapidly urea positive (within 4 hours). *Brucella* is also urea positive, but does not grow on MacConkey agar.
[Koneman 2005, p520]

187 c   *Enterobacteriaceae*, such as *E coli*, *Serratia* and *Enterobacter*, are oxidase negative. The only selection that is oxidase positive is *Aeromonas*. It is associated with wounds contaminated with water.
[Koneman 2005, p419]

188 d   The oxidase and urea reactions
MLS ONLY   differentiate *Bordetella pertussis* and *B parapertussis*. *B pertussis* is oxidase positive and urea negative.
[Mahon 2006, p499]

189 d   Both organisms are oxidase positive;
MLS ONLY   *Bordetella bronchiseptica* is urea positive in 4 hours.
[Mahon 2006, p499]

190 d   Media for isolation of *Legionella* should be incubated at 35°-37°C for at least 7 days.
[Mahon 2006, p488]

191 a   Both *Acinetobacter* and *Moraxella* display resistance to penicillin, and some species grow on MacConkey agar. *Acinetobacter* are oxidase negative, and *Moraxella* are oxidase positive.
[Mahon 2006, p570]

192 a   Growth at 42°C and pyocyanin production are classic tests for the identification of *Pseudomonas aeruginosa*. Gelatin hydrolysis separates *Pseudomonas putida* (negative) from *Pseudomonas fluorescence* (positive).
[Mahon 2006, pp571-571, 569]

193 a   *Francisella tularensis* is the causative agent of tularemia. It has a specific growth requirement for cysteine.
[Mahon 2006, p873]

194 b   "Pitting the agar" and the bleach smell of
MLS ONLY   the colonies are hallmark characteristics of *Eikenella corrodens*.
[Murray 2007, p615]

195 b   *Capnocytophaga* requires increased CO_2,
MLS ONLY   ferments glucose, sucrose, and lactose, and is a gram-negative bacillus. *Capnocytophaga* produces characteristic spreading colonies.
[Murray 2007, p612]

196 d   Buffered charcoal yeast extract agar is recommended for culture of specimens for *Legionella*.
[Murray 2007, p815]

197 d   Thiosulfate citrate bile salt agar is a selective media for *Vibrio*, and it also differentiates sucrose-fermenting species, such as *V cholerae* and *V alginolyticus*.
[Mahon 2006, p548]

198 **d**   The consumption of raw shell fish is a risk factor for *Vibrio vulnificus* and the biochemical reactions support a *Vibrio* species. *V vulnificus* is one of the only vibrios that ferments lactose.
MLS ONLY
[Mahon 2006, pp545-550]

199 **d**   Both organisms are gram-negative bacilli and grow on MacConkey agar. Neither ferments glucose. *Stenotrophomonas* is oxidase negative, while most other nonfermenters are oxidase positive.
[Mahon 2006, p569]

200 **a**   *Burkholderia cepacia* is associated with respiratory infections in cystic fibrosis patients, and the biochemicals are typical for this organism.
MLS ONLY
[Mahon 2006, pp569, 574-575]

201 **c**   The HACEK group of organisms are gram-negative bacilli that require increased CO_2 for growth. They are commonly associated with endocarditis, and include *Haemophilus* species (especially *H aphrophilus*), *Actinobacillus actinomycetemcomitans*, *Cardiobacterium hominis*, *Eikenella corrodens*, and *Kingella* species.
MLS ONLY
[Mahon 2006, pp470-476]

202 **d**   *Brucella* causes undulant fever and is a cause of fever of unknown origin. It is slow growing, and is associated with laboratory-acquired infections. It is also a potential agent of bioterrorism. Suspected *Brucella* isolates should not be tested in automated or manual identification systems.
[Murray 2007, pp798-801]

Aerobic Gram-Negative Cocci

203 **c**   *Neisseria gonorrhoeae* requires an enhanced CO_2 atmosphere for optimal growth.
[Mahon 2006, p439]

204 **b**   Of the possible types of meningitis listed, only *Neisseria meningitidis* is oxidase positive.
[Mahon 2006, p451]

205 **c**   Based on the biochemicals listed the most likely identification of the organism is *Neisseria gonorrhoeae*. *N gonorrhoeae* is most commonly isolated from the genitourinary tract.
[Mahon 2006, p446]

206 **d**   *Neisseria gonorrhoeae* requires an enhanced carbon dioxide atmosphere for optimal growth.
[Murray 2007, p604]

207 **b**   The *Neisseria* species listed all ferment several carbohydrates, *Moraxella catarrhalis* is biochemically inert and does not ferment carbohydrates.
[Mahon 2006, p454]

208 **b**   One of the less commonly used methods for identification of *Neisseria gonorrhoeae* grown in culture is coagglutination.
[Murray 2007, p611]

209 **a**   Penicillin resistance in *Streptococcus pyogenes* and *S agalactiae* have not been described. *Neisseria meningitidis* is rarely resistant to penicillin, which can be beta-lactamase mediated in some isolates. The primary mechanism of penicillin resistance in *N gonorrhoeae* is beta-lactamase.
[Mahon 2006, p345]

210 **d**   Since all *Neisseria* species are oxidase positive, they possess the enzyme to oxidize tetramethyl-phenylenediamine.
[Murray 2007, p608]

211 **b**   Clinical history does not distinguish *Neisseria gonorrhoeae* from *Chlamydia trachomatis*. Because of the presence of nonpathogenic *Neisseria* in the female genital tract, Gram stain does not differentiate these organisms from *N gonorrhoeae*. Culture of an appropriate genital tract specimen is required to confirm identification.
[Mahon 2006, p442]

212 **d**   Because of the presence of nonpathogenic *Neisseria* in the female genital tract, Gram stain does not differentiate these organisms from *N gonorrhoeae*. For this reason Gram stain results should not be reported on vaginal specimens.
MLS ONLY
[Mahon 2006, p443]

213 **c**   Both *Neisseria meningitidis* and *N lactamica* produce acid from maltose and grow on modified Thayer martin agar. *N lactamica* ferments lactose, *N meningitidis* does not.
[Mahon 2006, p458]

214 **d**   Of the choices provided, only fermentation of carbohydrates provides definitive identification of *Neisseria gonorrhoeae*.
[Mahon 2006, p449]

215 **b** *Neisseria gonorrhoeae* is oxidase positive and ferments glucose but not maltose.
[Mahon 2006, p449]

216 **b** *Moraxella catarrhalis* is an oxidase-positive gram-negative diplococcus that is usually beta-lactamase positive. It does not ferment carbohydrates.
[Mahon 2006, p454]

217 **b** Waterhouse-Friderichsen syndrome is a known complication of severe *Neisseria meningitidis* infection.
[Murray 2007, p603]

218 **b** *Neisseria sicca* is the only *Neisseria* species of those listed that ferments glucose, maltose and sucrose.
[Mahon 2006, p457]

Aerobic or Facultative Gram-Positive Bacilli

219 **d** Media containing potassium tellurite is used for the recovery of *Corynebacterium diphtheriae*.
[Mahon 2006, p413]

220 **c** *Bacillus cereus* is the etiologic agent of 2 distinct types of food poisoning syndromes. Spores can survive cooking and germinate. Vegetative cells multiply and produce toxin.
[Koneman 2005, p779]

221 **a** *Nocardia* are capable of growing on Lowenstein-Jensen agar within 7 days and demonstrate branching, beaded gram-positive bacilli on Gram stain. *Nocardia* are partially acid fast, and are stained best with the modified acid-fast stain.
[Mahon 2006, pp432-433]

222 **b** *Corynebacterium* and *Listeria* are catalase-positive and gram-positive bacilli. *Listeria* demonstrates "tumbling" motility that is best demonstrated following growth at 25°C. A few species of *Corynebacterium* species are motile when grown at 35°C.
[Mahon 2006, p419]

223 **c** In order to determine if an isolate of *Corynebacterium diphtheriae* produces toxin, testing for the presence of diphtheria toxin must be performed using methods such as the Elek test or PCR.
[Mahon 2006, p413]

224 **d** *Erysipelothrix rhusipathiae* is the only gram-positive bacillus that produces hydrogen sulfide when inoculated into triple sugar iron agar.
[Mahon 2006, p421]

225 **d** *Listeria* may be confused with some streptococci because *Listeria* is beta-hemolytic and is capable of hydrolyzing esculin.
[Mahon 2006, p419]

226 **c** *Bacillus anthracis* are large, rectangular gram-positive bacilli that produce colonies with an irregular edge (often described as a "medusa-head" appearance) on blood agar. Colonies are nonhemolytic, catalase positive and nonmotile.
[Mahon 2006, p427]

227 **d** *Nocardia asteroides* are partially acid fast, and do not hydrolyze the substrates casein, tyrosine, or xanthine.
[Mahon 2006, p433]

Anaerobes

228 **d** Anaerobic bacteria characteristically produce foul-smelling metabolic end products.
[Mahon 2006, pp593-594]

229 **d** The specimen Gram stain suggests the presence of *Bacillus* or *Clostridium*. Since no growth was observed aerobically, the specimen should be inoculated to media that are incubated anaerobically.
[Koneman 2005, p900]

230 **b** A probable anaerobe is the only organism growing so the microbiologist can proceed with identification.
[Mahon 2006, p614]

231 **c** Most infections involving anaerobes are polymicrobic and can include obligate aerobes, facultative anaerobes, microaerophilic bacteria in addition to anaerobic bacteria.
[Koneman 2005, p887]

Answers–Microbiology

Answers–Microbiology

232 c In this culture there is an aerobic or facultative gram-negative bacillus **and** a second organism growing in the TSB only (a gram-positive bacillus). This leads one to think it could be an anaerobe because it did not grow on any of the media incubated in 3%-5% CO_2. The aerotolerance test is the first step in determining if an anaerobe is present.
[Mahon 2006, p617]

233 a Kanamycin-vancomycin laked blood agar is a selective medium used for the isolation of *Bacteroides* or *Prevotella*.
[Murray 2007, p884]

234 a Anaerobes normally inhabit skin and mucous membranes as part of the normal flora. Distractors **b**, **c**, and **d** are virtually always unacceptable for anaerobic culture, because they normally contain anaerobic organisms. It is difficult to interpret culture results from these specimens and distinguish between pathogens and normal flora.
[Koneman 2005, p891]

235 d *Propionibacterium acnes* is part of the normal flora of the skin, so it is frequently isolated from improperly collected blood cultures.
[Mahon 2006, p627]

236 d The toxin produced by *Clostridium botulinum* is a neurotoxin that is excreted by the organism in food materials, and is then ingested.
[Mahon 2006, p596]

237 a *Corynebacterium* species and *Propionibacterium* species do not produce spores, and *Bacillus* is an aerobic organism.
[Mahon 2006, pp595-596]

238 b *Actinomyces* and *Eubacterium* are anaerobic gram-positive bacilli that do not form spores; *Bacillus* is not an anaerobic organism. *Clostridium perfringens* is a spore-forming anaerobe organism.
[Mahon 2006, p594]

239 b One must compare the sensitivity of latex agglutination that is currently used in the laboratory with the proposed EIA method for toxin A detection. The cell culture cytotoxin assay should be included as a gold standard for toxin detection.
[Koneman 2005, pp936-937]

240 a The reverse CAMP test, production of lecithinase, and demonstration of double zone hemolysis are tests and characteristics used for the identification of *Clostridium perfringens*.
[Koneman 2005, pp905, 932]

241 c SPS in blood culture media enhances recovery of most bacteria, including anaerobes. However, *Peptostreptococcus anaerobius* is inhibited by SPS.
[Koneman 2005, p892]

242 b Latex agglutination identifies the organism, but does not distinguish between toxigenic and nontoxigenic strains, while EIA can detect toxins. Fluorescent staining and HPLC are not used for detection of *C difficile* toxins.
[Murray 2007, p846; Koneman 2005, p937]

243 b *Bacillus cereus* is not an anaerobic organism; *Eubacterium* and *Bifidobacterium* are anaerobic gram-positive bacilli that do not form spores. *Clostridium septicum* forms subterminal spores.
[Koneman 2005, p936]

244 a Botulism infection is confirmed by reference laboratories such as the CDC by demonstrating toxin in serum, feces, gastric contents or vomitus.
[Koneman 2005, p938]

245 c Selective media are needed to isolate *Clostridium difficile* from stool and CCFA is also differential—fermentation of lactose produces classic colony morphology for this organism.
[Mahon 2006, p975]

246 c The Gram stain and double zone of hemolysis are characteristics of *Clostridium perfringens*. *C perfringens* is lecithinase positive on the egg yolk agar test for lecithinase and lipase.
[Mahon 2006, p620]

247 b *Propionibacterium acnes* is part of the normal flora on the skin and is a common blood culture contaminant. The Gram stain given is typical for *P acnes*, and it is catalase and indole positive.
[Mahon 2006, pp628-629]

248 a *Bacteroides* and *Fusobacterium* are anaerobic gram-negative bacilli and *Nocardia* is an aerobic gram-positive bacillus. Gram stain and colony morphology described are classic for *Actinomyces*.
[Mahon 2006, pp598, 626]

249 **a**   Anaerobic gram-negative bacilli
MLS
ONLY   predominate among anaerobes in clinical
infections. *Bacteroides fragilis* is the most
common isolated anaerobic bacteria in
clinical specimens.
[Mahon 2006, p627]

250 **d**   *Brucella* and *Pasteurella* are aerobic,
gram-negative bacilli, and *Actinomyces* is an
anaerobic gram-positive bacillus. *Bacteroides*
species are anaerobic, gram-negative bacilli.
[Koneman 2005, pp912-913]

251 **b**   *Bacteroides fragilis* grows on BBE
MLS
ONLY   agar and because it can hydrolyze esculin
produces black colonies. *B fragilis* is also
catalase positive and indole negative.
[Murray 2007, pp886-887; Koneman 2005, pp914-917]

252 **c**   *Prevotella*, *Porphyromonas* and *Veillonella*
MLS
ONLY   produce colonies that fluoresce brick red.
[Murray 2007, p886]

253 **c**   Both *Prevotella* and *Porphyromonas*
MLS
ONLY   colonies fluoresce brick red. *Porphyromonas*
is susceptible to vancomycin and can be
catalase positive.
[Koneman 2005, p916; Murray 2007, p886]

254 **c**   *Fusobacterium nucleatum* is classically
MLS
ONLY   described as a long, slender, gram-negative
bacillus with tapered ends. Inhibition of
growth by 20% bile and a positive indole
reaction narrow the selection process.
[Koneman 2005, p916]

255 **a**   *Bacteroides fragilis* is indole
MLS
ONLY   negative, unlike *Fusobacterium nucleatum*
and *Porphyromonas asaccharolytica*.
Proteus mirabilis is an indole negative, aerobic
organism.
[Mahon 2006, pp632-633]

256 **b**   Bile tolerant *Bacteroides* species will
MLS
ONLY   grow on agar with 20% bile (BBE agar), while
Fusobacterium, *Prevotella*, and *Porphyromonas*
are sensitive to 20% bile and will not grow
on BBE agar. This reinforces the usefulness
of bile esculin agar for differentiation of
anaerobic gram-negative bacilli.
[Mahon 2006, pp631-633; Koneman 2005, p916]

257 **b**   Several *Clostridium* species are obligate
anaerobes, and will only grow in an anaerobic
environment. The growth of one of these
Clostridium species would confirm that an
anaerobic environment has been achieved in
the anaerobic jar.
[Isenburg 1992, p2.2.6]

258 **c**   *Clostridium perfringens* is lecithinase
MLS
ONLY   positive. *Bacteroides*, *Fusobacterium* and
Clostridium sporogenes are lecithinase
negative.
[Murray 2007, p902]

Fungi

259 **a**   Macroscopic characteristics and
microscopic morphology are observations
used for the routine identification of molds.
[Larone 2002, p1]

260 **c**   Since fungi grow more slowly than
bacteria, a medium with antimicrobials is
included to assist in the recovery of fungi.
Chloramphenicol is an antibacterial agent
active against *Klebsiella* and most other
bacteria.
[Larone 2002, p301]

261 **d**   *Histoplasma capsulatum* is most
frequently transmitted by inhalation.
[Larone 2002, p148]

262 **b**   Calcofluor white binds to cellulose and
chitin present in fungal cell walls.
[Larone 2002, p316]

263 **d**   Many factors influence clinical response
MLS
ONLY   to an antifungal agent; studies have shown
that strains that are resistant in vitro are less
likely to show a clinical response in vivo.
[Murray 2007, p1982]

264 **c**   Interpretation of India ink preparations
MLS
ONLY   can be hindered if too much India ink is
added, blocking the transmission of light.
Equal parts of India ink and CSF should be
combined.
[Murray 2007, pp1687-1688]

265 **a**   *Cryptococcus neoformans* is a cause
of meningitis in immunocompromised
patients, and produces a polysaccharide
capsule.
[Larone 2002, p54]

266 **d**   *Candida albicans* produces germ tubes.
[Larone 2002, p116]

267 **a**   *Cryptococcus neoformans* is a cause
of meningitis in immunocompromised
patients, and produces a polysaccharide
capsule.
[Larone 2002, p54]

268 **d**   *Cryptococcus neoformans* is the only
MLS
ONLY   yeast that produces brown colonies (due to
melanin production) on birdseed agar.
[Larone 2002, pp130, 332]

Answers–Microbiology

269   **c**   *Cryptococcus* may not stain well on Gram stain. Rapid identification is important when yeast is detected in CSF, the presence of capsules seen in an India ink preparation would be presumptive for *C neoformans*.
[Larone 2002, p299]

270   **d**   *Cryptococcus neoformans* is the only
MLS ONLY   clinically encountered yeast that is phenol oxidase positive.
[Larone 2002, pp308-309]

271   **d**   Of the yeasts listed, only
MLS ONLY   *Candida glabrata* is urease negative and does not produce pseudohyphae.
[Larone 2002, pp116-117, 130-131]

272   **d**   Conventional tests, such as carbohydrate assimilation, must be performed for definitive identification of the yeast in this CSF specimen, especially in light of the fact that the yeast is both cryptococcal antigen and germ tube negative.
[Larone 2002, p306]

273   **a**   Cycloheximide is known to inhibit the growth of some fungal pathogens, including *Cryptococcus neoformans*.
[Larone 2002, p300]

274   **b**   *Malassezia furfur* causes catheter-related
MLS ONLY   sepsis, requires lipids for growth, and is a small yeast with a wide bud.
[Larone 2002, p136]

275   **d**   Chromogenic agar is extremely effective
MLS ONLY   in detecting mixed yeast populations in clinical specimens.
[Murray 2007, p1776]

276   **b**   CHROMagar™ produces the best color
MLS ONLY   development when incubated at 35°-37°C.
[Larone 2002, p335]

277   **c**   *Candida albicans* produce tubular
MLS ONLY   structure with no constrictions (germ tubes) when incubated in rabbit plasma.
[Larone 2002, p113]

278   **c**   Cryptococcal latex antigen test has been proven to be significantly more sensitive than staining methods.
[Larone 2002, p299]

279   **c**   *Candida albicans* (positive) and *C tropicalis* (negative) can be used as control organisms for quality control of the germ tube test.
[Murray 2007, p1774]

280   **b**   Several monomorphic molds resemble the filamentous phase of dimorphic molds, so conversion to yeast phase must be performed for identification of dimorphic molds.
[Larone 2002, p309]

281   **d**   The arthroconidia of *Coccidioides immitis* are highly infectious; cultures must be handled with care to minimize aerosols.
[Larone 2002, p259]

282   **a**   Cultures of *Coccidioides immitis* produce
MLS ONLY   alternating arthrospores.
[Larone 2002, p258]

283   **c**   The presence of tuberculate
MLS ONLY   macroconidia indicates a presumptive identification of *H capsulatum*. The identification must be confirmed using nucleic acid probes or exoantigen testing.
[Larone 2002, p150]

284   **b**   The characteristics listed define
MLS ONLY   *Sporothrix* and differentiate it from other dimorphic fungi.
[Larone 2002, p148]

285   **a**   Dimorphism differentiates *Sporothrix* from the other fungi listed.
[Larone 2002, p148]

286   **c**   Conversion of thermally dimorphic fungi
MLS ONLY   in culture requires the use of moist enriched (blood-containing) agar incubated at 35°C.
[Larone 2002, p309]

287   **d**   The microscopic morphology of the
MLS ONLY   yeast phase is characteristic of *Blastomyces*. The microscopic morphology of the mycelial phase of *Blastomyces* is round or pear-shaped small conidia attached to conidiophores of irregular lengths.
[Larone 2002, p152]

288   **a**   Nucleic acid probe test specific for
MLS ONLY   *Coccidioides immitis* can be completed in <4 hours.
[Larone 2002, p258]

289   **c**   *Penicillium marneffei* is a dimorphic fungi
MLS ONLY   that produces a diffusible red pigment.
[Larone 2002, p156]

290   **d**   Dermatophytes include 3 genera
MLS ONLY   that are generally differentiated by their macroconidia and microconidia formation.
[Larone 2002, p231]

291 **a**   Lactophenol cotton blue is used as the mounting medium, since lactic acid acts as a clearing agent, phenol acts as a killing agent, glycerol prevents drying, and cotton blue gives color to the structures.
[Larone 2002, pp303-304]

292 **b**   The absence of conidia differentiates
MLS ONLY
Microsporum audouinii from the other dermatophytes listed.
[Larone 2002, p232]

293 **d**   Smooth walled, club-shaped
MLS ONLY
macroconidia are characteristic of *Epidermophyton floccosum*.
[Larone 2002, p253]

294 **c**   Hair that fluoresces yellow-green under
MLS ONLY
a Woods lamp indicates the presence of a *Microsporum* species. The colony morphology and microscopic characteristics are consistent with *M audouinii*.
[Larone 2002, p232]

295 **c**   *Zygomycetes* grow rapidly and fill the dish with cotton candy-like growth.
[Larone 2002, p163]

296 **d**   Mucormycosis is an aggressive infection where biopsy, curettage or fine-needle aspiration is essential for diagnosis.
[Murray 2007, p1843]

297 **d**   Microscopic morphology (arrangement
MLS ONLY
of the conidia on the conidiophore) is used to differentiate *Penicillium* from *Aspergillus*.
[Larone 2002, pp268-269]

298 **d**   Elongated and tapered phialides
MLS ONLY
(tenpins) are characteristic of *Paecilomyces*.
[Larone 2002, p270]

299 **c**   *Fusarium* frequently cause cornea
MLS ONLY
infections and have sickle-shaped macroconidia.
[Larone 2002, p280]

300 **a**   *Pseudallescheria boydii* is a common cause
MLS ONLY
of eumycotic mycetoma.
[Larone 2002, p32]

301 **a**   Only *Fonsecaea pedrosoi* produces
MLS ONLY
cladiosporium, phialophora and fonsecaea types of sporulation simultaneously.
[Larone 2002, p183]

302 **c**   The microscopic characteristics
MLS ONLY
differentiate *Pseudallescheria boydii* from the other fungi listed.
[Larone 2002, p196]

303 **a**   Inhalation is a common mode of transmission for fungal spores. Specimens for fungal culture should be processed in a biological safety cabinet to minimize the potential for aerosol spread.
[Murray 2007, p1864]

Mycobacteria

304 **b**   Early-morning sputum specimens are optimal for AFB culture.
[Murray 2007, p553]

305 **a**   Mycobacteria use glycerol as a carbon source in the presence of mineral salts.
[Murray 2007, p544]

306 **d**   Many species of mycobacteria are slow growing, and may take up to 12 weeks for growth.
[Murray 2007, p559]

307 **d**   Specimens contaminated by normal flora must be decontaminated prior to inoculation of media; NaOH is the most common decontaminant.
[Murray 2007, p555]

308 **a**   Sabouraud dextrose is fungal media; mycobacterial media should have been inoculated.
[Murray 2007, p557]

309 **d**   The concentration of sodium hydroxide
MLS ONLY
may be too strong due to decreased recovery of AFB and lack of contaminated cultures.
[Murray 2007, pp554-555]

310 **b**   Lowenstein-Jensen is an egg based medium, 7H11 is an agar-based medium, and Lowenstein-Jensen Gruft is a selective egg-based medium.
[Murray 2007, p557]

311 **a**   The most widely used digestion-decontamination method is the N-acetyl-L-cysteine-2% NaOH method.
[Murray 2007, p555]

312 **d**   N-acetyl-L-cysteine (NALC) is a mucolytic agent; the concentration of NALC may be increased to digest thick, mucoid specimens.
[Murray 2007, pp554-555]

313 **b**   The counterstain acts as a quenching agent and reduces the background fluorescence of cellular debris.
[Murray 2007, p345]

314 **d** If exposed to light, agar-based media such as 7H11 may release formaldehyde, which is toxic to mycobacteria.
[Murray 2007, p557]

315 **d** The oxalic acid method is superior to alkali methods for processing specimens contaminated with *Pseudomonas*.
[Murray 2007, p565]

316 **b** Liquid medium is recommended to provide more rapid recovery of AFB than solid medium. Isolation rates of mycobacteria is also higher with liquid medium.
[Murray 2007, pp558-559]

317 **d** Specimens processed for mycobacterial culture must be processed in a biological safety cabinet to minimize aerosol transmission of the organism.
[Murray 2007, p100]

318 **d** Mycobacteria form stable complexes with Kinyoun carbol fuchsin.
[Murray 2007, p555]

319 **d** A positive niacin reaction differentiates *Mycobacterium tuberculosis* from *M leprae*, *M kansasii* and *M fortuitum*.
MLS ONLY
[Murray 2007, p574]

320 **c** *Mycobacterium tuberculosis* and *M bovis* cannot grow in the presence of NAP, while other mycobacteria can grow in the presence of NAP.
MLS ONLY
[Koneman 2005, p910]

321 **d** Growth rate, colony morphology and positive niacin differentiates *Mycobacterium tuberculosis* from other mycobacteria.
MLS ONLY
[Murray 2007, p574]

322 **c** A positive niacin test differentiates *Mycobacterium tuberculosis* from most other mycobacteria.
MLS ONLY
[Murray 2007, p574]

323 **d** Growth rate, colony morphology, niacin production, and nitrate reduction differentiate *Mycobacterium tuberculosis* from other mycobacteria.
MLS ONLY
[Murray 2007, p574]

324 **b** The niacin test can be repeated in several days from the initial tube rather than setting up new biochemicals that would take longer to grow.
MLS ONLY
[Murray 2007, pp574, 577]

325 **c** *Mycobacterium tuberculosis* can remain viable but dormant in macrophages for many years.
[Murray 2007, p545]

326 **b** *Mycobacterium tuberculosis* can remain viable but dormant in macrophages for many years. ?
[Murray 2007, p546]

327 **b** Several commercial PCR tests are available that identify *Mycobacterium tuberculosis* from positive respiratory specimens.
[Murray 2007, p563]

328 **b** If the molecular fingerprint is the same, the smear-negative culture should be considered a false positive, and the laboratory should review its processing procedures.
MLS ONLY
[Murray 2007, p562]

329 **a** Primary drugs for the treatment of *Mycobacterium tuberculosis* include isoniazid, rifampin, pyrazinamide, and ethambutol.
[Murray 2007, p1230]

330 **b** *Mycobacterium gordonae* is widely distributed in soil and water, and is generally considered nonpathogenic.
MLS ONLY
[Murray 2007, p549]

331 **d** *Mycobacterium scrofulaceum* is a scotochromogen.
MLS ONLY
[Murray 2007, p574., 595]

332 **b** Scotochromogens produce deep yellow or orange pigment when grown in either light or darkness.
[Murray 2007, p573]

333 **a** Photochromogens produce nonpigmented colonies only when grown in darkness, but pigmented colonies after exposure to light.
[Murray 2007, p573]

334 **b** *Mycobacterium leprae* cannot be cultured in vitro. A clinical diagnosis is made, supported by the presence of AFB in a biopsy specimen.
[Murray 2007, p547]

335 **c** Lowenstein-Jensen is an egg-based medium used to isolate AFB. The other media are not used for the isolation of AFB.
[Murray 2007, p557]

336 **b**   *Mycobacterium marinum* causes
MLS   infections as a result of trauma to the skin
ONLY   and exposure to contaminated fish tanks or
salt water. Its optimal growth temperature is
28°-30°C.
[Murray 2007, p548]

337 **d**   *Mycobacterium xenopi* grows best at
MLS   42°-45°C and is not pigmented.
ONLY
[Murray 2007, p549]

338 **b**   Pigment production is controlled by an
oxygen-dependent, light-inducible enzyme in
photochromogenic mycobacteria.
[Murray 2007, pp573-575]

339 **b**   The characteristics given differentiate
MLS   *Mycobacterium gordonae* from the other
ONLY   mycobacteria listed. *M szulgai* and
flavescens are nitrate reduction positive,
and *M scrofulaceum* is negative for Tween®
hydrolysis.
[Murray 2007, p574]

340 **b**   Tween® hydrolysis differentiates
MLS   *Mycobacterium gordonae* (Tween® positive)
ONLY   from *M scrofulaceum* (Tween® negative).
[Murray 2007, p574]

341 **d**   *Mycobacterium avium* and *M intracellulare*
have the same biochemical pattern, but can
be differentiated by the use of DNA probes.
[Murray 2007, p547]

342 **a**   Rapidly-growing mycobacteria such as
Mycobacterium fortuitum may be <10% acid
fast and may not stain with fluorochrome.
[Murray 2007, p555]

343 **c**   *Mycobacterium haemophilum* grows best
MLS   at 30°C, requires hemin or ferric ammonium
ONLY   citrate for growth, and causes subcutaneous
lesions presenting as multiple skin nodules.
[Murray 2007, p548]

344 **a**   *Mycobacterium malmoense* requires up to
MLS   12 weeks for growth.
ONLY
[Murray 2007, pp548, 559]

345 **c**   *Mycobacterium tuberculosis* is the
MLS   only mycobacterium listed that is nitrate
ONLY   reduction positive.
[Murray 2007, p577]

Viruses and Other Microorganisms

346 **b**   Antibiotics and antifungal agents are
added to viral transport medium to inhibit
the growth of bacteria and fungus.
[Murray 2007, p45]

347 **b**   In tissue smears or biopsy specimens,
the presence of virally infected cells is
indicated by intranuclear or intracytoplasmic
inclusions.
[Murray 2007, p1299]

348 **a**   Respiratory syncytial virus (RSV)
infected the ciliated respiratory epithelium
of the upper respiratory tract. A
nasopharyngeal swab or aspirate is the
optimal specimen for RSV recovery.
[Murray 2007, p1363]

349 **a**   Cytomegalovirus is a slow-growing
MLS   herpesvirus, and may require up to 3 weeks
ONLY   to grow in conventional viral culture.
[Murray 2007, p1555]

350 **b**   Human papilloma virus (HPV) infects
epithelial tissues throughout the body,
including skin, larynx, and anogenital tissue.
Persistent infection with oncogenic types of
HPV and integration of HPV DNA into the
cellular genome is a pathway leading to HPV-
induced neoplasia, such as cervical cancer.
[Murray 2007, pp1601-1603]

351 **b**   Herpes simplex virus is the most
common cause of fatal sporadic encephalitis
in the United States.
[Murray 2007, p1525]

352 **b**   Adenovirus infections are common. It
causes up to 5% of all respiratory infections,
and the prevalence of infection is higher (up
to 14%).
[Murray 2007, p1589]

353 **c**   The classic clinical syndrome associated
MLS   with Epstein-Barr virus (EBV) infection
ONLY   is infectious mononucleosis. However,
in immunocompromised patients,
EBV is associated with posttransplant
lymphoproliferative disorders, and
malignancies such as Burkitt lymphoma.
[Murray 2007, p1565]

354 **c**   *Chlamydia trachomatis, Neisseria
MLS   gonorrhoeae* and herpes simplex virus can
ONLY   all be isolated in culture. Direct culture of
Treponema pallidum on artificial media has
not been achieved. Darkfield microscopy and
serological techniques are used to diagnose
T pallidum infection.
[Murray 2007, p991]

355 **c**   Darkfield microscopy can be performed
MLS   to visualize *Treponema pallidum* in genital or
ONLY   skin lesions. Darkfield examination allows
for the visualization of *T pallidum*'s typical
morphology and motility.
[Murray 2007, p991]

Answers–Microbiology

356 **a** The presence of typical intracytoplasmic inclusions are particularly useful in diagnosing *Chlamydia trachomatis* inclusion conjunctivitis. Multinucleated giant cells are seen in cells infected with herpes simplex and varicella zoster virus. Cytomegalovirus produces large cells with intranuclear inclusions.
MLS ONLY
[Murray 2007, p1026]

357 **c** Iodine staining can be used to detect the glycogen-rich cytoplasmic inclusions in *Chlamydia trachomatis* infected cells. These inclusions stain brown with iodine.
MLS ONLY
[Murray 2007, p1028]

358 **c** Iodine staining can be used to detect the glycogen-rich cytoplasmic inclusions in *Chlamydia trachomatis* infected cells. These inclusions stain brown with iodine.
MLS ONLY
[Murray 2007, p1029]

359 **d** Bacterial L-forms are bacteria that lose their cell wall as a result of therapy with cell wall-active antibiotics, such as beta-lactam antibiotics. Unlike *Mycoplasma* species, which permanently lack a cell wall, the lack of a cell wall in L-forms is a result of environmental conditions. Once beta-lactam therapy is discontinued, an L-form has the capability to regrow the cell wall.
MLS ONLY
[Murray 2007, p1004]

360 **a** Relapsing fever is caused by *Borrelia recurrentis* and is transmitted by the human body louse. Relapsing fever is characterized by the acute onset of high fever lasting 3-7 days, interspersed with periods of no fever lasting days to weeks.
[Murray 2007, p972]

361 **b** *Chlamydophila psittaci*, the agent of psittacosis, is transmitted to humans via inhalation of nasal secretions, as well as infected fecal or feather dust, of psittacine birds (parrot family).
[Murray 2007, p1024]

362 **a** *Chlamydia trachomatis* is a well-known cause of sexually transmitted infections, including urethritis and cervicitis, as well as inclusion conjunctivitis and pneumonia in neonates. It also causes trachoma and lymphogranuloma venereum.
[Murray 2007, p1023]

363 **c** *Mycoplasma* are smaller than other bacteria and lack a cell wall. Instead, they possess a trilaminar cell membrane. Because they lack a cell wall, they cannot be stained with Gram stain.
[Murray 2007, p1004]

364 **d** *Leptospira* are spiral-shaped organisms with hooked ends. They are ubiquitous in water (eg, lakes, ponds) and associated with renal infection in animals. Leptospirosis is a zoonosis, and humans are usually infected via direct or indirect contact with the urine of infected animals (including rats). Between 5%-10% of patients with leptospirosis have the icteric form and develop jaundice, and may develop acute renal failure.
MLS ONLY
[Murray 2007, pp964-965]

365 **c** The clinical syndrome described is most likely the icteric form of *Leptospira interrogans*. The most commonly used medium for culture is Fletcher semisolid agar. Cultures are incubated in the dark for up to 6 weeks at 28°-30°C and examined weekly by darkfield microscopy.
MLS ONLY
[Murray 2007, pp352, 966]

366 **d** *Leptospira* cultures are incubated in the dark for up to 6 weeks in ambient air at 28°-30°C, and examined weekly by darkfield microscopy. Fletcher semisolid agar contains peptone, bee extract and rabbit serum, which create an enriched medium to support the growth of leptospires.
MLS ONLY
[Murray 2007, p352]

367 **b** *Leptospira* organisms can be readily detected by culturing blood during the first week of illness. After this time the organisms disappear from blood and are excreted from the urine for up to 1 month.
MLS ONLY
[Murray 2007, p966]

368 **d** Since viruses are intracellular organisms, the collection of cellular material is required to be able to demonstrate virus using stains or fluorescent techniques. Scrapings of the base of a vesicle are required to collect cellular material.
MLS ONLY
[Murray 2007, p1299]

369 **b** Up to 1/3 of patients with *Neisseria gonorrhoeae* infection are also co-infected with *Chlamydia trachomatis*. Patients with identified infection with one organism are usually treated for both infections.
MLS ONLY
[Murray 2007, p1023]

370 **a** *Ureaplasma urealyticum*, like other *Mycoplasma*, lacks a cell wall and possesses an extremely small genome. As a result, this organism has limited biosynthetic capability and fastidious growth requirements. Culture medium should contain serum (provides sterols), growth factors such as yeast extract, and a metabolic substrate.
MLS ONLY
[Murray 2007, p346]

371 d McCoy cells, in addition to buffalo green monkey kidney cells, are susceptible to infection with *Chlamydia trachomatis*, and are used routinely for the recovery of *C trachomatis* in culture.
[Murray 2007, p1011]

372 d
MLS
ONLY *Rickettsia* species infect and multiply within vascular endothelial cells.
[Murray 2007, p1036]

Parasites

373 d Pollen grains are common artifacts in stool specimens submitted for ova and parasite examination. Their appearance is similar to protozoan cysts.
[Provlab 2009]

374 c
MLS
ONLY Polyvinyl alcohol is an adhesive and is used in the preparation of smears for stains, such as trichrome.
[Murray 2007, p2014]

375 d
MLS
ONLY The recommended technique for culturing *Acanthamoeba* is the use of nonnutrient agar seeded with a lawn of *E coli*. Specimens with suspected *Acanthamoeba* are inoculated onto a freshly inoculated lawn of *E coli*, incubated and observed for 7 days. Identification is based on the characteristic patterns of locomotion and morphologic features of the trophic and cystic forms.
[Murray 2007, p2017]

376 d
MLS
ONLY *Naegleria fowleri* is the etiologic agent of primary amoebic encephalitis.
[Murray 2007, p2031]

377 d
MLS
ONLY Formed stool is unlikely to contain trophozoites so direct examination of the stool is not necessary. The stool should be preserved as soon as possible to preserve any cysts, ova or larvae that may be present in the specimen.
[Murray 2007, p2006]

378 d
MLS
ONLY Incomplete removal of mercuric chloride may cause the smear to contain refractive crystals. Since the 70% ethanol-iodine solution removes the mercury, it should be changed at least weekly to maintain the strong tea color.
[Isenburg 1992, p.7.3.6.5.VIII.D]

379 b
MLS
ONLY The increased amount of blood placed on the slide of a thick smear for blood parasites improves the sensitivity of the smear. Thick smears should be performed on all requests for blood parasites.
[Murray 2007, p2042]

380 a The most common cause of ring-enhancing brain lesions in a patient with HIV/AIDS is *Toxoplasma gondii*.
[Murray 2007, p2071]

381 c
MLS
ONLY The patient's history is suggestive of *Babesia* infection. *Babesia microti* ring forms are similar to *Plasmodium falciparum*. A travel history is helpful in determining the cause of infection.
[Murray 2007, pp2051-2053]

382 b The trophozoite of *Entamoeba histolytica* ranges in size from 12-60 µm, which is significantly larger than *Endolimax nana*. The nucleus of *E histolytica* displays evenly distributed peripheral chromatin unlike *E coli*, which has coarse peripheral chromatin and *I bütschlii*, which has none.
[Murray 2007, p2094]

383 d Trophozoites of *Entamoeba coli* demonstrate slow and undefined motility.
[Murray 2007, p2094]

384 b
MLS
ONLY *Entamoeba coli* is a nonpathogenic protozoan. Its presence indicates the ingestion of fecally contaminated food or water and should lead to a closer review of the specimen for pathogenic parasites or the collection of additional specimens.
[Murray 2007, p2094]

385 a
MLS
ONLY The cysts of *Entamoeba coli* and *E histolytica* may appear similar to the unexperienced technologist. *E coli* cysts are larger and contain more than 4 nuclei in each cyst.
[Murray 2007, p2094]

386 a
MLS
ONLY The image displays the cyst form of *Entamoeba coli*, a nonpathogenic parasite.
[Murray 2007, p2094]

387 b The image displays the trophozoite form of *Giardia lamblia*, a flagellated protozoan parasite.
[Murray 2007, p2100]

388 a Diarrhea associated with *Giardia lamblia* is caused by the consumption of contaminated water and results in greasy, foul-smelling stools.
[Murray 2007, p2100]

Answers–Microbiology

389 a Protozoan trophozoites are fragile and begin to disintegrate as soon as they are passed. Liquid stool specimens should be preserved within 30 minutes of passage in order to adequately preserve parasite morphology. If a liquid specimen cannot be properly preserved, another specimen should be collected.
[Murray 2007, p1998]

390 a
MLS
ONLY While *Entamoeba hartmanni* and *Endolimax nana* are a similar size, *E hartmanni* has similar peripheral chromatin to *E histolytica,* while *E nana* has none. *E histolytica* cysts are larger and round when compared to *E nana. Chilomastix* is a flagellated protozoan, and has only 1 nucleus.
[Murray 2007, p2094]

391 d
MLS
ONLY *Strongyloides stercoralis* rhabditiform larvae are capable of transforming into filariform (infective) larvae in the intestines of immunocompromised patients. This establishes an autoinfective cycle.
[Murray 2007, p2152]

392 b The ova of *Enterobius vermicularis* cannot be demonstrated in a routine ova and parasite examination. The adult female *Enterobius* worm migrates out of the anus, and lays her eggs in the perianal folds. A scotch tape preparation of the skin of the perianal folds is used to collect ova.
[Murray 2007, p2027]

393 c The ova of *Enterobius vermicularis* cannot be demonstrated in a routine ova and parasite examination. The adult female *Enterobius* worm migrates out of the anus, and lays her eggs in the perianal folds. A scotch tape preparation of the skin of the perianal folds is used to collect ova.
[Isenburg 1992, p7.6.1.II]

394 c
MLS
ONLY *Onchocerca volvulus* is the only microfilaria that is detected in the skin snips of patients with raised skin nodules. The microfilaria of *Wuchereria, Brugia* and *Loa loa* are found in the blood of infected patients.
[Murray 2007, p2161]

395 c The most common sign of *Enterobius vermicularis* infection is intense perianal itching.
[Murray 2007, p2149]

396 d The ova of *Enterobius vermicularis* cannot be demonstrated in a routine ova and parasite examination. The adult female *Enterobius* worm migrates out of the anus and lays her eggs in the perianal folds. A scotch tape preparation of the skin of the perianal folds is used to collect ova.
[Murray 2007, p2027]

397 c
MLS
ONLY The diagnostic stages of *Strongyloides, Entamoeba* and *Ancylostoma* can be detected in the stool of infected patients. The diagnostic stage of *Echinococcus granulosus* is not detected in an infected patient's stool.
[Murray 2007, pp2033, 2172]

398 a Humans may become infected with *Taenia solium* by either ingesting the larval form or ova. If ova are ingested the parasite cannot complete the life cycle, and cysticerci encyst in various tissues including the brain.
[Murray 2007, p2171]

399 d Of the organisms listed, only *Paragonimus* and *Hymenolepis* can be identified to the species level by the appearance of their ova in stool.
[Murray 2007, p2168, 2185]

400 a The scolex of *Taenia saginata* is square with 4 suckers and no hooks.
[Murray 2007, p2168]

401 c
MLS
ONLY Adult *Paragonimus* worms live in cystic cavities in the lungs. Eggs are laid by the adult and transferred to the bronchial tree with sputum. Ova may be found in sputum or swallowed and passed in stool.
[Murray 2007, p2183]

402 b The rhabditiform larvae of hookworm and *Strongyloides stercoralis* can be differentiated by the size of their genital primordium. *Strongyloides* has a prominent genital primordium and a small buccal cavity. Hookworm larvae have a longer buccal cavity, and the genital primordium is not evident. *S. stercoralis* larvae have a notched tail whereas hookworm larvae have a tapering tail.
[Murray 2007, p2144]

Molecular Biology

The following items have been identified generally as appropriate for both entry level medical laboratory scientists and medical laboratory technicians. Items that are appropriate for medical laboratory scientists **only** are marked with an "MLS ONLY."

Molecular Science

1
MLS ONLY
Which nucleotide pair has a high frequency of mutation in human chromosomal DNA?

  a CC
  b CG
  c CA
  d CT

2   During the G2 phase of the cell cycle, the DNA content of a cell is:

  a haploid
  b diploid
  c triploid
  d tetraploid

3   Intervening sequences are found in:

  a heteronuclear RNA
  b mature mRNA
  c ribosomal RNA
  d transfer RNA

4
MLS ONLY
Which is considered an epigenetic modification of DNA?

  a a transversion of an A nucleotide to a T in an exon of a gene
  b a transition of an A to a G in an intron of a gene
  c methylation of CpG islands in the promoter region of a gene
  d insertion of a nucleotide into the coding region of a gene

5   A metaphase chromosome with primary constriction that gives the chromosome clearly defined short and long arms is considered:

  a acrocentric
  b submetacentric
  c metacentric
  d telocentric

6
MLS ONLY
Reverse transcriptase would best be described as a:

  a DNA-dependent DNA polymerase
  b DNA-dependent RNA polymerase
  c RNA-dependent DNA polymerase
  d RNA-dependent RNA polymerase

7   The 2 alleles for a sex-linked recessive disease are X and x. The mutant allele is x. What is the
      percentage of male offspring that would be expected to be affected by the disease from parents
      who have the following genotypes?

     mother: Xx
     father: xY

a   0
b   25
c   50
d   100

8   The term that best describes males regarding X-linked genes is:

a   heterozygous
b   homozygous
c   haplozygous
d   hemizygous

9   The mode of inheritance of mitochondrial DNA is:

a   dominant
b   recessive
c   codominant
d   maternal

Molecular Techniques

10   Which statement concerning the resolution of DNA on an agarose gel is true?
MLS
ONLY a   the polymerization of agarose is initiated by adding TEMED and ammonium persulfate to
            agarose monomer in solution
      b   agarose gel electrophoresis can resolve smaller molecules of DNA compared to acrylamide gel
            electrophoresis
      c   as the concentration of agarose in the gel increases, the smaller the size of DNA that can be
            resolved on the gel
      d   DNA must be denatured before being loaded into the sample wells of an agarose gel

11   An RFLP is most likely detected using which of the following methods?
MLS
ONLY a   Northern blot
      b   Southern blot
      c   Western blot
      d   Southwestern blot

12   The methodology of performing a reverse dot blot is best described as:
MLS
ONLY a   attaching many patient DNA samples to a nitrocellulose membrane and hybridizing the patient
            samples with a single labeled probe
      b   attaching multiple patient samples to a nitrocellulose membrane and hybridizing multiple
            labeled probes to the patient samples
      c   attaching multiple labeled probes to a nitrocellulose membrane and hybridizing a patient
            sample to the multiple labeled probes
      d   attaching multiple probes to a nitrocellulose membrane and then hybridizing a single labeled
            patient sample to the multiple probes

13   Which condition has the highest stringency for washing a Southern blot after hybridization has
MLS   been completed?
ONLY
      a   low temperature, low salt concentration
      b   high temperature, low salt concentration
      c   high temperature, high salt concentration
      d   low temperature, high salt concentration

14 The Klenow fragment of *E coli* DNA polymerase I is used:
MLS
ONLY
   a to make cDNA from an RNA template
   b to label DNA probes by random primer labeling
   c in quantitative real time PCR
   d to label a DNA probe by nick translation

15 What is a solution hybridization method for the detection of nucleic acid:protein interactions?
MLS
ONLY
   a RNase protection assay
   b gel mobility shift assay
   c strand displacement amplification assay
   d hybrid capture assay

16 Which probe is most often used to detect trisomy 21 by interphase FISH?
MLS
ONLY
   a locus-specific probe
   b alpha satellite DNA probe
   c chromosome paint probe
   d spectral karyotyping probe

17 How many volumes of ethanol are added to 1 volume of a DNA:salt solution to cause the DNA
MLS
ONLY to precipitate?

   a 1
   b 1.5
   c 2
   d 2.5

18 Chelex® 100 resin is used to:

   a purify mRNA from total RNA
   b extract total RNA from cells
   c extract DNA from cells
   d remove unincorporated primers from PCR reactions prior to gel analysis of PCR products

19 The fluorescent dye that exhibits the greatest sensitivity for quantization of DNA is:

   a ethidium bromide
   b Hoechst 33258
   c propidium iodide
   d SYBR® Green

20 When quantifying the amount of genomic DNA in a sample by spectrophotometry, an OD 260 of
1.0 corresponds to what concentration of DNA?

   a 10 µg/mL
   b 20 µg/mL
   c 50 µg/mL
   d 100 µg/mL

21 A RNA sample is isolated from peripheral blood cells of a patient. When performing
MLS
ONLY spectrophotometric analysis to determine the yield of RNA in the sample you find the
1:40 dilution of the 0.5 mL sample gives an OD 260 reading of 0.03125 and an OD 280 reading
of 0.01760. What is the total amount of RNA contained in the 0.5 mL sample?

   a 50 µg
   b 25 µg
   c 12.5 µg
   d 5 µg

22 Which statement is true concerning the analysis of short tandem repeats (str)?
MLS
ONLY
   a str are detected by RT-PCR
   b str alleles are determined by Southern blotting
   c str alleles are determined by PCR product size
   d str analysis requires that high molecular weight genomic DNA be available in samples to be tested

23 Which reagent generates a signal during the annealing stage of a quantitative real time
MLS
ONLY
PCR reaction?

   a SYBR® Green
   b TaqMan® probe
   c molecular beacon
   d Scorpion™ probe

24 Denaturation of DNA during a PCR reaction refers to breaking:

   a hydrogen bonds between nitrogenous bases in base-paired nucleotides
   b phosphodiester bonds between nitrogenous bases in base-paired nucleotides
   c covalent bonds between nitrogenous bases in base-paired nucleotides
   d peptide bonds between nitrogenous bases in base-paired nucleotides

25 What is the most critical step in determining the specificity of a PCR reaction?

   a denaturation temperature
   b annealing temperature
   c extension temperature
   d number of cycles in the PCR reaction

26 A PCR reaction in which 4 different sets of primers are used to simultaneously amplify 4 distinct loci in the same reaction tube is known as a:

   a multiplex PCR reaction
   b heteroplex PCR reaction
   c polyplex PCR reaction
   d quadraplex PCR reaction

27 A variation of a standard PCR reaction that can increase the sensitivity and specificity of a low
MLS
ONLY
copy number target in a patient sample is known as:

   a branched PCR
   b RT-PCR
   c nested PCR
   d cleavage-based PCR

28 Probes are often used during real time PCR to quantitate the formation of specific amplicons
MLS
ONLY
during the reaction. Which system involves the use of 2 distinct probes to generate a fluorescent signal?

   a TaqMan®
   b molecular beacon
   c FRET
   d Scorpion™

29 Which technique employs the amplification of the signal resulting from probe:target
MLS
ONLY
hybridization rather than by amplifying the target or the probe?

   a branched DNA analysis
   b polymerase chain reaction
   c ligase chain reaction
   d nucleic acid sequence-based amplification

30
MLS
ONLY
Refer to the figure. An amplicon for gene X is 176 base pairs (bp) in size. A variant allele x, gives the same size amplicon but has an Alwl restriction enzyme recognition site that is not present in the amplicon arising from allele X. A PCR reaction is run on a DNA sample isolated from 3 patients. The sample is digested with Alwl after the PCR is complete and products of the digestion are resolved on a 4.0% agarose gel (– = no Alwl digestion, + = Alwl digested).

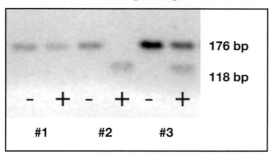

Assuming all appropriate controls have worked correctly, what is the interpretation of the genotype of patient #3 with regards to alleles X and x?

a patient is homozygous for X
b patient is heterozygous for X and x
c patient is homozygous for x
d patient's genotype cannot be determined

31
MLS
ONLY
Methylation of cytosine residues is involved in the alteration of gene expression in a number of cancers. Which sequencing technique is best suited to determine if methylation of cytosine residues has taken place in the promoter region of a given gene?

a Maxam/Gilbert chemical cleavage
b Sanger dideoxyterminator
c bisulfite sequencing
d pyrosequencing

32
MLS
ONLY
Which method is best suited to screen for mutations in a gene having multiple possible mutations?

a comparative genome hybridization
b allele-specific PCR
c real time PCR
d single-strand conformational polymorphism

33
MLS
ONLY
What is the purpose of the enzyme uracil-N-glycolase in a molecular diagnostics laboratory?

a to lower the melting temperature of RNA:DNA hybrids in Northern blot analysis
b to remove any previously generated amplicons containing dUTP from PCR reactions
c to remove contaminating genomic DNA from an RT-PCR reaction
d to melt double-stranded DNA to single-stranded DNA during a Southern blot procedure

34
MLS
ONLY
What is the best method to rule out the possibility of genomic DNA giving a false-positive result in an RT-PCR reaction?

a use of upstream and downstream primers that span an exon-intron-exon region of the target
b treatment of RNA that will be used in the RT reaction with RNase
c addition of uracil-N-glycolase to the RT reaction
d omission of Taq DNA polymerase from the PCR reaction

Applications of Molecular Testing

35
MLS
ONLY
Monitoring the load of HIV circulating in a patient's plasma would best be accomplished using which method?

   a PCR
   b DNA sequencing
   c NABSA
   d bDNA

36
MLS
ONLY
A common use for pulsed-field gel electrophoresis is:

   a DNA fingerprinting
   b mitochondrial DNA typing
   c epidemiological typing of bacterial strains
   d tumor cell phenotyping

37
MLS
ONLY
When genotyping strains of bacteria by PFGE, what is the minimum number of genetic differences that must be observed between a reference strain and a test strain before it can be determined that the test strain is unrelated to the reference strain?

   a 1
   b 2
   c 3
   d 4

38
MLS
ONLY
A human actin gene may be used as an amplification control when performing PCR testing for *Mycoplasma pneumoniae* in a bronchoalveolar lavage taken from a human patient. The type of amplification control is described as:

   a homologous extrinsic
   b homologous intrinsic
   c heterologous extrinsic
   d heterologous intrinsic

39
MLS
ONLY
Molecular-based testing was performed on a nasopharyngeal swab sample taken from a patient. Results are reported as positive for IS481 and negative for IS1000. These results indicate the patient's nasopharynx is colonized with:

   a *Bordetella pertussis*
   b *Bordetella holmesii*
   c *Bordetella parapertussis*
   d *Bordetella* sp

40
MLS
ONLY
DNA-based testing for the presence of MRSA uses PCR with primers specific for which gene?

   a *vanA*
   b *inhA*
   c *mecA*
   d *rpoB*

41
A translocation in which chromosome pair creates a *BCR/ABL1* fusion gene product associated with CML?

   a 11;18
   b 14;18
   c 9;22
   d 9;14

42
MLS
ONLY
The molecular-based diagnostic test for *Mycobacterium tuberculosis* uses ribosomal RNA as the target. Primers are made to be specific for which RNA subunit?

    a 5.8S
    b 16S
    c 18S
    d 28S

43
MLS
ONLY
A PCR-based assay is performed to determine the clonality of B cells in a patient using a forward primer specific for the innermost framework region and a reverse primer complimentary to the joining region (of the immunoglobulin heavy chain). When run on an agarose gel containing ethidium bromide, the patient sample exhibits a smear of staining over a wide range in the patient sample lane along with one distinct band approximately a third of the way down from the sample loading well. Assuming all controls worked properly for the assay, what is your interpretation of the results for this patient?

    a patient is normal
    b patient has mononucleosis
    c patient has a polyclonal population of B cells
    d patient has a monoclonal population of B cells

44
MLS
ONLY
After performing interphase FISH with X chromosome-specific and Y chromosome-specific alpha satellite probes, it is determined that nuclei in cells from your phenotypic female exhibit only 1 bright fluorescent spot with the X chromosome-specific probe and do not react at all with the Y-specific probe. Assuming all controls have worked correctly, what is the most likely diagnosis for this patient?

    a patient is a genetically normal female
    b patient is a female with Turner syndrome
    c patient is a female with fragile X syndrome
    d patient is a male who suffers from androgen insensitivity syndrome due to the lack of a Y chromosome

45
MLS
ONLY
A Robertsonian translocation may be associated with which genetic disorder?

    a Turner syndrome
    b Down syndrome
    c Angelman syndrome
    d Cri du chat syndrome

46
MLS
ONLY
A molecular-based test commonly used in testing donors and recipients prior to organ transplantations is:

    a sequence-specific PCR
    b allele-specific PCR
    c real time PCR
    d reverse transcriptase PCR

47
MLS
ONLY
The results of str typing of a child, the child's mother and 3 alleged fathers (AF) of the child are listed in the table below.

Locus name	Child genotype	Mother genotype	AF1 genotype	AF2 genotype	AF3 genotype
CSF1PO	10,12	12,12	11,12	10,12	12,13
TPOX	9,9	9,11	8,9	9,11	9,11
TH01	7,9	7,9.3	7,8	7,9	7,9.3
F13A01	6,9	9,9	6,9	6,6	9,9
FESFPS	10,11	11,13	11,14	7,10	10,9
vWA	14,18	18,19	13,18	13,14	15,18

Which of the statements below is correct concerning the alleged fathers?

a AF1 is most likely the father of the child.
b AF2 is most likely the father of the child.
c AF3 is most likely the father of the child.
d None of the alleged fathers is likely the father of the child.

48
MLS
ONLY
DNA sequencing of hypervariable regions I and II is used to:

a detect polymorphisms in human TP53
b genotype strains of *Mycoplasma*
c to monitor chemotherapy for B cell lymphoma
d detection of polymorphisms in human mitochondrial DNA

49
MLS
ONLY
Which locus is used to identify the gender of the individual from whom a DNA sample is obtained?

a amelogenin
b CSF1PO
c TPOX
d vWA

50
MLS
ONLY
Which statement is true concerning molecular-based paternity testing?

a paternity testing is typically performed using VNTR loci in the mother, child and alleged father
b single mismatch between an allele in the child (that must have come from the father of the child) and the alleged father is sufficient to exclude the alleged father
c match between the alleged father and the child at a rare allele carries less weight in paternity than does a match involving a higher frequency allele
d paternity index is calculated for the alleged father using all loci tested, even if one of the loci does not directly match the child

1	b	19	d	37	c
2	d	20	c	38	d
3	a	21	b	39	a
4	c	22	c	40	c
5	b	23	c	41	c
6	c	24	a	42	b
7	c	25	b	43	d
8	d	26	a	44	b
9	d	27	c	45	b
10	c	28	c	46	a
11	b	29	a	47	b
12	d	30	b	48	d
13	b	31	c	49	a
14	b	32	d	50	d
15	b	33	b		
16	b	34	a		
17	c	35	c		
18	c	36	c		

Molecular Science

1
MLS ONLY
b Spontaneous deamination of methyl-cytosine results in thymine formation; it occurs 2.5× more frequently than any other single nucleotide mutation.
[Nussbaum 2007, p178]

2 **d** The G2 phase of the cell cycle follows the S phase, where DNA content goes from 2N to 4N or from diploid to tetraploid.
[Buckingham 2007, p334]

3 **a** Heteronuclear RNA is made up of newly transcribed mRNA that still contains intervening sequences.
[Buckingham 2007, p32]

4
MLS ONLY
c Methylation of CpG islands is an epigenetic mechanism of gene silencing.
[Buckingham 2007, p311]

5 **b** Chromosomes with clearly defined short and long arms are known as submetacentric chromosomes.
[Buckingham 2007, p159]

6
MLS ONLY
c RT synthesizes a DNA molecule from an RNA template.
[Nussbaum 2007, p546]

7 **c** One X chromosome is passed on to all sons by the mother; since she is a carrier of a mutant X allele, 50% of her sons will be affected.
[Nussbaum 2007, p132]

8 **d** Males are hemizygous for X-linked alleles because they have only one copy of the X chromosome.
[Buckingham 2007, p130]

9 **d** All mitochondria are passed on from a mother to her children, but not by a father to his children.
[Buckingham 2007, p320]

Molecular Techniques

10
MLS ONLY
c The greater the concentration of agarose, the smaller the size of DNA that can be resolved.
[Buckingham 2007, p82]

11
MLS ONLY
b RFLP analysis is performed on DNA. Southern blotting is the method used to separate DNA fragments by size, transfer the DNA fragments to a solid support, and then hybridize with a probe specific for the gene of interest.
[Buckingham 2007, p101]

12
MLS ONLY
d A reverse dot blot allows for the screening of several different mutations at one time by putting probes specific for different mutations on the membrane and then hybridizing a labeled patient DNA sample to the membrane.
[Buckingham 2007, pp179-180]

13
MLS ONLY
b High temperature and low salt concentration in the wash buffer favors dissociation of the probe: DNA targets that are not completely base-paired along the length of the probe. This will give the lowest nonspecific or background hybridization.
[Buckingham 2007, p107]

14
MLS ONLY
b Klenow fragment lacks $5' \rightarrow 3'$ exonuclease activity and is therefore used for random primer labeling.
[Buckingham 2007, p10]

15
MLS ONLY
b A gel mobility shift assay involves mixing a labeled oligonucleotide with a protein extract to see if specific protein: nucleic acid interaction occurs. The oligonucleotide will exhibit an apparent increase in molecular size on a gel due to its association with a protein should such an interaction occur.
[Buckingham 2007, pp117-118]

16
MLS ONLY
b Alpha satellite probes are centromere-specific and can be used to identify specific chromosomes. A chromosome 21-specific alpha satellite probe would give 3 distinct dots in interphase cells. Chromosome paint probes have greater utility in metaphase spreads to detect translocations or other alterations in chromosome structure. A unique sequence probe specific for chromosome 21 could also theoretically be used, but would give a weaker signal compared to the alpha satellite probe due to the highly repetitive nature of the alpha satellite sequence.
[Buckingham 2007, p84]

17
MLS ONLY
c 2 volumes of ethanol are used to precipitate DNA, whereas 2.5 volumes are used to precipitate RNA.
[Buckingham 2007, p68]

18 **c** Chelex® resin is often used to extract DNA from forensic samples, but may also be used for clinical samples.
[Buckingham 2007, p71]

19 **d** SYBR® Green is the most sensitive of the listed dyes.
[Buckingham 2007, pp77-78]

20 **c** The absorptivity constant for DNA is 50 µg/mL.
[Buckingham 2007, p77]

21 **b** (OD260 × 40 × 40)/2 =
MLS ONLY (0.03125 × 40 × 40)/2 =50/2 = 25 µg.
[Buckingham 2007, p77]

22 **c** Str at a particular locus differ in size.
MLS ONLY [Buckingham 2007, p213]

23 **c** Reporter and quencher fluorochromes
MLS ONLY are separated from one another when the beacon anneals its target.
[Buckingham 2007, p140]

24 **a** Hydrogen bonds hold the 2 strands of DNA together in a double-stranded DNA molecule.
[Nussbaum 2007, p7]

25 **b** Annealing temperature determines the amount of mismatch tolerated between the primers and the target.
[Buckingham 2007, p123]

26 **a** PCR reactions in which multiple loci are amplified in the same reaction by multiple sets of primers are known as multiplex PCR.
[Buckingham 2007, p134]

27 **c** When target sequences are limited, 2
TECH ONLY successive PCR reactions can be performed using primer pairs that are 3′ to the first set of primers in the second round of PCR. This is called a nested PCR reaction.
[Buckingham 2007, p136]

28 **c** FRET stands for fluorescent resonance
MLS ONLY energy transfer. One probe has a donor fluorophore at its 5′ end and the other has a reporter fluorophore at its 3′ end. When both probes anneal to one strand of an amplicon, the donor and reporter fluorophores achieve the correct geometry to generate a signal.
[Buckingham 2007, p142]

29 **a** Branched DNA analysis is performed
MLS ONLY by capturing a target nucleic acid onto a microtiter plate and then adding an amplifier probe to greatly increase the signal resulting from the captured nucleic acid. PCR and NASB amplifications amplify the target nucleic acid sequence, whereas the ligase chain reaction amplifies the amount of probe in the reaction when the target is present.
[Buckingham 2007, p147]

30 **b** The amplicon from X would not be
MLS ONLY digested by Alwl because it lacks the enzyme recognition site and thus remains 176 bp in size. The amplicon for allele x would give the 118 bp and 58 bp fragments. Since the patient has bands of all 3 sizes on the gel he/she must be heterozygous, having one X allele and one x allele.
[Buckingham 2007, p189]

31 **c** Bisulfite sequencing is a modified chain
MLS ONLY terminator method specifically designed to detect methylated nucleotides.
[Buckingham 2007, p216]

32 **d** SSCP is a screening test in which the
MLS ONLY exact nature of a mutation does not need to be known in order to detect the presence of a mutation.
[Buckingham 2007, p193]

33 **b** UNG digests amplicons containing
MLS ONLY dUTP as part of a system to prevent contamination of PCR products generated in previous rounds of PCR in a lab.
[Buckingham 2007, p133]

34 **a** When primers span an in exon-intron-
MLS ONLY exon boundary, amplicons generated from genomic DNA would be larger than the specific amplicon generated from a mature mRNA.
[Coleman 2006, p110]

Applications of Molecular Testing

35 **c** The HIV genome is RNA, so only NABSA
MLS ONLY would allow direct detection.
[Buckingham 2007, p296]

36 **c** PFGE after digestion of bacterial
MLS ONLY chromosomes with restriction enzymes is used to determine similarity between bacterial isolates.
[Buckingham 2007, pp285-286]

37 **c** Bacterial genotyping by PFGE follows
MLS
ONLY the rule of three, so 3 or more differences
indicate the test strain is different from
the reference strain.
[Buckingham 2007, p286]

38 **d** Human DNA (extrinsic to the target
MLS
ONLY DNA) would be expected to be collected
along with the *Mycoplasma* DNA (intrinsic to
the sample).
[Buckingham 2007, p267]

39 **a** IS481 is found in both *B pertussis* and
MLS
ONLY *B homesii* and IS1001 is found in *B homesii*
and *B parapertussis*, but not in *B pertussis*.
IS481 is not found in *B parapertussis*.
[Buckingham 2007, p273]

40 **c** *mecA* is the gene responsible for
MLS
ONLY resistance in *Staph aureus*; *vanA* for
vancomycin resistance in *Enterococcus*; *inhA*
for isoniazid in *Mycobacterium tuberculosis*;
and *rpoB* for rifampin in *Mycobacterium
tuberculosis*.
[Buckingham 2007, p282]

41 **c** The 9;22 translocation creates the
BCR/ABL1 fusion gene in CML.
[Rodak 2007, p418]

42 **b** Only 16S ribosomal RNA is found in
MLS
ONLY prokaryotes and is the target; the others
listed are eukaryotic RNA subunits.
[Buckingham 2007, p272]

43 **d** The presence of a distinct band along
MLS
ONLY with the smear indicates at least 1% of
the patient's B cells have a monoclonal
rearrangement of the Ig heavy chain.
[Buckingham 2007, p352]

44 **b** Turner syndrome females have a
MLS
ONLY 45X genotype.
[Nussbaum 2007, p108]

45 **b** Robertsonian translocations involving
MLS
ONLY chromosome 21q account for about 4% of
the cases of Down syndrome.
[Buckingham 2007, p91]

46 **a** Sequence-specific PCR in 96-well plates
MLS
ONLY is commonly performed to determine
polymorphisms in class I and class II *DRB*
and *DRQ* genes.
[Buckingham 2007, p390]

47 **b** AF2 could possibly have contributed all
MLS
ONLY of the alleles inherited by the child after the
alleles the child inherited from the mother
have been considered.
[Buckingham 2007, p239]

48 **d** HV1 and HV2 are portions of the
MLS
ONLY mitochondrial genome that are sequenced
to determine mitochondrial inheritance.
[Buckintgham 2007, p254]

49 **a** Amelogenin gives different sized
MLS
ONLY amplicons based on whether it is amplified
from the X or Y chromosomes, so males
would have 2 bands on a gel at the
amelogenin locus, while females would
have only 1.
[Buckingham 2007, pp234-235]

50 **d** A paternity index is calculated even
MLS
ONLY with 1 or 2 mismatches because germ line
mutations could have occurred during the
formation of sperm in the father.
[Buckingham 2007, p239]

Urinalysis and Body Fluids

*The following items have been identified generally as appropriate for both entry level medical laboratory scientists and medical laboratory technicians. Items that are appropriate for medical laboratory scientists **only** are marked with an "MLS ONLY."*

Urinalysis: Pre-Analytical Examination

1   After receiving a 24-hour urine for quantitative total protein analysis, the technician must first:

 a subculture the urine for bacteria
 b add the appropriate preservative
 c screen for albumin using a dipstick
 d measure the total volume

protein (mg/dL) × dL in total sample

2   False results in urobilinogen testing may occur if the urine specimen is:

 a exposed to light
 b adjusted to a neutral pH
 c cooled to room temperature
 d collected in a nonsterile container

3   A clean-catch urine is submitted to the laboratory for routine urinalysis and culture. The routine urinalysis is done first, and 3 hours later, the specimen is sent to the microbiology department for culture. The specimen should:

 a be centrifuged, and the supernatant cultured
 b be rejected due to the time delay
 c not be cultured if no bacteria are seen
 d be processed for culture only if the nitrate is positive

4   Which of the following urine results is most apt to be changed by prolonged exposure to light?

 a pH
 b protein
 c ketones
 d bilirubin

5   Urine samples should be examined within 1 hour of voiding because:

 a RBCs, leukocytes and casts agglutinate on standing for several hours at room temperature
 b urobilinogen increases and bilirubin decreases after prolonged exposure to light
 c bacterial contamination will cause alkalinization of the urine
 d ketones will increase due to bacterial and cellular metabolism

6 The following results were obtained on a urine specimen at 8:00 AM:

MLS
ONLY

pH:	5.5
protein:	2+
glucose:	3+
ketones:	3+
blood:	negative
bilirubin:	positive
nitrite:	positive

If this urine specimen was stored uncapped at 5°C without preservation and retested at 2 PM, which of the following test results would be changed due to these storage conditions?

a glucose
b ketones
c protein
d nitrite

7 A urine specimen comes to the laboratory 7 hours after it is obtained. It is acceptable for culture only if the specimen has been stored:

a at room temperature
b at 4°-7°C
c frozen
d with a preservative additive - *by SBMF standards*

8 Which of the following would be affected by allowing a urine specimen to remain at room temperature for 3 hours before analysis?

a occult blood
b specific gravity
c pH
d protein

9 A 24-hour urine from a man who had no evidence of kidney impairment was sent to the laboratory for hormone determination. The volume was 600 mL, but there was some question as to the completeness of the 24-hour collection. The next step would be to:

MLS
ONLY

a perform the hormone determination, since 600 mL is a normal 24-hour urine volume
b check the creatinine level; if it is <1 g, do the procedure
c report the hormone determination in mg/dL in case the specimen was incomplete
d check the creatinine level; if it is >1 g, do the procedure

10 Failure to observe RBC casts in a urine specimen can by caused by:

a staining the specimen
b centrifuging an unmixed specimen - *left in bottom of container*
c mixing the sediment after decantation
d examining the sediment first under low power

11 eGFR calculated by the MDRD formula takes into account the age, BUN, race, albumin and what else for its calculations?

MLS
ONLY

a urea
b ammonia
c creatinine
d cystatin C

12 The creatinine clearance is reported in: *CREATININE CLEARANCE FORMULA:*

a mg/dL
b mg/24 hours
c mL/min
d mL/24 hours

13   Microalbumin can be measured by a random urine collection. An increased microalbumin is predictive of:

    a   diabetes mellitus
    b   nephropathy   **✱✱**
    c   hypertension
    d   nephrotic syndrome

Urinalysis: Physical Examination

14   A patient with uncontrolled diabetes mellitus will most likely have:

    a   pale urine with a high specific gravity ↑ *specific gravity due to sugar; pale = polyuria*
    b   concentrated urine with a high specific gravity
    c   pale urine with a low specific gravity
    d   dark urine with a high specific gravity

15   While performing an analysis of a baby's urine, the technologist notices the specimen to have a "mousy" odor. Of the following substances that may be excreted in urine, the one that **most** characteristically produces this odor is:

    a   phenylpyruvic acid *(PKU - mousy odor)*
    b   acetone - *fruity*
    c   coliform bacilli - *ammonia*
    d   porphyrin - *no smell*

16   An ammonia-like odor is characteristically associated with urine from patients who:
MLS ONLY

    a   are diabetic
    b   have hepatitis
    c   have an infection with *Proteus* sp
    d   have a yeast infection

17   Urine that develops a port wine color after standing may contain:

    a   melanin - *black*
    b   porphyrins - *port wine*
    c   bilirubin - *amber to brown*
    d   urobilinogen

18   Acid urine that contains hemoglobin will darken on standing due to the formation of:
MLS ONLY

    a   myoglobin
    b   sulfhemoglobin
    c   methemoglobin
    d   red blood cells

19   Urine from a 50-year-old man was noted to turn dark red on standing. This change is caused by:

    a   glucose
    b   porphyrins
    c   urochrome - *yellow*
    d   creatinine

20   The clarity of a urine sample should be determined:

    a   using glass tubes only; never plastic
    b   following thorough mixing of the specimen
    c   after addition of sulfosalicylic acid
    d   after the specimen cools to room temperature

21   Milky urine from a 24-year-old woman would most likely contain:

     a spermatozoa
     (b) many white blood cells
     c red blood cells
     d bilirubin

22   A brown-black urine would most likely contain:

     a bile pigment – *green/brown*
     b porphyrins – *wine red*
     (c) melanin
     d blood cells – *red or white*

23   The yellow color of urine is primarily due to:

     (a) urochrome pigment
     b methemoglobin
     c bilirubin
     d homogenistic acid

(24)   Red urine may be due to:

     a bilirubin
     b excess urobilin
     (c) myoglobin
     d homogenistic acid – *dark urine on standing*

25   A urine specimen collected on an apparently healthy 25-year-old man shortly after he finished
MLS ONLY   eating lunch was cloudy but showed normal results on a multiple reagent strip analysis. The most
      likely cause of the turbidity is:

     a fat
     b white blood cells
     c urates
     (d) phosphates – *more alkaline urine after eating*

26   In which of the following metabolic diseases will urine turn dark brown to black upon standing?
MLS ONLY

     a phenylketonuria
     (b) alkaptonuria
     c maple syrup disease
     d aminoaciduria

27   Urine osmolality is related to:

     a pH
     b filtration
     (c) specific gravity
     d volume

28   Urine specific gravity is an index of the ability of the kidney to:

     a filter the plasma
     (b) concentrate the urine
     c alter the hydrogen ion concentration
     d reabsorb sodium ions

29   Osmolality is a measure of:

     (a) dissolved particles, including ions
     b undissociated molecules only
     c total salt concentration
     d molecule size

30 A patient urine sample has an increased protein and a high specific gravity. Which of the following
MLS
ONLY would be a more accurate measure of urine concentration?

    a osmolality
    b ketones
    c refractive index
    d pH

31 To prepare a solution appropriate for quality control of the refractometer, a technician should use:

    a urea with a specific gravity of 1.040
    b water with a specific gravity of ~~1.005~~ 1.000
    c sodium chloride with a specific gravity of 1.022   *positive control: 6.5% NaCl*
    d calcium chloride with an osmolarity of 460   *always 1.022*

32 A urine's specific gravity is directly proportional to its:

    a turbidity
    b dissolved solids
    c salt content
    d sugar content

33 Isosthenuria is associated with a specific gravity which is usually:
MLS
ONLY
    a variable between 1.001 and 1.008
    b variable between 1.015 and 1.022
    c fixed around 1.010   *↑ hyper; ↓ hypo*
    d fixed around 1.020

34 The fluid leaving the glomerulus normally has a specific gravity of:
MLS
ONLY   *isosthenuric*
    a 1.001
    b 1.010
    c 1.020
    d 1.030

35 An antidiuretic hormone deficiency is associated with a:
MLS
ONLY
    a specific gravity around 1.031
    b low specific gravity
    c high specific gravity
    d variable specific gravity

36 Use of a refractometer over a urinometer is preferred due to the fact that the refractometer uses:

    a large volume of urine and compensates for temperature
    b small volume of urine and compensates for glucose
    c small volume of urine and compensates for temperature   *affects by proteins and sugars*
    d small volume of urine and compensates for protein

37 Calibration of refractometers is done by measuring the specific gravity of distilled water and:
MLS
ONLY
    a protein
    b glucose
    c sodium chloride
    d urea

38 The method of choice for performing a specific gravity measurement of urine following
administration of x-ray contrast dyes is:

    a reagent strip   *** not affected*
    b refractometer
    c urinometer
    d densitometer

39 Which of the following urinary parameters are measured during the course of concentration
MLS ONLY and dilution tests to assess renal tubular function?

    a urea, nitrogen and creatinine
    b osmolality and specific gravity
    c sodium and chloride
    d sodium and osmolality

40 Refractive index is a comparison of:
MLS ONLY

    a light velocity in solutions to light velocity in solids
    b light velocity in air to light velocity in solutions
    c light scattering by air to light scattering by solutions *cytometry*
    d light scattering by particles in solution

Urinalysis: Chemical Examination

41 Which of the following can give a <u>false-negative urine protein</u> reading?
MLS ONLY

    a contamination with vaginal discharge
    b heavy mucus
    c presence of blood
    d very dilute urine

42 The pH of a urine specimen measures the:
MLS ONLY

    a free sodium ions
    b free hydrogen ions
    c total acid excretion
    d volatile acids

43 Upon standing at room temperature, a urine pH typically: ✱✱

    increase caused by:
    a decreases   *breakdown of urea into ammonia*
    b increases   *by urease producing bacteria*
    c remains the same   *and loss of CO_2*
    d changes depending on bacterial concentration

44 Urine reagent strips should be stored in a(n):

    a refrigerator (4°-7°C)
    b incubator (37°C)
    c cool dry area
    d open jar exposed to air

45 The principle of the reagent strip test for urine protein depends on:
MLS ONLY

    a an enzyme reaction
    b protein error of indicators
    c copper reduction
    d the toluidine reaction

46 The protein section of the urine reagent strip is **most** sensitive to:

    a albumin - *most abundant; points to nephropathy*
    b mucoprotein
    c Bence Jones protein
    d globulin

47 Routine screening of urine samples for glycosuria is performed primarily to detect:

MLS
ONLY

   a glucose
   b galactose
   c bilirubin
   d ketones

48 Which of the following reagents is used to react with ketones in the urine?

   a sodium nitroprusside
   b acetoacetic acid
   c acetone
   d beta-hydroxybutyric acid

→ all ketone subtypes ✱

49 A test area of a urine reagent strip is impregnated with only <u>sodium nitroprusside</u>. This section

MLS
ONLY

will react with: *ketones*

   a acetoacetic (diacetic) acid
   b leukocyte esterase
   c beta-hydroxybutyric acid
   d ferric chloride

50 A reagent strip area impregnated with stabilized, <u>diazotized</u> 2,4-dichloroaniline will yield a positive reaction with:

   a bilirubin – *diazo reaction*
   b hemoglobin
   c ketones – *sodium nitroprusside*
   d urobilinogen

51 Which of the following factors will **not** interfere with the reagent strip test for leukocytes?

MLS
ONLY

   a ascorbic acid
   b formaldehyde
   c nitrite
   d urinary protein level of 500 mg/dL

52 Excess urine on the reagent test strip can turn a normal pH result into a falsely acidic pH when

MLS
ONLY

which of the following reagents runs into the pH pad?

   a tetrabromphenol blue – *pH color indicator*
   b citrate <u>buffer</u>
   c glucose oxidase – *glucose*
   d alkaline copper sulfate – *reducing substances*

53 When employing the urine reagent strip method, a false-positive protein result may occur in the presence of:

   a large amounts of glucose
   b x-ray contrast media
   c Bence Jones protein   ✱✱
   d highly alkaline urine

54 A 17-year-old girl decided to go on a starvation diet. After 1 week of starving herself, what substance would most likely be found in her urine?

   a protein
   b ketones – *fat metabolism*
   c glucose
   d blood

55   A 2-year-old child had a positive urine ketone. This would most likely be caused by:

    (a) vomiting
    b anemia
    c hypoglycemia
    d biliary tract obstruction

56   A patient's urinalysis revealed a positive bilirubin and a decreased urobilinogen level. These results
MLS ONLY   are associated with:

    a hemolytic disease
    (b) biliary obstruction
    c hepatic disease
    d urinary tract infection

57   A urine specimen with an elevated urobilinogen and a negative bilirubin may indicate:
MLS ONLY

    a obstruction of the biliary tract
    b viral hepatitis
    (c) hemolytic jaundice
    d cirrhosis

58   Microscopic analysis of a urine specimen yields a moderate amount of red blood cells in spite of a negative result for occult blood using a reagent strip. The technologist should determine if this patient has taken:

    (a) vitamin C *– inhibits peroxidase tests*
    b a diuretic
    c high blood pressure medicine
    d antibiotics

59   The purpose for routinely screening diabetes mellitus patients for microalbuminuria is to monitor
MLS ONLY   the development of:

    a urinary tract infection
    (b) renal disease
    c yeast infections
    d diabetes insipidus

60   The principle of the reagent strip test for microalbuminuria is:
MLS ONLY

    ~~a~~ a diazo reaction
    b the protein error of indicators   **✱✱**
    (c) a dye-binding reaction *– dye highly sensitive to albumin*
    ~~d~~ the release of hydrogen ions to an indicator

61   The reason that an albumin:creatinine ratio can be run on a random specimen is:
MLS ONLY

    (a) creatinine corrects for over or under body hydration *– constant rate; not affected*
    b a first morning specimen may be too concentrated   *by hydration*
    c albumin corrects for over or under body hydration
    d the reaction is sensitive to any level of albumin

(62) To prepare the reagent used in confirmatory protein testing, a technician would:

    (a) dissolve 3 g sulfosalicylic acid in 100 mL of water *3% SSA – protein confirmatory*
    b dissolve 5 g trichloroacetic acid in 100 mL of water   *test*
    c combine 3 mL of hydrochloric acid and 97 mL of water
    d combine 5 mL of glacial acetic acid and 95 mL of water

63   A positive result for bilirubin on a reagent strip should be followed up by:

    a notifying the physician
    b requesting a new specimen
    (c) performing an Ictotest
    d performing a urobilinogen

64 Ammonium sulfate was added to red urine. The urine had a positive reaction for blood, but no RBCs were seen on microscopic examination. After centrifugation the supernatant fluid is red. The abnormal color is caused by:

   a pyridium
   b hemoglobin   *Ammonium sulfate* **
   c porphyrins
   ⓓ myoglobin – *supernatant remains red; hemoglobin precipitates out*

65 A urine tested with Clinitest® exhibits a passthrough reaction and is diluted by adding 2 drops of urine to 10 drops water. This is a dilution of:

   a 1:4
   b 1:5
   ⓒ 1:6
   d 1:8

66 When performing a routine urinalysis, the technologist notes a 2+ protein result. He should:

   a request another specimen
   ⓑ confirm with the acid precipitation test
   c test for Bence Jones protein
   d report the result obtained without further testing

67 The confirmatory test for a positive protein result by the reagent strip method uses:

   a Ehrlich reagent – *urobilinogen*   *
   b a diazo reaction – *bilirubin*   **
   ⓒ sulfosalicylic acid – *protein*
   d a copper reduction tablet – *reducing substances*

68 A urine specimen is analyzed for glucose by a glucose oxidase reagent strip and a copper reduction test. If both results are positive, which of the following interpretations is correct?

   a galactose is present
   ⓑ glucose is present
   c lactose is not present
   d sucrose is not present

69 A woman in her ninth month of pregnancy has a urine sugar which is negative with the urine
MLS ONLY reagent strip, but gives a positive reaction with the copper reduction method. The sugar most likely responsible for these results is:

   a maltose
   ~~b~~ galactose
   ~~c~~ glucose
   ⓓ lactose – *pregnant women lactating*

70 An urinalysis performed on a 2-week-old infant with diarrhea shows a negative reaction with the glucose oxidase reagent strip. A copper reduction tablet test should be performed to check the urine sample for the presence of:

   a glucose
   ⓑ galactose
   c bilirubin
   d ketones

71 When using the sulfosalicylic acid test, false-positive protein results may occur in the presence of:
MLS ONLY
   a ketones
   b alkali
   c glucose
   ⓓ radiographic contrast media

72 Which of the following is the primary reagent in the copper reduction tablet?

MLS
ONLY
   a sodium carbonate
   b copper sulfate
   c glucose oxidase
   d polymerized diazonium salt

Urinalysis: Microscopic Examination

73 In most compound light microscopes, the ocular lens has a magnification of:

   a 10×
   b 40×
   c 50×
   d 100×

74 The best way to lower the light intensity of the microscope is to:

   – **a** lower the condenser
   b adjust the aperture diaphragm
   c lower the rheostat (*light adjustment*)
   d raise the condenser

75 The advantage to using phase microscopy in urinalysis is to:

   a provide higher magnification
   b enhance constituents with a low refractive index
   c allow constituents to stain more clearly
   d provide a larger field of view

76 The presence of leukocytes in urine is known as:

   a chyluria
   b hematuria
   c leukocytosis
   d pyuria

77 Oval fat bodies are:

   a squamous epithelial cells that contain lipids   ✳✳
   b renal tubular epithelial cells that contain lipids
   c free-floating fat droplets
   d white blood cells with phagocytized lipids

78 A microscopic examination of urine sediment reveals ghost cells. These red blood cells seen in urine with a:

   a >2% glucose concentrations (*hypotonic*)
   b specific gravity <1.007 — *dilute urine; caused by osmosis*
   c large amounts of ketone bodies   *cells swell by absorbing water,*
   d neutral pH   *lyse and spill hemoglobin contents*

79 Glitter cells are a microscopic finding of:

   a red blood cells in hypertonic urine
   b red blood cells in hypotonic urine
   c white blood cells in hypertonic urine
   d white blood cells in hypotonic urine → *swell*

80   What cell is **most** commonly associated with vaginal contamination?

   a white
   b transitional
   c squamous
   d glitter

81   A reagent strip test for blood has been reported positive. Microscopic examination fails to yield red blood cells. This patient's condition can be called:

   a hematuria
   b hemoglobinuria – *caused by lysed RBC's; (+) due to hemoglobin in urine, not RBC's*
   c oliguria
   d hemosiderinuria

82   Ghost red blood cells are seen in urine that is:

   a acidic and dilute
   b alkaline and dilute
   c acidic and concentrated
   d alkaline and concentrated

83   The possibility of detecting glitter cells is associated with urine that is:

   a acidic
   b dilute
   c alkaline
   d concentrated

84   *MLS ONLY* — An eosinophil count may be requested on urine from a patient with suspected:

   a acute glomerulonephritis
   b cystitis
   c renal lithiasis
   d acute interstitial nephritis – *caused by allergic reaction*

85   Clue cells are a form of:

   a squamous epithelial cell
   b urothelial cell
   c white blood cell
   d renal tubular epithelial cell

86   Which of the following cells is most likely to be seen in the urine sediment following a catheterization procedure?

   a squamous epithelial cell
   b urothelial cell – *line bladder*
   c white blood cell
   d renal tubular epithelial cell

87   A patient admitted following an accident involving massive crush injuries has the following urinalysis results:

		Microscopic findings	
color:	red brown	renal tubular epithelial:	5-10
clarity:	(clear)	renal tubular cell casts:	1-2
specific gravity:	1.011		
pH:	6.0		
protein:	1+		
blood:	large −		
glucose:	negative		
ketones:	negative		
nitrite:	negative		
leukocytes:	negative		
bilirubin:	negative		
urobilinogen:	negative		

The discrepancy between the large amount of blood and the absence of RBCs on microscopy is caused by:

a   failure to mix the specimen before centrifuging
b   mistaking RBCs for RTE cells
c   contaminating oxidizing detergents in the container
d   the presence of myoglobin in the urine specimen – *myoglobin = muscle destruction (crush injuries)*

88   What is the most likely diagnosis given this microscopic finding?

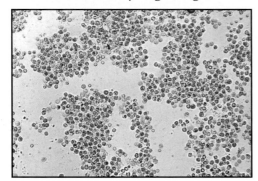

✳✳✳

a   glomerulonephritis – *RBC casts*
b   pyelonephritis – *WBC casts*
c   nephrotic syndrome – *lipids and fatty casts*
d   cystitis – *no casts; WBC's, bacteria, possibly RBC's*

89   Identify the formed element in this photomicrograph:

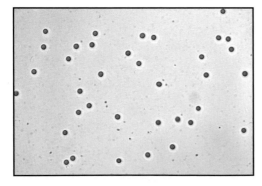

a   RBC
b   WBC
c   epithelial cell
d   yeast

90   All casts typically contain:

   a   albumin
   b   globulin
   c   immunoglobulins G and M
   d   Tamm-Horsfall glycoprotein ✳

91   Hyaline casts are usually found:

   a   in the center of the coverslip
   b   under subdued light
   c   under very bright light
   d   in the supernatant

92   Which of the following casts is most likely to be found in healthy people?

   a   hyaline
   b   red blood cell
   c   waxy
   d   white blood cell

93   Which of the following casts is most indicative of end stage renal disease?

   a   hemoglobin
   b   granular
   c   cellular
   d   waxy — *bread casts* ✳

94   A technologist performed a STAT microscopic urinalysis and reported the following:

MLS ONLY

   WBC: 10-13
   RBC: 2-6
   hyaline casts: 5-7
   bacteria: 1+

The centrifuge tube was not discarded and the urine sediment was reevaluated microscopically 5 hours after the above results were reported. A second technologist reported the same results, except 2+ bacteria and no hyaline casts were found. The most probable explanation for the second technologist's findings is:

   a   sediment was not agitated before preparing the microscope slide
   b   casts dissolved due to decrease in urine pH
   c   casts dissolved due to increase in urine pH
   d   casts were never present in this specimen

95   Which of the following aids in differentiating a spherical transitional cell from a round renal tubular cell?

   a   spherical transitional cell is larger
   b   eccentrically-placed nucleus in the renal tubular cell ✳
   c   eccentrically-placed nucleus in the spherical transitional cell
   d   round renal tubular cell is larger

96   The urine microscopic constituents that best differentiate between cystitis and pyelonephritis are:

   a   WBCs
   b   bacteria
   c   RBCs
   d   WBC casts

97   Epithelial cell casts are most indicative of:

MLS ONLY

   a   glomerulonephritis
   b   nephrotic syndrome
   c   tubular necrosis
   d   pyelonephritis

98   Granular casts found in the urine of a football player admitted to the hospital with a broken leg occurring during the game can be the result of:

   a excessive bruising
   b strenuous exercise
   c excess power drink ingestion
   d bone fracture

99   Which of the following casts most frequently appears to have a brittle consistency?

   a hyaline
   b granular
   c waxy
   d fatty

100   To distinguish between a clump of WBCs and a WBC cast, it is important to observe:

   a the presence of free-floating WBCs
   b a positive leukocyte reaction
   c a positive nitrite reaction
   d the presence of a cast matrix

101   Spherical urothelial cells may be confused with:

   a oval fat bodies
   b renal tubular epithelial cells – *nucleus off-center*
   c glitter cells
   d lymphocytes

102   Prior to reporting a red blood cell cast, it is important to observe:

   a free-floating RBCs
   b hyaline casts
   c granular casts
   d increased white blood cells

103   In a specimen with a large amount of bilirubin, which of the following sediment constituents would be most noticeably bile-stained?

   a squamous epithelial cells
   b white blood cell casts
   c cystine crystals
   d renal tubular epithelial cell casts – *absorb filtrate; bilirubin stains them*

104   What is the most likely diagnosis given this microscopic finding?

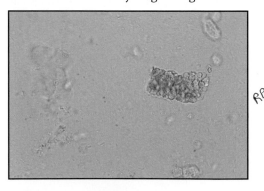

RBC Cast

   a glomerulonephritis
   b pyelonephritis
   c nephrotic syndrome
   d cystitis

105 A white precipitate in a urine specimen with a pH of 7.5 would most probably be caused by:

 a amorphous urates – *acidic*
 b WBCs – *no precipitate*
 c amorphous phosphates – *alkaline*
 d bacteria – *no precipitate*

106 Which of the following is an abnormal crystal described as a hexagonal plate?

 a cystine – *hexagons*
 b tyrosine – *thin needles*   ✳✳
 c leucine – *round*
 d cholesterol – *flat with notched corners*

107 The primary component of most urinary calculi is:

MLS ONLY

 a calcium
 b uric acid
 c leucine
 d cystine

108 After warming, a cloudy urine clears. This is due to the presence of:

 a urates – *dissolve when warmed*
 b phosphates – *need acid to dissolve*
 c WBCs
 d bacteria

109 Tiny, colorless, dumbbell-shaped crystals were found in an <u>alkaline</u> urine sediment. They most likely are:

 a calcium oxalate
 b calcium carbonate – *dumb-bell shaped*
 c calcium phosphate
 d amorphous phosphate

110 Which of the following crystals may be found in acidic urine?

 a calcium carbonate
 b calcium oxalate
 c calcium phosphate
 d triple phosphate

111 Using polarized light microscopy, which of the following urinary elements are birefringent?

MLS ONLY

 a cholesterol
 b triglycerides
 c fatty acids
 d neutral fats

112 Which of the following crystals appear as fine, silky needles?

 a cholesterol
 b leucine
 c hemosiderin – *dark clumps*
 d tyrosine

113 Which of the following crystals is seen in an amber urine with a positive bilirubin?

 a ammonium biurate
 b cystine   ✳✳
 c tyrosine/ *leucine → liver disorders*
 d uric acid

114 Following ingestion of ethylene glycol (antifreeze) numerous crystals are found in the urine. The shape of these crystals is:

    a flat with notched corners
    b oval/dumbbell – *calcium oxide = ethylene glycol*
    c coffin-lid
    d rosettes/rhomboid

115 Cholesterol crystals will most likely be observed in urine that contains:

    a 3+ glucose
    (b) 4+ protein
    c WBC casts
    d triple phosphate crystals

Cholesterol crystals = ~~nephrotic~~ nephrotic syndrome
↑ protein

116 The finding of a large amount of uric acid crystals in a urine specimen from a 6-month-old boy:

MLS ONLY

    a may actually be diaper fibers
    (b) could indicate Lesch-Nyhan syndrome – *purine metabolism disorder*
    c should not be reported   *uric acid crystals = incomplete metabolism*
    d may indicate improper feeding

117 The following crystal is found in:

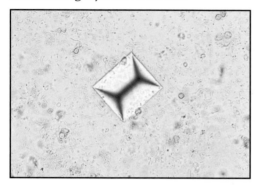

Triple phosphate crystals "coffin lids"

    a acid pH and is nonpathologic
    (b) alkaline pH and is nonpathologic
    c acid pH and is pathologic
    d alkaline pH and is pathologic

(118) Identify this crystal:

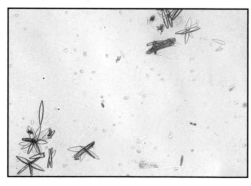

uric acid – many shapes

    (a) uric acid
    b calcium phosphate
    c calcium carbonate
    d triple phosphate acid –

119 Alkaline urine showed this microscopic finding.

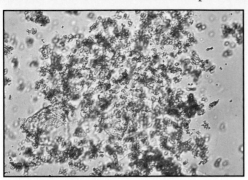

** amorphous phosphates = acetic acid

The technologist should:

a   dilute with saline
b   request a new sample
c   culture for bacteria
d dissolve with acetic acid

120 Polarized light can often be used to differentiate between:

a fibers and mucus clumps – *contaminants polarized light*
b hyaline and waxy casts
c   squamous and transitional epithelial cells
d   red blood cells and white blood cells

121 Which of the following contaminants has a dimpled center and will polarize?

a starch – *maltese cross*
b   oil droplets
c   air bubbles
d   pollen grains

122 The presence of this element in urine indicates the presence of:

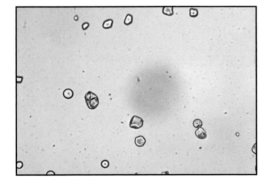

a   a UTI
b powder
c   carbohydrate deficiency
d   high urine amylase

123 Identify the formed element in this photomicrograph:

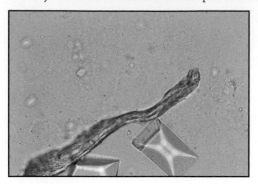

- (**a**) cloth fiber
- **b** hyaline cast
- **c** granular cast
- **d** waxy cast

124 A technologist is having trouble differentiating between red blood cells, oil droplets and yeast cells on a urine microscopy. Acetic acid should be added to the sediment to:

- **a** lyse the yeast cells
- (**b**) lyse the red blood cells
- **c** dissolve the oil droplets
- **d** crenate the red blood cells

125 A urine specimen is tested and has the following results:

Reagent strip	**Microscopic findings**
glucose: 3+	>100 WBCs/hpf
protein: 1+	many yeast cells

This is indicative of:

- (**a**) diabetes mellitus
- **b** contamination
- **c** pyelonephritis
- **d** diabetes insipidus

126 When identifying urinary crystals, which reagent strip result is most important?

- **a** protein
- (**b**) pH
- **c** specific gravity
- **d** nitrite

127 Bacteria are considered significant in the urine sediment when the:

- (**a**) nitrite is positive *(may be contaminant in poorly processed specimen)*
- **b** protein is positive
- **c** specimen is cloudy
- (**d**) leukocytes is positive = *infection*

128 Which of the following exhibits rapid motility in urine sediment?

- **a** spermatozoa – *urine is toxic!*
- (**b**) *Trichomonas vaginalis*
- **c** *Gardnerella vaginalis*
- **d** *Enterobius vermicularis*

129 Which of the following positive chemical reactions is most closely associated with the presence of yeast in the urine sediment?

    a nitrite
    b protein
    (c) glucose
    d blood

130 What of the following is consistent with this urine microscopic finding?

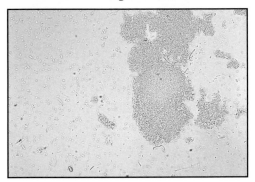

    a ketone
    b glucose
    c specific gravity
    (d) nitrate

131 A 21-year-old woman had glucose in her urine with a normal blood sugar. These findings are most consistent with:

    (a) renal glycosuria – *inherited disorder – no sugar receptors in renal tubules proximal convoluted tubules or renal tubule damage*
    b diabetes insipidus
    c diabetes mellitus
    d alkaline tide

Urinalysis: Complete Examination

132 A 59-year-old man is evaluated for back pain. Urine studies (urinalysis by multiple reagent
_{MLS ONLY} strip) include:

Urinalysis

specific gravity:	1.017
pH:	6.5
protein:	negative
glucose:	negative
blood:	negative

Microscopic findings
rare epithelial cells

Urine protein electrophoresis
monoclonal spike in gamma globulin region *(Bence-Jones protein → immunoglobulin)*

Which of the following statements best explains these results?

    a urine protein is falsely negative due to the specific gravity
    (b) urine protein is falsely negative because the method is not sensitive for Bence Jones protein
    c microscopic examination is falsely negative due to the specific gravity
    d electrophoresis is incorrect and should be repeated

133 The results of a urinalysis on a first morning specimen are:

specific gravity: 1.024
pH: 8.5
protein: negative
glucose: negative

Microscopic findings
uric acid crystals

The next step is to repeat the:

a microscopic examination
b protein and glucose
c specific gravity
d pH and microscopic examination

134 The following urinalysis results were obtained from an 18-year-old woman in labor:

pH: 6.5
protein: 30 mg/dL
glucose: 250 mg/dL
ketones: negative
bilirubin: small (color slightly abnormal)
blood: negative
nitrite: negative
urobilinogen: 0.1 EU/dL
specific gravity: 1.025
copper reduction test: 1.0 g/dL

Which of the following is the **most** likely explanation for the patient's positive copper reduction test?

a only glucose is present
b only lactose is present
c glucose and possibly other reducing substances/sugars are present *(possibly lactose)*
d results are false positive due to the presence of protein

135 The following urine results were obtained on a 25-year-old female:

pH:	7.0	**Microscopic findings**	
color:	yellow	bacteria:	many
appearance:	cloudy	WBC casts:	0-3/lpf
protein:	1+	WBC/hpf:	30-40
glucose:	negative		
blood:	small		
specific gravity:	1.015		

These results are most compatible with:

a glomerulonephritis – *RBC casts*
b renal calculus
c cystitis – *bacteria, WBC's*
d pyelonephritis – *WBC casts*

136 A urinalysis performed on a 27-year-old woman yields the following results:

		Microscopic findings	
specific gravity:	1.008	WBC/hpf:	10-15
pH:	5.0	RBC/hpf:	30-55
protein:	2+	casts/lpf:	hyaline, 5-7; RBC, 2-5;
glucose:	negative		granular, 2-3
ketones:	negative	uric acid crystals: moderate	
bilirubin:	negative		
blood:	3+		
nitrite:	negative		
leukocytes:	positive		
urobilinogen:	0.1 EU/dL		

These findings are **most** consistent with:

a yeast infection
b pyelonephritis
c bacterial cystitis
d glomerulonephritis *- WBC, RBC and protein = glomerular damage*   *RBC CASTS*

137 A 62-year-old patient with hyperlipoproteinemia has a large amount of protein in his urine. Microscopic analysis yields moderate to many fatty, waxy, granular and cellular casts. Many oval fat bodies are also noted. This is most consistent with:

a nephrotic syndrome
b viral infection
c acute pyelonephritis
d acute glomerulonephritis

138 A patient has 2 separate urinalysis reports, which contain the following data:

Test	Report A	Report B
specific gravity	1.004	1.017
pH	5.5	7.0
protein	negative	1+
glucose	negative	negative
blood	negative	small
microscopy	rare epithelial cells	1-2 granular cast/lpf
		2-3 hyaline cast/lpf
		moderate epithelial cells

Which of the following statements best explains these results?

a protein, glucose and microscopy of A are false negatives because of the specific gravity
b protein and glucose are false positives in B due to the specific gravity
c microscopic of A is false negative because of the pH
d microscopic of B is false positive because of the pH

139 A 4-year-old girl develops edema following a recent immunization. Laboratory studies reveal:

MLS ONLY

serum albumin:	1.8 g/dL (18 g/L)
serum cholesterol:	450 mg/dL (11.66 mmol/L)
serum urea nitrogen:	20 mg/dL (7.14 mmol/L)
urinalysis:	protein 4+; hyaline, granular and fatty casts

These findings are most compatible with:

a acute poststreptococcal glomerulonephritis
b minimal change disease
c acute pyelonephritis
d diabetes mellitus

140 A specimen with a negative nitrate reaction and a positive leukocytes reaction that has WBCs, WBC casts, and no bacteria in the sediment will be seen in cases of:

  a cystitis   ✳✳
  b pyelonephritis
  c acute interstitial nephritis *— allergic reaction, causing inflammation*
  d acute glomerulonephritis   *NOT INFECTION*

141 Urinalysis results on a female patient who brings a urine specimen to the physician's office for her annual physical are:

		Microscopic findings	
color:	yellow	squamous epithelial cells:	moderate
clarity:	cloudy	WBC/hpf:	0-2
specific gravity:	1.020	bacteria:	heavy
pH:	7.0		
protein:	trace		
glucose:	negative		
ketones:	negative		
blood:	negative		
bilirubin:	negative		
urobilinogen:	0.2 mg/dL		
nitrite:	positive		
leukocytes:	negative		

What action should be taken?

  a place the patient on a broad spectrum antibiotic for 7 days
  (b) ask the patient to collect another specimen at the office
  c tell the patient she will be called when the culture and sensitivity reports are back
  d have the patient return in a week with a new specimen

142 A patient with lupus erythematosus has the following urinalysis results:

MLS ONLY

		Microscopic findings	
color:	red	WBC/hpf:	5-10
clarity:	cloudy	RBC/hpf:	40-50
specific gravity:	1.011	casts/lpf:	hyaline, 2-4; RBC, 3-5
pH:	6.0		
protein:	3+		
glucose:	negative		
ketones:	negative		
blood:	large		
bilirubin:	negative		
urobilinogen:	1.0 mg/dL		
nitrite:	negative		
leukocytes:	trace		

These results would be associated with:

  —**(a)** chronic glomerulonephritis
  b chronic pyelonephritis
  c acute interstitial nephritis
  d acute tubular necrosis *— tubular epi's*

143 The sediment of a urine specimen with a reagent strip glucose of 250 mg/dL (13.8 mmol/L) and a pH of 5.5 is ideal for the presence of:

  a cystine crystals
  b *Trichomonas vaginalis*
  (c) *Candida albicans*
  d thorny apple crystals

144 A patient with severe back pain has the following urinalysis results:

		Microscopic findings	
color:	dark yellow	RBC/hpf:	10-20
clarity:	hazy	squamous epithelial cells:	moderate
specific gravity:	1.030	calcium oxalate crystals:	moderate
pH:	6.0		
protein:	trace		
glucose:	negative		
ketones:	negative		
blood:	small		
bilirubin:	negative		
urobilinogen:	0.4 mg/dL		
nitrite:	negative		
leukocytes:	negative		

In addition to the presence of blood, what other reagent strip result relates to the patient's symptoms?   *KIDNEY STONE: back pain, blood*

a specific gravity *— dehydration favors kidney stone formation*
b pH
c protein
d urobilinogen

Urine Physiology

145 The normal renal threshold for glucose in the adult is approximately:

a 50 mg/dL (2.8 mmol/L)
b 100 mg/dL (5.5 mmol/L)   *160-180 mg/dL*
c 160 mg/dL (8.8 mmol/L)
d 300 mg/dL (16.5 mmol/L)

146 The volume of urine excreted in a 24-hour period by an adult patient was 300 mL. This condition would be termed: *1200 mls normal volume*

a anuria *— not*   *oligo → scanty*
b oliguria *— scanty*   ✱ ✱
c polyuria *— many*
d dysuria *— pain*

147 A patient has glucosuria, hyperglycemia and polyuria. These findings are most consistent with:

a renal glucosuria
b diabetes mellitus
c emotional stress ⎫ *transient glucosuria*
d eating a heavy meal ⎭

148 The normal glomerular filtration rate is:

a   1 mL/min   *tubular reabsorption — returns*
b   120 mL/min   *all but 1 ml*
c   660 mL/min
d   1,200 mL/min

149 Normal urine primarily consists of:

a water, protein and sodium
b water, urea and protein
c water, urea and sodium chloride
d water, urea and bilirubin

150 An abdominal fluid is submitted from surgery. The physician wants to determine if this fluid could be urine. The technologist should:

   a perform a culture

   b smell the fluid   ✳✳

   (**c**) test for urea and creatinine

   d test for protein, glucose and pH

151 Antidiuretic hormone regulates the reabsorption of:

   (**a**) water

   b glucose

   c potassium

   d calcium

152 Which of the following components are present in serum but **not** present in the glomerular filtrate?

   a glucose

   b amino acids

   c urea

   (**d**) large molecular weight proteins ✳

153 Polyuria is usually correlated with:

   a acute glomerulonephritis

   (**b**) diabetes mellitus

   c hepatitis

   d tubular damage

154 Cessation of urine flow is defined as:

   a azotemia– *azo- = nitrogenous*

   b dysuria – *pain*

   c diuresis– *double = di*

   (**d**) anuria

155 The reason for performing a Clinitest® on a newborn's urine is to check for:

   a fructose

   (**b**) galactose

   c glucose

   d lactose

156 Ketones in urine are due to:

   a complete utilization of fatty acids

   (**b**) incomplete fat metabolism

   c high carbohydrate diets

   d renal tubular dysfunction

157 Reagent strip tests for ketones measure primarily:

   a acetone– *needs glycine*

   (**b**) acetoacetic acid ·

   c cholesterol

   d beta-hydroxybutyric acid

158 Bilirubinuria may be associated with:

   a strenuous exercise

   b increased destruction of platelets

   (**c**) viral hepatitis

   d hemolytic anemia

159 Myoglobinuria is **most** likely to be noted in urine specimens from patients with which of
the following disorders?

    a hemolytic anemia
    b lower urinary tract infection
    (c) myocardial infarction
    d paroxysmal nocturnal hemoglobinuria

160 A patient with renal tubular acidosis would most likely excrete a urine with a:

    a low pH
    (b) high pH
    c neutral pH
    d variable pH

161 Glycosuria may be due to:

    a hypoglycemia
    b increased renal threshold
    (c) renal tubular dysfunction
    d increased glomerular filtration rate

* glucose reabsorbed by proximal convoluted tubule (PCT)

162 The area of the nephron that is impermeable to water is the:

    a proximal convoluted tubule
    b descending loop of Henle
    (c) ascending loop of Henle
    d distal convoluted tubule

163 The urinary tract structures responsible for renal concentration are the:

    a renal pelvis
    b cortical nephrons
    c renal papillae
    (d) juxtamedullary nephrons

164 The most accurate test to determine renal concentration is:

    (a) osmolarity *– number of particles*
    b glomerular filtration rate
    c specific gravity *– number and density of particles*
    d tubular reabsorption rate

165 Failure of the nephron to produce ammonia will result in urine with a:

    a low specific gravity
    b positive nitrite
    (c) high pH
    d positive protein

Other Body Fluids

166 To avoid falsely elevated spinal fluid cell counts:

    a use an aliquot from the first tube collected
    b use only those specimens showing no turbidity
    c centrifuge all specimens before counting
    (d) select an aliquot from the last tube collected

167 A turbid cerebrospinal fluid is most commonly caused by increased:

   (a) white blood cells
   b protein
   c glucose
   d bacterial organisms

168 The normal concentration of proteins in cerebrospinal fluid, relative to serum protein, is:

   (a) <1%
   b 5%-10%
   c 25%-30%
   d 50%-60%

Normal serum protein: 7 g/dL
Normal CSF protein: 15 mg/dL
(less by 1,000)

169 To prepare the reagent used for mucin clot determination of synovial fluid, water is mixed with:

   a hydrochloric acid
   b sodium hydroxide
   c trichloroacetic acid
   (d) glacial acetic acid

170 In addition to the sperm count in a fertility study, analysis of seminal fluid should also include:

   (a) time of liquefaction, estimation of motility, morphology
   b motility, morphology, test for alkaline phosphatase
   c time of liquefaction, test for acid phosphatase, qualitative test for hemoglobin
   d time of liquefaction, qualitative test for hemoglobin and motility

171 The following lab values were obtained on a body fluid sample:

protein:	3 g/dL (30 g/L) – *high protein (CSF mg/dL)* *+ urine*
albumin:	2.1 g/dL (21 g/L)
hyaluronate:	0.4 g/dL (4 g/L) – *synovial fluid*
glucose:	80 mg/dL (4.4 mmol/L)
lactate:	10 mg/dL (1.1 mmol/L)

The sample is:

   a pleural fluid
   (b) synovial fluid
   c urine
   d cerebrospinal fluid

172 A physician attempts to aspirate a knee joint and obtains 0.1 mL of slightly bloody fluid. Addition of acetic acid results in turbidity and a clot. This indicates that:

   (a) the fluid is synovial fluid
   b plasma was obtained
   c red blood cells caused a false-positive reaction
   d the specimen is not adequate

173 Synovial fluid is analyzed with a polarizing microscope. Strongly birefringent needles are seen. This most likely indicates:

   (a) monosodium urate crystals *(MSU) → needles*
   b calcium pyrophosphate crystals *→ (CPPC) → rhomboid*
   c corticosteroid crystals – *only if history*
   d talc crystals – *contaminant*

174 A sperm count is diluted 1:20 and 50 sperm are counted in 2 large squares of the Neubauer counting chamber. The sperm count in mLs is:

   a   5,000
   b   50,000
   c   500,000
   d 5,000,000

*   *   cells × dilution × 10 . 1,000*
               squares   (micro to mls)

175 The principal mucin in synovial fluid is:
(handwritten: → lubrication of joints)

MLS ONLY

    (a) hyaluronate

    b albumin

    c orosomucoid

    d pepsin

176 The synovial fluid easily forms small drops from the aspirating syringe. This viscosity is:
(handwritten: ↓ decreased = arthritis)

MLS ONLY

    a normal

    b increased

    (c) associated with inflammation

    d associated with hypothyroidism

177 Pleural transudates differ from pleural exudates in that transudates have:
(handwritten: oozes out; large molecules ↑; infection / outside blood vessels in tissues / by pressure, filtrate of blood; ↓ (thin))

MLS ONLY

    a protein values of >4 g/dL

    b specific gravity values of >1.020

    c LD values of >200 IU *(handwritten: ✳)*

    (d) relatively low cell counts

178 Pleural fluid from a patient with congestive heart failure would be expected to:

MLS ONLY

    a contain bacteria

    b have a high protein content

    c be purulent

    (d) appear clear and pale yellow

179 Monosodium urate (MSU) and calcium pyrophosphate dehydrate (CPPD) crystals can be distinguished by using a red compensator in a polarizing microscope. When the crystal is aligned with the slow vibration of the compensator, which is true?

MLS ONLY

    a MSU are blue *(handwritten: (perpendicular blue))*

    (b) MSU are yellow *(handwritten: (aligned - uric acid yellow))*

    c CPPD are blue

    d corticosteroids are yellow

180 False-positive results can occur for fecal occult blood due to the ingestion of

    a ascorbic acid *(handwritten: - false negative)*

    (b) horseradish *(handwritten: - false positive)*   *(handwritten: ✳✳ - reacts with peroxidase)*

    c acetaminophen

    d blueberries

181 The chromogen for the fecal occult blood test is:

    (a) gum guaiac *(handwritten: - chromogen, hydrogen peroxide → reagent / principle: oxidation of guaiac)*

    b NADH

    c o-toluidine

    d p-aminocinnamaldehyde

182 A build up of fluid in a body cavity is called:

    (a) an effusion *(handwritten: - build-up of fluid)*

    b a transudate

    c an exudate

    d metastasis

183 A fluid sample was collected by thoracentesis. A serum sample was collected immediately afterward. The LD fluid to serum ratio was 0.9. There were 5,000 WBC/µL, with 75% PMNs. Which of the following describes this fluid?

MLS ONLY

    (a) pleural effusion exudate

    b pericardial effusion exudate

    c pleural effusion transudate

    d pericardial effusion transudate

184 Ascites is collected by: *accumulation of fluid in the ~~abdomel~~ abdomenal cavity (paritoneal)*

   a thoracentesis
   b lumbar puncture
   c amniocentesis
   (d) paracentesis

185 Amniotic fluid is tested for the concentration of lamellar bodies. This test determines:

   (a) fetal lung maturity (FLM)   *(phospholipeds produced by maturing Lungs of baby)*
   b hemolytic disease of the newborn (HDN)
   c alpha-fetoprotein (AFP)
   d trisomy 21   *counted by platelet counter*

186 Amniocentesis should be performed to:

   ~~(a)~~ screen for Down syndrome - *never for a screen*
   (b) to <u>confirm</u> a high maternal serum alpha-fetoprotein (MSAFP)
   c to test bilirubin levels for an Rh positive mother
   d test folic acid levels in fetal blood

187 A sweat chloride >60 mEq/L (60 mmol/L) is indicative of:

   a multiple sclerosis
   b muscular dystrophy
   c respiratory distress syndrome
   (d) cystic fibrosis - *defective ion channel*

188 The most common genetic defect associated with cystic fibrosis is called:

   (a) delta-F508
   b trisomy 21 - *down's*
   c Philadelphia chromosome - *leukemia (acute myeloid)*
   d fragile X - *additional X*

189 The presence of oligoclonal bands in the CSF but not in the serum is associated with:

   a spina bifida
   b hydrocephalus
   c Reye syndrome
   (d) multiple sclerosis ↑ *IgG (gamma protein)*

190 Normal CSF has a relative abundance of which of the following proteins when compared to serum?

   a transferrin
   (b) prealbumin - *absent in serum*
   c albumin
   d fibrinogen

191 A CSF was collected from a 5-year-old with a fever, and 3 tubes were transported to the lab. Tube 1 had 50,000 RBC/mL and 48 WBC/mL. Tube 3 had 10 RBC/mL and 0 WBC/mL. What is the most likely explanation for the discrepancy?

   a tube 3 was QNS
   b bacterial meningitis
   c subarachnoid hemorrhage
   (d) traumatic tap

192 An increased IgG index indicates:

   a antibody response to bacteria
   (b) synthesis of IgG in the CNS
   c brain tumor
   d breach of the blood brain barrier

193 The appearance of normal CSF is:

   a pale yellow and clear
   b colorless and clear
   c opalescent
   d xanthochromic

194 A CSF was hazy and the WBC was too high to perform undiluted. The technologist took 50 mL of sample and added 500 mL of saline. The cell count on the diluted sample was 200 WBC per mL. This should be multiplied by:

   a 10
   b 11
   c 1/10
   d 1/11

195 The finding of hemosiderin laden macrophage in a CSF sample indicates:

   a bacterial infection
   b viral infection
   c previous hemorrhage
   d traumatic tap

196 Which CSF results are most consistent with bacterial meningitis?

CSF sample	Glucose	Protein	Lactate
A	↓20 mg/dL (1.1 mmol/L)	↑50 mg/dL (500 mg/L)	increased
B	75 mg/dL (4.1 mmol/L)	20 mg/dL (200 mg/L)	increased
C	20 mg/dL (1.1 mmol/L)	45 mg/dL (450 mg/L)	decreased
D	75 mg/dL (4.1 mmol/L)	120 mg/dL (1,200 mg/L)	decreased

   a sample A   *glucose: decreased (60% of serum glucose)*
   b sample B   *lactate: increased*
   c sample C   *protein: slightly increased (15-45)*
   d sample D

197 Which of the following is the <u>best indicator</u> of Reye syndrome for CSF (hepatic encephalopathy)?

   a glutamine – *by-product of ammonia; more stable*   ✳
   b ammonia – *hard to test due to instability*
   c ALT
   d bilirubin

198 The <u>tau isoform of transferrin</u> is a carbohydrate deficient protein found only in:

   a CSF
   b sweat   ✳
   c amniotic fluid
   d semen

199 Which marker can be used to identify a body fluid as semen?

   a PSA   ✳
   b alkaline phosphatase – *bone/liver; acid phosphatase → semen*
   c fructose – *major carbohydrate in semen; not unique*
   d hyaluronic acid – *synovial*

200 Which stain is used to measure sperm viability?

   a eosin nigrosin – *live and dead sperm* ✳
                (blue)   *(red)*
   b Wright
   c toluidine blue
   d Papanicolaou

201 The dimensions of a hemacytometer are:

    (a) $3 \times 3 \times 0.1$ mm
    b $1 \times 1 \times 10$ mm
    c $3 \times 10 \times 1$ mm
    d $1 \times 1 \times 0.3$ mm

202 Rapid forward progression of sperm is rated as:

    a 1.0
    b 2.0
    c 3.0
    (d) 4.0

203 Laboratory characteristics of malabsorption syndrome due to pancreatic insufficiently include:
MLS ONLY

    (a) increased fecal fat
    b fecal leukocytes
    c positive Clinitest®
    d fecal occult blood

204 Pilocarpine iontophoresis refers to the specific process of:

    (a) inducing sweat
    b separating proteins in CSF
    (c) measuring ions in sweat
    d measuring pilocarpine in CSF

205 During sweat collection, a consideration that can result in a falsely high result is:
MLS ONLY

    a high ambient temperature
    (b) evaporation - *concentrated ions*
    c preparation of area with type 1 water
    d high sweat rate

206 Methods used as screening tests for cystic fibrosis include:

    a coulometric Cl measurement— *confirmatory methods*
    b Cl selective electrodes —   ✱
    (c) sweat conductivity - *screening*
    (d) pilocarpine iontophoresis

207 Which pair does not match with respect to amniotic fluid?

    a colorless—normal
    b dark red-brown—fetal death
    (c) dark green—~~hemolytic disease of the newborn~~ *meconium → fetal distress*
    d blood-streaked—traumatic tap

208 Amniotic fluid is evaluated using a Liley graph and change in absorbance at 450 nm. What is being evaluated, and why?

    (a) bilirubin, which increases in HDN *(Delta - OD50) - spec @ 450 nm → absorbance change*
    b AFP, which increases in spina bifida
    c HCG, which increases in Down syndrome
    d lamellar bodies, which increase with fetal lung maturity

209 Which assay for fetal lung maturity using amniotic fluid gives a ratio of surfactant to albumin?
MLS ONLY

    a Amniostat
    (b) L/S
    c lamellar bodies
    (d) fluorescence polarization assay

210 Triglycerides (chyle) can be identified in body fluids by their ability to:

    a polarize light
    (b) stain with Sudan III
    c sediment upon standing
    d glitter

211 Peritoneal lavage is used to: *✳*

    (a) detect intra-abdominal bleeding in blunt injury
    b dialyze patients with end stage renal disease (ESRD)
    c replace ascites with saline
    d perform therapeutic thoracentesis

212 Tumor markers that can be measured on body fluids include all except:

    a CEA
    b CA 125
    (c) ANA-*not a tumor marker*
    d CYFRA 21-1

213 Which semen result is abnormal?

    a sample pours in droplets after 60 minutes *- 30-60 minutes normal*
    b >50% are motile within 1 hour of collection
    c pH 7.5 *(7.2-8.0 normal)*
    (d) motility of 1.0 *(2.0 or > normal)*

214 Increased CSF lactate is found in:

    (a) bacterial meningitis *↑ hypoxia*
    b Reye encephalopathy
    c spina bifida
    d multiple sclerosis

215 Decreased CSF protein can be found in:

    a meningitis
    b hemorrhage
    c multiple sclerosis
    (d) CSF leakage

216 What calculation is used to determine if there is a breach in the blood-brain barrier?   *✳✳*

    a IgG index - *IgG synthesized in CSF*
    (b) CSF/serum albumin index *< 9 = intact blood/brain barrier*
    c fluid/serum LD ratio = *transudate or exudate* *<0.6 >0.6*
    d albumin gradient- *effusion of hepatic origin*

1	d	59	b	117	b	175	a
2	a	60	c	118	a	176	c
3	b	61	a	119	d	177	d
4	d	62	a	120	a	178	d
5	c	63	c	121	a	179	b
6	b	64	d	122	b	180	b
7	b	65	c	123	a	181	a
8	c	66	b	124	b	182	a
9	d	67	c	125	a	183	a
10	b	68	b	126	b	184	d
11	c	69	d	127	d	185	a
12	c	70	b	128	b	186	b
13	b	71	d	129	c	187	d
14	a	72	b	130	d	188	a
15	a	73	a	131	a	189	d
16	c	74	c	132	b	190	b
17	b	75	b	133	d	191	d
18	c	76	d	134	c	192	b
19	b	77	b	135	d	193	b
20	b	78	b	136	d	194	b
21	b	79	d	137	a	195	c
22	c	80	c	138	a	196	a
23	a	81	b	139	b	197	a
24	c	82	b	140	c	198	a
25	d	83	b	141	b	199	a
26	b	84	d	142	a	200	a
27	c	85	a	143	c	201	a
28	b	86	b	144	a	202	d
29	a	87	d	145	c	203	a
30	a	88	d	146	b	204	a
31	c	89	a	147	b	205	b
32	b	90	d	148	b	206	c
33	c	91	b	149	c	207	c
34	b	92	a	150	c	208	a
35	b	93	d	151	a	209	d
36	c	94	c	152	d	210	b
37	c	95	b	153	b	211	a
38	a	96	d	154	d	212	c
39	b	97	c	155	b	213	d
40	b	98	b	156	b	214	a
41	d	99	c	157	b	215	d
42	b	100	d	158	c	216	b
43	b	101	b	159	c		
44	c	102	a	160	b		
45	b	103	d	161	c		
46	a	104	a	162	c		
47	a	105	c	163	d		
48	a	106	a	164	a		
49	a	107	a	165	c		
50	a	108	a	166	d		
51	c	109	b	167	a		
52	b	110	b	168	a		
53	d	111	a	169	d		
54	b	112	d	170	a		
55	a	113	c	171	b		
56	b	114	b	172	a		
57	c	115	b	173	a		
58	a	116	b	174	d		

Urinalysis: Pre-Analytical Examination

1 **d** Measure the total volume of the sample before removing an aliquot. To calculate the total protein, measure the protein of an aliquot to learn the mg/dL. Then multiply that answer by the number of dL in the 24-hour collection.
[Strasinger 2008, p36]

2 **a** Urobilinogen is degraded by light.
[Strasinger 2008, p69]

3 **b** It is common practice to share samples between the microbiology department and urinalysis. Ideally, the culture is set up first to prevent contamination. If that is not feasible timewise, the sample should be aliquotted using aseptic technique, and refrigerated until it can be cultured.
[Strasinger 2008, p36]

4 **d** Bilirubin is degraded by light. The other analytes will not be affected.
[Strasinger 2008, p69]

5 **c** Evaluate each statement. **a** is incorrect because these cells don't agglutinate. **b** is partially correct, but urobilinogen decreases in light. **c** is true, bacterial overgrowth does lead to an alkaline urine. **d** is false, ketones are produced by fat metabolism in the patient.
[Strasinger 2008, pp56, 69]

6 **b** The sample is mistreated by being
MLS ONLY uncapped. It is refrigerated, which will prevent bacteria from reproducing (so **d** is incorrect), and from metabolizing glucose (so **a** is incorrect). Ketones can evaporate, but protein will not.
[Strasinger 2008, p65]

7 **b** Storage must inhibit bacterial growth but not kill the bacteria. Freezing and additives are not acceptable. The most commonly used method of preservation is refrigeration.
[Strasinger 2008, p33]

8 **c** Consider whether a substance can increase or decrease outside the body. No more blood can be produced. Although the RBC may rupture, they will still make a positive result on a biochemical strip. The amount of solutes won't change, so specific gravity won't change. pH is affected by metabolism of the urine components by bacteria, and room temperature is warm enough for this to occur. Protein will not increase or decrease.
[Strasinger 2008, p33]

9 **d** The reader should know the
MLS ONLY approximate volume of a daily void, which is approximately 1,500 mL, but can range from 600-2,000 mL. In order to determine if 600 is the actual volume, or some sample was missed, evaluate the creatinine. Creatinine is excreted at approximately 1.2 mg/24 hour. Now evaluate the choices. **a** could be correct, but it is not sufficient, since 600 mL is unusually low. **b** is incorrect, because the creatinine is too low. **c** is incorrect, because it does not answer the medical question, and it bills the patient. This leaves **d**, which is the correct answer.
[McBride 1999]

10 **b** Larger sediment constituents sink to the bottom of the specimen container. Without prior mixing, the sediment in the container may not be poured into the centrifuge tube.
[Strasinger 2008, p83]

11 **c** Several methods have been described
MLS ONLY to estimate glomerular filtration. The creatinine clearance test uses plasma creatinine vs urine creatinine. However, it is unwieldy and time consuming for the patient. The new estimated formula, called the modification of diet in renal disease (MDRD) uses ethnicity, serum creatinine, BUN and serum albumin.
[Strasinger 2008, p21]

12 **c** The creatinine clearance is a filtration rate, and is reported in minutes. The sample is a 24-hour urine, which is entered into the calculation as the volume in milliliters, and the factor of 1,440 minutes per 24 hours is applied.
[Strasinger 2008, p20]

13 **b**   Patients with hypertension and diabetes mellitus are at risk for kidney disease. Detection of small amounts of albumin in the urine predict eventual kidney disease. The advantage of this sensitive detection is that patients with microalbuminuria can be treated with anti-hypertensive medications and followed up more intensely to delay nephropathy.
[Strasinger 2008, p58]

Urinalysis: Physical Examination

14 **a**   The high specific gravity is due to the glucose in the urine. Patients with diabetes mellitus have polyuria, so that the volume of urine dilutes the urochrome (color), making the urine pale.
[Strasinger 2008, p42]

15 **a**   Phenylketonuria is a genetic disorder that results in a urine with a mousy odor. Acetone has a fruity odor. Bacteria can produce an ammonia odor. Porphyrin has no odor, but a characteristic red color.
[Strasinger 2008, p49]

16 **c**   Ammonia is the byproduct of urea
MLS ONLY breakdown. *Proteus* is urease positive.
[Strasinger 2008, p49]

17 **b**   Colors associated with urine are due to pigments. Melanin is black. Porphyrin is port wine (red). Bilirubin is amber to brown.
[Strasinger 2008, pp43, 44]

18 **c**   Hemoglobin may be converted to
MLS ONLY methemoglobin in an acid urine. This will cause the sample to darken on standing.
[Strasinger 2008, p43]

19 **b**   The 2 pigments are porphyrin and urochrome. Urochrome is "urine color," which is yellow. Porphyrin is red.
[Strasinger 2008, p42]

20 **b**   **a** is false, you don't use glass tubes in urinalysis. **b** is true—clarity or haziness is due to solids and cells in the solution. These settle to the bottom of the tube; therefore, the sample should be well mixed. It is not necessary to add anything to view clarity. Furthermore, adding SSA will precipitate urines with positive protein. Allowing the specimen to cool to room temperature may cause amorphous crystals to form, so **d** is false.
[Strasinger 2008, pp44, 45]

21 **b**   The 2 items listed that produce a white color are white blood cells and semen. It is more likely that a woman would have a UTI with many WBC than enough post coital sperm contamination to make the urine white.
[Strasinger 2008, p45]

22 **c**   Match the color to the pigment. Bile is green/brown. Porphyrins are red. Melanin is black. Blood cells are red or white.
[Strasinger 2008, p44]

23 **a**   The only normal pigment/substance listed here is urochrome.
[Strasinger 2008, p42]

24 **c**   Match the color to the pigment. Bilirubin is amber. Myoglobin is red, like hemoglobin. Homogentisic acid will produce a dark urine on standing.
[Strasinger 2008, pp42-43]

25 **d**   Since the patient is healthy, assume
MLS ONLY the turbidity is caused by something nonpathologic. After meals, urine is more alkaline; this is referred to as the alkaline tide. Due to this pH, amorphous phosphates may be found.
[McBride 1999, p63]

26 **b**   In alkaptonuria, the acid urine will turn
MLS ONLY black on standing.
[Strasinger 2008, p44]

27 **c**   Both osmolality and specific gravity measure solutes in a solution.
[Strasinger 2008, p22]

28 **b**   Specific gravity gives the concentration for the sample relative to water. It does not give specific information about H^+ or Na^+ ions.
[Strasinger 2008, p46]

29 **a**   Osmolality measures the number of particles in a solution. Salts will dissociate into ions, and each ion contributes to the osmolality.
[Strasinger 2008, p22]

30 **a**   Only 2 of the answers, osmolality
MLS ONLY and refractive index, measure urine concentration. Refractive index is disproportionately affected by protein, so the correct answer is osmolality.
[McBride 1999, p58]

31 **c** An easy to make control for urinalysis is 6.5% NaCl. This has a specific gravity of 1.022, so **c** is correct. **b** is false, since the specific gravity of water is 1.000. **d** refers to osmolality, which is not measured by refractometry.
[Strasinger 2008, p48]

32 **b** Dissolved solids, including salt, sugar, urea, etc, contribute to specific gravity. Turbidity is caused by cells and crystals, which do not dissolve, and do not contribute to specific gravity.
[McBride 1999, p57]

33
MLS
ONLY
c Isosthenuric urine has a specific gravity of 1.010. A specific gravity less than that is termed hyposthenuric, and one greater than that is hypersthenuric.
[Strasinger 2008, p48]

34
MLS
ONLY
b Fluid leaving the glomerulus is isosthenuric.
[Strasinger 2008, p48]

35
MLS
ONLY
b Diuretics cause people to lose water as urine. Antidiuretic hormone has the opposite effect, that of retaining water. A deficiency of ADH results in a loss of water in the urine. The amount of solutes (salts and sugars) is not altered, but they are diluted, resulting in a low specific gravity.
[Strasinger 2008, p149]

36 **c** Although few labs (if any) use a urinometer, all of them should have a refractometer. These use 1 drop of sample, and compensate for temperature. A pitfall is that they are disproportionately affected by glucose and protein.
[Strasinger 2008, p47]

37
MLS
ONLY
c Distilled water is used to calibrate the refractometer. Since protein and glucose cause refractometer error, these should not be used as calibrators. Urea is susceptible to urease from bacterial contamination. NaCl is cheap and reliable.
[Strasinger 2008, p48]

38 **a** The reagent strip is not affected by contrast dye. The refractometer reads the darker solution as density. A densitometer is a chemistry instrument, not a urinalysis instrument. A urinometer is not generally used in the modern lab.
[Strasinger 2008, p49]

39
MLS
ONLY
b Osmolality and specific gravity are both measures of the concentration of urine.
[Strasinger 2008, p22]

40
MLS
ONLY
b Light bends when it hits the surface of the liquid, because the liquid slows down its velocity. This is called refraction. The degree that the light bends is the refractive index.
[Strasinger 2008, p47]

Urinalysis: Chemical Examination

41
MLS
ONLY
d **a**, **b**, and **c** may give false-positive results. A false-negative can result from a dilute urine, so **d** is correct.
[Strasinger 2008, p149]

42
MLS
ONLY
b Both **b** and **c** refer to pH; however, a urine pH is a number, not a concentration per unit of urine, so **c** is incorrect.
[Strasinger 2008, p56]

43 **b** The change in pH is due to breakdown of urea to ammonia by urease producing bacteria, and loss of CO_2.
[Strasinger 2008, p33]

44 **c** Reagent strips must be handled carefully to prevent them from picking up excess moisture. Heating or refrigeration is not appropriate. They work optimally at room temperature. They should be stored in a dark, tightly capped bottle, not exposed to light.
[Strasinger 2008, p55]

45
MLS
ONLY
b Two pH indicators are incorporated in the strip. Protein accepts H^+ ions from the pad, resulting in a pH and, therefore, color change.
[Strasinger 2008, p58]

46 **a** Albumin is the most abundant plasma protein and it is relatively small. In nephropathy, albumin will be the most abundant protein in the urine. This test is done to look for nephropathy (ie, kidney disease).
[Strasinger 2008, p58]

47
MLS
ONLY
a The 2 sugars in these distractor answers are glucose and galactose. Galactosuria is relatively rare genetic condition. The glucose biochemical strip is specific for glucose and will not detect galactose. Glucose is found in diabetes mellitus as well as other diseases.
[Strasinger 2008, p61]

48 **a** The only reagent listed is in **a**. The other answers are forms of ketones.
[Strasinger 2008, p665]

49
MLS
ONLY
a You should recognize that sodium nitroprusside is the reagent for ketones. It reacts with acetoacetic acid, not beta-hydroxybutyric acid.
[Strasinger 2008, p65]

50 **a** The student should memorize the chemical reactions for each of the dipstick biochemicals. Diazo reagent is used for bilirubin.
[Strasinger 2008, p68]

51
MLS
ONLY
c Nitrite is produced by bacteria, and WBCs are found when there is a bacterial infection. If nitrite interfered with the WBC reaction, then the dipstick would be worthless when testing patients with UTIs.
[Strasinger 2008, p74]

52
MLS
ONLY
b The protein pad of the biochemical strip is held at an acid pH by citrate buffer. If the strip is not blotted, the acid buffer can "run over" to the pH pad and cause a falsely acidic pH. Tetrabromphenol blue is a pH indicator, not an acid. Glucose oxidase is the reagent on the glucose strip. Copper sulfate is the reagent of the reducing substances (Benedict) test.
[Strasinger 2008, p56]

53 **d** The protein pad must be held at a pH of 3 in order to see the effect that protein has on the double indicators. In alkaline urine, the pH of 3 may be neutralized, and the indicators change color.
[Strasinger 2008, p51]

54 **b** Ketones are byproducts of fat metabolism. During low carbohydrate or starvation diets, ketones can be found in the urine.
[Strasinger 2008, p64]

55 **a** Vomiting leads to dehydration and utilization of fat for energy. Fat metabolism produces ketones.
[Strasinger 2008, p64]

56
MLS
ONLY
b Biliary obstruction inhibits the normal flow of conjugated bilirubin into the intestine, and it backs up into the blood. From there, it will be filtered into the urine. Urobilinogen is a product of bacterial reduction of bilirubin in the intestine. Some urobilinogen is reabsorbed into the bloodstream and will be filtered into the urine. In biliary obstruction, less bilirubin reaches the intestine, and less is converted into urobilinogen.
[Strasinger 2008, pp68-70]

57
MLS
ONLY
c Each answer is a different live/biliary condition. In hemolytic jaundice, the total bilirubin goes up, but the direct/conjugated bilirubin does not.
[Strasinger 2008, p70]

58 **a** Ascorbic acid inhibits reactions that use peroxidase.
[Strasinger 2008, p67]

59
MLS
ONLY
b Microalbuminuria refers to the urinary excretion of amounts of albumin that cannot be detected by routine reagent strips. Persons with diabetes mellitus are at risk for end-stage renal disease if the damage occurring to the glomerulus is not detected in its early stages.
[Strasinger 2008, p60]

60
MLS
ONLY
c The reagent strip test for microalbuminuria uses a dye binding technique. As opposed to the conventional protein error of indicators principle used in routine reagent strips, the dye is highly sensitive and specific for albumin.
[Strasinger 2008, p61]

61
MLS
ONLY
a Including a reagent strip reaction for creatinine, along with the reaction of microalbuminuria, the amount of creatinine that is excreted at a constant rate can correct for the hydration or dehydration in a patient's urine.
[Strasinger 2008, p61]

62 **a** 3% SSA is used to confirm positive protein tests. 3% implies 3 g in 100 mL.
[Campbell 1997, p136]

63 **c** The bilirubin dipstick pad can show a false positive from a colored urine. All positives should be confirmed with an ictotest.
[Strasinger 2008, p68]

64 **d** Both hemoglobin and myoglobin will produce a red urine without RBC. Hemoglobin will be precipitated by ammonium sulfate, but myoglobin will not. Myoglobin will remain in the supernate after centrifugation.
[Strasinger 2008, p67]

65 **c** When 2 drops of urine are added to 10 drops of water, it is a 2/12 proportion. 12 is the total volume. This is the same as a 1:6 dilution.
[Strasinger 2008, p63]

66 **b** It is not uncommon to find a urine specimen with positive protein. It is necessary to confirm positive protein if the urine pH is elevated, but this is not one of the choices. The choice of **b** will allow all results to be correct, but the choice of **d** would cause some of the results to be wrong.
[Strasinger 2008, p59]

67 **c** Sulfosalicylic acid will precipitate protein. Ehrlich reagent is for urobilinogen. Diazo is for bilirubin, and copper reduction is for reducing substances.
[Strasinger 2008, p59]

68 **b** A positive glucose oxidase is specific for glucose. Glucose will also cause copper reduction (a positive Clinitest®).
[Strasinger 2008, p64]

69 **d** The 2 keys here are that the dipstick
MLS ONLY glucose is negative, so the answer is not glucose; and that the woman is pregnant, and about to deliver. This implies that she may be making milk. Lactose is the most likely answer.
[Strasinger 2008, p64]

70 **b** Children with failure to thrive may have galactosuria. In this case, only **a** and **b** are reducing substances. Since the reagent strip for glucose is negative, this leaves galactose.
[Strasinger 2008, p64]

71 **d** Radiographic dye will precipitate in SSA.
MLS ONLY [Strasinger 2008, p60]

72 **b** The Clinitest® is a copper reduction test,
MLS ONLY utilizing copper sulfate as the reactant. In the presence of a reducing substance, such as a sugar, and heat and alkali, the copper is reduced, producing a change in color from blue to orange/red.
[Strasinger 2008, p63]

Urinalysis: Microscopic Examination

73 **a** The ocular lens has a magnification of 10x. This multiplied by the magnification of the objectives 10× (low power), 40× (high power), etc, equals the total magnification.
[Strasinger 2008, p88]

74 **c** Adjusting the condenser of the diaphragm of the microscope also affects image resolution. Adjusting the main light source only changes the light intensity.
[Strasinger 2008, p89]

75 **b** The diffracted light in phase microscopy enhances slight variations in the refractive indices of constituents with low refractive indices. Staining is not required to enhance low refractive index constituents when using phase microscopy.
[Strasinger 2008, p90]

76 **d** The prefix *py-* means pus (leukocytes). The suffix *-uria* means pertaining to urine.
[Masters 2003, p149]

77 **b** Renal tubular epithelial cells lining the tubules absorb the urinary filtrate. In disorders producing fat in the filtrate, the fat is absorbed into the cells. When the cells slough from the tubules, they appear as oval fat bodies.
[Strasinger 2008, p99]

78 **b** Osmosis occurs through the red blood cell membrane. In dilute urine, the cells absorb water and swell, lyse, and release hemoglobin.
[Strasinger 2008, p92]

79 **d** White blood cells absorb water when they are in hypotonic (low specific gravity) urine, and swell. Granules in the WBCs then exhibit Brownian movement, producing the glittering effect in the cells.
[Strasinger 2008, p94]

80 **c** Squamous epithelial cells line the female vagina and urethra, but only the distal part of the male urethra. In females, they may also indicate perianal contamination.
[Brunzel 2004, p195]

81 **b** The reagent strip test for blood is positive for hemoglobin from lysed red blood cells, filtered hemoglobin from intravascular hemolysis, and myoglobin. With no RBCs present, the terminology is hemoglobinuria, indicating the presence of filtered hemoglobin.
[Strasinger 2008, p65]

82 **b** RBCs absorb water when in dilute urine, and are also less preserved in alkaline urine. Therefore, as the cells swell in the alkaline urine, the cell membrane allows hemoglobin to leak from the cell, resulting in the empty cell membrane and the pale appearance.
[Strasinger 2008, p92]

83 **b** In a hypotonic urine, WBCs will absorb water and swell. This results in the granules in the granulocytic WBCs to exhibit Brownian movement.
[Strasinger 2008, p94]

84 **d** Acute interstitial nephritis is
MLS
ONLY caused by an allergic reaction resulting
in inflammation of the renal tubules.
The reaction is frequently caused by a
medication. As a result of the allergic
reaction, eosinophils are increased. An
eosinophil count can aid in confirming
the diagnosis.
[Strasinger 2008, p151]

85 **a** Clue cells represent the attachment
of the bacterium *Gardnerella vaginalis* to
squamous epithelial cells. *Gardnerella* causes
vaginal infections, and the cells lining
the vagina are the squamous epithelial cells.
[Strasinger 2008, p97]

86 **b** Urothelial/transitional epithelial cells
line the bladder, renal pelvis and ureters.
These can be dislodged from the walls of the
bladder during a catheterization procedure.
[Strasinger 2008, p97]

87 **d** Myoglobin is a product of muscle
destruction as occurs with crush injuries.
The reagent strip reaction for blood
is positive with the presence of RBCs,
hemoglobin, and myoglobin. Both
hemoglobin and myoglobin are toxic to
the renal tubules, resulting in decreased
urine flow, favoring cast formation and the
sloughing of the damaged cells. Notice also
that the specimen is clear.
[Strasinger 2008, p66]

88 **d** Some key findings for each condition
are: **a** glomerulonephritis—red blood cell
casts, **b** pyelonephritis—white blood cell
casts, **c** nephrotic syndrome—lipids and
fatty casts, and **d** cystitis (urinary tract
infection)—white blood cells, bacteria,
possible RBCs. This image has no casts, just
WBCs, bacteria, and RBCs.
[Strasinger 2008, p95]

89 **a** RBCs are smooth, circular, greenish
objects. They can be confused with yeast
and fat globules. To distinguish yeast from
RBC, react an aliquot with water. RBCs will
lyse, but yeast will not. Fat globules can be
stained with Sudan III, turning them orange.
RBCs should produce a positive blood result
on a biochemical strip.
[Strasinger 2008, p34]

90 **d** Tamm-Horsfall protein is continuously
excreted by the renal tubular cells. In
conditions that cause urine stasis, the
excreted protein aggregates into fibrils that
mesh to form the matrix of casts.
[Strasinger 2008, p102]

91 **b** Hyaline casts have a low refractive
index, and may not be visible under bright
light. Urine microscopic analysis is first
performed under reduced light, and the
edges of the coverslip examined for the
casts. Casts are larger than other sediment
constituents and are pushed to the edges
of the coverslip.
[Strasinger 2008, pp102-103]

92 **a** Hyaline casts may be excreted by
healthy people following strenuous exercise
or normal condition that produces decreased
urine flow. Red cell, white cell, and waxy
casts indicate a pathogenic condition
within the nephron.
[Strasinger 2008, p103]

93 **d** Broad casts indicate extreme stasis
of urine flow through the nephron. Stasis
allows casts to form in the larger collecting
ducts. Damage to the walls of the distal
convoluted tubules also causes broader
casts to form.
[Strasinger 2008, p109]

94 **c** Multiplication of bacteria present in
MLS
ONLY the specimen caused an increase in the urine
pH during the 5-hour delay, resulting in
the casts dissolving.
[Strasinger 2008, p102]

95 **b** Centrally-placed nuclei are characteristic
of spherical transitional cells.
[Strasinger 2008, p98]

96 **d** Pyelonephritis is an inflammation/
infection of the renal tubules. Therefore,
white blood cell casts would indicate the
location of the source of the inflammation/
infection. Cystitis is an infection of
the bladder.
[Strasinger 2008, p105]

97 **c** Damage to the renal tubules causes
MLS
ONLY sloughing of the cells lining the tubules,
making these cells the most prominent in
the cast formation. Although casts are seen
in each of the other listed disorders, each
has its own most prominent cast feature
ie, red blood cells, fat, and white blood cells.
[Strasinger 2008, p149]

98 **b** Formation of a cast matrix is not
uncommon following strenuous exercise,
due primarily to dehydration resulting in
decrease urine flow. Increased metabolism
by the renal tubular cells results in excess
excretion of lysomes that become attached
to the cast matrix, resulting in the
appearance of granular casts.
[Strasinger 2008, p108]

99 **c** Waxy casts are seen with extreme stasis of urine flow, indicating they have remained in the tubles for an extended time. These aging casts are more refractile, and often contain notches and jagged edges as the result of granular disintegration.
[Strasinger 2008, p109]

100 **d** White blood cells are often attached to the cast matrix as well as being imbedded in the matrix. White blood cells frequently occur in clumps and could can resemble a cast, but no cast matrix is observed. WBC casts indicate a more serious tubular infection, whereas WBC clumps can be seen in cystitis.
[Strasinger 2008, p106]

101 **b** Spherical urothelial cells appear similar to round tubular epithelial cells. The eccentric placement of the nucleus in renal tubular cells differentiates them from spherical urothelial cells, which have a centrally-placed nucleus.
[Strasinger 2008, p97]

102 **a** Before reporting a red blood cell cast, it is essential to observe free-floating RBCs in the sediment. A coarsely granular cast may sometimes resemble a red blood cell cast. Without the presence of free red blood cells, a red blood cell cast could not have formed in the tubules.
[Strasinger 2008, p105]

103 **d** The renal tubular cells lining the tubules absorb the urinary filtrate, and therefore will appear bile-stained.
[Strasinger 2008, p107]

104 **a** RBC casts, protein and RBCs together are indicative of glomerulonephritis. RBC casts form when there is bleeding in the glomerulus and tubules.
[Strasinger 2008, p29]

105 **c** Amorphous phosphates are found in alkaline urine. Under conditions such as refrigeration, they produce a white precipitate. Urates produce a pink precipitate, and WBCs and bacteria do not precipitate.
[Strasinger 2008, p115]

106 **a** Cystine crystals appear as hexogonal plates, frequently in clumps. Tyrosine crystals are needle-shaped, leucine crystals are round, and cholesterol crystals are flat with notched corners.
[Strasinger 2008, p116]

107 **a** Approximately 75% of renal calculi are composed of calcium compounds (oxalate, phosphate and others). Magnesium ammonium phosphate makes up about 15% of the calculi.
MLS ONLY
[Brunzel 2004, p261]

108 **a** Amorphous urates will dissolve when the specimen is briefly warmed. Amorphous phosphates are dissolved by the addition of acid, which will also destroy other sediment constituents.
[Strasinger 2008, p113]

109 **b** Calcium carbonate crystals are small dumbell-shaped or round crystals often seen in clumps. With careful examination, dumbell-shaped forms can be distinguished.
[Strasinger 2008, p116]

110 **b** Calcium oxalate crystals are found in acidic and neutral urine, but not in alkaline urine.
[Strasinger 2008, p113]

111 **a** Cholesterol is the only one of these lipids capable of polarizing light. The other lipids will stain with Sudan III.
MLS ONLY
[Strasinger 2008, p85]

112 **d** Tyrosine crystals are fine needles often seen in clumps. Leucine crystals are spherical with concentric striations. Cholesterol crystals are flat plates with notched corners. Hemosiderin granules are dark, and often clumped.
[Strasinger 2008, p117]

113 **c** Urinary crystals associated with liver disorders include bilirubin, tyrosine, and leucine.
[Strasinger 2008, p118]

114 **b** Calcium oxide monohydrate crystals are most frequently seen following ingestion of ethylene glycol/antifreeze. Unlike the more commonly seen envelope-shaped dihydrate crystals, they are oval or dumbbell shaped.
[Strasinger 2008, p113]

115 **b** Increased lipids in the urine is a characteristic of the nephrotic syndrome. Massive amounts of protein also are associated with the nephrotic syndrome. The crystals form more readily in urine that has been refrigerated.
[Strasinger 2008, p116]

116 **b** Lesch-Nyhan syndrome is an inherited
MLS
ONLY disorder of purine metabolism. The
first indication of this disorder may be
the presence of uric acid indicating the
incomplete metabolism of dietary purines.
[Strasinger 2008, p170]

117 **b** Triple phosphates crystals, nicknamed
"coffin lids" are nonpathologic. They are
found in alkaline urines, usually urines with
bacterial overgrowth.
[Strasinger 2008, p113]

118 **a** Uric acid has many shapes, is found
in acid urine, and is nonpathologic.
The reader should become familiar with
the different shapes.
[Strasinger 2008, p44]

119 **d** The crystals are amorphous phosphates.
These can be dissolved in dilute acetic acid,
in order to view other formed elements that
are obscured.
[Strasinger 2008, p113]

120 **a** Contaminants frequently contain
substances capable of polarizing light.
None of the other listed constituents are
capable of polarizing light.
[Strasinger 2008, p120]

121 **a** Starch granules are very refractile and
produce a Maltese cross under polarized
light. Oil, air bubbles and pollen grains
do not polarize.
[Strasinger 2008, p120]

122 **b** These are starch crystals, a contaminant
from powder.
[Strasinger 2008, p120]

123 **a** Cloth fiber is a contaminant. It should
not be confused with a cast. Fiber can have
a rough and stringy appearance. Vegetable
fibers have intricate repeating detail.
[Strasinger 2008, pp120-121]

124 **b** Acetic acid lyses red blood cells, but not
oil droplets and yeast. Acetic acid will also
lyse other formed elements and should be
added to an aliquot of the sediment.
[Strasinger 2008, p93]

125 **a** Yeast cells are commonly seen in urine
specimens from persons with diabetes
mellitus, because the high glucose content
provides an excellent growth media for yeast.
[Strasinger 2008, p100]

126 **b** Urine crystal formation is associated
with the optimal pH needed for their
formation (acid, alkaline or neutral).
[Strasinger 2008, p110]

127 **d** Based on the time between collection
and analysis of a urine specimen and the
method of preservation, bacteria can be
a heavy contaminant of urine. A positive
LE test indicating the presence of WBCs
confirms the actual presence of an infection.
[Strasinger 2008, p100]

128 **b** The flagellate *Trichomonas vaginalis*
moves rapidly through the sediment. If not
moving, it may resemble a WBC, and careful
examination of phase microscopy is needed
to visualize the flagellum. Urine is toxic
to spermatozoa.
[Strasinger 2008, p100]

129 **c** Yeast cells are commonly seen in urine
specimens from persons with diabetes
mellitus, because the high glucose content
provides an excellent growth media for yeast.
[Strasinger 2008, p100]

130 **d** Many bacteria produce nitrites from
nitrate. If the biochemical strip is positive
for nitrite, you should find bacteria in
the sediment.
[Strasinger 2008, p72]

131 **a** Glucose in the urine of a person with
a normal blood glucose is indicative of renal
tubule damage or the inherited disorder,
renal glycosuria, in which transport
receptors are absent in the proximal
convoluted tubules.
[Strasinger 2008, p149]

Urinalysis: Complete Examination

132 **b** Reagent strip tests for protein
MLS
ONLY are primarily sensitive to albumin.
The monoclonal spike in the gamma region
indicates the presence of Bence Jones
protein that is an immunoglobulin rather
than albumin.
[Strasinger 2008, p59]

133 **d** Uric acid crystals are seen in acid
urine. The reagent strip pH may have been
recorded wrong. Uric acid crystals have
many shapes, and an artifact may have been
mistaken for the uric acid crystals.
[Strasinger 2008, p112]

134 c The reagent strip glucose test using glucose oxidase is specific for glucose; therefore, glucose must be present in the sample. The copper reduction test is positive with many sugars, including glucose. The copper reduction test has a lower sensitivity than the reagent strip; therefore, the higher reading on the copper reduction test indicates the presence of an additional sugar. In the case of a nursing mother, the most likely additional sugar is lactose.
[Strasinger 2008, p64]

135 d Pyelonephritis is an infection involving the renal tubules. Therefore, the presence of WBC casts and bacteria aids in the diagnosis. Cystitis is an infection of the bladder and does not affect the tubules. RBC casts are the prominent finding with glomerulonephritis.
[Strasinger 2008, p150]

136 d The presence of RBC casts is consistent with glomerulonephritis. WBCs, RBCs and protein are present as a result of the glomerular damage.
[Strasinger 2008, p147]

137 a Damage to the electrical charges of the glomerular membrane, allowing the passage of high molecular-weight proteins and lipids occurs in nephrotic syndrome. This results in markedly increased urine protein levels, and the appearance of fatty casts and oval fat bodies that are characteristic of nephrotic syndrome.
[Strasinger 2008, p144]

138 a A specimen with a specific gravity of 1.004 is very dilute. This will result in the concentration of urine constituents being too low, below the ability to be detected by chemical and microscopic examination.
[Strasinger 2008, p34]

139 b
MLS
ONLY
Minimal change disease is seen primarily in children, often following allergic reactions or immunizations. Classic laboratory results include markedly elevated urine protein, fatty casts, elevated serum lipids, decreased serum albumin, and normal BUN.
[Strasinger 2008, p146]

140 c Acute interstitial nephritis is caused by an allergic reaction, resulting in inflammation, not infection, of the renal tubules. Bacteria are not present in an inflammation.
[Strasinger 2008, p151]

141 b The presence of heavy bacteria with a negative leukocyte esterase and normal WBC numbers indicates the specimen has been collected >2 hours before being tested. Testing a fresh specimen will determine if bacterial multiplication has occurred in the first specimen.
[Strasinger 2008, p33]

142 a
MLS
ONLY
A major cause of glomerular disorders is the deposition of immune complexes on the glomerular membrane, producing damage to the membrane. The presence of RBC casts is indicative of glomerulonephritis. WBC casts would be present in chronic pyelonephritis and acute interstitial nephritis, and renal tubular epithelial cells are present in tubular necrosis.
[Strasinger 2008, p144]

143 c The ideal conditions for the growth of *Candida albicans* are an acid pH and the presence of glucose. *Candida* is a frequent cause of urinary tract infections in diabetic patients.
[Strasinger 2008, p101]

144 a
MLS
ONLY
The high specific gravity indicates the patient is in a dehydrated state that favors the formation of the renal calculi, producing the back pain and presence of red blood cells resulting from irritation to the urinary tract caused by the calculi.
[Strasinger 2008, p153]

Urine Physiology

145 c The renal threshold is the plasma level at which a substance, such as glucose, is not longer reabsorbed by the proximal convoluted tubules. The plasma level for glucose ranges from 160-180mg/dL.
[Strasinger 2008, p62]

146 b The prefix *oligo-* means scanty. Knowing that the normal daily urine volume is around 1200mL, 300mL is scanty. The prefix *an-* means not, *poly-* means many, and *dys-* means pain.
[Masters 2003, p147]

147 b The combination of these results is consistent with diabetes mellitus. The polyuria occurs due to the need to excrete the excess dissolved glucose in the urinary filtrate. Hyperglycemia is not present with renal glucosuria. Both stress and a heavy meal can cause transient glucosuria.
[Strasinger 2008, p62]

148 **b**   Although the normal glomerular filtration rate is 120mL/min, tubular reabsorption returns normally all but 1 mL to the plasma.
[Strasinger 2008, p20

149 **c**   Normal plasma constituents that can be filtered by the glomerulus are water, urea and sodium chloride. Protein molecules are too large to normally pass the glomerulus. Bilirubin is not a normal constituent of plasma.
[Strasinger 2008, p13]

150 **c**   Urine is the only body fluid containing large amounts of the waste products urea and creatinine. These 2 constituents are used to determine if an unknown fluid is urine.
[Strasinger 2008, p31]

151 **a**   Based on the body's state of hydration,
MLS
ONLY   antidiuretic hormone regulates the permeability of the walls of the collecting ducts to water. When the body is dehydrated, ADH is released by the pituitary gland, reducing the permeability of the walls to water.
[Brunzel 2004, p51]

152 **d**   The intact structure of the glomerular membrane does not permit passage of high-molecular-weight substances, such as protein molecules.
[Strasinger 2008, p13]

153 **b**   The increased plasma glucose seen in diabetes mellitus results in excess glucose in the glomerular filtrate. Increased amounts of water are required for excretion of the excess glucose in the filtrate. As a result, increased fluid intake is characteristic of persons with diabetes mellitus.
[Strasinger 2008, p31]

154 **d**   The prefix *an-* means not, or without. The prefix *azo-* stands for nitrogenous, *dys-* means pain, and *di-* means double.
[Masters 2003, p146]

155 **b**   Galactosuria is an inborn error of metabolism, resulting in the failure to inherit the one of the enzymes needed to metabolize dietary galactose to glucose. Byproducts of this metabolic failure are toxic, and can result in severe mental retardation. Early detection and dietary changes can prevent the toxicity.
[Strasinger 2008, p170]

156 **b**   Ketones are intermediate components of fat metabolism. When access to carbohydrates normally broken down to supply energy is limited, fats are broken down for energy, and the intermediate ketone products (acetone, acetoacetic acid and beta-hydroxybutyric acid) can be detected in the urine.
[Strasinger 2008, p64]

157 **b**   The nitroprusside/ferricyanide reagent strip reaction reacts with acetoacetic acid. Glycine must be present for the reaction to include acetone. beta-hydroxybutyric acid is present in the largest amount, but does not react with nitroferricyanide.
[Strasinger 2008, p65]

158 **c**   Bilirubin is a product of hemoglobin degradation. It occurs in both unconjugated and conjugated forms. Only conjugated bilirubin can pass through the glomerulus, because unconjugated bilirubin is bound to albumin. Conjugation of bilirubin takes place in the liver, and liver damage interfers with the continued degradation to urobilinogen.
[Strasinger 2008, p68]

159 **c**   Myoglobin is a product of muscle
MLS
ONLY   destruction. Myocardial infarctions damage the heart muscle.
[Brunzel 2004, p134]

160 **b**   Renal tubular acidosis is the inability to
MLS
ONLY   produce an acid urine even when in acidosis. The hydrogen ions needed to produce an acid urine are easily reabsorbed. To remove them, tubular secretion of the ions, combined with ammonium ions produced in the proximal and distal convoluted tubules, is needed.
[Brunzel 2004, p256]

161 **c**   The majority of the filtered glucose is reabsorbed by active transport in the proximal convoluted tubules (PCT). Damage to the PCTs results in glycosuria and a normal plasma glucose.
[Strasinger 2008, p62]

162 **c**   To maintain the high concentration
MLS
ONLY   of solutes in the renal medulla that result in the ability to concentrate urine, water cannot be removed from the filtrate as it passes through to ascending loop of Henle.
[Strasinger 2008, p17]

163 d The juxtaglomerular nephron have
MLS
ONLY long loops of Henle, and the urinary filtrate
passes through the renal medulla with its
high osmotic gradient, causing reabsorption
of water in the descending loop of Henle.
Cortical nephrons are located in the renal
cortex and have short loops of Henle that do
not reach the medulla.
[Strasinger 2008, p12]

164 a Osmolarity measures the number of
particles in a solution, whereas specific
gravity is influenced not only by the number
of particles but also their density. Renal
concentration is concerned with smaller
molecules, such as sodium and chloride.
Each of these molecules will contribute the
same to an osmolarity reading as a large
molecule of glucose.
[Strasinger 2008, p22]

165 c The production of ammonia is essential
MLS
ONLY for the removal of hydrogen ions from the
glomerular filtrate. Lack of ammonia results
in a lack of hydrogen ions in the filtrate and
a high pH.
[Strasinger 2008, p20]

Other Body Fluids

166 d The lumbar tap may be traumatic,
which will produce blood. Blood cells in the
CSF will not be due to a central nervous
system defect in that case. Do the cell count
on the last tube; it is the least likely to be
contaminated by a bloody tap.
[Strasinger 2008, p179]

167 a Protein and glucose are dissolved
MLS
ONLY substances and don't contribute to turbidity.
Bacteria and WBCs are solids that make the
CSF turbid. When bacteria are present, so
are WBCs. The large WBCs contribute more
to turbidity than the smaller bacteria.
[Strasinger 2008, p180]

168 a Consider that a normal serum protein
MLS
ONLY is approximately 7 **g**/dL, and a normal CSF
protein is 15 **mg**/dL. The units are different
by 1,000. This indicates that the CSF protein
is <1% of serum protein.
[Strasinger 2008]

169 d Diluting cells for counting should
not disturb them osmotically. Saline is
the best choice. Water can lyse the cells,
trichloroacetic acid will precipitate the
sample, and acetic acid will form a clot with
hyaluronic acid in the sample.
[Strasinger 2008, p213]

170 a It is not necessary to test alkaline
MLS
ONLY phosphatase, acid phosphatase or
hemoglobin for fertility. Sperm should
be motile, have normal morphology, and
the sample should have normal viscosity.
Therefore **a** is the only correct choice.
[Strasinger 2008, p201]

171 b Urine and CSF are ruled out because of
MLS
ONLY the high protein value. Urine and CSF have
proteins in the mg/dL range. Hyaluronate is
a component of synovial fluid, not pleural
fluid. The best answer is synovial fluid.
[Strasinger 2008, p201]

172 a Hyaluric acid clots in the presence
MLS
ONLY of acetic acid. Synovial fluid has
hyaluronic acid.
[Strasinger 2008, p213]

173 a **a**, **b**, and **c** are possibilities, but the most
MLS
ONLY likely cause is monosodium urate (MSU).
MSU (uric acid) are needles, whereas calcium
pyrophosphate crystals are rhomboid
and square. Corticosteroid crystals are
birefringent and needle shaped but will only
be present if the patient has been treated
with corticosteroid injections. Talc crystals
are found as contaminants, and are not
needle shaped.
[Strasinger 2008, p215]

174 d Use the formula of cells × dilution × 10
MLS
ONLY divided by the number of secondary squares.
Then remember to convert from microliters
to milliliters by multiplying by 1,000.
[Strasinger 2008, p205]

175 a Hyaluronic acid is also known as
MLS
ONLY *hyaluronate*. It is the principal mucin in
synovial fluid, and its role is lubrication of
the joints. A low hyaluronic acid leads to
decreased viscosity of the synovial fluid,
and inflammation.
[Strasinger 2008, p213]

176 c A normal synovial fluid is viscous,
MLS
ONLY and will form a string of 4-6 cm when
expressed from the syringe. If the fluid
forms small drops, the viscosity is decreased.
This is associated with arthritis; hence,
inflammation is the correct answer.
[Strasinger 2008, p213]

177 **d** Transudates are thin, watery effusions
MLS
ONLY with low LD, low protein, and low cell
counts. Exudates are inflammatory or
infectious effusions with high LD, protein,
and WBC.
[Strasinger 2008, p223]

178 **d** Congestive heart failure is a buildup of
MLS
ONLY fluid because of poor heart pumping. The
fluid is watery, not infected.
[Strasinger 2008, p223]

179 **b** Uric acid produces a yellow color when
MLS
ONLY the crystal is aligned with the compensator,
but the color is blue when the crystal is
perpendicular to the compensator. CPPD,
calcium pyrophosphate has the opposite
color results. This difference is due to the
molecular stacking within the crystals.
[Strasinger 2008, pp216-217]

180 **b** False positives for fecal occult blood
occur when patient diet includes food that
produces peroxidase. Horseradish, broccoli,
radishes, melons, and other foods can cause
a false positive. Patients that take aspirin
may have some occult bleeding that is
not associated with colorectal cancer, but
acetaminophen is not a cause of bleeding.
Ascorbic acid at high doses can interfere
with the test and cause a false-negative.
[Strasinger 2008, p251]

181 **a** The principle of occult blood testing
is based on the oxidation of guaiac. This
occurs in the presence of hydrogen peroxide
(the reagent) and the enzyme peroxidase.
Hemoglobin has a pseudoperoxidse activity
that drives the reaction, making oxidized
guaiac, which is blue in color.
[Strasinger 2008, p250]

182 **a** A small amount of fluid fills the cavity
between the cavity wall (the parietal
membrane) and the organ (visceral
membrane). An increase in the fluid can
be due to infection, inflammation, cancer,
and defects in hydrostatic and colloidal
pressure. An accumulation of fluid is called
an effusion.
[Strasinger 2008, p222]

183 **a** The thorax is the chest. Fluid from
MLS
ONLY the chest, surrounding the lungs, is called
pleural fluid. An increase in this fluid is a
pleural effusion. When the fluid/serum LD
ratio is over 0.6, and/or the WBC is over
1,000/μL, the fluid is an exudate.
[Strasinger 2008, pp223, 284]

184 **d** Accumulation of fluid in the peritoneal
cavity is called ascites, and it is collected
by paracentesis.
[Strasinger 2008, pp229, 282]

185 **a** Amniotic fluid can be collected to test
for birth defects such as trisomy 21 (Down
syndrome), spina bifida (increased AFP and
acetylcholinesterase), hemolytic disease
of the newborn (bilirubin), and fetal lung
maturity (FLM). FLM can be determined
by increased lamellar body production in
the amniotic fluid. Lamellar bodies are
phospholipids produced by the maturing
pneumocytes. They are approximately the
size of small platelets, and can be counted by
instruments that are used to count platelets.
[Strasinger 2008, p241]

186 **b** Amniocentesis is an invasive procedure,
and should not be used as a screen. In
women with a high MSAFP, amniocentesis
is used to collect fluid to detect levels of
AFP and acetylcholinesterase. High levels
are predictive of neural tube disorders, such
as spina bifida and anencephaly. Neural
tube disorders are linked to a low folic acid
level in the mother in early pregnancy. **c** is
a distractor in that, while Rh– women may
have an Rh+ fetus with hemolytic disease,
Rh+ women do not have that complication.
[Strasinger 2008, p237]

187 **d** Cystic fibrosis is a caused by a defective
ion channel, which causes an accumulation
of chloride in the sweat.
[Burtis 2001, p437]

188 **a** All of the answers are mutations.
Delta-F508 is the deletion of phenylalanine
at position 508 of the CFTR protein.
Trisomy 21 is a third copy of chromosome
21, associated with Down syndrome.
The Philadelphia chromosome is a gene
translocation associated with acute
myelocytic leukemia. Fragile X is a form of
mental retardation caused by an increased
number of nucleotide repeats.
[Buckingham 2007, p319]

189 **d** The synthesis of IgG in the central
MLS
ONLY nervous system is associated with some
neurologic disorders, most predominantly
multiple sclerosis. The other conditions are
also CNS disorders, but do not cause an
increased gamma protein.
[Strasinger 2008, p191]

190 **b**   If one compares CSF electrophoresis to
MLS
ONLY
serum electrophoresis, there is an obvious
band seen in CSF that is absent in serum.
This band runs ahead of albumin, and
is prealbumin.
[Strasinger 2008, p190]

191 **d**   A traumatic tap is a collection of a body
fluid that has blood contamination. The first
tube will have most of the contamination,
so that subsequent tubes will show fewer
blood cells. Cell counts should routinely be
performed on the last tube, to minimize
the amount of cellular contamination due
to the tap.
[Strasinger 2008, pp179-180]

192 **b**   The IgG index is used to determine if
MLS
ONLY
increased IgG in CSF is due to increased
production in the CNS or contamination
from a breach to the blood-brain barrier.
The calculation includes the CSF IgG/serum
IgG ratio, and is normalized by dividing that
by the CSF albumin/serum albumin.
[Strasinger 2008, p191]

193 **b**   CSF looks like water. If it is yellow
or pink it is called xanthochromic.
This indicates a previous bleed into the CNS.
Opalescence is a haziness, usually due to
the presence of lipids.
[Strasinger 2008, p18]

194 **b**   To calculate the dilution, take the
amount of sample and divide it by the
total of the new solution. So the dilution
is 50 μL divided by 500 + 50 μL. This is a
1/11 dilution. To correct the final answer,
multiply by the inverse of the dilution,
or 11.
[Strasinger 2008, p181]

195 **c**   Hemosiderin is an indication that RBCs
have been processed and degraded. The
presence of hemosiderin, then, indicates
bleeding, which limits the answers to **c** and
d. The degradation of RBCs to hemosiderin
takes time, so that a traumatic tap would
not show hemosiderin, but a previous
hemorrhage would.
[Strasinger 2008, p184]

196 **a**   Normal CSF glucose is approximately
60% of plasma glucose. Glucose is decreased
in bacterial meningitis, and lactate is
produced. Normal protein in CSF is 15-45
mg/dL. Protein is slightly elevated in
bacterial meningitis.
[Strasinger 2008, p193]

197 **a**   In hepatic encephalopathy, ammonia
levels in the plasma building up, and
ammonia can be found in the spinal
fluid. Ammonia is volatile, and not easily
measured. Glutamine is a byproduct
of ammonia, and is stable, making it a
better choice.
[Strasinger 2008, p192]

198 **a**   Tau transferrin is found only in CSF.
[Strasinger 2008, p190]

199 **a**   Consider each answer, and determine if
it is are unique to a particular site:
a   PSA is used to screen for prostate
cancer, because it is high in secretions from
the prostate; therefore, semen is high in
PSA. PSA can be used forensically to identify
a fluid as semen.
b   Alkaline phosphatase is found
predominantly in bone and liver. On the other
hand, acid phosphatase, not a choice, is high in
prostate secretions, and semen.
c   Fructose is the major carbohydrate
found in semen, but it is not unique
to semen.
d   Hyaluronic acid is associated with
synovial fluid.
[Burtis 2001, pp344-345]

200 **a**   All of these stains can be used to view
sperm; however, the eosin-nigran stain is
differential between live and dead sperm.
Living cells will stain bluish white, dead cells
stain red.
[Strasinger 2008, p205]

201 **a**   The total volume of the 9 large cells is
0.9 μL. Counting 10 of the large cells is the
equivalent of 1 μL.
[Rodak 2007, p161]

202 **d**   The WHO rating for sperm motility is:
   0 = no movement
   1.0 = no forward movement
   2.0 = slow forward/lateral movement,
   3.0 = faster speed, some lateral movement
   4.0 = rapid, straight line movement.
[Strasinger 2008, p203]

203 **a**   Pancreatic insufficiency can lead
MT
ONLY
to increased fecal fat and to the finding
of undigested muscle in the stool. Fecal
leukocytes are associated with pathogenic
bacteria, and a positive Clinitest® is due
to the presence of sugars, usually from an
osmotic diarrhea, as in lactose intolerance.
Fecal occult blood is associated with
colorectal cancer, and is positive in other
gastrointestinal bleeding. It is not associated
with pancreatic insufficiency.
[Strasinger 2008, pp248-249]

204 **a**   Sweat chloride is measured to diagnose
cystic fibrosis. Sweating is induced by
stimulating local sweat glands by driving
pilocarpine into the skin, using a process
called pilocarpine iontophoresis.
[Burtis 2001, p437]

205 **b**   Evaporation of the sample will
MLS
ONLY
concentrate the ions. This can happen in
a patient with a low sweat rate, or with a
prolonged collection time.
[Burtis 2001, p437]

206 **c**   Sweat conductivity testing is relatively
easy to perform, and used as a screening
method. A positive should be confirmed
with a chloride measurement by coulometry
or by ion-selective electrode. Pilocarpine
iontophoresis is used to stimulate sweat
production, not to measure it.
[Burtis 2001, p437]

207 **c**   Dark green amniotic fluid indicates the
presence of meconium. This is the infant's first
bowel movement, and indicates fetal distress.
[Strasinger 2008, p238]

208 **a**   A fetus with hemolytic disease will have
increased bilirubin in the amniotic fluid.
Bilirubin absorbs light at 450 nm. The change
in absorbance between the expected and
observed value is plotted on a Liley graph, and
used to assess the fetus. This is also called a
Delta-OD 450.
[Strasinger 2008, p239-240]

209 **d**   The amount of surfactant (phospholipids)
MLS
ONLY
in amniotic fluid increases during gestation,
and is an indicator of fetal lung maturity.
The value is compared to albumin, as
albumin concentration remains constant
during gestation. Fluorescent dye binds to
surfactants and to albumin in this assay;
when it is bound to the surfactant, it has a low
polarization. As surfactant increases during
lung maturation, the fluorescence polarization
of the sample decreases.
[Strasinger 2008, p241]

210 **b**   Neutral fats, such as triglycerides, stain
MLS
ONLY
orange with Sudan III. They do not polarize
light. Fats are lighter than body fluids, so they
do not sediment. They do not glitter.
[Strasinger 2008, p224]

211 **a**   A patient with blunt trauma, such as
a car accident, may have internal bleeding.
Peritoneal lavage introduces a fixed volume
of saline into the peritoneal cavity, and
withdraws an aliquot. RBC are counted.
Counts greater than 100,000/μL indicate
blunt trauma.
[Strasinger 2008, p229]

212 **c**   The only acronym listed here that is not a
tumor marker is ANA. This stands for
anti-nuclear antibody.
[Strasinger 2008, p228]

213 **d**   Semen should liquefy and pour in
droplets after 30-60 minutes. The normal pH
is 7.2-8.0. Within an hour after collection,
more than 50% should be motile, and their
motility grade should be 2.0 or greater.
[Strasinger 2008, p201]

214 **a**   Lactate is increased in the CSF in
conditions that cause hypoxia. The highest
lactate values (>35 mg/dL) are found in
patients with bacterial meningitis. Viral,
tubercular and fungal meningitis have lactate
levels above normal, but not as high as
bacterial meningitis.
[Strasinger 2008, p193]

215 **d**   Meningitis, hemorrhage, and neurologic
diseases, such as MS, will increase CSF
protein. Decreased protein can be found due
to CSF leakage, recent puncture, and rapid
CSF production.
[Strasinger 2008, p190]

216 **b**   The CSF/serum albumin ratio with a
value of <9 indicates an intact blood-brain
barrier. The other distractors have different
purposes: **a** the IgG index compares IgG in
CSF and serum to determine if IgG is being
synthesized in the CNS; **c** the fluid/serum
LD ratio is used to determine if a body fluid
is a transudate or an exudate; **d** the albumin
gradient is used to determine if an effusion
is of hepatic origin.
[Strasinger 2008, p191]

Laboratory Operations

*The following items have been identified generally as appropriate for both entry level medical laboratory scientists and medical laboratory technicians. Items that are appropriate for medical laboratory scientists **only** are marked with an "MLS ONLY."*

Quality Assessment

1 The laboratory manager receives a complaint from the ICU about turnaround times for coagulation tests. The first step in problem solving should be:

MLS ONLY

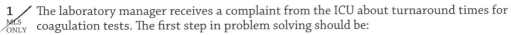

   a gather data on current times by shift
   b talk to staff about various solutions   *TAT*
   c perform root cause analysis
   d draw a process map to send to the ICU explaining why it takes so long

2 Which action by the phlebotomist will comply with the College of American Pathologists (CAP) Patient Safety Goal "to improve patient and sample identification at the time of specimen collection" and The Joint Commission Patient Safety Goal to "improve the accuracy of patient identification"?

   a match the name and room number on the patient's ID bracelet to the name and room number on the preprinted collection label
   b match the name and medical record number on the patient's ID bracelet to the name and medical record number on the preprinted collection label
   c verify patient information by stating the patient's name when approaching the patient
   d label the collection tubes prior to the blood draw at the patient's bedside

3   A swab and requisition are received in the microbiology laboratory with the following information:

Label on specimen
Patient name:	Mary Jane Smith
MR#:	400567
Location:	emergency department
Doctor:	Henry Jones
Specimen type:	lesion on left ankle
Collection:	@ 2 PM by nurse MB

Requisition
Patient name:	Nancy Ann Smith
MR#:	400443
Location:	emergency department
Doctor:	Henry Jones
Specimen type:	lesion on left ankle
Collection:	@ 2 PM by nurse MB

The laboratory receiving clerk notes a discrepancy between the patient identifiers on the requisition and the specimen label, and questions the emergency department nurse MB. This is the fourth specimen this week that has had a specimen discrepancy. What action is the most appropriate to prevent this type of error in the future?

a correct the error in the laboratory when the nurse communicates the appropriate patient name
b ask nurse MB to correct discrepancy and read the procedure for specimen labeling
c document error and communicate to laboratory supervisor so that the risk manager conducts a root cause analysis
d discard the specimen and call the emergency department for a recollect

4   Preanalytical variables in laboratory testing include:

a result accuracy
b report delivery to the ordering physician
c test turnaround time
d specimen acceptability

5   The first procedure to be followed if the blood gas instrument is out-of-control for all parameters is:

a recalibrate, then repeat control
b repeat control on the next shift
c replace electrodes, then repeat control
d report patient results after duplicate testing

6 Refer to the following graph:

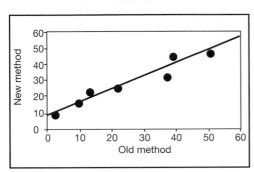

A new methodology for amylase has been developed and compared with the existing method as illustrated in the graph shown above. The new method can be described as:

a poor correlation with constant bias
b good correlation with constant bias
c poor correlation with no bias
d good correlation with no bias

7 Refer to the following diagram:

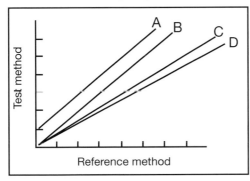

The line that demonstrates a proportional error relationship is:

a line A
b line B
c line C
d line D

8   Refer to the following illustration:

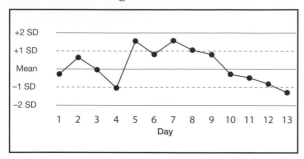

Shown above is a Levy-Jennings quality control chart, which represents control values for 13 consecutive analyses for a particular serum constituent. If the 14th value is below the −2 SD limit, which of the following should be done?

  a   control should be repeated to see if it will fall within the established interval
  b   analysis system should be checked for a deteriorating component
  c   analysis system should be checked for a change in reagent lot number
  d   no action is needed

9   The precision of an instrument is validated by:
_{MLS ONLY}

  a   running the same sample multiple times
  b   performing serial dilutions
  c   processing unknown specimens
  d   monitoring normal and abnormal controls

10   The mean value of a series of hemoglobin controls was found to be 15.2 g/dL, and the standard deviation was calculated at 0.20. Acceptable control range for the laboratory is ±2 standard deviations. Which of the following represents the allowable limits for the control?

  a   14.5-15.5 g/dL
  b   15.0-15.4 g/dL
  c   15.2-15.6 g/dL
  d   14.8-15.6 g/dL

11   In quality control, ±2 standard deviations from the mean includes what percent
_{MLS ONLY} of the sample population?

  a   50
  b   75
  c   95
  d   98

12   Upon completion of a run of cholesterol tests, the technician recognizes that the controls are not within the 2 standard deviations confidence range. What is the appropriate course of action?

  a   report the results without any other action
  b   run a new set of controls
  c   run a new set of controls and repeat specimens
  d   recalibrate instrument and run controls

13   The following data were calculated on a series of 30 determinations of serum uric acid control: mean = 5.8 mg/dL, 1 standard deviation = 0.15 mg/dL. If confidence limits are set at ±2 standard deviations, which of the following represents the allowable limits for the control?

  a   5.65-5.95 mg/dL
  b   5.35-6.25 mg/dL
  c   5.50-6.10 mg/dL
  d   5.70-5.90 mg/dL

14   An index of precision is statistically known as the:

   a median
   b mean
   c standard deviation
   d coefficient of variation

15   The term used to describe reproducibility is:

   a sensitivity
   b specificity
   c accuracy
   d precision

16   The ability of a procedure to measure only the component(s) it claims to measure is called:

   a specificity
   b sensitivity
   c precision
   d reproducibility

17   The extent to which measurements agree with the true value of the quantity being measured is known as:

   a reliability
   b accuracy
   c reproducibility
   d precision

18   Diagnostic specificity is defined as the percentage of individuals:

   a with a given disease who have a positive result by a given test   ✳✳
   b without a given disease who have a negative result by a given test
   c with a given disease who have a negative result by a given test
   d without a given disease who have a positive result by a given test

19   If the correlation coefficient (r) of 2 variables is 0:
MLS
ONLY
   a there is complete correlation between the variables
   b there is an absence of correlation
   c as one variable increases, the other increases
   d as one variable decreases, the other increases

20   Employees are guaranteed the right to engage in self-organization and collective bargaining through representatives of their choice, or to refrain from these activities by which of the following?

   a Civil Rights Act
   b Freedom of Information Act
   c Clinical Laboratory Improvements Act (CLIA)
   d National Labor Relations Act

21   Which of the following organizations was formed to encourage the voluntary attainment of uniformly high standards in institutional medical care?

   a Centers for Disease Control (CDC)
   b Health Care Finance Administration (HCFA)
   c The Joint Commission (JCAHO)
   d Federal Drug Administration (FDA)

22   The process by which an agency or organization uses predetermined standards to evaluate and recognize a program of study in an institution is called:

   a regulation
   b licensure
   (c) accreditation
   d credentialing

23   CLIA was established to provide oversight to:

   a research labs
   b point-of-care testing by nonlaboratory personnel
   c CAP-accredited labs
   (d) any lab performing patient testing

24   Which statement about Proficiency Testing (PT) is true?
MLS
ONLY

   a results can be compared to another hospital prior to submission if that hospital is in your system
   b results between 2 technologists can be averaged
   c CAP requires duplicate testing to ensure good instrument performance
   d it is necessary to assess results even if a PT challenge is ungraded

25   Which of the following is part of The Joint Commission's National Patient Safety Goals?
MLS
ONLY

   a communication of critical results
   b documentation of lab QC
   c trending of instrument problems
   d reconciliation of lab orders and results in the medical record

26   If your lab performs a test for which there is no commercially available control of Proficiency Test
MLS
ONLY   material, which of the following is acceptable for documentation of test accuracy?

   a perform the test in duplicate
   b you do not have to do anything if there is nothing available
   c make an internal lab control from a previous negative and positive
   d have 2 technologists perform the test independently

27   CAP requires refrigerator temperatures to be recorded:

   (a) daily
   b weekly
   c monthly
   d periodically

28   A paper or electronic report of lab results must include:

   a the name of the person who collected the specimen
   b the test price
   c a pathologist's signature
   (d) the name and address of the testing laboratory

29   CAP requires that glassware cleaning practices include periodic testing for:
MLS
ONLY

   a chemical residues
   b silicates
   (c) detergents
   d heavy metals

30 Prior to implementing a new lab test, the analytical measurement range (AMR) must be verified. This is to verify a value that can be:

MLS ONLY

    a directly measured on a specimen without any dilution or concentration
    b reported after specimen pretreatment
    c reported up to a 1:100 dilution
    d sent out to a reference lab for verification

31 HIPAA is a federal law that requires:

    a confidentiality of patients' health care information between 2 organizations
    b reporting of errors in laboratory results
    c access to patient records when there is a lawsuit
    d unannounced inspections by accreditation agencies

32 Your friend calls and asks you to access his test results. Which of the following does this violate?

    a CAP
    b The Joint Commission
    c HIPAA
    d CLIA

33 An ICD-9 code is related to:

MLS ONLY

    a patient charges
    b diagnosis ✱
    c lab accreditation
    d test methodology

Safety

34 A technician is asked to clean out the chemical reagent storeroom and discard any reagents not used in the past 5 years. How should the technician proceed?

    a discard chemicals into biohazard containers where they will later be autoclaved
    b pour reagents down the drain, followed by flushing of water
    c consult MSDS sheets for proper disposal
    d pack all chemicals for incineration

35 Using a common labeling system for hazardous material identification such as HMIS® or NFPA 704, the top red quadrant represents which hazard?

    a reactivity - yellow
    b special reactivity - white
    c health - blue
    d flammability

36 If the HMIS® or NFPA 704 hazardous material identification system has a number 4 in the left blue quadrant, it represents a:

    a high health hazard
    b low health hazard
    c high reactivity hazard
    d low reactivity hazard

37 Which chemical is a potential carcinogen?

    a potassium chloride
    b formaldehyde
    c mercury
    d picric acid

38   Compressed gas cylinders should:

     a   be stored with flammable materials
     b   be transported by rolling or dragging
     c   have safety covers removed when pressure regulators are unattached
     (d)   be secured upright to the wall or other stable source

39 A chemical that is extremely volatile, flammable, and capable of forming explosive peroxides upon
MLS
ONLY long-term contact with atmospheric oxygen, is:

     a   ethyl alcohol
     b   ethyl acetate
     (c)   diethyl ether
     d   xylene

40   The HMIS® or NFPA 704 hazardous material identification system rating for a slightly toxic
chemical would be:

     a   1 in the yellow quadrant
     b   4 in the blue quadrant
     (c)   1 in the blue quadrant
     d   4 in the yellow quadrant

41   A chemical that causes immediate visible destruction or irreversible alterations of human tissue
at the contact site is best classified as a(n):

     a   carcinogenic
     b   toxic
     c   ignitable
     (d)   corrosive

42 Labels on shipped chemicals from manufacturers, importers or distributors are required
MLS
ONLY to include information on:

     a   physical properties of the chemical
     b   accident instructions
     (c)   appropriate hazard warnings
     d   exposure limits

43   When hazardous chemicals are transferred from the original appropriately labeled container(s)
to a secondary container for immediate use by the person performing the transfer, it:

     a   must be labeled with an emergency response phone number(s)
     b̸   must be labeled with the identity or contents of the hazardous chemical(s)
     c   must be labeled with hazard warnings related to the effect on involved target organs
     (d)   does not require labeling   ✳

44 Which hazardous chemical combinations are incompatible and should not be stored together?
MLS
ONLY
     a   acetone and xylene
     (b)   chlorine and ammonia
     c   ethanol and acetone
     d   sodium and potassium

45   A technologist spilled 10 gallons of formaldehyde on the floor. After determining the chemical
poses a significant health hazard, the first action step would be to:

     a   notify emergency assistance
     b̸   control the spill with appropriate absorbent material
     (c)   evacuate the area
     d   don appropriate personal protective equipment

46 A gallon of xylene waste should be:

MLS ONLY

  a flushed down the sink
  b allowed to evaporate in an open room
  c disposed of with nonincinerated regulated medical waste
  d disposed of as an EPA hazardous waste through a licensed waste hauler

47 A technologist, who has been routinely working with hazardous chemicals, begins to notice
MLS ONLY symptoms of persistent headaches after exposure to these chemicals. What is the first action
the technologist should take?

  a seek independent medical consultation and evaluation
  b continue to perform work assignment to see if symptoms persist
  c acquire involved MSDS to investigate signs and symptoms
  d report situation to supervisor

48 When an employee reports signs and symptoms of a chemical exposure, the employer should
MLS ONLY suggest a medical consultation and evaluation, which is paid by the:

  a employee using the employee's personal benefit time
  b employer using the employee's personal benefit time
  c employer on work time without loss of pay
  d employee on work time without loss of pay

49 When initial or baseline chemical exposure monitoring required by OSHA for substances like
MLS ONLY formaldehyde or xylene is performed and the results are within permissible exposure limits,
repeat monitoring should be performed:

  a when procedures or equipment surrounding use of the specific chemical change
  b annually
  c twice a year
  d every 2 years

50 An example of personal protective equipment (PPE) for handling hazardous chemicals is:

MLS ONLY

  a eyewash or safety shower
  b fume hood
  c latex or vinyl gloves
  d neoprene or nitrile gloves

51 One of the elements of a written laboratory chemical hygiene plan is to:

  a require employees who handle chemicals to have annual medical evaluations
  b prohibit use of carcinogens
  c designate a laboratory chemical hygiene officer
  d perform chemical monitoring every 6 months for OSHA regulated substances

52 The purpose of the OSHA Hazard Communication, General Industry Standard, 29 CFR,
Subpart Z, 1910.1200, is to require employers to establish a program ensuring personnel are
provided with information regarding the workplace dangers of:

  a bloodborne pathogens
  b environmental hazards
  c general safety hazards
  d hazardous chemicals

53   Refer to the following illustration:

This symbol indicates which of the following hazards?

a flammable
b electrical
c radiation
d biohazard

54   When working with sharp equipment and objects, use a:

a double-glove technique with specimen handling gloves
b mechanical device
c paper towel or gauze as a barrier
d two-handed technique

55   For safe operation of a centrifuge:

a clean with soap/detergent when maintenance is performed or spills occur
b open the centrifuge cover when it is in the process of slowing down
c leave liquid specimen tubes uncovered during centrifugation
d ensure proper balance is maintained

56   For safe use and handling of liquid nitrogen:
MLS
ONLY

a use chemically resistant gloves
b shield all skin and use a face shield
c store cylinders away from ventilation
d store cylinders in a horizontal position in a cool dry place

57   Incident reports for occupational injury or illness should:

a include information on the employee's past medical history
b be filed only for incidents involving serious injury or illness
c be filed for all incidents including near miss incidents
d not be retained after review by a safety committee or officer

58   According to OSHA, what type of warning sign should be posted in an area where an <u>immediate</u> hazard exists and where special precautions are necessary?

a red, black and white "Danger" sign
b yellow and black "Caution" sign
c green and white "Safety Instruction" sign
d orange and black "Biohazard" sign

59   All laboratory instruments should:

a have repairs conducted while connected to facility wiring
b be grounded or double insulated
c have safety checks performed initially and then every 6 months
d be connected to multiple outlet adapters

60   If areas of the laboratory are designated as "clean" or "contaminated," it is appropriate for a technologist to:

    a clean technical area bench tops after spills and on a weekly basis
    b wear a lab coat in the break or lunch room
    c apply lip balm in a contaminated area
    d touch a "contaminated" area phone with ungloved hands if hands are washed afterward

61   For fire safety and prevention:

    a fire drills should be announced and practiced in advance
    b hallways and corridors should be clear and free of obstruction at all times
    c only one exit is necessary in laboratories that contain an explosion hazard
    d hazard evaluations only need to be done prior to initiation of clinical operations

62   What type of identification system does this symbol represent?

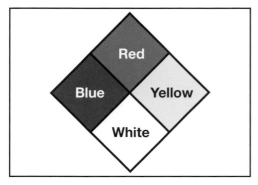

    a transmission-based precautions
    b physical environmental hazards
    c chemical hazardous materials
    d radiation hazards

63   Flammable and combustible liquids in containers ≥5 gallons should be stored in a(n):

    a flammable safety cabinet vented to room air
    b nonexplosion proof refrigerator
    c fume hood
    d approved safety can

64   After receiving appropriate training, the first step in using a fire extinguisher is to:

    a sweep the flow of the hose from side to side
    b pull the pin
    c squeeze the top handle or lever
    d aim the hose at the base of the fire

65   To help prevent electrical fires in healthcare facilities:

    a use multiple outlet or gang plug adapters
    b change circuit breakers annually
    c tape over worn wiring with certified electrical tape
    d use only UL or other safety-agency-rated electrical equipment

66   In addition to keeping the load close to your body and tightening your abdominal muscles when lifting heavy boxes of supplies, it is important to bend at the:

    a waist; lift with legs and buttocks
    b knees and hips; lift with legs and buttocks
    c knees and hips; lift with arms and back
    d waist; twist your body when lifting

67 The best way to prevent or relieve symptoms of carpal tunnel syndrome is to:

MLS ONLY
- **a** raise arms and bend wrists downward
- **b** redesign facilities
- **c** bend back and neck slightly forward
- **(d)** maintain wrists in a neutral position

68 A fire occurs in the laboratory. The first course of action is to:

- **a** evacuate the entire area
- **b** pull the fire alarm box
- **(c)** remove persons from immediate danger
- **d** contain the fire by closing doors

69 An electrical equipment fire breaks out in the laboratory. Personnel have been removed from immediate danger, the alarm has been activated. What is the next action to be taken?

- **a** evacuate the facility
- **(b)** contain the fire by closing doors
- **c** extinguish fire with type A extinguisher
- **d** lock all windows and doors in the immediate area

70 Class C fires involve:

- **a** grease and oil (B)
- **b** xylene and alcohol (B)   ✳ ✳
- **c** paper, wood and plastics (A)
- **d** electrical equipment (C)

71 A laboratory employee identifies arm and neck pain after performing repetitive movements

MLS ONLY
during his/her work assignment. What is the best first action to be taken?

- **(a)** report to and discuss issue with supervisor
- **b** continue to perform work assignment and see if it improves
- **c** make an appointment with his/her personal physician
- **d** change or adjust his/her workstation

72 A technologist splashed a corrosive chemical in his/her eyes. To prevent permanent injury, the first action should be to:

- **a** bandage the eyes and seek immediate emergency medical assistance
- **b** flush eyes with a chemical of opposite pH to neutralize the injury
- **(c)** use the eyewash station to flush eyes with water for 15 minutes
- **d** seek immediate emergency medical assistance

73 A technologist spilled concentrated hydrochloric acid on his/her clothing and skin, affecting a large portion of the body. After removing involved clothing, the next first aid treatment step would be to:

- **a** seek immediate emergency medical assistance
- **(b)** use emergency safety shower and flush body with water
- **c** apply burn ointment to affected skin
- **d** pour baking soda on the skin and bandage

74 An example of personal protective equipment (PPE) is a(n):

- **a** biological safety cabinet
- **b** emergency safety shower
- **c** eyewash station
- **(d)** lab coat

75   Gloves worn in the laboratory for specimen processing must be removed and hands washed when:

    a answering the telephone in the technical work area
    b carrying a specimen outside the technical work area through "clean" areas
    c answering the telephone in a designated "clean" area
    d after handling specimens from known isolation precaution patients

76   Safety glasses, face shields or other eye and face protectors must be worn when:

    a working with caustic or toxic materials
    b present in technical work area
    c viewing microbiology culture plates
    d processing specimens using a splash barrier

77   To prevent injury, a safe lab work practice is to:

    a secure long hair and jewelry
    b store well-wrapped food in the supply refrigerator
    c wear contact lenses for eye protection
    d wear comfortable, rubber-bottomed, open-weaved shoes

78   Safe handling and disposal of laboratory generated infectious waste require:

    a disinfection of all waste
    b thorough mixing of infectious and noninfectious waste
    c separation of infectious and noninfectious waste
    d incineration of all waste

79   Which of the following is the best choice for decontaminating bench tops contaminated by the AIDS virus?

    a sodium hypochlorite bleach
    b formalin
    c a quaternary ammonium compound
    d 100% alcohol

80   The safest method of disposing of hypodermic needles is:

    a recap the needle with its protective sheath prior to discarding
    b cut the needle with a special device before disposal
    c discard the needle in an impermeable container without other handling immediately after use
    d drop the needle in the waste basket immediately after use

81   Precautions for health care workers dealing with patients or patient specimens include:

    a mouth pipetting when specimens lack a "Precaution" label
    b reinserting needles into their original sheaths after drawing blood from a patient
    c wearing a mask and disposable gown to draw blood
    d prompt cleaning of blood spills with a disinfectant solution such as sodium hypochlorite

82   Infection rate is highest for laboratory professionals exposed to blood and body fluids containing:

    a hepatitis A
    b hepatitis B
    c CMV
    d HIV

83   Which of the following forms of exposure places a technologist at the highest risk for infection with human immunodeficiency virus (HIV)?

    a aerosol inhalation (eg, AIDS patient's sneeze)
    b ingestion (eg, mouth pipetting of positive serum)
    c needlestick (eg, from AIDS contaminated needle)
    d splash (eg, infected serum spill onto intact skin)

84 Which disinfectant inactivates HIV and HBV?

    a alcohol
    b iodine
    c phenol
    (d) sodium hypochlorite

85 Filters generally used in biological safety cabinets to protect the laboratory worker from particulates and aerosols generated by microbiology manipulations are:

    a fiberglass
    (b) HEPA
    c APTA   ✳
    d charcoal

86 What is the single most effective method to prevent nosocomial spread of infection?

    a wear mask, gown and gloves
    b require infectious patients to mask
    c wear an N95 respirator mask
    (d) perform frequent and appropriate hand hygiene

87 Contaminated needles and syringes without safety self-sheathing devices should be:

    a sheared by a needle cutter or bent
    b re-capped using a two-handed technique
    (c) discarded directly into an appropriate sharps container
    d removed from the syringe/needle holder

88 Use of "standard" (universal) precautions minimizes exposure to:

    (a) bloodborne pathogens
    b chemical hazards
    c radiation hazards
    d environmental hazards

89 After an accidental needle stick with a contaminated needle, the first action should be to:

    a apply antiseptic ointment to the wound
    b seek immediate medical assistance
    c bandage the wound
    (d) thoroughly wash the wound with soap and water

90 What is the most likely mode of transmission for bloodborne pathogens in laboratory-acquired infections?

    (a) parenteral inoculation of blood
    b contact with intact skin
    c airborne transmission
    d fecal-oral transmission

91 Which infectious agent is considered to be the primary occupational health hazard regarding transmission of <u>bloodborne pathogens?</u>

    a human immunodeficiency virus
    (b) hepatitis B
    c tuberculosis
    d methicillin-resistant *Staphylococcus aureus*

92   When processing specimens for mycobacterial testing, what specific engineering control must be used?

    a horizontal laminar flow hood
    b barrier protection only
    c biological safety cabinet
    d fume hood

93   Hepatitis B vaccine is:

    a administered as a single 1-time injection
    b required for all healthcare employees
    c must be provided by the employer free of charge
    d recommended only when an exposure incident occurs

94   When cleaning up a small (5 mL) blood spill on the counter-top, the first step after donning appropriate personal protective equipment is to:

    a flood the area with an appropriate intermediate to high-level disinfectant
    b absorb the spill with disposable absorbent material
    c evacuate the area for 30 minutes   ✳
    d clean the area with an aqueous detergent solution

95   The most effective <u>disinfectant</u> recommended for bloodborne pathogens is:

    a sodium hypochlorite ✳
    b isopropyl alcohol
    c chlorhexidine gluconate
    d povidone-iodine

96   Which of the following microbial agents do not respond to the general rules regarding microbial inactivation and decontamination?
MLS
ONLY

    a *Mycobacterium tuberculosis*
    b transmissible spongiform encephalopathy agents (prions)
    c agents of bioterrorism (smallpox, *Bacillus anthracis*)
    d *Coccidioides immitis*

97   When processing patient blood specimens and handling other potentially infectious material, the best choice of gloves is:

    a reusable utility gloves
    b latex gloves only
    c single use and disposable gloves
    d cut-resistant gloves

98   While processing patient specimens, a technologist splashes a few small drops of a bronchial wash specimen on his/her gloves. The first action should be to:

    a wash the gloves with antiseptic/soap and water
    b continue to wear the gloves until grossly contaminated or leaving the area
    c wash the gloves with an appropriate disinfectant
    d change gloves and wash hands with antiseptic/soap and water

99   This symbol represents a:

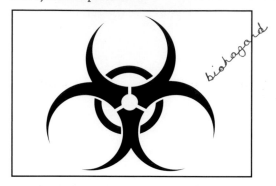

biohazard

   a   biohazard
   b   radiation hazard
   c   chemical hazard
   d   environmental hazard

100   Regulated medical waste refers to:
   a   chemical waste
   b   infectious waste
   c   radioactive waste
   d   all waste from healthcare facilities

Management

101   A technologist repeatedly misses tubercle bacilli when examining stained smears for acid-fast
bacilli. What plan of action should the supervisor **first** take to correct this problem?

   a   issue a written warning
   b   send the employee to a workshop to improve his/her knowledge
   c   review the diagnostic criteria with the employee and monitor progress
   d   reassign employee to another part of the laboratory

102   Which of the following is considered to be a variable cost in a clinical laboratory?
   a   overtime pay
   b   health insurance premiums
   c   FICA
   d   pension contributions

103   Direct, indirect and overhead costs incurred during the production of tests per unit time
are classified as:

   a   total costs
   b   actual costs
   c   standard costs
   d   controllable costs

104   An advantage of reagent lease/rental agreements is:
   a   less time spent by a laboratory manager justifying new instrumentation
   b   increased flexibility to adjust to changes in workload
   c   flexibility in reagent usage from 1 manufacturer to another
   d   less expenditures over life expectancy of instrument

105 The number of hours used to calculate the annual salary of a full-time employee is:

   a 1,920
   b 1,950
   (**c**) 2,080
   d 2,800

106 The overtime budget for the laboratory is $38,773, but $50,419 has already been spent.
What percent over budget does this represent?

   (**a**) 30%
   b 70%
   c 77%
   d 100%

$$\frac{50,419}{38,773} = 130\% - 100\% = 30\%$$

107 Matching the content and requirements of the task with the skills, abilities and needs of
the worker is a function of:

   a leadership
   (**b**) job design
   c recruitment
   d reward systems

108 The most important part of any effective behavior modification system is:

   (**a**) feedback to employees
   b salary structure
   c job enrichment
   d tactful discipline

109 Disciplinary policy is generally developed as a series of steps with each step more strict than
the previous. Normally, the first step in the process is to:

   a send the employee a warning letter
   b send the employee a counseling memo
   (**c**) counsel the employee verbally
   d dismiss less serious infractions

110 A supervisor notices that a technologist continues to mouth pipet liquids when making reagents.
The supervisor's best course of action is to:

   a allow the technologist to continue this practice as long as it is not done when dealing
        with specimens
   (**b**) discuss this problem with the employee immediately
   c order a mechanical device (bulb pipet) for employee to use
   d compliment the employee on his rapid pipetting technique

111 On repeated occasions, the day shift supervisor has observed a technologist on the night
shift sleeping. Which of the following is the most appropriate **initial** course of action for
the day supervisor?

   a ignore the repeated incidents
   (**b**) discuss the incidents with the technologist's immediate supervisor
   c notify the personnel department
   d advise the laboratory director

112 A workload reporting system is an important part of laboratory management because it:

   a tells exactly how much should be charged per test
   b keeps personnel busy in their free time
   c counts only tests done and specimens received in the laboratory without inflating these figures
        by adding in quality control and standardization efforts
   (**d**) helps in planning, developing, and maintaining efficient laboratory services with
        administrative and budget controls

113 Which one of the following questions can be legally asked on an employment application?

    a Are you a US citizen?
    b What is your date of birth?
    c Is your wife/husband employed full-time?
    d Do you have any dependents?

114 Which of the following topic areas can be discussed with a prospective employee during
MLS ONLY a job interview?

    a have you ever been arrested
    b number of dependents
    c previous employment that the applicant disliked
    d if they are a US citizen

115 An effective program of continuing education for medical laboratory personnel should first:
MLS ONLY
    a find a good speaker
    b motivate employees to attend
    c determine an adequate budget
    d identify the needs

116 In general, 70% of the operating expenses of laboratories are:
MLS ONLY
    a labor or labor related
    b reagents and supplies
    c equipment replacement and maintenance
    d safety supplies and disposables

117 Legal pre-employment questions on an application are:

    a medical history of an employee
    b place of birth
    c felonies unrelated to job requirements
    d name and address of person to notify in case of emergency

118 A requirement for a job is to be able to stand for long periods of time. If you have a current
MLS ONLY employee who comes to work with a doctor's letter stating that they can no longer stand to do
their job due to a disability, what is the manager's responsibility?

    a find the employee a desk job
    b make a reasonable accommodation for them to alternate sitting and standing if possible
    c you are not legally required to do anything
    d let the employee go

119 Which of the following is a tool that can be used to follow the progression of a project?
MLS ONLY
    a Pareto analysis
    b fishbone diagrams
    c Gantt charts
    d FIFO (first in, first out)

120 Which of the following is an indirect cost?
MLS ONLY
    a equipment rental
    b office supplies
    c PT test material
    d IT support

121 Which of the following activities is <u>not</u> under the direction or control of the lab manager?

    a number of employees
    b direct test costs
    c skill mix
    d military leave

122 ABN (Advanced Beneficiary Notice) is required when:

MLS
ONLY

   (a) a test may not be covered by insurance
   b when there is no CPT code associated with a test   *Medicare*
   c when an HMO submits any lab test
   d when there is automatic reflex testing for a screen

123 Data for a new procedure is as follows:

MLS
ONLY

number of procedures per year:	10,000	
equipment cost:	$97,000	*13,857.14*
expected useful life:	7 years	*20,000.00*
reagent cost:	$20,000 per year	
CAP units per procedure:	30.0	
average wage:	$10.75 per hour	

The cost per procedure is:

   a $2.00
   b $5.38
   c $7.38
   (d) $8.77

124 A new clinic in the area is sending a very large number of additional chemistry tests to the

MLS
ONLY

laboratory. The existing chemistry instrument is only 2 years old and works well; however, there is a need to acquire a high throughput instrument. Which one of the following is the appropriate "Justification Category"?

   a replacement
   (b) volume increase
   c reduction of FTEs
   d new service

125 A general term for the formal recognition of professional or technical competence is:

MLS
ONLY

   a regulation
   b licensure
   c accreditation
   (d) credentialing

126 Evaluating the performance of employees should be done:

MLS
ONLY

   a annually
   b semiannually
   c as needed in the judgment of management
   (d) in the form of immediate feedback and at regular intervals

Laboratory Mathematics

127 An automated CK assay gives a reading that is above the limits of linearity. A dilution of the serum sample is made by adding 1 mL of serum to 9 mL of water. The instrument now reads 350 U/L. The correct report on the undiluted serum should be:

   a 2,850 U/L
   b 3,150 U/L
   (c) 3,500 U/L
   d 3,850 U/L

128 The unit of measure for a standard solution is:

  a g/L
  b %
  c mg/%
  (d) mg/mL

129 A glucose determination was read on a spectrophotometer. The absorbance reading of the standard was 0.30. The absorbance reading of the unknown was 0.20. The value of the unknown is:

  (a) ⅔ of the standard
  b ⅗ of the standard
  c the same as the standard
  d 1½× the standard

$ratio = \dfrac{.20}{.30}$

130 A technician is asked by the supervisor to prepare a standard solution from the stock standard. What is the glassware of choice for this solution?

  (a) graduated cylinder
  b volumetric flask
  c acid-washed beaker
  d graduated flask

131 How many mL of red blood cells are to be used to make 25 mL of a 4% red cell suspension?

  a 0.25 mL
  b 0.5 mL
  (c) 1 mL
  d 2 mL

132 The volume of 25% stock sulfosalicylic acid needed to prepare 100 mL of 5% working solution is:

  a 1.25 mL
  b 5 mL
  (c) 20 mL
  d 50 mL

$\_\_ \cdot 25 = 100 \times 5$

133 To prepare 25 mL of 3% acetic acid, how much glacial acetic acid is needed?

MLS ONLY

  (a) 0.75 mL
  b 1.5 mL
  c 3.0 mL
  d 7.5 mL

134 How many grams of sodium chloride are needed to prepare 1 L of 0.9% normal saline?

  a 0.9
  b 1.8
  (c) 9.0
  d 18.0

0.9 gr/100 mls of saline

$\dfrac{0.9}{100} = \dfrac{X}{1000}$

135 To prepare 40 mL of a 3% working solution, a technician would use what volume of stock solution?

MLS ONLY

  a 0.9 mL
  b 1.2 mL
  c 1.5 mL
  d 3.0 mL

136 A technician is preparing a 75% solution. What volume of stock solution should be used to prepare 8 mL?

MLS
ONLY

   a 4.5 mL
   b 6.0 mL
   c 7.5 mL
   d 9.4 mL

137 A new method is being evaluated. A recovery experiment is performed with the following results:

MLS
ONLY

0.9 mL serum sample + 0.1 mL H_2O	89 mEq/L
0.9 mL serum sample + 0.1 mL analyte standard at 800 mEq/L	161 mEq/L

The percent recovery of the added analyte standard is:

   a 55%
   b 81%
   c 90%
   d 180%

138 Which of the following is the formula for standard deviation?

   a square root of the mean
   b square root of (sum of squared differences)/(N-1)
   c square root of the variance
   d square root of (mean)/(sum of squared differences)

139 The acceptable limit of error in the chemistry laboratory is 2 standard deviations. If you run the normal control 100 times, how many of the values would be out of the control range due to random error?

   a 1
   b 5
   c 10
   d 20

140 A mean value of 100 and a standard deviation of 1.8 mg/dL were obtained from a set of glucose measurements on a control solution. The 95% confidence interval in mg/dL would be:

   a 94.6-105.4
   b 96.4-103.6
   c 97.3-102.7
   d 98.2-101.8

141 When 0.25 mL is diluted to 20 mL, the resulting dilution is:

   a 1:20
   b 1:40
   c 1:60
   d 1:80

$$\frac{.25}{20} = \frac{1}{X}$$

142 When the exact concentration of the solute of a solution is known and is used to evaluate the concentration of an unknown solution, the known solution is:

   a standard
   b normal
   c control
   d baseline

143 A serum glucose sample was too high to read, so a 1:5 dilution using saline (dilution A) was made. Dilution A was tested and was again too high to read. A further 1:2 dilution was made using saline (dilution B). To calculate the result, the dilution B value must be multiplied by:

   a 5
   b 8
   c 10
   d 20

144 In performing a spinal fluid protein determination, the specimen is diluted 1 part spinal fluid to 3 parts saline to obtain a result low enough to measure. To calculate the protein concentration, the result must be:

   a multiplied by 3
   b multiplied by 4
   c divided by 3
   d divided by 4

145 How many mL of anti-D reagent are needed to prepare 5 mL of a 1:25 dilution?
MLS ONLY

   a 0.1
   b 0.2
   c 0.25
   d 0.5

146 To make 1 L of 1.0 N NaOH from a 1.025 N NaOH solution, how many mL of the NaOH should be used?
MLS ONLY

   a   950.0
   b   975.6
   c   997.5
   d 1,025.0

147 If 0.5 mL of a 1:300 dilution contains 1 antigenic unit, 2 antigenic units would be contained in 0.5 mL of a dilution of:

   a 1:150
   b 1:450
   c 1:500
   d 1:600

148 A 2% saline erythrocyte suspension contains how many mL of packed erythrocytes per 5 mL of isotonic saline solution?
MLS ONLY

   a 0.1
   b 0.2
   c 0.5
   d 1.0

149 A 600 mg/dL glucose solution is diluted 1:30. The concentration of the final solution in mg/dL is:
MLS ONLY

   a   2
   b   20
   c   180
   d 1,800

150 How many mL of 30% bovine albumin are needed to make 6 mL of a 10% albumin solution?
MLS ONLY

   a 1
   b 2
   c 3
   d 4

151 Which of the following is the formula for calculating the dilution of a solution?
(V = volume, C=concentration)

   a $V1 + C1 = V2 + C2$
   b $V1 + C2 = V2 + C1$
   c $V1 \times C1 = V2 \times C2$
   d $V1 \times V2 = V1 \times C2$

152 A colorimetric method calls for the use of 0.1 mL of serum, 5 mL of reagent and 4.9 mL of water. What is the dilution of the serum in the final solution?

   a 1:5
   b 1:10   .1 : 10
   c 1:50
   d 1:100

153 Four mL of water are added to 1 mL of serum. This represents which of the following serum dilutions?

   a 1:3
   b 1:4
   c 1:5
   d 1:6

154 Which of the following is the formula for calculating a percent (w/v) solution?

   a grams of solute/volume of solvent × 100
   b grams of solute × volume of solvent × 100
   c volume of solvent/grams of solute × 100
   d (grams of solute × volume of solvent)/100

155 A solution contains 20 g of solute dissolved in 0.5 L of water. What is the percentage of this solution?

                                      grams per 100 mls
   a 2% $\frac{20}{.5} = \frac{x}{100}$
   b 4%
   c 6%
   d 8%

156 How many grams of sulfosalicylic acid (MW = 254) are required to prepare 1 L of a 3% (w/v) solution?

                         3 grams per 100 mls
   a   3 $10 \cdot 100 = 1$ liter
   b 30
   c 254
   d 300

157 How many mL of a 3% solution can be made if 6 grams of solute are available?

   a 100 mL $3 = 100$ mls
   b 200 mL
   c 400 mL
   d 600 mL

158 The following results were obtained from a set of automated white blood cell counts performed
MLS
ONLY
on 40 samples:

standard deviation: 153.2/µL
mean value: 12,450/µL

The coefficient of variation.

a 0.01%
b 1.2%
c 2.5%
d 8.1%

159 The following 5 sodium control values in unit (mEq/L) were obtained:

140, 135, 138, 140, 142

Calculate the coefficient of variation.

a 1.9%
b 2.7%
c 5.6%
d 6.1%

160 The statistical term for the average value is the:

a mode
b median
c mean
d coefficient of variation

161 The most frequent value in a collection of data is statistically known as:

a mode
b median
c mean
d standard deviation

162 The middle value of a data set is statistically known as the:

a mean
b median
c mode
d standard deviation

163 Which of the following is the formula for arithmetic mean?

a square root of the sum of values
b sum of values × number of values
c number of values/sum of values
d sum of values/number of values

164 Given the following values:

100, 120, 150, 140, 130

What is the mean?

a 100
b 128
c 130
d 640

165 Which of the following is the formula for coefficient of variation?

    a (standard deviation × 100)/standard error
    b (mean × 100)/standard deviation
    c (standard deviation × 100)/mean
    d (variance × 100)/mean

166 A cholesterol QC chart has the following data for the normal control:

× (mean of data)	=	137 mg/dL
#x	=	1,918 mg/dL
2 SD	=	6 mg/dL
N	=	14

The coefficient of variation for this control is:

    a 1.14%
    b 2.19%
    c 4.38%
    d 9.49%

167 The sodium content (in grams) in 100 grams of NaCl is approximately:
(atomic weights: Na = 23.0, Cl = 35.5)

    a 10
    b 20
    c 40
    d 60

168 Given the following results, calculate the molar absorptivity:
MLS ONLY

absorbance:	0.500
light path:	1.0 cm
concentration:	0.2 M/L

    a 0.4
    b 0.7
    c 1.6
    d 2.5

169 Absorbance (A) of a solution may be converted to percent transmittance (%T) using the formula:
MLS ONLY

    a 1 + log %T
    b 2 + log %T
    c 1 – log %T
    d 2 – log %T

170 Which of the following is the formula for calculating the unknown concentration based on Beer's law? (A = absorbance, C = concentration)
MLS ONLY

    a (A unknown/A standard) × C standard
    b C standard × A unknown
    c A standard × A unknown
    d (C standard)/(A standard) × 100

171 Which of the following is the formula for calculating the gram equivalent weight of a chemical?

    a MW × oxidation number
    b MW/oxidation number
    c MW + oxidation number
    d MW – oxidation number

172 80 grams of NaOH (MW = 40) are how many moles?

    a 1
    b 2
    c 3
    d 4

173 A serum potassium (MW = 39) is 19.5 mg/100 mL. This value is equal to how many mEq/L?

    a 3.9
    b 4.2
    c 5.0
    d 8.9

174 Which of the following is the formula for calculating the number of moles of a chemical?

    a g/GMW
    b g × GMW
    c GMW/g
    d (g × 100)/GMW

175 A 1 molal solution is equivalent to:

    a a solution containing 1 mole of solute per kg of solvent
    b 1,000 mL of solution containing 1 mole of solute
    c a solution containing 1 gram equivalent weight of solute in 1 L of solution
    d a 1 L solution containing 2 moles of solute

176 Which of the following is the formula for calculating the molarity of a solution?

    a number of moles of solute/L of solution
    b number of moles of solute × 100
    c 1 GEW of solute × 10
    d 1 GEW of solute/L of solution

177 What is the molarity of a solution that contains 18.7 g of KCl (MW = 74.5) in 500 mL of water?
MLS
ONLY
    a 0.1
    b 0.5
    c 1.0
    d 5.0

178 25 grams of NaOH (MW = 40) are added to 0.5 L of water. What is the molarity of this solution if
MLS
ONLY
an additional 0.25 L of water are added?

    a 0.25 M
    b 0.50 M
    c 0.75 M
    d 0.83 M

179 What is the normality of a solution that contains 280 grams of NaOH (MW = 40) in 2,000 mL
MLS
ONLY
of solution?

    a 3.5 N
    b 5.5 N
    c 7.0 N
    d 8.0 N

180 How many grams of H_2SO_4 (MW = 98) are in 750 mL of 3N H_2SO_4?
MLS
ONLY
    a 36 g
    b 72 g
    c 110 g
    d 146 g

181 How many mL of 0.25 N NaOH are needed to make 100 mL of a 0.05 N solution of NaOH?

    a 5 mL
    b 10 mL
    c 15 mL
    d 20 mL

182 A pH of 7.0 represents a H+ concentration of:
MLS
ONLY

    a 70 mEq/L
    b 10 µmol/L
    c   7 nmol/L
    d 100 nmol/L

183 The predictive value of a positive test is defined as:
MLS
ONLY

    a (true positives + true negatives)/true positives × 100
    b true positives/(true positives + false positives) × 100
    c (true positives + true negatives)/true negatives × 100
    d true negatives/(true negatives + false positives) × 100

Instrumentation and General Laboratory Principles

184 The reliability of a test to be positive in the presence of the disease it was designed to detect is known as:

    a accuracy
    b sensitivity
    c precision
    d specificity

185 Which of the following parameters of a diagnostic test will vary with the prevalence of a given disease in a population?

    a precision
    b sensitivity
    c accuracy
    d specificity

186 Package inserts may be used:

    a instead of a typed procedure
    b as a reference in a procedure
    c at the bench but not in the procedure manual
    d if initialed and dated by the laboratory director

187 An evaluation of a new POC instrument shows the following comparisons.

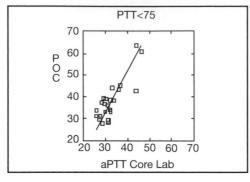

aPTT

Best-fit values

slope	1.894 ± 0.2750
y-intercept	−23.59 ± 8.969
x-intercept	12.45
1/slope	0.5281

95% confidence intervals

slope	1.326-2.461
y-intercept when X=0.0	−42.10 to −5.073

Goodness of fit

r^2	
Sy.x	6.018

The best course of action would be to:

a establish a different reference range for the POC test
b do not implement the POC test as there is no correlation
c implement the POC test after informing physicians that the whole blood test is just different
d implement the test since the slope and confidence intervals are acceptable

188 The following target shows a set of results that show a high degree of:

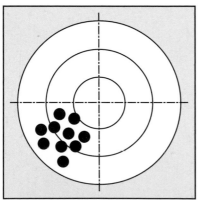

a accuracy
b precision
c sensitivity
d specificity

189 Which of the following is the advantage for adding point-of-care testing?

MLS
ONLY
    a higher test accuracy
    b lower costs
    c faster TAT
    d more skilled test personnel

190 The first step to be taken when attempting to repair a piece of electronic equipment is:

    a check all the electronic connections
    b reset all the printed circuit boards
    c turn the instrument off
    d replace all the fuses

191 The methodology based on the amount of energy absorbed by a substance as a function of its concentration and using a specific source of the same material as the substance analyzed is:

    a flame emission photometry
    b atomic absorption spectrophotometry
    c emission spectrography
    d x-ray fluorescence spectrometry

192 Which of the following wavelengths is within the ultraviolet range?

    a 340 nm
    b 450 nm
    c 540 nm
    d 690 nm

193 One means of checking a spectrophotometer wavelength calibration in the visible range is by using a:

    a quartz filter
    b diffraction grating
    c quartz prism
    d didymium filter

194 In spectrophotometry, the device that allows for a narrow band of wavelengths is the:

    a hollow cathode lamp
    b monochromator
    c refractometer
    d photodetector

195 What is the first step in preparing a spectrophotometer for an assay?

MLS
ONLY
    a adjust wavelength selector
    b zero with deionized water
    c read standard absorbance
    d place a cuvette in the well

196 The nanometer is a measurement of:

    a wavelength of radiant energy
    b specific gravity
    c density
    d intensity of light

197 In a double-beam photometer, the additional beam is used to:

    a compensate for variation in wavelength
    b correct for variations in light source intensity
    c correct for changes in light path
    d compensate for variation in slit-widths

198 The source of radiant energy in atomic absorption spectrophotometry is:

MLS
ONLY

   a hollow anode lamp
   b hollow cathode lamp
   c halogen vapor lamp
   d deuterium lamp

199 A spectrophotometer is being considered for purchase by a small laboratory. Which of the following specifications reflects the spectral purity of the instrument?

MLS
ONLY

   a photomultiplier tube
   b dark current
   c band width
   d galvanometer

200 A chemistry assay utilizes a bichromatic analysis. This means that absorbance readings are taken at:

MLS
ONLY

   a 2 wavelengths so that 2 compounds can be measured at the same time
   b 2 wavelengths to correct for spectral interference from another compound
   c the beginning and end of a time interval to measure the absorbance change
   d 2 times and then are averaged to obtain a more accurate result

201 Nephelometers measure light:

   a scattered at a right angle to the light path
   b absorbed by suspended particles
   c transmitted by now-particulate mixtures
   d reflected back to the source from opaque suspensions

202 A technologist is asked to write a procedure to measure the Evan blue concentration on a spectrophotometer. The technologist is given 4 standard solutions of Evan blue:

     Std A = 0.8 mg/dL
     Std B = 1.6 mg/dL
     Std C = 2.4 mg/dL
     Std D = 4.0 mg/dL

The first step is to:

   a calculate the slope of the calibration curve
   b determine the absorbance of the 4 standards
   c find the wavelength of the greatest % transmittance for Evan blue
   d find the wavelength of the greatest absorbance for Evan blue

203 Which of the following is used to verify wavelength settings for narrow bandwidth spectrophotometers?

   a didymium filter
   b prisms
   c holmium oxide glass
   d diffraction gratings

204 Which of the following statements about fluorometry is true?

   a a compound fluoresces when it absorbs light at 1 wavelength and emits light at a second wavelength
   b the detector in a fluorometer is positioned at 180° from the excitation source
   c fluorometry is less sensitive than spectrophotometry
   d an incandescent lamp is commonly used in a fluorometer

205 The measurement of light scattered by particles in the sample is the principle of:

   a spectrophotometry
   b fluorometry
   c nephelometry
   d atomic absorption

206 In a spectrophotometer, light of a specific wavelength is isolated from the light source by the:

   a double beam
   b monochromator
   c aperture
   d slit

207 A mass spectrometer detects which property of ionized molecules?

   a column retention time
   b charge to mass ratio
   c mass to charge ratio
   d fluorescence

208 Chromatography is based on the principle of:

   a differential solubility
   b gravity
   c vapor pressure
   d temperature

209
MLS
ONLY
 Gel filtration chromatography is used to separate:

   a polar and nonpolar compounds
   b compounds on the basis of molecular weight and size
   c isomers of the same compound
   d compounds on the basis of different functional groups

210
MLS
ONLY
 An R_f value of 0.5 in thin-layer chromatography means:

   a solute moves twice as far as solvent front
   b solute moves half the distance of solvent front
   c solute moves with solvent front
   d solvent moves half the distance of solute

211
MLS
ONLY
 An HPLC operator notes that the column pressure is too high, is rising too rapidly and the recorder output is not producing normal peaks. The most probable cause of the problem is:

   a not enough sample injected
   b bad sample detector
   c effluent line obstructed
   d strip chart motor hanging up

212 To be analyzed by gas liquid chromatography a compound must:

   a be volatile or made volatile
   b not be volatile
   c be water-soluble
   d contain a nitrogen atom

213 A true statement about column chromatography methods, including high-performance liquid and gas chromatography, is that it:

   a all utilizes a flame ionization detector
   b requires derivation of nonvolatile compounds
   c can be used to separate gases, liquids or soluble solids
   d can be used for adsorption, partition, ion-exchange and steric-exclusion chromatography

214 In thin-layer chromatography, the R_f value for a compound is the:

    a ratio of distance moved by compound
    b rate of movement of compound through the adsorbent
    c difference in distance between the compound spot and solvent front
    d distance moved by compound from the origin

215 In electrophoretic analysis, buffers:

    a stabilize electrolytes
    b maintain basic pH
    c act as a carrier for ions
    d produce an effect on protein configuration

216 On electrophoresis, distorted zones of protein separation are usually due to:

    a presence of therapeutic drugs in serum sample
    b dirty applicators
    c overloading of serum sample
    d prestaining with tracer dye

217 An ion-selective electrode (ISE) measures the:

    a activity of one ion only
    b concentration of one ion only
    c activity of one ion much more than other ions present
    d activity of only H^+ ions

218 The selectivity of an ion-selective electrode is determined by the:

    a properties of the membrane used
    b solution used to fill the electrode
    c magnitude of the potential across the membrane
    d internal reference electrode

219 A centrifuge head has a diameter of 60 cm and spins at 3,000 RPM. What is the maximum achievable G force?
($G = 0.00001 \times$ radius in cm $\times (RPM)^2$)

    a   1.8 G
    b 2,700 G
    c 27,000 G
    d 90,000 G

220 In a centrifugal analyzer, centrifugal force is used to:

    a add reagents to the rotor
    b transfer liquids from the inner disc to the outer cuvette
    c measure changes in optical density in the centrifugal force field
    d counteract the tendency of precipitates to settle in the cuvette

221 Which of the following is the best guide to consistent centrifugation?

    a potentiometer setting
    b armature settings
    c tachometer readings
    d rheostat readings

222 A benefit of microassays, such as point-of-care methods, include:

    a increased analytical reliability
    b reduced sample volume
    c increased diagnostic specificity
    d reduced numbers of repeated tests

223 In the proper use of cobalt treated-anhydrous $CaCl_2$, the desiccant should be:

    a changed when it turns pink
    b changed when it turns blue
    c kept in the dark
    d kept in the cold

224 Enzyme-multiplied immunoassay techniques (EMIT) differ from all other types of enzyme immunoassays in that:

    a lysozyme is the only enzyme used to label the hapten molecule
    b no separation of bound and free antigen is required
    c inhibition of the enzyme label is accomplished with polyethylene glycol
    d antibody absorption to polystyrene tubes precludes competition to labeled and unlabeled antigen

225 Which of the following statements about immunoassays using enzyme labeled antibodies or antigens is correct?

    a inactivation of the enzyme is required
    b the enzyme label is less stable than an isotopic label
    c quantitation of the label can be carried out with a spectrophotometer
    d the enzyme label is not an enzyme found naturally in serum

226 Which of the following immunoassay labels offer the greatest detection limit?

    a fluorescence
    b electrochemiluminescence
    c radioactivity
    d chemiluminescence

Education and Communication

227 The objective, "The student will be able to perform daily maintenance on the Hematology analyzer" is an example of which behavioral domain?
MLS ONLY

    a psychomotor
    b affective
    c intellectual
    d cognitive

228 To be effective, criticism should be:
MLS ONLY

    a specific to the behavior
    b related to general laboratory performance
    c focused on the person, not the behavior
    d repeatedly discussed for reinforcement

229 The first step in the development of long-term objectives for a laboratory continuing education program must include:
MLS ONLY

    a total cost of the program
    b total number of hours in the program
    c a list of topics to be covered
    d a statement of competencies to be achieved

230 Given the following objective:

MLS ONLY

"After listening to the audioconference, the student will be able to describe the interaction between T and B lymphocytes in the immune system, to the satisfaction of the instructor."

Which of the following test questions reflects the intent of this objective?

  a how are T and B lymphocytes separated in vitro?
  b how many T lymphocytes does a normal person have in peripheral blood?
  c what are the morphological characteristics of B lymphocytes?
  d how are antibodies produced after a viral infection?

231 Higher levels of employee motivation occur when the supervisor:

MLS ONLY

  a collaborates to set goals to be accomplished
  b provides all the details of the task
  c constantly monitors progress
  d immediately corrects every error

232 Several complaints have been received from parents of children in the pediatric wing about the anxiety that venipuncture causes their children. An informal staff meeting with the phlebotomists reveals that they feel both parents and pediatric nurses are less than supportive and frequently make the task of venipuncture in children worse with their own anxiety. The best course of action would be to:

  a have pediatric nurses do venipuncture on children as they are more familiar with the children
  b limit physicians to only one draw per day on children
  c prepare written pamphlets for parents and in-service education for nursing personnel
  d take no action as parents will always overreact where their children are concerned

233 A major laboratory policy change that will affect a significant portion of the laboratory personnel is going to take place. In order to minimize the staff's resistance to this change, the supervisor should:

  a announce the policy change the day before it will become effective
  b discuss the policy change in detail with all personnel concerned, well in advance of implementation
  c announce only the positive aspects of the policy change in advance
  d discuss only the positive aspects of the policy with those concerned

234 When employees are going to be responsible for implementing a change in procedure or policy, the manager should:

  a make the decision and direct the employees to implement it
  b solicit the employee input but do what he/she thinks should be done
  c involve the employees in the decision-making process from the very beginning
  d involve only those employees in the decision-making process who would benefit from the change

235 The best way to motivate an ineffective employee would be to:

MLS ONLY

  a confirm low performance with subjective data
  b set short-term goals for the employee
  c transfer the employee to another department
  d ignore failure to meet goals

236 A technologist has an idea that would possibly decrease the laboratory turnaround time for reporting results. In order to begin implementation of this idea, he/she should:

MLS ONLY

  a encourage the staff to utilize the idea
  b discuss it with his/her immediate supervisor
  c try out the idea on himself/herself on an experimental basis
  d present the idea to the laboratory director

237 The most important aspect of supervision is:
MLS
ONLY
   a balancing the budget
   b performing technical procedures
   c writing accurate job descriptions
   d dealing with people

238 A course of instruction is being planned to teach laboratory employees to recognize, troubleshoot
MLS
ONLY
and correct simple malfunctions in selected laboratory instruments. In writing the objectives for this course, which one of the following would be most appropriate?

   a learn how to repair 9 of 10 simple instrument malfunctions
   b correctly answer 9 of 10 test questions dealing with simple instrument malfunctions
   c recognize, detect and correct 9 of 10 simple instrument malfunctions
   d document corrective action procedure for 9 of 10 simple instrument malfunctions

239 The ability to make good decisions often depends on the use of a logical sequence of steps that include:

   a defining problem, considering options, implementing decisions
   b obtaining facts, considering alternatives, reviewing results
   c defining problem, obtaining facts, considering options
   d obtaining facts, defining problem, implementing decision

240 In planning an instructional unit, the term "goal" has been defined as a:

   a plan for reaching certain objectives
   b set of specific tasks
   c set of short- and long-term plans
   d major purpose or final desired result

241 Delegation is a process in which:
MLS
ONLY
   a interpersonal influence is redefined
   b authority of manager is surrendered
   c power is given to others
   d responsibility for specific tasks is given to others

242 What action should be taken when dealing with a long-term problem?
MLS
ONLY
   a ignore the problem
   b seek more information
   c base decision on available information
   d refer the problem to another level of management

243 A major laboratory policy change that will affect a significant portion of the laboratory employees
MLS
ONLY
is going to take place. In order to minimize the resistance to change the supervisor should:

   a announce the change one day after it goes into effect
   b discuss the change in detail with all concerned, well in advance
   c announce only the positive aspects in advance
   d discuss only the positive aspects with those concerned

244 Which of the following actions will facilitate group interactions at staff meetings?
MLS
ONLY
   a adhering strictly to an agenda
   b treating every problem consistently
   c encouraging input from all staff
   d announcing the assignments for upcoming projects

245 As information is reported upward through an organization, the amount of detail communicated
MLS
ONLY
will generally:

   a decrease to facilitate the flow of information
   b increase to allow consideration of all options
   c remain the same to ensure consistency in reporting
   d remain the same to ensure goal accomplishment

246 To sustain the highly motivated employee the evaluation should include:

MLS
ONLY

a performance feedback
b retraining opportunities
c quality of performance discussions
d competency-based tasks

247 Communication is enhanced by:

a a planned strategy that includes listening skills and ensuring an understanding with questions
b relying on e-mail, memos and voice mail to communicate new information
c formal, hierarchical patterns instead of informal networking patterns
d assumptions if there are questions about the intent of the message

248 In its guidelines, CAP stresses that communication must be effective and efficient. An effective component to enhance a multifaceted communication plan in the clinical laboratory is:

a posting department goals on communication bulletin boards
b daily meetings with a question to foster conversation and focus the discussion
c written e-mail to communicate all new changes in processes and procedures
d posting errors on communication bulletin boards to prevent repeat errors

Laboratory Information Systems

249 Identify the first step a laboratory manager must take in the selection of a laboratory information system.

MLS
ONLY

a write a request for proposal (RFP)
b select a computer vendor
c select an LIS team
d decide on services needed

250 Laboratory results can be sent to a hospital's electronic medical record by:

MLS
ONLY

a autofax
b HL-7 interface
c internet routing
d backup server

251 The use of security systems such as firewalls and data encryption for electronic transmission of patient data from a laboratory information system to a remote location are required for:

a LOINC
b HIPAA
c ICD-9
d CLIA

252 CODE 128, ISBT 128, CODE 39 and Interleaved 2 of 5 symbologies are used by laboratory information systems to create which of the following?

a barcode labels
b worklists
c instrument download files
d patient reports

253 A standard electronic file format recommended for transmitting data from the laboratory information system to an electronic medical record is:

a Health Level 7
b ISBT 128
c FTP
d SNOMED

254 Auto-verification of test results requires all of the following to be established by the laboratory **except**:

    a patient results entered into the LIS via an instrument interface
    b patient results evaluated based on validated rules defined in the LIS
    c successful quality control testing obtained prior to releasing patient results
    d review of results by a qualified technologist or technician

255 Validation of calculated test results performed by a laboratory information system must be performed:

    a every 6 months
    b annually
    c biannually
    d only upon initial LIS installation

256 The Hematology laboratory is evaluating new instruments for purchase. The supervisor wants to ensure that the instrument they select has bidirectional interface capabilities. The instrument specification necessary to meet this requirement is:

    a 9,600 baud rate
    b on-board test selection menu
    c HL-7 file format
    d host query mode

257 The Chemistry department has requested that a new test be defined in the LIS to run on the existing analyzer. The new test set up is completed by the LIS coordinator. A few days later, the accessioning department receives a request for the new test but an error is displayed when they try to place the order. All other tests can be successfully ordered. The most likely cause of the error is the:

    a instrument interface for the Chemistry analyzer is down
    b test was not defined on the Chemistry worklist
    c database did not properly update with the new test information
    d ADT interface with the hospital system is down

258 The process of testing and documenting changes made to a laboratory information system is known as:

    a validation
    b quality engineering
    c customization
    d hazard analysis

259 Performance of laboratory information system back-up procedures includes all of the following **except**:

    a creating an exact copy of LIS data
    b off-site storage of the data media
    c shutting down the LIS and bringing it back up
    d completion at regularly defined intervals

260 A large hospital has implemented an outreach program, which will involve processing samples
MLS received with a variety of barcode labels that are not compatible with the hospital's LIS.
ONLY The laboratory does not have the staff to re-label every specimen received from their outreach clients. Which of the following solutions would be the most appropriate for the LIS coordinator to consider?

    a mandate that the outreach clients modify their LIS to print compatible barcode labels
    b purchase a middleware product to manage samples containing different barcode formats
    c install a new LIS in the hospital that is compatible with the outreach clients' systems
    d manually process all samples received from the outreach clients

Answer Key–Laboratory Operations

1 a	59 b	117 d	175 a	233 b
2 b	60 d	118 b	176 a	234 c
3 c	61 b	119 c	177 b	235 b
4 d	62 c	120 d	178 d	236 b
5 a	63 d	121 d	179 a	237 d
6 b	64 b	122 a	180 c	238 c
7 d	65 d	123 d	181 d	239 c
8 b	66 b	124 b	182 d	240 d
9 a	67 d	125 d	183 b	241 d
10 d	68 c	126 d	184 b	242 b
11 c	69 b	127 c	185 c	243 b
12 c	70 d	128 d	186 b	244 c
13 c	71 a	129 a	187 a	245 a
14 d	72 c	130 b	188 b	246 a
15 d	73 b	131 c	189 c	247 a
16 a	74 d	132 c	190 c	248 b
17 b	75 c	133 a	191 b	249 c
18 b	76 a	134 c	192 a	250 b
19 b	77 a	135 b	193 d	251 b
20 d	78 c	136 b	194 b	252 a
21 c	79 a	137 c	195 a	253 a
22 c	80 c	138 b	196 a	254 d
23 d	81 d	139 b	197 b	255 c
24 d	82 b	140 b	198 b	256 d
25 a	83 c	141 d	199 c	257 c
26 d	84 d	142 a	200 b	258 a
27 a	85 b	143 c	201 a	259 c
28 d	86 d	144 b	202 d	260 b
29 c	87 c	145 b	203 c	
30 a	88 a	146 b	204 a	
31 a	89 d	147 a	205 c	
32 c	90 a	148 a	206 b	
33 d	91 b	149 b	207 c	
34 c	92 c	150 b	208 a	
35 d	93 c	151 c	209 b	
36 a	94 b	152 d	210 b	
37 b	95 a	153 c	211 c	
38 d	96 b	154 a	212 a	
39 c	97 c	155 b	213 d	
40 c	98 d	156 b	214 a	
41 d	99 a	157 b	215 c	
42 c	100 b	158 b	216 c	
43 d	101 c	159 a	217 c	
44 b	102 a	160 c	218 a	
45 c	103 b	161 a	219 b	
46 d	104 b	162 b	220 b	
47 d	105 c	163 d	221 c	
48 c	106 a	164 b	222 b	
49 a	107 b	165 c	223 a	
50 d	108 a	166 b	224 b	
51 c	109 c	167 c	225 c	
52 d	110 b	168 d	226 b	
53 a	111 b	169 d	227 a	
54 b	112 d	170 a	228 a	
55 d	113 a	171 b	229 d	
56 b	114 c	172 b	230 d	
57 c	115 d	173 c	231 a	
58 a	116 a	174 a	232 c	

Quality Assessment

1 **a**   Evaluation of turn-around times is an
MLS
ONLY   important part of the laboratory's quality
assurance program and is a good way to
assess the laboratory's performance in
the overall testing process. The laboratory
manager is responsible for determining the
overall testing process and schedules that
will be the most cost effective and provide
reliable test results within a clinically
appropriate time frame.
[Garcia 2004, p382]

2 **b**   The Joint Commission requires 2
patient identifiers when providing care,
treatment, or service.
[LabQ 2008, pp118-122]

3 **c**   The focus must center on a root cause
analysis of such errors to prevent them from
occurring in the clinical setting.
[Lab Medicine 2008a, pp395-400]

4 **d**   Preanalytical (ie, pre-examination)
variables include all steps in the process
prior to the analytic phase of testing,
starting with the physician's order.
Examples include accuracy of transmission
of physicians' orders, specimen transport
and preparation, requisition accuracy,
quality of phlebotomy services, specimen
acceptability rates, etc. This list is neither all-
inclusive nor exclusive. The variables chosen
should be appropriate to the laboratory's
scope of care.
[CAP 2009, GEN 20348]

5 **a**   If multiple controls are out of range and
the instrument and reagents are verified,
recalibration or calibration verification is
required before subsequent control analysis.
[Clarke 2006, p149]

6 **b**   The y-intercept, which should be close
MLS
ONLY   to 0 if the methods are comparable, provides
an assessment of constant bias.
[Clarke 2006, p54]

7 **d**   If the error in a method is consistently
MLS
ONLY   low or high by an amount proportional to
the concentration of the analyte, it is called
proportional error, and it is monitored by
the slope of the equation of the line.
[Kaplan 2003, p411]

8 **b**   Repeating a QC measurement on a new
sample of QC material may establish that
the alert was caused by a deteriorated QC
material rather than a method problem.
[Clarke 2006, p148]

9 **a**   Validation is the confirmation by
MLS
ONLY   objective evidence that the requirement
for the specified use of the instrument/
procedure is consistently fulfilled.
[Kaplan 2003, p415]

10 **d**   Standard deviation is a measure of the
dispersion of data around the mean.
[Campbell 1997, p309]

11 **c**   The probability of an observation having
MLS
ONLY   a value within ±2 standard deviations of the
mean in a normal distribution is 95.5%.
[Campbell 1997, p313]

12 **c**   Repeating a QC measurement on a new
sample of QC material may establish that
the alert was caused by a deteriorated QC
material rather than a method problem.
[Clarke 2006, p148]

13 **c**   Standard deviation is a measure of the
dispersion of data around the mean.
[Campbell 1997, p309]

14 **d**   Precision is the closeness of agreement
among replicate measurements, or
reproducibility. The coefficient of variation,
a more useful measure of reproducibility,
is the measure of relative random error
expressed as a percentage.
[Clarke 2006, p53]

15 **d**   Precision is the reproducibility of
analytical results, or the degree to which
results of multiple analyses of the same
specimen agree.
[Clarke 2006, p32]

16 **a**   Specificity is defined as negativity in the
absence of disease.
[Clarke 2006, p35]

17 **b**   Accuracy or trueness is the closeness of
agreement with the true value.
[Clarke 2006, p53]

18 **b**   Specificity is defined as negativity in the
absence of disease.
[Clarke 2006, p35]

19 **b**   A correlation coefficient, or r-value, of 0
MLS
ONLY   indicates that there is no correlation between
the methods, while an r-value of +1 and
−1 indicate a perfect positive and negative
correlation between methods, respectively.
[Kaplan 2003, p416]

20 **d**   National Labor Relations Act (NLRA)
includes the right to form or join unions,
freedom to bargain collectively with the employer
and the right to engage in group activity.
[Garcia 2004, p354]

21   **c**   JCAHO sets standards by which healthcare is measured and accredits institutions and laboratories worldwide.
[JCAHO 2009]

22   **c**   Accreditation is the approval of an institution or program based on a review by one or more independent examiners that specific requirements or predetermined standards are met.
[Garcia 2004, p815]

23   **d**   CLIA was established to ensure quality standards for laboratory testing.
[Garcia 2004, p75]

24
MLS
ONLY   **d**   CAP General Checklist 11226: "Does the laboratory have a procedure for assessing its performance on PT challenges that were not graded..."
[CAP 2009, GEN 11226]

25
MLS
ONLY   **a**   National Patient Safety Goal (NPSG) 02.03.01: The [organization] measures, assesses, and, if needed, takes action to improve the timeliness of reporting and the timeliness of receipt of critical tests and critical results and values by the responsible licensed caregiver.
[NPSG 2009, 02.03.01]

26
MLS
ONLY   **d**   "GEN 10500: For tests for which CAP does not require enrollment in PT, does the laboratory at least semi-annually 1) participate in external PT, or 2) exercise an alternative performance assessment system for determining the reliability of analytic testing?" **Note**: Appropriate alternative performance assessment procedures may include: split sample analysis with reference or other laboratories, split samples with an established in-house method, assayed material, regional pools, clinical validation by chart review, or other suitable and documented means. It is the responsibility of the laboratory director to define such alternative performance assessment procedures, as applicable, in accordance with good clinical and scientific laboratory practice. As an example, the biannual CAP CED educational challenge in esoteric coagulation testing offers an opportunity to compare test results with other participants. Participation in ungraded/educational proficiency testing programs also satisfies this checklist question.
[CAP 2009, GEN 10500]

27   **a**   "GEN 41042: Are refrigerator/freezer temperatures checked and recorded daily?"
[CAP 2009, GEN 41042]

28   **d**   "GEN 41096:
Does the paper or electronic report include the following elements?
1. Name and address of testing laboratory (see note below)
2. Patient name and identification number, or unique patient identifier
3. Name of physician of record, or legally authorized person ordering test, as appropriate
4. Date and time of specimen collection, when appropriate
5. Date of release of report (if not on the report, this information should be readily accessible)
6. Time of release of report, if applicable (if not on the report, this information should be readily accessible)
7. Specimen source, when applicable
8. Test result(s) (and units of measurement, when applicable)
9. Reference intervals, as applicable (see note below)
10. Conditions of specimen that may limit adequacy of testing."
[CAP 2009, GEN 41096]

29
MLS
ONLY   **c**   "GEN 41770: Are there appropriate documented procedures for handling and cleaning glassware, including methods for testing for detergent removal?"
[CAP 2009, GEN 41770]

30
MLS
ONLY   **a**   "GEN 42085: The ANALYTICAL MEASUREMENT RANGE (AMR) is the range of analyte values that a method can directly measure on the specimen without any dilution, concentration, or other pretreatment not part of the usual assay process."
[CAP 2009, GEN 42085]

31   **a**   HIPAA protects health insurance coverage for workers and their families when they change or lose their jobs, and also addresses the security and privacy of health data.
[Garcia 2004, pp144-145]

32   **c**   HIPAA protects health insurance coverage for workers and their families when they change or lose their jobs, and also addresses the security and privacy of health data.
[Garcia 2004, pp144-147]

33 **d** The official CMS system for assignment
MLS of codes for clinical conditions associated
ONLY with consequent medical procedures,
including laboratory testing.
[Garcia 2004, p562]

Safety

34 **c** MSDS is an OSHA required document
that provides information such as physical
data (melting point, boiling point, flash
point etc), toxicity, health effects, first aid,
reactivity, storage, disposal, protective
equipment, and spill/leak procedures.
[McClatchey 1994, p63]

35 **d** The correct answer is **d**, flammability.
For distractor **a**, reactivity is the right yellow
quadrant. For distractor **b**, special reactivity
is the lower white quadrant. For distractor **c**,
health is the left blue quadrant.
[Forbes 2007, p48]

36 **a** The correct answer is **a**, high health
hazard. The ratings range for both systems is
0-4 with 0 being no hazard and 4 being the
most severe hazard. The other distractors
are incorrect due to the hazard type or
number rating.
[Forbes 2007, p48]

37 **b** The correct answer is **b**, formaldehyde.
The other distractors are hazardous
chemicals, but are not considered to be
potential or actual carcinogens.
[Gile 2004, p208]

38 **d** The correct answer is **d**, be secured
upright to the wall or other stable source.
The other distractors are incorrect practices.
Compressed gas tanks should be stored
away from flammable materials, have safety
covers on when pressure regulators are
unattached and transported chained to a
hand cart or dolly.
[Gile 2004, pp197-202; Forbes 2007, p49]

39 **c** The correct answer is **c**, diethyl ether.
MLS The other distractors do not form explosive
ONLY peroxides upon long-term contact with
atmospheric oxygen.
[Gile 2004, pp122-123]

40 **c** The correct answer is **c**, 1 in the blue
quadrant. The ratings range for both
systems is 0-4 with 0 being no hazard and 4
being the most severe hazard. The left blue
quadrant represents a health hazard and a
toxic chemical causes a health hazard. The
rating of 1 would be a low or slight health
hazard. The other distractors are incorrect
due to the hazard type or rating.
[Forbes 2007, p48]

41 **d** The correct answer is **d**, corrosive, which
causes immediate damage to human tissue,
such as a burn. Distractors **a** and **b** are
health hazards, but generally do not cause
immediate tissue damage. For distractor
c, ignitable chemicals are both flammable
and combustible and only will cause tissue
damage if accidental flame or explosion
occurs.
[Gile 2004, p107]

42 **c** The correct answer is **c**, hazard warnings
MLS related to effect on involved target organs.
ONLY The other distractors are not required to be
listed on the label of hazardous chemicals.
[Gile 2004, p123]

43 **d** The correct answer is **d**, does not require
labeling. The other distractors are incorrect
and are only required on the original
containers or secondary containers, which
are not used immediately or by a different
person.
[OSHA 2004; Woodcock 2004; NFPA 1981]

44 **b** The correct answer is **b**, chlorine and
MLS ammonia, which combine to form an
ONLY extremely toxic hydrochloric gas. The other
distractors represent compatible storage
combinations.
[Gile 2004, p108]

45 **c** The correct answer is **c**, evacuate the
area. The other distractors are secondary
responses after evacuating the area.
[Gile 2004]

46 **d** The correct answer is **d**, disposed of
MLS as an EPA hazardous waste through a
ONLY licensed waste hauler. Distractors **a** and
b are prohibited as unsafe disposal and
work practices. Distractor **c**, xylene, is not
a regulated medical waste. However, if
regulated medical waste and chemicals are
mixed together in processing, the resulting
waste should be disposed of as incinerated
regulated medical waste.
[Gile 2004, pp128-129]

47
MLS
ONLY
d   The correct answer is **d**, report situation to supervisor, which always is the first step in any potential workplace exposure of any kind. For distractor **a**, it is the employer's responsibility to provide a medical consultation and evaluation free of charge to employees, who are involved in potential workplace exposures. For distractor **b**, early recognition, evaluation and treatment is key to preventing further exposure and exacerbation of symptoms. For distractor **d**, acquiring the MSDS would be part of the supervisor-directed investigation and secondary to reporting the situation to supervisor.
[OSHA 2004; Woodcock 2004]

48
MLS
ONLY
c   The correct answer is **c**, paid by the employer on work time without loss of pay.
[Gile 2004, p124]

49
MLS
ONLY
a   The correct answer is **a**, when procedures or equipment surrounding use of the specific chemical change. If the baseline monitoring was not within permissible exposure or action limits initially, periodic subsequent monitoring would be required. However, since the permissible limits in this case were not exceeded, subsequent monitoring only needs to be performed again if changes are made. Therefore, the other distractors are incorrect.
[Gile 2004, pp208-209]

50
MLS
ONLY
d   The correct answer is **d**, neoprene or nitrile gloves, which are chemically resistant. Distractor **c** gloves are not chemically resistant. Distractors **a** and **b** are engineering controls and not personal protective equipment.
[Gile 2004, p54]

51   **c**   The correct answer is **c**, designate a laboratory chemical hygiene officer.
[Gile 2004, p110]

52   **d**   The correct answer is **d**, hazardous chemicals.
[Gile 2004, p93]

53   **a**   Healthcare workers must be knowledgeable of chemical safety signage as they may be using chemicals as preservatives in specimens for transport. The flammable sign is from the Department of Transportation Hazardous Materials Warning Signs.
[Garza 2008, p89]

54   **b**   The correct answer is **b**, use a mechanical device. Distractors **a** and **c** do not afford adequate protection and **d** leads to recapping injuries vs using a one-handed technique.
[Fleming 2006, pp348-350]

55   **d**   The correct answer is **d**, ensure proper balance is maintained. For distractor **a**, a disinfectant should be used. For distractor **b**, the cover should not be opened until the centrifuge comes to a complete stop. For distractor **c**, all specimen tubes need to be covered to prevent aerosol formation.
[Woodcock 2004]

56
MLS
ONLY
b   The correct answer is **b**, shield all skin and use a face shield. For distractor **a**, cryogenic gloves, such as Zetex gloves, should be used. Chemically-resistant gloves are not protective against liquid nitrogen. For distractor **c**, cylinders should be stored near good ventilation. For distractor **d**, cylinders should be stored in an upright position.
[Gile 2004, p200]

57   **c**   The correct answer is **c**, be filed for all incidents, including near miss incidents. For distractor **a**, employee's medical history is confidential. For distractor **b**, all incidents require an incident report be filed. For distractor **d**, incidents reports need to be maintained for a defined period of time.
[Fleming 2006, p212]

58   **a**   The correct answer is **a** and the other distractors are incorrect and used for other purposes as listed in the answers. The word *immediate* is the key to this answer.
[Gile 2004, p94]

59   **b**   The correct answer is **b**, be grounded or double insulated. For distractor **a**, repairs should not be conducted while connected to facility wiring. For distractor **c**, safety checks should be performed initially, annually and when ever repairs are made. For distractor **d**, multiple outlet adapters are unsafe and should not be used.
[Gile 2004, p186]

60   **d**   The correct answer is **d**, touch a "contaminated" area phone with ungloved hands if hands are washed afterward. For distractor **a**, bench tops are to be cleaned after spills and at the end of each shift. For distractor **b**, personal protective equipment, such as a lab coat, is to be removed prior to leaving a "contaminated" area. For distractor **c**, cosmetics and lip balm are not to be applied in a "contaminated" area.
[Gile 2004, p30]

61   **b**   The correct answer is **b**, hallways and corridors should be clear and free of obstruction at all times. For distractor **a**, fire drills should not be announced or practiced in advanced. For distractor **c**, laboratories larger than 1,000 square feet and/or contain explosion hazards require 2 exits.
[Gile 2004, p180]

62   **c**   The symbol in the figure represents a common labeling system for hazardous material identification, such as HMIS® or NFPA 704 and the correct answer is **c**, chemical hazardous materials. All other distractors are incorrect. Distractors **a** and **b** do not use the NFPA hazard label at all, and there is more appropriate signage for radiation. If a chemical is radioactive, there would be a radioactive symbol in the bottom white area.
[Gile 2004, p115; Forbes 2007, p48]

63   **d**   The correct answer is **d**, approved safety can. For distractor **a**, flammable safety cabinets should not be vented to room air. For distractor **b**, flammable and combustible liquids that require refrigeration are only to be stored in an explosion-proof refrigerator. For distractor **c**, hazardous substances, particularly of that volume, are not to be stored in a fume hood.
[Gile 2004, p180]

64   **b**   The correct answer is **b**, pull the pin. The sequence of actions should be pull the pin, aim the hose, squeeze the lever, and sweep the flow.
[Gile 2004, p182]

65   **d**   The correct answer is **d**, use only UL or other safety agency-rated electrical equipment. For distractor **a**, multiple outlet or gang plug adapters are not to be used. For distractor **b**, there is no requirement to change circuit breakers annually. For distractor **c**, worn wiring is to be replaced and not taped over.
[Gile 2004, pp186-187; Forbes 2007, p49]

66   **b**   The correct answer is **b**, bend at the knees and hips, lift with legs and buttocks. For distractors **a** and **d**, you should not bend at the waist. For distractor **c**, you should not lift with your back. For distractor **d**, you should not twist.
[Gile 2004, pp90-91]

67   **d**   The correct answer is **d**, maintain wrists
MLS ONLY   in a neutral position. Distractors **a** and **c** are not ergonomically correct positions. For distractor **b**, the first course of action would be to evaluate posture, body mechanics and adjustment of chair and keyboard prior to facility redesign.
[Gile 2004, p91]

68   **c**   The correct answer is **c**, remove persons from immediate danger. The other distractors are correct, but are secondary actions. The sequence of actions after removing persons from immediate danger is to pull the fire alarm, contain the fire and evacuate the area, if required.
[Gile 2004, p180; Forbes 2007, p49]

69   **b**   The correct answer is **b**, contain the fire by closing the doors. For distractor **a**, it is the last action to be taken and only if indicated. For distractor **c**, a type A extinguisher is for paper, wood and plastics fires, not electrical fires. Also, fire extinguishers only should be used by those who have received appropriate training. For distractor **d**, it is unnecessary and unacceptable to lock windows and especially doors, which would block access to firefighters.
[Gile 2004, p180; Forbes 2007, p49]

70   **d**   The correct answer is **d**, electrical equipment. Distractors **a** and **b** would be class B fires, and distractor **c** would be class A fires.
[Gile 2004, p182; Forbes 2007, p48]

71 **a** The correct answer is **a**, report to and
MLS
ONLY discuss issue with supervisor. For distractor
b, pain should never be ignored and early
intervention with ergonomic injuries is
important. For distractor **c**, this appears to
be a work-related issue and the employee is
entitled to an employer-provided medical
evaluation, if indicated. For distractor **d**,
this action is a secondary action and should
be done in consultation with the supervisor
and a trained ergonomics specialist.
[CLSI 2007]

72 **c** The correct answer is **c**, use eyewash
station to flush eyes with water for 15
minutes. Distractors **a** and **d** are secondary,
not the primary actions. Distractor **b** is
incorrect and completely unsafe.
[Gile 2004, p129]

73 **b** The correct answer is **b**, use emergency
safety shower and flush body with water.
Distractor **a** is secondary, not a primary
first aid action step. Distractors **c** and **d**
are incorrect and not appropriate first aid
actions.
[Gile 2004, p130]

74 **d** The correct answer is **d**, lab coat.
The other distractors are examples of
engineering controls, not PPE.
[Gile 2004, p43; Forbes 2007, p56]

75 **c** The correct answer is **c**, answering the
telephone in a designated "clean" area.
For distractor **a**, gloves do not need to be
removed. For distractor **b**, it is essential
to keep gloves on during specimen
transportation, even through "clean" areas,
such as the hallways. Care should be taken
not to touch anything in the clean areas.
For distractor **d**, gloves do not need to be
changed after these patients unless known
contamination has occurred, which is
the same for any patient specimen under
"standard precautions."
[Gile 2004, p30]

76 **a** The correct answer is **a**, working with
caustic or toxic materials. For the other
distractors, it is not required practice to
use eye and face protection during these
activities.
[Gile 2004, p53]

77 **a** The correct answer is **a**, secure long hair
and jewelry. These items should be secured
to avoid contamination with biohazards or
physical injury. The other distractors are
not safe or acceptable work practices. Food
should not be stored in supply refrigerators
at all, contact lenses should not be worn in
laboratories and open weaved shoes are a
spill hazard.
[Gile 2004, pp27-28]

78 **c** Knowledgeable personnel separate
waste into designated categories (ie,
chemical, routine, infectious, etc) at the
point of generation to reduce disposal
costs and minimize employee exposure to
hazardous materials.
[Garcia 2004, p458]

79 **a** A 10% solution of bleach is an effective
and economical disinfectant, which
inactivates HBV in 10 minutes and HIV in 2
minutes.
[Henry 2006, p9]

80 **c** The simplest method of disposing of
needles is to dispose of the entire collection
device into a container reserved for sharps.
[McClatchey 1994, p56]

81 **d** Blood spills must be cleaned up and
decontaminated by personnel using the
proper PPE.
[McClatchey 1994, p66]

82 **b** Hepatitis B infection is a global public
health problem and is one of the most
common infectious diseases in the world.
[Murray 2007, p1643]

83 **c** The 3 modes of HIV transmission are
through intimate sexual contact, contact
with blood, and perinatal. Needlestick injury
falls under the second mode, and poses, on
average, a 0.3% risk of transmission.
[Stevens 2003, p347]

84 **d** A 10% solution of bleach is an effective
and economical disinfectant, which
inactivates IIBV in 10 minutes and IIIV in 2
minutes.
[Henry 2006, p9]

85 **b** Microbiological hazards are contained
using a biological safety cabinet with the air
exhausting through a HEPA filter.
[Henry 2006, p9]

86   **d**   The correct answer is **d**, perform frequent and appropriate hand hygiene. The other distractors are methods for preventing spread of infection but are not the most effective method.
[Gile 2004, p30]

87   **c**   The correct answer is **c**, discard directly into an appropriate sharps container, to avoid undo contact with the sharp. Distractor **a** is a prohibited practice. For distractors **b** and **d**, needle re-capping or removal is not preferred, but if required, it must be done using mechanical devices or for re-capping only using a one-handed technique.
[Gile 2004, p31]

88   **a**   The correct answer is **a**, bloodborne pathogens.
[Fleming 2006, p347; Gile 2004, pp11-12; Forbes 2007, p54]

89   **d**   The correct answer is **d**, thoroughly wash the wound with soap and water. The other distractors are secondary, not primary actions.
[Fleming 2006]

90   **a**   The correct answer is **a**, parenteral inoculation of blood. The other distractors are not likely transmission modes for bloodborne pathogens.
[Fleming 2006]

91   **b**   The correct answer is **b**, hepatitis B.
[Forbes 2007, p52]

92   **c**   The correct answer is **c**, biological safety cabinet. Distractor **a** is used for pharmacy and other "clean room" functions. Distractor **b** does not provide adequate respiratory protection, and distractor **d** is used for chemical not biohazard control.
[Forbes 2007, p55]

93   **c**   The correct answer is **c**, must be provided by the employer free of charge. For distractor **a**, it is a series of 3, not a single injection. For distractor **b**, it is recommended, but not a mandatory vaccination. For distractor **d**, the vaccine is recommended for high-risk employees upon initial employment, not just when an exposure occurs.
[Gile 2004, p29; Forbes 2007, p51]

94   **b**   The correct answer is **b**, absorb the spill with disposable absorbent material. For distractor **a**, immediately flooding the area with disinfectant may create aerosolization. For distractor **c**, it is unnecessary to evacuate the area for 30 minutes due to the size and nature of the spill. For distractor **d**, the area should be first cleaned with a disinfectant, not a detergent.
[Gile 2004, pp145-146]

95   **a**   The correct answer is **a**, sodium hypochlorite, which is a disinfectant. The other distractors are antiseptics, not disinfectants.
[Gile 2004, p145]

96   **b**   The correct answer is **b**, transmissible
MLS ONLY   spongiform encephalopathy agents (prions), such as Creutzfelt-Jakob disease. These agents are not disinfected or inactivated through conventional means for other microbial agents, such as the distractors listed above.
[Fleming 2006, pp379-380]

97   **c**   The correct answer is **c**, single use and disposable gloves. For distractor **a**, reusable utility gloves are not ideal or the best choice, but could be used if properly decontaminated after use and inspected for punctures or tears prior to reuse. Latex gloves should be avoided because of potential sensitization to the latex and the development of a latex allergy.
[Fleming 2006]

98   **d**   The correct answer is **d**, change gloves and wash hands with antiseptic soap and water. The other distractors are inappropriate practices.
[Fleming 2006, pp353-354]

99   **a**   The correct answer is **a**, biohazard.
[Fleming 2006]

100   **b**   The correct answer is **b**, infectious
MLS ONLY   waste.
[Gile 2004, p225]

Management

101 **c**   Guidelines when appraising a
MLS ONLY poor performer include reviewing the
performance standard for the task and
then list specific changes and time frame
in which the behavior (improvement) must
be corrected. An improvement plan may be
added to the appraisal form to assist the
employee improve their performance. The
improvement plan can include attending
workshops or continuing education
programs or working with an experienced
technologist.
[Garcia 2004, pp286, 299]

102 **a**   Variable costs are indirect or direct
MLS ONLY costs that vary in direct proportion to test
volume.
[Garcia 2004, pp49, 673]

103 **b**   A cost is an expense that includes the
MLS ONLY money spent on supply, overhead and labor
to produce a product or service.
[Henry 2006, p122]

104 **b**   The decision to lease or buy equipment
MLS ONLY is based on the least costly alternative given
the expense to provide this service and the
anticipated revenue for offering the service.
[Garcia 2004, p678]

105 **c**   FTE (full-time equivalent) is 2,080
MT ONLY hours per year (based on 8 hours/day × 5
days/week × 52 weeks/year).
[Garcia 2004, p535]

106 **a**   Converting a fraction into a percentage:
MLS ONLY 50,419/38,773 × 100 = 130%; 130% – 100%
= 30% over budget.
[Campbell 1997, p20]

107 **b**   A job description is a written delineation
MLS ONLY of the title, duties, responsibilities and
reporting relationships of a position and the
requisite qualifications needed.
[Garcia 2004, p280]

108 **a**   Communication between employers
MLS ONLY and employees is key in the retention of
employees as well as in giving a successful
performance appraisal. Feedback lets
employees know what is expected of them
and what is expected from the employer.
They will be more satisfied with their job and
likely be more productive as well.
[Garcia 2004, pp285, 299]

109 **c**   The first step in progressive counseling
MLS ONLY is verbal counseling.
[Garcia 2004, p286]

110 **b**   The first step in progressive counseling
MLS ONLY is verbal counseling.
[Garcia 2004, p286]

111 **b**   The first step in progressive counseling
MLS ONLY is verbal counseling.
[Garcia 2004, p286]

112 **d**   A workload recording system is
MLS ONLY important in understanding the resource
requirements for each patient "sector" and is
used to determine staffing needs.
[Garcia 2004, p329]

113 **a**   Questions that could be discriminatory
in nature (eg, nationality, marital status,
dependents, religion, affiliations, sexual
orientation, or physical or mental
disabilities) should be avoided on the
employment application or during the
interview process, unless the question is
relevant or pertinent to the particular job;
otherwise, it can be considered illegal.
[Darrah 2007, p30]

114 **c**   Questions that could be discriminatory
MLS ONLY in nature (eg, nationality, marital
status, dependents, religion, affiliations,
sexual orientation or physical or mental
disabilities) should be avoided on the
employment application or during the
interview process, unless the question is
relevant or pertinent to the particular job;
otherwise, it can be considered illegal.
[Darrah 2007, p30]

115 **d**   Continuing education for medical
MLS ONLY laboratory personnel is undertaken
for many reasons (ie, improving job
performance; mandates by regulatory
agencies; satisfaction of intellectual curiosity
or enhancement of professional skills).
[Baer 2001]

116 **a**   Labor comprises approximately 70% of
MLS ONLY a healthcare organization's budget.
[Garcia 2004, p537]

117 **d**   Questions that could be discriminatory
in nature (eg, nationality, marital status,
dependents, religion, affiliations, sexual
orientation, or physical or mental
disabilities) should be avoided on the
employment application or during the
interview process, unless the question is
relevant or pertinent to the particular job;
otherwise, it can be considered illegal.
[Darrah 2007, p30]

118 **b**   An employer is required to make
MLS ONLY reasonable accommodations unless it creates an undue hardship (financially or logistically) to the business.
[Garcia 2004, p87]

119 **c**   Definition of a Gantt chart.
MLS ONLY [Lock 2007]

120 **d**   Indirect costs are all costs that are not
MLS ONLY directly related to the test, but are a part of total laboratory expenses.
[Garcia 2004, p830]

121 **d**   Manageable and unmanageable cost components for a laboratory manager. While it is under a manager's control to schedule and train employees, "acts of God" (eg, military leave, pregnancy, injury) are not under their control and affect their ability to schedule employees.
[Garcia 2004, p514]

122 **a**   ABN (advanced beneficiary notice) is a
MLS ONLY notification given to medicare beneficiaries prior to receiving a service that may not be covered by insurance and that the beneficiary may be required to assume financial responsibility.
[Garcia 2004, p572]

123 **d**   Unit cost of production of an individual
MLS ONLY test result and represents both fixed and variable direct costs as well as allocations of certain indirect costs most closely associated with production of the test result.
[Garcia 2004, p679]

124 **b**   The decision of whether or not to
MLS ONLY acquire new equipment requires analysis and supporting documentation to include: purpose, importance, projected client demand and utilization, estimated useful life, estimated total acquisition cost, estimated associated yearly cast out-flows, and estimated yearly cash inflows or savings.
[Garcia 2004, p677]

125 **d**   Credentialing or certification is
MLS ONLY demonstration of qualification or competence in a particular area of practice. It recognizes an individual as meeting predetermined criteria set by the administering organization, usually a professional association.
[Garcia 2004, p90]

126 **d**   Performance appraisals are done to
MLS ONLY provide ongoing performance feedback.
[Garcia 2004, pp292-293]

Laboratory Mathematics

127 **c**   To correct for having used a dilution, multiply the answer obtained times the reciprocal of the dilution made.
[Campbell 1997, p114]

128 **d**   Commonly used units for standard solutions are mg/mL.
[Campbell 1997, p232]

129 **a**   The value of the unknown is a ratio of the absorbance reading of the unknown to the absorbance reading of the standard.
[Campbell 1997, p126]

130 **b**   Volumetric flasks are used to measure exact volumes and are primarily used in preparing solutions of known concentrations.
[Tietz 2006, p18]

131 **c**   The most commonly used equation for preparing suspension solutions is $V1 \times C1 = V2 \times C2$. A 4% red cell suspension contains 4 mL of red cells per 100 mL (1 dL) of solution. Therefore, $(25) \times (4) = (100) \times (x)$. Solve for x.
[Kaplan 2003, p35]

132 **c**   The most commonly used equation for preparing suspension solutions is $V1 \times C1 = V2 \times C2$. In this case, $(100) \times (5) = (x) \times (25)$. Solve for x.
[Kaplan 2003, p35]

133 **a** $V1 \times C1 = V2 \times C2$. A 3% acetic acid
MLS ONLY solution contains 3 mL of acetic acid per 100 mL (1 dL) of solution. Therefore, $(25) \times (3) = (100)(x)$. Solve for x.
[Kaplan 2003, p35]

134 **c**   This is a ratio calculation. 0.9% normal saline contains 0.9 grams NaCl in 100 mL solution. $0.9/100 = x/1{,}000$ Solve for x to determine how much NaCl is needed to prepare 1 L (1,000 mL).
[Kaplan 2003, p35]

135 **b** $V1 \times C1 = V2 \times C2$. A 3% solution
MLS ONLY contains 3 mL solution A per 100 mL (1 dL) of solution B. Therefore, $(40) \times (3) = (100)(x)$. Solve for x.
[Kaplan 2003, p35]

136 **b**   This is a ratio calculation. $75/100 = x/8$.
MLS ONLY Solve for x.
[Kaplan 2003, p34]

137 **c**   Recovery is calculated as concentration
MLS
ONLY of the initial sample × volume of the
initial sample = concentration of the
final sample × volume of the final sample.
Therefore (800)×(0.1) = (x) × (1). Then
observed (recovery/x) × 100.
[Clarke 2006, p48]

138 **b**   Standard deviation is a measure of the
dispersion of data around the mean. It is
calculated by taking the square root of the
summation of the squared differences of the
observed × values from their mean divided
by n.
[Clarke 2006, p25]

139 **b**   The probability of an observation having
a value within ±2 standard deviations of
the mean in a normal distribution is 95.5%.
Therefore, 5 control values out of 100 would
be out of control due to random error.
[Clarke 2006, p27]

140 **b**   The probability of an observation having
a value within ±2 standard deviations of
the mean in a normal distribution is 95.5%.
Therefore, 100 ± 2 × 1.8 = 95% confidence
interval.
[Clarke 2006, p27]

141 **d**   Simple dilutions are ratios of 2 volumes,
which involve a single substance diluted
with one other substance. In this case,
0.25 mL solution A is added to 19.75 mL
solution B (ratio 0.25/19.75), for a total
volume of 20 mL. This represents a dilution
of 0.25/20. To convert a 0.25/20 dilution to
a 1-in-something dilution, set up a ratio-
proportion calculation: 0.25 is to 20 as 1 is
to x, and solve for x.
[Campbell 1997, p94]

142 **a**   Definition of a standard.
[Tietz 2006, pp3-4]

143 **c**   To correct for having used a dilution,
multiply the answer obtained times the
reciprocal of the dilution made.
[Campbell 1997, p114]

144 **b**   To correct for having used a dilution,
multiply the answer obtained times the
reciprocal of the dilution made.
[Campbell 1997, p114]

145 **b**   1/25 = x/5. Solve for x.
MLS
ONLY [Kaplan 2003, p35]

146 **b** $C1 \times V1 = C2 \times V2$. Therefore $1 \times 1 =$
MLS
ONLY $1.025 \times x$. Solve for x.
[Kaplan 2003, p34]

147 **a**   This is a ratio calculation. 1:300 dilution
equals 1 antigenic unit in 0.5mL. Therefore,
2 antigenic units in 0.5mL equals a 1:150
dilution.
[Kaplan 2003, p34]

148 **a**   This is a ratio calculation. A 2% saline
MLS
ONLY erythrocyte suspension contains 2 mL of
an erythrocyte suspension per 100 mL total
solution. Therefore 2/100 = x/5. Solve for x.
[Kaplan 2003, p34]

149 **b**   The original concentration of a
MLS
ONLY solution × dilution made = concentration of
resulting solution.
[Campbell 1997, p96]

150 **b** $C1 \times V1 = C2 \times V2$. Therefore $(30) \times (x) =$
MLS
ONLY $(10)\times(6)$. Solve for x.
[Kaplan 2003, p34]

151 **c**   The most common equation for
preparing dilutions is $V1 \times C1 = V2 \times C2$,
where V1 is the volume, C1 is the
concentration of solution 1, and V2 and C2
are the volume and concentration of the
diluted solution.
[Kaplan 2003, p34]

152 **d**   Simple dilutions are ratios of 2
volumes, which involve a single substance
diluted with one other substance. In this
case, 0.1 mL solution A is added to 9.9
mL solution B (ratio 0.1/9.9), for a total
volume of 10 mL. This represents a dilution
of 0.1/10. To convert a 0.1/10 dilution to
a 1-in-something dilution, set up a ratio-
proportion calculation: 0.1 is to 10 as 1 is
to x, ie, 0.1/10=1/x, and solve for x.
[Campbell 1997, p93]

153 **c**   Simple dilutions are ratios of 2 volumes,
which involve a single substance diluted
with one other substance. In this case,
1 mL solution A is added to 4 mL solution B
(ratio 1/4), for a total volume of 5 mL. This
represents a dilution of 1/5.
[Campbell 1997, p93]

154 **a**   The most frequently used expression,
concentrations of m/v are reported as grams
percent (g%) or g/dL, as well as mg/dL and
µg/dL. When percent concentration is
expressed without a specified form, it is
assumed to be weight per unit volume.
[Kaplan 2003, p35]

155 **b**   The concentration of a weight/unit
volume solution is expressed as grams/100 mL.
Therefore, 20 grams in 0.5 L = 4 grams in
100 mL = 4% solution.
[Campbell 1997, p135]

156 **b** The concentration of a weight/unit volume solution is expressed as grams/100 mL. A 3% (w/v) solution contains 3 grams in 100 mL therefore 1 L contains 30 grams.
[Campbell 1997, p136]

157 **b** This is a ratio calculation. 3/100 = 6/x. Solve for x.
[Campbell 1997, p136]

158 **b** The coefficient of variation % = (standard deviation/mean) × 100.
MLS ONLY
[Clarke 2006, p53]

159 **a** The mean = sum of values/number of values; standard deviation = square root of the sum of (observed values – mean) squared / number of samples; coefficient of variation % = (standard deviation/mean) × 100. Therefore, (2.64/139) × 100 = 1.9%.
[Clarke 2006, p53]

160 **c** The *mean* (often called the *average*) is the most widely recognized descriptive statistic. The mean of a set of data can be calculated in several ways, but in each case the result is, in general, an indication of the central point of the data.
[Clarke 2006, p23]

161 **a** The *mode* is the most frequently occurring value in a set of data.
[Clarke 2006, p24]

162 **b** The *median* is the value in the middle of a data set in which all the values are ranked from lowest to highest. This descriptive statistic is useful in sets of data that are heavily skewed or unevenly distributed, where the mean can be a misleading statistic.
[Clarke 2006, p24]

163 **d** The *arithmetic mean* is the quantity that is most familiar and is ordinarily meant when we refer to the mean or average of a set of data. It is calculated as the sum of values divided by the number of values.
[Clarke 2006, p23]

164 **b** The mean = sum of values/number of values.
[Clarke 2006, p23]

165 **c** Imprecision is the measure of random error commonly expressed as the standard deviation. A more useful measure, the coefficient of variation (CV), is the measure of relative random error usually expressed as a percentage: CV (%) = (standard deviation/mean) × 100.
[Clarke 2006, p53]

166 **b** The coefficient of variation % = (standard deviation/mean) × 100.
[Clarke 2006, p53]

167 **c** This is a ratio calculation. 100 (g of NaCl) to 58.5 (gram equivalent weight of NaCl) = 1.709. 23 (gram equivalent weight of Na) × 1.709 = grams of Na in 100g NaCl.
[Kaplan 2003, p35]

168 **d** Absorbance = (molar absorptivity coefficient) × (light path) × (concentration). Therefore (molar absorptivity) = (absorbance)/(light path) × (concentration).
MLS ONLY
[Kaplan 2003, p38]

169 **d** Absorbance, A, is a measure of the amount of light stopped, or absorbed, by a solution, and the absorbance of light is a logarithmic function. Hence, the A scale is a logarithmic scale. On the other hand, transmittance, T, is a measure of the amount of light allowed to pass through a solution. Because the following relationship is true, A = light stopped and T = light passed through, A and T are inversely related. They are also logarithmically related, because the absorption of light is a logarithmic function.
MLS ONLY
[Campbell 1997, p212]

170 **a** This is a ratio calculation: (absorbance of the unknown)/(concentration of the unknown) = (absorbance of the standard)/(concentration of the standard).
MLS ONLY
[Kaplan 2003, p38]

171 **b** By definition, a gram equivalent weight of an element or compound is the mass that will combine with or replace 1 mole of hydrogen.
[Campbell 1997, p143]

172 **b** Moles = grams / molecular weight.
[Campbell 1997, p138]

173 **c** Electrolyte equivalents can be calculated from the equation: mg/dL × 10 = 10 mg/L. Because mg/mEq weight is the millimolar weight in mg/valence, mg/L / mg/mEq = mEq/L.
[Kaplan 2003, p36]

Answers–Laboratory Operations

174 a Moles = grams/molecular weight.
[Campbell 1997, p138]

175 a Molality is the number of moles of solute per 1 kg of solvent.
[Campbell 1997, p142]

176 a Molarity is a number that expresses the number of moles of substance in 1 L of solution.
[Campbell 1997, p138]

177 b Molarity (M) equals (grams/GMW)/L.
MLS ONLY [Campbell 1997, p139]

178 d Molarity (M) equals (grams/GMW)/L.
MLS ONLY [Campbell 1997, p139]

179 a A 1 Normal solution contains 1 gram
MLS ONLY equivalent of solute in 1,000 mL of solution.
[Campbell 1997, p144]

180 c A 1 Normal solution contains 1 gram
MLS ONLY equivalent of solute in 1,000 mL of solution.
[Campbell 1997, p144]

181 d $C1 \times V2 = C2 \times V2$. Therefore $(0.25) \times (x) = (100) \times (0.05)$. Solve for x.
[Campbell 1997, p144]

182 d $pH = \log(1/[H^+]) = b - \log(a)$. The
MLS ONLY relationship between a and b is such that b may be any value and the $[H^+]$ will always be the same. To work out these problems, assign b the value that is the smallest whole number that is equal to or greater than the pH. In this problem, b =7. Therefore, $7 = 7 - \log(a)$;
$\log(a) = 7 - 7; \log(a) = 0; a = 1;$
$[H^+] = (a) \times (10^{-b})$.
In this problem, $H^+ = 1 \times 10^{-7}$, or 100 nanomoles/L.
[Campbell 1997, p195]

183 b The predictive value of a positive test
MLS ONLY indicates the probability that a laboratory result outside the reference interval reflects the true presence of disease.
[Clarke 2006, p36]

Instrumentation and General Laboratory Principles

184 b A method used for screening must have a high degree of sensitivity to detect everyone with the disease.
[Arneson 2007, p63]

185 c Accuracy is the comparison of a result with the true value.
[Arneson 2007, p52]

186 b The use of manufacturer inserts is not acceptable in place of a procedure manual.
[CAP 2007, p17, CHM 11000]

187 a Laboratory evaluation of methods to
MLS ONLY gather the appropriate data and interpret the method validation results in order to judge the acceptability of the method.
[Kaplan 2003, pp415-422]

188 b Precision describes the reproducibility
MLS ONLY of a method. The narrower the distribution of results, the smaller the standard deviation.
[Kaplan 2003, pp348-349]

189 c The key advantage to POCT is faster
MLS ONLY turnaround time.
[Garcia 2004, p407]

190 c Safety guidelines indicate that before attempting to solve any trouble shooting steps for any equipment, it is necessary to turn the power off for the instrument. This step is necessary to prevent any possible electric shock.
[Bishop 2005, p43]

191 b Definition of atomic absorption.
[Tietz 2006, p73]

192 a Visual vs ultraviolet wavelength.
[Tietz 2006, p62]

193 d Visual wavelength calibration.
[Tietz 2006, p71]

194 b Spectrophotometer wavelength.
[Tietz 2006, p66]

195 a For maximal light absorption of the
MLS ONLY measured chromogen.
[Kaplan 2003, p86]

196 a Nanometer is the unit for wavelength.
[Kaplan 2003, p85]

197 b Other distractors do not describe double beam-in-space.
[Tietz 2006, p64]

198 b Hollow cathode lamp emitting the line
MLS ONLY spectrum of the pure metal of the measured element.
[Tietz 2006, p1226]

199 c Bandwidth refers to the range of
MLS ONLY wavelengths that pass through the exit slit.
[Kaplan 2003, p90]

200 b Definition of bichromatic analysis.
MLS ONLY [Kaplan 2003, p432]

201 a Principle of nephelometry.
[Kaplan 2003, p101]

202 d To obtain the maximum absorbance of the measured chromogen.
[Kaplan 2003, p92]

203 c Wavelength accuracy is an essential performance parameter to be tested for the spectrophotometer. For the narrow-spectral bandwidth instruments, holmium oxide glass may be scanned over the range of 280-650 nm. The material shows very sharp absorbance peaks at the well defined wavelengths. Prism and diffraction gratings are monochromatic devices. The didymium filter is used with broader bandwidth instruments.
[Tietz 2006, p67]

204 a Fluorescence occurs when a molecule absorbs light at one wavelength and emits light of a longer wavelength. The detector in a fluorometer is usually at right angles to the incident light source. A xenon or mercury vapor lamp emits enough UV light to be useful as a light source in a fluorometer.
[Bishop 2005, pp98-99; Arneson 2007, p113]

205 c Nephelometric methods are based upon light scatter being proportional to the number of particles in suspension, such as antigen-antibody complexes, which are physically larger than uncomplexed molecules.
[Arneson 2007, p111]

206 b Light from the lamp or light source of a photometer is reduced to a specific wavelength by the monochromator. In spectrophotometers, a diffraction-grate is used as a monochromator.
[Bishop 2005, p94; Arneson 2007, p105]

207 c Mass spectrometers detect mass to charge ratios of ionized molecules.
[Clarke 2006, p106]

208 a Basis of chromatography.
[Tietz 2006, p141]

209 b Principle of separation by size exclusion.
MLS ONLY [Tietz 2006, p144]

210 b Definition of retention factor (R_f) in
MLS ONLY thin-layer chromatography.
[Tietz 2006, p147]

211 c Backflow causes increased pressure and
MLS ONLY bad chromatography.
[Tietz 2006, p157]

212 a Samples to be analyzed by gas-liquid chromatography must be volatile or become volatile upon heating. The vaporized sample then flows, with the inert carrier gas, through the column.
[Bishop 2005, p111; Arneson 2007, p127]

213 d Steric-exclusion chromatography is based upon smaller molecules being trapped by the porous column material, but larger molecules are carried along by the mobile phase.
[Bishop 2005, pp108-109; Arneson 2007, p125]

214 a In thin-layer chromatography, the
MLS ONLY retention factor (R_f) is the distance the leading edge of a sample component moves divided by total distance the solvent moves; eg, sample moves 5 cm and solvent moves 10 cm, $R_f = 0.5$.
[Bishop 2005, p109]

215 c Electrophoresis involves the migration of a charged molecule or particle in a liquid medium under the influence of an electric field. The 3 roles of the buffer are 1) to carry the applied current; 2) to establish the pH for the electrophoresis procedure and 3) to determine the electrical charge on the solute.
[Tietz 2006, p125]

216 c A commonly encountered problem in
MLS ONLY electrophoresis is holes seen in staining patterns. This is due to the analyte being present in too high a concentration. The corrective action is to apply a less concentrated sample.
[Kaplan 2003, p213]

217 c Ion-selective electrodes (ISE) are a potentiometric method of analysis. ISEs respond to individual ions present in a sample.
[Bishop 2005, p102; Arneson 2007, pp115, 221]

218 a Ion-selective electrodes portend their selectivity properties through the use of particular membranes, as the selected ions interact with the membranes used in ion-selective electrodes.
[Tietz 2006, p986]

219 b To determine the g factor, use 0.0001×30 cm $\times (3,000)^2$. Remember that the radius is half the diameter.
[Strasinger 2008, p83]

220 b Other distractors do not apply to centrifugal force.
[Tietz 2006, p266]

221 c The devices listed are electronic, but the only device that measures rpm is a tachometer. RPM must be consistent to produce adequate G force.
[Strasinger 2003, p316]

222 b Point-of-care testing devices use a small volume of sample and are therefore particularly useful in neonates, small babies, and those with increased risk from phlebotomy.
[Clarke 2006, p183]

223 a Dry cobalt-treated $CaCl_2$ is blue.
[Kaplan 2003, p9]

224 b Enzyme-multiplied immunoassay is a homogeneous enzyme immunoassay used to quantitate drugs, hormone, etc. Unlike the heterogeneous assays, the free-labeled reactant does not have to be separated from the bound-labeled reactant.
[Bishop 2005, pp189-190]

225 c Enzymes are one of the several labels used in labeled immunoassays. The catalytic property of the enzyme is used to detect and quantitate the immunological reaction. Alkaline phosphatase and horseradish peroxidase are examples of enzymes used. The product of the enzymatic activity is monitored spectrophotometrically.
[Bishop 2005, p152]

226 b Chemiluminescent labels are based on the emission of light produced during a chemical reaction. These labels are very useful because they provide very low levels of detection (2×10^{-20} mol/L) with little or no background interference.
[Clarke 2006, p122]

Education and Communication

227 a Psychomotor objective: The learner
MLS
ONLY must perform the task.
[Hudson 2003, pp248-249]

228 a It is important to reward job excellence
MLS
ONLY and identify unacceptable behavior in an employee evaluation.
[Hudson 2003, pp33, 41]

229 d The employer may identify an
MLS
ONLY educational need during the annual competency evaluations.
[Hudson 2003, pp241-243]

230 d The intent of objective: What does the
MLS
ONLY instructor want the student to do at the conclusion of the unit.
[Hudson 2003, p248]

231 a All employees need feedback to sustain
MLS
ONLY motivation.
[Hudson 2003, p34]

232 c Patient education can alleviate anxiety.
[Hudson 2003, p100]

233 b Informative communication shares knowledge about laboratory processes and policies.
[Hudson 2003, p69]

234 c The employee moved into a participating situation.
[Hudson 2003, p79]

235 b Employee motivation.
MLS
ONLY [Hudson 2003, pp73-77]

236 b Scalar principle (the chain of command).
MLS
ONLY [Hudson 2003, pp80-81]

237 d Employee correction and discipline.
MLS
ONLY [Hudson 2003, p41]

238 c An objective is a specific statement of
MLS
ONLY what is expected of the learner after a period of instruction. There are 3 questions that educational objectives must address. What does the instructor want the student to do? Under what conditions should the learner accomplish the objective? What is the criterion that signifies achievement?
[Hudson 2003, p248]

239 c Problem solving includes 3 steps: define problem, write down the facts, examine solution (consider options).
[Hudson 2003, pp184-186]

240 d A goal targets the purpose of an educational unit. The objective specifies what a learner is expected to know or do.
[Hudson 2003, pp247-248]

241 d   Delegation should be used as an
MLS
ONLY opportunity for subordinate learning. When
a task is delegated, the authority transfers to
the one to whom the task is delegated.
[Hudson 2003, p80]

242 b   A collaborative approach can be used
MLS
ONLY for a long-term problem. To work together
to solve an issue, both views of the issue are
important.
[Hudson 2003, p92]

243 b   If a change is mandated, the manager
MLS
ONLY should provide information to the
employees regarding the necessity of
change.
[Hudson 2003, p51]

244 c   Team development constant
MLS
ONLY communication between team members
should be fostered by leaders.
[Hudson 2003, p86]

245 a   Downward communication is used
MLS
ONLY primarily to state objectives, disseminate
policies or changes, provide directives and
convey general information to subordinates.
Upward communication flows up through
the ranks to top management and is used to
report and convey information.
[Turnbull 2005]

246 a   All employees need feedback to sustain
MLS
ONLY motivation.
[Hudson 2003, p34]

247 a   Personal communication should be
planned: P=plan your communication,
L= listen to others, A=avoid assumptions/
ensure communication is understood,
N=network.
[Lab Medicine 2008b, pp261-264]

248 b   A daily "line-up" can be conducted
at a time of day that is convenient to the
department. Providing a question for
discussion is an effective way to foster
conversation.
[Castor 2006]

Laboratory Information Systems

249 c   The first step in choosing a laboratory
MLS
ONLY information system is the selection of an LIS
team.
[Hudson 2003, pp212-214]

250 b   HL-7 interface is the standard for
MLS
ONLY healthcare information management.
[Garcia 2004, p399]

251 b   HIPAA patient confidentiality
requirements state that patient data is
secure from unauthorized access at all levels
of communication of that data.
[Kasoff 2008, p26-36]

252 a   LIS systems use barcode labels for
positive sample identification for many of
the processes in the lab. Each LIS vendor
will specify which of several barcode label
formats are compatible with their system.
[Kasoff 2009]

253 a   Health Level 7 (HL-7) is the
organization that specifies requirements for
electronic data transmission formatting. It
is considered to be the industry standard.
[Kasoff 2009]

254 d   Patient results can be automatically
released to the patient record as long as
they meet selected criteria defined and
validated by the users. Auto-verification
does not apply to manually entered results
and results cannot be released unless QC has
been performed and was within limits prior
to releasing.
[CLSI 2006, AUTO 10-A]

255 c   The CAP requires documentation that
calculated values that generate a patient
report are reviewed every 2 years, or when
a system change is made that may affect the
calculations. This requirement applies to
values calculated by the LIS or middleware.
[CAP 2007, GEN 43450]

256 d   The Host Query mode of an
instrument is a two-way communication
process whereby the instrument reads
the specimen barcode and queries the
LIS for the orders. The tests to be run are
sent to the instrument (ie, bidirectional
communication). Once results are obtained,
they are sent back to the LIS.
[Kasoff 2009]

257 c   Test definitions, as well as all types of
stored master files, are contained in the
database.
[Cowan 2005, pp1-20]

258 **a**   Validation of the LIS is required by various accrediting agencies in order to prove that the system is performing as expected. This must be done at implementation and over time as changes are made to the LIS.
[Cowan 2005, pp43-58]

259 **c**   System back-up procedures are mandated by accrediting agencies and include creating an exact copy of sensitive LIS data at regularly defined intervals and storage of the backed-up data at a separate location.
[Cowan 2005, pp59-86]

260 **b**   Middleware applications have become
MLS readily available, are capable of supporting
ONLY changes in laboratory workflow, and provide enhanced data management tools without having to upgrade or change the LIS.
[Vail 2008, pp26-36]

AABB [2007] *Practical Guide to Transfusion Medicine*, 2nd ed. Bethesda, MD: AABB Press.

AABB [2008a] *Standards for Blood Banks and Transfusion Services*, 25th ed. Bethesda, MD: AABB Press.

AABB [2008b] *Technical Manual*, 16th ed. Brecher ME, ed. Bethesda, MD: AABB Press.

Abbott [2008] *PRISM HBsAg (Package Insert).* Germany: Abbott Diagnostics Division.

Abbus AK, Lichtman AH, Pillai S [2007] *Cellular and Molecular Immunology*, 6th ed. Philadelphia: WB Saunders,

Alberts B [2008] *Molecular Biology of the Cell*, 4th ed. New York: Garland.

Arneson WL, Brickell JM [2007] *Clinical Chemistry: A Laboratory Perspective*. Philadelphia: FA Davis.

Arkin CF [2001] *Procedure for the Determination of Fibrinogen in Plasma: Approved Guideline*, 2nd ed. H30-A2. Wayne, PA: Clinical and Laboratory Standards Institute.

Baer DM [2001] Continuing education—whose responsibility? *Lab Med* 32:423-428.

Baron EJ et al [2005] *Cumitech 1C, Blood Cultures IV*. Washington DC: ASM Press.

Benjamin E, Coico R, Sunshine G [2000] *Immunology: A Short Course*, 4th ed. New York: Wiley-Liss.

Blaney KD, Howard PR [2009]. *Concepts of Immunohematology*, 2nd ed. St Louis, MO: Mosby.

Bick, R [1992] *Hereditary Coagulation Protein Defects*. Ch6: Disorders of thrombosis and hemostasis. Chicago: ASCP Press.

Bishop ML, Fody EP, Schoeff LE [2005] *Clinical Chemistry Principles, Procedures, Correlations*, 5th ed. Baltimore: Lippincott Williams & Wilkins.

Brunzel NA [2004] *Fundamentals of Urine and Body Fluid Analysis*. Philadelphia: WB Saunders.

Buckingham L, Flaws ML [2007] *Molecular Diagnostics: Fundamentals, Methods and Clinical Applications*. Philadelphia: FA Davis.

Burtis CA, Ashwood ER, Border BG [2001] *Tietz Fundamentals of Clinical Chemistry*, 5th ed. Philadelphia: WB Saunders.

Campbell JB, Campbell JM [1997] *Laboratory Mathematics: Medical and Biological Applications*, 5th ed. Philadelphia: Mosby.

CAP [2007] *Chemistry & Toxicology Checklist*. Northfield, IL: College of American Pathologists.

CAP [2009] *Laboratory Inspection Checklist*. Northfield, IL: College of American Pathologists.

CAP, Glassy EF [1998] *Color Atlas of Hematology: An Illustrated Field Guide Based on Proficiency Testing*. Northfield, IL: College of American Pathologists.

Castellone D [2007] *Overview of Hemostasis and Platelet Physiology*. Philadelphia: FA Davis.

Castor R [2006] Developing an effective communication plan in the clinical laboratory. *ASCP Tech Sample: Generalist.* Chicago: ASCP Press.

Ciesla, B [2007] *Hematology in Practice*. Philadelphia: FA Davis.

Clarke W, Dufour DR [2006] *Contemporary Practice in Clinical Chemistry*. Washington, DC: AACC Press.

CLSI [2006] *Autoverification of Clinical Laboratory Test Results, Approved Guidelines*. Wayne, PA: Clinical and Laboratory Standards Institute.

CLSI [2006] *Performance Standards for Antimicrobial Disk Susceptibility Tests; Approved Standard*, 9th ed. CLSI document M2-A9. Wayne, PA: Clinical and Laboratory Standards Institute.

CLSI [2007] *Laboratory Design: Approved Guideline GP18-A2*. Villanova, PA: Clinical Laboratory Standards Institute.

CLSI [2008] *Performance Standards for Antimicrobial Susceptibility Testing*, 15th Infl Suppl. CLSI document M100-S18. Wayne, PA: Clinical and Laboratory Standards Institute.

Coleman WB, Tsongalis GJ [2006] *Molecular Diagnostics: For the Clinical Laboratorian*, 2nd ed. Totowa, NJ: Humana Press.

Cowan DF [2005] *Informatics for the Clinical Laboratory*. New York: Springer.

Darrah J [2007] How to answer illegal questions. *Advance Medical Lab Prof* 19:14.

Detrick B, Hamilton RG, Folds JD [2006] *Manual of Molecular and Clinical Laboratory Immunology*, 7th ed. Washington, DC: ASM Press.

Fleming DO, Hunt DL [2006] *Biological Safety: Principles and Practices*, 4th ed. Washington, DC: ASM Press.

Folds JD, Normansell DE [1999] *Pocket Guide to Clinical Immunology*. Washington, DC: ASM Press.

Forbes BA, Sahm DF, Weissfeld AS [2007] *Bailey and Scott's Diagnostic Microbiology*, 12th ed. St Louis, MO: Mosby.

Garcia LS [2004] *Clinical Laboratory Management*. Washington, DC: ASM Press.

Garza D, Becan-McBride K [2008] *Phlebotomy Simplified*. New Jersey: Prentice Hall.

Gile TJ [2004] *Complete Guide to Laboratory Safety*. Marblehead, MA: HCPro.

Goldsby RA, Kindt TJ, Kuby J, Osborne BA [2003] *Kuby Immunology*, 5th ed. Oxford: WH Freeman.

Gorbach SL, Bartlett JG, Blacklow NR [2003] *Infectious Diseases*, 3rd ed. Philadelphia: Lippincott Williams & Wilkins.

Gulati G, Caro J [2007] *Blood Cells: An Atlas of Morphology with Clinical Relevance*. Chicago: ASCP Press.

Harmening DM [2002] *Clinical Hematology and Fundamentals of Hemostasis*, 4th ed. Philadelphia, FA Davis.

Harmening DM [2005]. *Modern Blood Banking and Transfusion Practices*, 5th ed. Philadelphia: FA Davis.

Henry JB [2006] *Clinical Diagnosis and Management by Laboratory Methods*, 21st ed. Philadelphia: WB Saunders.

Hudson J [2003] *Principles of Clinical Laboratory Management*. Upper Saddle River, NJ: Prentice Hall.

Isenberg HD [1992] *Clinical Microbiology Procedures Handbook*, 1st ed. Washington DC: ASM Press

JCAHO [2009] http://www.jointcommission. org/Standards/facts_about_accreditation_ standards.htm, last accessed April 28, 2009.

Kaplan LA, Pesce AJ, Kazmierczak S [2003] *Clinical Chemistry: Theory, Analysis, Correlation*, 4th ed. Philadelphia: Mosby.

Kasoff J [2008] Advances in LIS functionality. *Advance Admin Lab* 17:2.

Kasoff J [2009] Laboratory information systems (LIS). *Clin Lab Products* January 2009.

Kindt TJ, Goldsby RA, Osborne BA [2007] *Kuby Immunology*, 6th ed. New York: WH Freeman.

Koepke J [1991] *Practical Laboratory Hematology*. New York: Churchill Livingstone.

Koneman EW [2005] *Koneman's Color Atlas and Textbook of Diagnostic Microbiology*, 6th ed. Baltimore: Lippincott Williams & Wilkins.

Lab Medicine [2008a] Interpersonal Communications, pp261-264.

Lab Medicine [2008b] *Root Cause Analysis of Specimen Misidentification in Surgical Pathology Accession and Grossing, Lab Med* 39:497-502.

LabQ [2008a] *Patient Safety Goals*. Chicago: ASCP Press.

Lapchak J [2008] Specimen discrepancies in a clinical setting. *Lab Med* 39:395-400.

Larone DH [2002] *Medically Important Fungi: A Guide to Identification*, 4th ed. Washington, DC: ASM Press.

Larsen SA [1998] *A Manual of Tests for Syphilis*, 9th ed. Washington, DC: American Public Health Association.

Lee GR, Foerster J, Lukens J, et al [1999] *Wintrobe's Clinical Hematology*, 10th ed. Baltimore: Lippincott Williams & Wilkins.

Lock D [2007] *Project Management*, 9th ed. Aldershot: Ashgate.

Mahon C, Manuselis G, Lehman D [2006] *Textbook of Diagnostic Microbiology*, 3rd ed. Philadelphia: WB Saunders.

Mahon CR, Tice D [2006] *Clinical Laboratory Immunology*, Upper Saddle River, NJ: Pearson Prentice Hall.

Mandell GL et al [2005] *Principles and Practice of Infectious Diseases*, 6th ed. Philadelphia: Churchill Livingstone.

Marlar R, Potts R, Marlar A [2006] Effect on routine and special coagulation testing values of citrate anticoagulant adjustment in patients with high hematocrit values. *Am J Clin Pathol* 126:400-405.

Marques MB, Fritsma MG [2007] *Quick Guide to Transfusion Medicine*. Washington, DC: AACC Press.

Masters RM, Glyls BA [2003] *Medical Terminology Specialties*. Philadelphia: FA Davis.

McBride L [1999] *Textbook of Urinalysis and Body Fluids*. Philadelphia: Lippincott.

McKenzie SB [2004] *Clinical Laboratory Hematology*. Upper Saddle River, NJ: Pearson Prentice Hall.

McPherson R, Pincus M [2007] *Henry's Clinical Diagnosis and Management by Laboratory Methods*, 21st ed. Philadelphia: Saunders Elsevier.

Miller LE, Ludke HR, Peacock JE, Tomar RH [1991] *Manual of Laboratory Immunology*, 2nd ed. Philadelphia: Lea & Febiger.

Morris MW, Williams WJ, Nelson DA [2006] Automated blood cell counting. In: Beutler E, Lichtman MA, Coller BS et al. *Williams' Hematology*, 7th ed. New York: McGraw-Hill.

Murray PR, Baron EJ, Jorgensen JH et al [2007] *Manual of Clinical Microbiology*, 9th ed. Washington, DC: ASM Press.

NCCLS [1997] *Determination of Factor Coagulant Activities; Approved Guideline*, H48-A, vol 17, no 4. Wayne, PA: National Committee for Clinical Laboratory Standards.

Nester EW et al [2001] *Microbiology: A Human Perspective*, 3rd ed. New York: McGraw-Hill.

NFPA [1981] Prudent practice for handling hazardous chemicals in the laboratories. *NFPA Standards* - 10, 30, 45, 49, 70, 99, 321 325M, 704. Quincy, MA: National Fire Protection Agency; National Research Council, National Academy Press.

NPSG [2009] *The Joint Commission National Patient Safety Goals*. http://www.jointcommission.org/PatientSafety/NationalPatientSafetyGoals. Last accessed April 28, 2009.

Nussbaum RL, McInnes RR, Willard HF [2007] *Thompson & Thompson Genetics in Medicine*, 7th ed. Washington, DC: WB Saunders.

O'Gorman MRG, Donnenberg AD [2008] *Handbook of Human Immunology*, 2nd ed. Boca Raton, FL: Taylor and Francis, CRC Press.

OSHA [2004] *Laboratory Standard*: 29 CFR 1910.1200; 1910.1030; 1910.1048; 1910.1450, subpart Z. Washington, DC: US Department of Labor, Occupational Safety and Health Administration.

Provlab [2009] *Fact or artifact?* http://secure.provlab.ab.ca/bugs/webbug/parasite/artifact/artifacts.htm. Last accessed May 5, 2009.

Rodak BF, Fritsma GA, Doig K [2007] *Hematology: Clinical Principles and Applications*, 3rd ed. Philadelphia: Saunders Elsevier.

Rose NR, Hamilton RG, Detrick B [2002] *Manual of Clinical Laboratory Immunology*, 6th ed. Washington, DC: ASM Press.

Rudmann SV [2005] *Textbook of Blood Banking and Transfusion Medicine*, 2nd ed. Philadelphia: Elsevier Saunders.

Steine-Martin EA, Lotspeich-Steininger CA, Koepke JA [1998] *Clinical Hematology: Principles, Procedures, Correlations*, 2nd ed. Philadelphia: Lippincott-Raven.

Stevens, CD [1996] *Clinical Immunology and Serology*. Philadelphia: FA Davis.

Stevens, CD [2003] *Clinical Immunology and Serology*, 2nd ed. Philadelphia: FA Davis.

Strasinger SK, DiLorenzo MS [2008] *Urinalysis and Body Fluids*, 5th ed. Philadelphia: FA Davis.

Stone JE [1998] Urine analysis in the diagnosis of mucopolysaccharide disorders. *Ann Clin Biochem* 2:207-225.

Tietz N, Burtis C, Ashwood ER, Bruns D [2006] *Tietz Textbook of Clinical Chemistry & Molecular Diagnostics*, 4th ed. Philadelphia: WB Saunders.

Turgeon ML [2005] *Clinical Hematology: Theory and Procedures*, 4th ed. Philadelphia: Lippincott Williams & Wilkins.

Turgeon, ML [2009] *Immunology and Serology in Laboratory Medicine*, 4th ed. St Louis, MO: Mosby.

Turnbull DC [2005] Communicating successfully in the workplace. *Lab Med* 36:205-208.

Vail GR [2008] Middleware augments the LIS. *Advance Admin Lab* 17:2.

Woodcock, SM [2004] Approved guideline GP17-A2. *Clinical Laboratory Safety*, 2nd ed. Villanova: Clinical Laboratory Standards Institute.

Wu AHB [2006] *Tietz Clinical Guide to Laboratory Tests*, 4th ed. Philadelphia: Saunders.